Breast Cancer: A Multidisciplinary Approach

Editorial Advisor

JOEL J. HEIDELBAUGH

ELSEVIER

1600 John F. Kennedy Boulevard • Suite 1800 • Philadelphia, Pennsylvania, 19103-2899

http://www.theclinics.com

CLINICS COLLECTIONS
ISSN 2352-7986, ISBN-13: 978-0-443-34300-1

Editors: John Vassallo (j.vassallo@elsevier.com); Megan Ashdown (m.ashdown@elsevier.com)

Clinics Collections (ISSN 2352-7986) is published by Elsevier Inc., 360 Park Avenue South, New York, NY 10010-1710. Business and editorial offices: 1600 John F. Kennedy Boulevard, Suite 1800, Philadelphia, PA 19103-2899. **POSTMASTER:** Send address changes to *Clinics Collections*, Elsevier Health Sciences Division, Subscription Customer Service, 3251 Riverport Lane, Maryland Heights, MO 63043. **Customer Service: Telephone: 1-800-654-2452** (U.S. and Canada); **1-314-447-8871** (outside U.S. and Canada). **Fax: 314-447-8029. E-mail: journalscustomerserviceusa@elsevier.com** (for print support); **journalsonlinesupport-usa@ elsevier.com** (for online support).

Reprints. For copies of 100 or more of articles in this publication, please contact the Commercial Reprints Department, Elsevier Inc., 360 Park Avenue South, New York, NY 10010-1710. Tel.: 212-633-3874; Fax: 212-633-3820; E-mail: reprints@elsevier.com.

Printed in the United States of America.

Contributors

EDITOR

JOEL J. HEIDELBAUGH, MD, FAAFP, FACG
Clinical Professor, Departments of Family Medicine and Urology, Director of Medical Student Education and Clerkship Director, Department of Family Medicine, University of Michigan Medical School, Ann Arbor, Michigan, USA

AUTHORS

JAMES ABDO, MD
General Surgeon, Marshfield Medical Center, Marshfield, Wisconsin, USA

SALMA A. ABDOU, MD
Resident, Department of Plastic Surgery, MedStar Plastic and Reconstructive Surgery, Washington, DC, USA

BEATRIZ ELENA ADRADA, MD, FSBI
Professor, Department of Breast Imaging, The University of Texas MD Anderson Cancer Center, Houston, Texas, USA

ROBERT ALLEN, MD
Clinical Professor of Plastic Surgery, Plastic and Reconstructive Surgery, Department of Surgery, Louisiana State University, New Orleans, Louisiana, USA

ANDERSON BAUER, MD
Radiation Oncologist, Radiation Oncology Department, Marshfield Clinic Health System, Marshfield, Wisconsin, USA

MICHAEL BORRERO, MD
Resident, Plastic and Reconstructive Surgery, Department of Surgery, Louisiana State University, New Orleans, Louisiana, USA

OTIS W. BRAWLEY, MD, MACP, FRCP(L)
Bloomberg Distinguished Professor, Department of Oncology, Johns Hopkins School of Medicine, Department of Epidemiology, Johns Hopkins Bloomberg School of Public Health, Baltimore, Maryland, USA

ELIZABETH J. CATHCART-RAKE, MD
Assistant Professor, Department of Oncology, Mayo Clinic, Rochester, Minnesota, USA

CAROLINE F. CENTENO, BS
Medical Student, Department of Psychiatry and Neurobehavioral Sciences, UVA Cancer Center, University of Virginia School of Medicine and Health System, Charlottesville, Virginia, USA

KARINA CHARIPOVA, MD
Resident Physician, Department of Plastic Surgery, MedStar Plastic and Reconstructive Surgery, Washington, DC, USA

ASHLEY CIMINO-MATHEWS, MD
Associate Professor, Departments of Pathology and Oncology, Johns Hopkins School of Medicine, Baltimore, Maryland, USA

NICHOLAS W. CLAVIN, MD
Assistant Professor, Department of Plastic Surgery, Atrium Health, Charlotte, North Carolina, USA

LAURA C. COLLINS, MD
Vice Chair of Anatomic Pathology, Professor, Department of Pathology, Beth Israel Deaconess Medical Center, Harvard Medical School, Boston, Massachusetts, USA

AMY CORDOVA, MSN, APRN-CNP, OCN
Survivorship Program Coordinator, Reflections Breast Health Center, Cleveland Clinic Akron General, Akron, Ohio, USA

CHANDLER S. CORTINA, MD, MS, FSSO
Assistant Professor, Department of Surgery, Division of Surgical Oncology, Medical College of Wisconsin, Milwaukee, Wisconsin, USA

AMY E. CYR, MD
Assistant Professor, Department of Medicine, Washington University, St. Louis, Missouri, USA

LESLY A. DOSSETT, MD, MPH
Associate Professor, Department of Surgery, Institute for Healthcare Policy and Innovation, University of Michigan, Ann Arbor, Michigan, USA

NICKI DOWNES, DO
Surgical Breast Oncology Fellow, Cleveland Clinic Akron General, Akron, Ohio, USA

LEISHA C. ELMORE, MD, MPHS
Assistant Professor, Department of Surgery, University of Pennsylvania, Perelman School of Medicine, Philadelphia, Pennsylvania, USA

LEISHA A. EMENS, MD, PhD
Professor, Department of Oncology, UPMC Hillman Cancer Center/Magee Women's Hospital, Pittsburgh, Pennsylvania, USA

OLUWADAMILOLA M. FAYANJU, MD, MA, MPHS, FACS
Helen O. Dickens Presidential Associate Professor, Chief, Division of Breast Surgery, Hospital of the University of Pennsylvania, Philadelphia, Pennsylvania, USA

ANDREW FENTON, MD, FACS
Executive Medical Director, McDowell Cancer Center, Surgical Director, Reflections Breast Health Center, Cleveland Clinic Akron General, Professor of Surgery, Northeast Ohio Medical University, Akron, Ohio, USA

AMY M. FOWLER, MD, PhD, FSBI
Associate Professor, Section of Breast Imaging and Intervention, Department of Radiology, University of Wisconsin-Madison School of Medicine and Public Health, University of Wisconsin Carbone Cancer Center, Department of Medical Physics, University of Wisconsin-Madison, Madison, Wisconsin, USA

FRANCIS D. GRAZIANO, MD
Division of Plastic and Reconstructive Surgery, Department of Surgery, Icahn School of Medicine, Mount Sinai, New York, New York, USA

VICTORIA L. GREEN, MD, JD, MBA
Professor, Department of Gynecology and Obstetrics, Emory University, Winship Cancer Institute at Grady Memorial Hospital, Atlanta, Georgia, USA; Medical Director, Gynecology Comprehensive Breast Center, Avon Breast Center, San Francisco, California, USA

MENG S. GUO, MD
Plastic Surgeon, Department of Plastic Surgery, Medical College of Wisconsin, Milwaukee, Wisconsin, USA

HUGO ST. HILAIRE, MD
Division Chairman, Plastic and Reconstructive Surgery, Department of Surgery, Louisiana State University, New Orleans, Louisiana, USA

JULIE IMANI, MSN, APRN-CNS, OCN
Hematology Oncology Clinical Nurse Specialist, Cleveland Clinic Akron General McDowell Cancer Center, Akron, Ohio, USA

GEETHA JAGANNATHAN, MBBS
Surgical Pathology Assistant, Department of Pathology, Johns Hopkins School of Medicine, Baltimore, Maryland, USA

STEPHEN R.D. JOHNSTON, MA, FRCP, PhD
Professor of Breast Cancer Medicine, Department of Medicine, Royal Marsden NHS Foundation Trust, Chelsea, London, United Kingdom

NOLAN S. KARP, MD
Plastic Surgeon, Hansjörg Wyss Department of Plastic Surgery, NYU Langone Health, New York, New York, USA

KAITLYN KENNARD, MD
Breast Surgical Oncology Fellow, Department of Surgery, Washington University, St. Louis, Missouri, USA

AMANDA L. KONG, MD, MS, FACS, FSSO
Professor, Department of Surgery, Division of Surgical Oncology, Medical College of Wisconsin, Milwaukee, Wisconsin, USA

DINA GEORGE LANSEY, MSN, RN
Assistant Professor, Department of Oncology, Johns Hopkins School of Medicine, Baltimore, Maryland, USA

GINGER P. LAYNE, MD
Breast Imaging Fellowship Director, Associate Professor of WVU Department of Radiology, West Virginia University School of Medicine, Morgantown, West Virginia, USA

MARLA LIPSYC-SHARF, MD
Fellow, Department of Medical Oncology, Dana-Farber Cancer Institute, Boston, Massachusetts, USA

JOCELYN LU, MD
Plastic Surgeon, Division of Plastic and Reconstructive Surgery, Department of Surgery, Icahn School of Medicine, Mount Sinai, New York, New York, USA

KATHY LUKITY, RN, BSN, CBCN
Care Coordinator, Reflections Breast Health Center, Cleveland Clinic Akron General, Akron, Ohio, USA

AMANDA MENDIOLA, MD, FACS
Program Director, Breast Surgery Oncology Fellowship, Cleveland Clinic Akron General, Akron, Ohio, USA

ELENA MICHAELS, MD
Internal Medicine Specialist, Department of Medicine, University of Chicago, Chicago, Illinois, USA

KRISLYN N. MILLER, DO
Breast Surgical Oncology Fellow, Department of Surgery, Duke University Medical Center, Durham, North Carolina, USA

STEFANIA MORGANTI, MD
Clinical Research Fellow, Medical Oncology, Dana-Farber Cancer Institute, Breast Oncology Program, Dana-Farber Brigham Cancer Center, Harvard Medical School, Broad Institute of MIT and Harvard, Boston, Massachusetts, USA; Medical Oncology Fellow, Department of Oncology and Hemato-Oncology, University of Milan, Istituto Europeo di Oncologia, Milan, Italy

SAIMA MUZAHIR, MD, FCPS, FRCPE
Assistant Professor of Radiology, Enterprise Theranostic Lead, Division of Nuclear Medicine and Molecular Imaging, Department of Radiology and Imaging Sciences, Emory University Hospital, Atlanta, Georgia, USA

ANAND K. NARAYAN, MD, PhD
Vice Chair of Equity, Associate Professor, Department of Radiology, University of Wisconsin-Madison, Madison, Wisconsin, USA

SARAH NIELSEN, DO
Section Head–Breast Imaging, Department of Radiology, Marshfield Clinic Health System, Marshfield Clinic–Wausau Center, Wausau, Wisconsin, USA

HOLLY ORTMAN, MD
General Surgeon, Marshfield Medical Center, Marshfield, Wisconsin, USA

ANN H. PARTRIDGE, MD, MPH
Vice Chair, Department of Medical Oncology, Founder and Director of the Program for Young Adults with Breast Cancer, Director of the Adult Survivorship Program, Eric P. Winer Chair in Breast Cancer Research, Dana-Farber Cancer Institute, Professor of Medicine, Harvard Medical School, Boston, Massachusetts, USA

MIRAL M. PATEL, MD
Assistant Professor, Department of Breast Imaging, The University of Texas MD Anderson Cancer Center, Houston, Texas, USA

ANNE WARREN PELED, MD
Co-Director, Sutter Health California Pacific Medical Center Breast Cancer Program, San Francisco, California, USA

DAVID R. PENBERTHY, MD, MBA
Associate Professor of Radiation Oncology, Medical Director of Radiation Oncology, Department of Radiation Oncology, Penn State Cancer Institute, Penn State Health Milton S. Hershey College of Medicine, Hershey, Pennsylvania, USA

JENNIFER KIM PENBERTHY, PhD
Chester F. Carlson Professor of Psychiatry and Neurobehavioral Sciences, Department of Psychiatry and Neurobehavioral Sciences, UVA Cancer Center, University of Virginia School of Medicine and Health System, Charlottesville, Virginia, USA

JENNIFER K. PLICHTA, MD, MS
Director of the Breast Risk Assessment Clinic, Associate Professor, Department of Surgery, Duke Cancer Institute, Department of Population Health Sciences, Duke University Medical Center, Durham, North Carolina, USA

GAIANE M. RAUCH, MD, PhD, FSBI, FSABI
Professor, Departments of Abdominal Imaging and Breast Imaging, The University of Texas MD Anderson Cancer Center, Houston, Texas, USA

ELIZABETH O. RIORDAN, MD
Breast Surgery Specialist, Marshfield Medical Center, Marshfield, Wisconsin, USA

MARK ROBSON, MD
Chief, Breast Medicine Service, Department of Medicine, Attending Physician, Memorial Hospital for Treatment of Cancer and Allied Disease, Member, Memorial Sloan Kettering Cancer Center, Professor of Medicine, Weill Cornell Medical College, New York, New York, USA

NATALIA RODRIGUEZ, MD
General Surgery Resident, Marshfield Medical Center, Marshfield, Wisconsin, USA

MARGUERITE M. ROONEY, BS
Medical Student, Department of Surgery, Duke University Medical Center, Durham, North Carolina, USA

KATHRYN J. RUDDY, MD, MPH
Professor, Department of Oncology, Mayo Clinic, Rochester, Minnesota, USA

JENNIFER RUSIECKI, MD, MS
Assistant Professor of Medicine, Department of Medicine, University of Chicago, Chicago, Illinois, USA

ARA A. SALIBIAN, MD
Plastic Surgeon, Division of Plastic and Reconstructive Surgery, University of California, Davis, Sacramento, California, USA

HANI SBITANY, MD
Chief, Division of Plastic and Reconstructive Surgery, Professor, Department of Surgery, Icahn School of Medicine, Mount Sinai, New York, New York, USA

DAVID M. SCHUSTER, MD, FACR
Professor of Radiology and Imaging Sciences and Urology, GRA Distinguished Cancer Scientist, Director, Division of Nuclear Medicine and Molecular Imaging, Department of Radiology and Imaging Sciences, Emory University Hospital, Atlanta, Georgia, USA

ANNA SEYDEL, MD, FACS
Director, Surgical Breast Services, Marshfield Medical Center, Marshfield, Wisconsin, USA

CIMMIE L. SHAHAN, MD
Medical Director of the Betty Puskar Breast Care Center, Section Chief of Breast Imaging, WVU Department of Radiology, Assistant Professor of Radiology, West Virginia University School of Medicine, Morgantown, West Virginia, USA

DAVID H. SONG, MD, MBA, FACS
Physician Executive Director, Department of Plastic Surgery, MedStar Plastic and Reconstructive Surgery, Washington, DC, USA

ANNE LOUISE STEWART, MD
Assistant Professor, Department of Psychiatry and Neurobehavioral Sciences, UVA
Cancer Center, University of Virginia School of Medicine and Health System,
Charlottesville, Virginia, USA

SAM Z. THALJI, MD
Surgery Resident, Department of Surgery, Division of Surgical Oncology, Medical College
of Wisconsin, Milwaukee, Wisconsin, USA

RACHEL TILLMAN, MD
Resident Physician, Marshfield Medical Center, Marshfield, Wisconsin, USA

SARA M. TOLANEY, MD, MPH
Chief of the Division of Breast Oncology, Medical Oncology, Dana-Farber Cancer
Institute, Breast Oncology Program, Dana-Farber Brigham Cancer Center, Harvard
Medical School, Boston, Massachusetts, USA

GARY A. ULANER, MD, PhD, FACNM
James and Pamela Muzzy Endowed Chair in Molecular Imaging and Therapy, Hoag
Family Cancer Institute, Newport Beach, California, USA; Clinical Professor of Radiology
and Translational Genomics, Department of Radiology, Department of Translational
Genomics, University of Southern California, Los Angeles, California, USA

TON WANG, MD, MS
Surgical Oncologist, Department of Surgery, Cedars-Sinai Medical Center, Los Angeles,
California, USA

HANNAH Y. WEN, MD, PhD
Director of Breast Pathology Fellowship, Associate Attending Pathologist, Department of
Pathology and Laboratory Medicine, Memorial Sloan Kettering Cancer Center, New York,
New York, USA

MARISSA J. WHITE, MD
Assistant Professor, Department of Pathology, Johns Hopkins School of Medicine,
Baltimore, Maryland, USA

REBECA ORTIZ WORTHINGTON, MD, MS
Assistant Professor of Medicine, Department of Medicine, University of Chicago,
Chicago, Illinois, USA

RENA R. XIAN, MD
Assistant Professor, Departments of Pathology and Oncology, Johns Hopkins School of
Medicine, Baltimore, Maryland, USA

Contents

Genetic testing plays an important role in assessing breast cancer risk and often the risk of other types of cancers. Accurate risk assessment and stratification represents a critical element of identifying who is best served by increased survelllance and consideration of other prevention or treatment options while also limiting overtreatment and unnecessary testing. The indications for testing will likely continue to expand, and ideally, more women with a genetic predisposition to breast cancer will be identified before they are diagnosed with breast cancer and thus have the option to consider effective screening and prevention management strategies.

The era of genomic medicine provides an opportunity for pathologists to offer greater detail about the molecular underpinnings of a patient's cancer and thereby more targeted therapeutic options. In this review article, the role of genomics in breast cancer pathology is discussed, as it pertains to risk management, classification of special tumor types, predictive and prognostic testing, identification of actionable therapeutic targets, and monitoring for disease progression or development of treatment resistance.

Among women, breast cancer remains the second leading cause of cancer death in the United States. Mammography remains the only validated screening tool to reduce breast cancer mortality. The American Society of Breast Surgeons recommends that average-risk women undergo breast cancer screening every year starting at age 40. This article reviews the fundamentals of mammography screening, current age-based mammography screening recommendations, supplemental breast cancer screening recommendations in high-risk women, and novel imaging technologies. This review summarizes recommendations from the American Society of Breast Surgeons and published guidelines from major societies to reflect a range of evidence-based perspectives regarding mammographic screening.

When *BRCA1* and *BRCA2* were first identified, the initial models for delivering testing were shaped by concepts of genetic exceptionalism and a lack of data regarding therapeutic implications and the effectiveness of risk reduction. Since then, interventions have been effective, and treatment implications have become clear. The sensitivity of guideline-based testing is incomplete, leading to calls for universal testing. Completely universal testing, however, is not necessary to identify the great majority of *BRCA1* or *BRCA2* variants. Broader testing (both in terms of eligibility and genes tested) will identify more variants, particularly in moderate penetrance genes, but the clinical implications remain less clear for these variants

Predictive biomarker testing on metastatic breast cancer is essential for determining patient eligibility for targeted therapeutics. The National Comprehensive Cancer Network currently recommends assessment of specific biomarkers on metastatic tumor subtypes, including hormone receptors, HER2, and *BRCA1/2* mutations, on all newly metastatic breast cancers subtypes; programmed death-ligand 1 on metastatic triple-negative carcinomas; and *PIK3CA* mutation status on estrogen receptor-positive carcinomas. In select circumstances mismatch repair protein deficiency and/or microsatellite insufficiency, tumor mutation burden, and *NTRK* translocation status are also testing options. Novel biomarker testing, such as detecting *PIK3CA* mutations in circulating tumor DNA, is expanding in this rapidly evolving arena.

Primary Care

Multiple tools exist to assess a patient's breast cancer risk. The choice of risk model depends on the patient's risk factors and how the calculation will impact care. High-risk patients—those with a lifetime breast cancer risk of $\geq 20\%$—are, for instance, eligible for supplemental screening with breast magnetic resonance imaging. Those with an elevated short-term breast cancer risk (frequently defined as a 5-year risk $\geq 1.66\%$) should be offered endocrine prophylaxis. High-risk patients should also receive guidance on modification of lifestyle factors that affect breast cancer risk.

Breast cancer is the most commonly diagnosed cancer in women. Associated psychological symptoms include stress, adjustment difficulties, anxiety, depression, impaired cognitive function, sleep disturbances, altered body image, sexual dysfunction, and diminished overall well-being. Distress screening and assessment identifies women who will benefit from therapeutic interventions. Addressing these symptoms improves compliance with treatment and outcomes including disease-related outcomes, psychological symptoms, and quality of life. The most effective treatments include teaching coping skills such as expressing emotion, along with other structured cognitive behavioral, interpersonal, and mindfulness approaches. Patients should be provided these psychosocial supports throughout their cancer journey.

There has been a 40% decline in breast cancer age-adjusted death rate since 1990. Black American women have not experienced as great a decline; indeed, the Black-White disparity in mortality in the United States is greater today than it has ever been. Certain states (areas of residence), however, do not see such dramatic differences in outcome by race. This latter finding suggests much more can be done to reduce disparities and prevent deaths. Interventions to get high-quality care (screening, diagnostics, and treatment) involve understanding the needs and concerns of the patient and addressing those needs and concerns. Patient navigators are 1 way to improve outcomes.

Diagnosis

This review provides an outline of a risk-based approach to breast cancer screening and prevention. All women should be assessed for breast cancer risk starting at age 18 with identification of modifiable and non-modifiable risk factors. Patients can then be stratified into average, moderate, and high-risk groups with personalized screening and prevention plans. Counseling on breast awareness and lifestyle changes is recommended for all women, regardless of risk category. High-risk individuals may benefit from additional screening modalities such as MRI and chemoprevention and should be managed closely by a multidisciplinary team.

Breast cancer is the most commonly diagnosed nonskin cancer in women. To decrease the breast cancer burden, conserve resources, and decrease unnecessary treatments, guidelines suggest interventions be reserved for those women at greatest risk for disease. Risk assessment incorporating breast cancer risk factors and risk assessment models is of paramount importance in identifying women who have the greatest benefit from risk reduction strategies. Principles of shared decision-making should guide practitioners to incorporate patients' values, goals, and objectives in decisions around genetic testing, pharmacologic intervention, enhanced surveillance, and other risk reduction strategies.

In the last several decades, breast imaging has undergone transformation. Technological advances in mammography and ultrasound and the development and increased availability of imaging modalities used in

Breast cancer (BC) remains one of the leading causes of death among women. The management and outcome in BC are strongly influenced by a multidisciplinary approach, which includes available treatment options and different imaging modalities for accurate response assessment. Among breast imaging modalities, MR imaging is the modality of choice in evaluating response to neoadjuvant therapy, whereas F-18 Fluorodeoxyglucose positron emission tomography, conventional computed tomography (CT), and bone scan play a vital role in assessing response to therapy in metastatic BC. There is an unmet need for a standardized patient-centric approach to use different imaging methods for response assessment.

Chemotherapy

There is now a deeper understanding of the biology of hormone receptor-positive (HR+) early breast cancer (EBC) that can be used to inform assessment of risk and prognosis, and also guide more effective adjuvant systemic therapies. For postmenopausal HR+ EBC endocrine therapy remains the mainstay of treatment with extended duration up to 10 years for some, the addition of targeted CDK 4/6 inhibitors for those with node-positive high-risk disease, and de-escalation of chemotherapy use for those in whom it is unlikely to be of benefit. As such, systemic adjuvant therapy is now highly tailored and individualized.

For women with triple-negative breast cancer, the addition of pembrolizumab to chemotherapy has become a standard of care in the early-stage and first-line metastatic setting. However, many questions persist. Different chemotherapy backbones and sequencing strategies have been evaluated, but evidence supporting the superiority of one over the other is weak. Although many have been investigated, programmed cell death ligand 1 (PDL1) is the only approved biomarker. Since immunotherapy has been associated with potentially severe and permanent toxicities, the identification of better predictive biomarkers is essential. New strategies are needed to increase the proportion of patients who might benefit from immunotherapy.

Surgical Treatment

Although surgery of the breast and axilla is generally well-tolerated by patients, the breast surgeon recognizes that complications can occur even when operating with experience on the lowest risk patients. The operative repertoire ranges from breast conserving surgery, mastectomy (including skin-sparing and nipple-sparing types), to modified radical mastectomy, with each procedure carrying a different expected surgical morbidity.

Patients and families who are fully informed of potential complications before their operation describe greater trust in their surgeon and are better able to co-manage complications with the surgical team, when they occur.

Anne Warren Peled and Nicholas W. Clavin

As breast oncologic surgical procedures and approaches have evolved in recent years, so have breast reconstruction techniques. Newer advances focus on expanding the options of reconstructive approaches and patient selection, optimizing quality of life, and helping improve postsurgical survivorship. These advances span from techniques to expand criteria for nipple-sparing mastectomies, optimizing and enhancing oncoplastic surgery, evolving autologous reconstruction options, and preserving and restoring sensation after mastectomy.

Ara A. Salibian and Nolan S. Karp

The modern approach to implant-based breast reconstruction encompasses an evolution in surgical techniques, patient selection, implant technology, and use of support materials. Successful outcomes are defined by teamwork throughout the ablative and reconstructive processes as well as appropriate and evidence-based utilization of modern material technologies. Patient education, focus on patient-reported outcomes, and informed and shared decision-making are the key to all steps of these procedures.

Francis D. Graziano, Jocelyn Lu, and Hani Sbitany

Prepectoral breast reconstruction has gained popularity due to numerous benefits in properly selected patients. Compared with subpectoral implant reconstruction, prepectoral reconstruction offers preservation of the pectoralis major muscle in its native position, resulting in decreased pain, no animation deformity, and improved arm range of motion/strength. Although prepectoral reconstruction is safe and effective, the implant sits closer to the mastectomy skin flap. Acellular dermal matrices play a critical role, allowing for precise control of the breast envelope and providing long-term implant support. Careful patient selection and intraoperative mastectomy flap evaluation are critical to obtaining optimal results with prepectoral breast reconstruction.

Salma A. Abdou, Karina Charipova, and David H. Song

The latissimus dorsi flap with immediate fat transfer is a viable option for fully autologous breast reconstruction in patients who are not candidates for free flap reconstruction. Technical modifications described in this article allow for high-volume and efficient fat grafting at the time of reconstruction to augment the flap and mitigate complications associated with the use of an implant.

Marla Lipsyc-Sharf and Ann H. Partridge

Fertility and sexual health may be impaired by early breast cancer treatment in young women, and these issues should be addressed at diagnosis and through survivorship. Future fertility interest and risk should be considered and communicated, and early referral made to an infertility specialist for those interested. Data regarding safety of fertility preservation options as well as pregnancy after breast cancer are overall reassuring. Patients should be counseled about the impact of systemic therapies and breast surgeries on sexual health outcomes and educated about and referred as needed for available strategies for prevention and management of impairment.

Preface
A Modern Day Approach to Breast Cancer

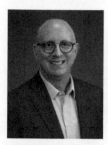

Joel J. Heidelbaugh,
MD, FAAFP, FACG
Consulting Editor

According to the National Breast Cancer Foundation, one in eight women in the United States will be diagnosed with breast cancer in her lifetime. In 2023, an estimated 297,790 women and 2800 men were diagnosed with invasive breast cancer. When detected in its earliest and localized stages, the 5-year relative survival rate approaches 99%. As a testament to screening guidelines and advances in diagnostics and therapeutics, there are currently over 3.8 million breast cancer survivors in the United States.

This issue of *Clinics Collections* provides an in-depth overview that spans many aspects of breast cancer from screening to the care of the patient that has been diagnosed with breast cancer. The issue highlights articles that encompass elements of pathology, primary care, oncology, surgery, and psychology. This comprehensive guide to breast cancer commences with information presented on genetics and genomics, screening guidelines and techniques, and novel options for testing in patients with metastatic breast cancer. As primary care providers play an integral role in screening patients for potential breast cancer, detailed articles highlight provisions for risk assessment and primary prevention as well as guides to advances in breast imaging on both the molecular and the radiographic levels.

The scope of our issue on breast cancer is significantly enhanced with articles that discuss how to incorporate value-based decisions in treatment algorithms, the role of the patient navigator in care coordination, and the importance of addressing inequalities and disparities in breast cancer care delivery. Current strategies in therapeutics spanning chemotherapy, radiation therapy, and surgery, including reconstructive surgery, are presented by leading experts in their respective fields. Last, yet perhaps most importantly, quality-of-life issues in the patient with breast cancer are presented

Clinics Collections 14 (2024) xvii–xviii
https://doi.org/10.1016/j.ccol.2024.02.001
2352-7986/24/© 2024 Published by Elsevier Inc.

incorporating issues following treatment, evidence-based guidelines for survivorship, and fertility and sexual health issues in young women with early-stage breast cancer.

The paradigms for diagnosis and treatment of breast cancer have evolved substantially in recent decades, and advances in technology and health care delivery will continue to drive this important topic forward. We hope that you will find this issue dedicated to breast cancer highly useful in your respective practices.

DISCLOSURES

The author has no conflicts of interest to disclose.

Joel J. Heidelbaugh, MD, FAAFP, FACG
Departments of Family Medicine and Urology
Department of Family Medicine
University of Michigan Medical School
200 Arnet, Suite 200
Ypsilanti, MI 48198, USA

E-mail address:
jheidel@umich.edu

Pathology

Genetics of Breast Cancer

Risk Models, Who to Test, and Management Options

Marguerite M. Rooney, BS[a], Krislyn N. Miller, DO[a],
Jennifer K. Plichta, MD, MS[a,b,c],*

KEYWORDS

- Breast cancer risk • Breast cancer genetics • Genetic testing
- Breast cancer prevention • Breast cancer screening

KEY POINTS

- Women age ≥25 years old should undergo breast cancer risk assessment, particularly those with a family history of cancer.
- Multiple risk models exist to help evaluate a patient's risk of developing breast cancer, and they differ based on the risk factors included and the types of risk calculations provided.
- Not all risk models are appropriate for assessing breast cancer risk for every patient.
- Depending on risk level or known genetic mutation, increased imaging surveillance may be recommended.
- Depending on risk level or known genetic mutation, bilateral risk-reducing mastectomy may be considered.

INTRODUCTION

Breast cancer is the most common noncutaneous cancer in women, with more than 285,000 estimated cases to be diagnosed in 2022 in the United States.[1] Efforts to improve breast cancer treatment and increase survival focus not only on treatment development and early detection but also on the identification of patients at a higher risk of developing breast cancer. Breast cancer risk factors can include hormonal and lifestyle factors, family history, and/or known germline mutations in a breast-cancer-related gene.[2] Current research has identified several germline mutations that contribute to a patient's risk of developing breast cancer.[3,4] In addition to known genetic mutations, patients can also be considered high risk based on family history alone.[5]

This article previously appeared in *Surgical Clinics* volume 103 Issue 1 February 2023.
^a Department of Surgery, Duke University Medical Center, Durham, NC 22710, USA; ^b Duke Cancer Institute, Duke University Medical Center, Durham, NC 22710, USA; ^c Department of Population Health Sciences, Duke University Medical Center, Durham, NC 27710, USA
* Corresponding author. Department of Surgery, Duke University Medical Center, DUMC 3513, Durham, NC 22710.
E-mail address: jennifer.plichta@duke.edu

In all, approximately 5% to 10% of breast cancers are from identifiable germline genetic causes.[6] As such, many breast cancer risk models have been developed to combine risk factors to estimate an individual's risk of developing breast cancer, risk of carrying a *BRCA1* or *BRCA2* mutation, or the risk of both. These tools can assist clinicians when selecting which patients to refer for genetic counseling and when patients may qualify for genetic testing, increased imaging surveillance, and/or consideration of other medical or surgical interventions, thus helping to guide testing, treatment, and screening recommendations for these patients. Several organizations, including the National Comprehensive Cancer Network (NCCN), recommend genetic risk evaluation for selected patients. The American Society for Breast Surgeons (ASBrS) recommends that all women aged 25 years or more undergo formal risk assessment for breast cancer with updates based on changes in family or personal medical history.[7] The United States Preventive Services Task Force, meanwhile, recommends risk assessment only for patients with a personal or family history of breast, ovarian, tubal, or peritoneal cancers, or for those with ancestry associated with mutations, such as Ashkenazi Jews.[8,9]

At present, the NCCN does not recommend universal germline genetic testing for all patients with breast cancer, although the ASBrS does recommend offering genetic testing to all patients with breast cancer, recognizing insurance coverage may not consistently support this universal approach. The NCCN guidelines describe criteria for genetic testing based on a family history of several different cancers with associated ages at diagnosis for the affected family members. If patients do not meet the criteria set forth by the NCCN but do have a greater than 5% probability of a *BRCA1/2* mutation based on risk models, testing may still be indicated, and it may even be considered for those patients with a 2.5% to 5% probability of a *BRCA1/2* mutation based on these models.[10] Although there are many models, this article describes several of the most relevant and validated (**Table 1**).

MODELS: BREAST CANCER AND GENETIC RISK
Family History Assessment Tool

The Family History Assessment Tool (FHAT) is a validated scoring tool initially developed to help clinicians identify which patients would most benefit from a referral to genetic counseling based on family cancer history.[11] As expected with a first-pass screening tool, FHAT has high sensitivity (94%; specificity 51%), and as such does typically identify several false-positives.[12] Unlike the other models discussed later, this tool does not provide a percent likelihood of developing breast cancer but rather has a scoring threshold after which genetic counseling is recommended.

Breast Cancer Risk Assessment Tool

One of the earliest breast cancer risk models, Breast Cancer Risk Assessment Tool (BCRAT), based on the Gail Model, estimates the risk of developing invasive breast cancer in the next 5 years and through age 90 years (lifetime risk) for women older than 35 years using personal reproductive history and family history of first-degree relatives.[13] This model uses hormonal risk factors (age at menarche, age at first live birth) and pathologic (personal history of breast disease and breast biopsy). This model was initially developed on 280,000 white women aged 35 to 74 years in the Breast Cancer Detection Demonstration Project and Surveillance, Epidemiology, and End Results Program as a joint National Cancer Institute and American Society of Breast Cancer screening study.[14] Later, it was extended via smaller studies (ranging from 1563–3244 patients) to include risk assessment for black, Asian, Pacific Islander, and Hispanic women.[15–17] However, it is thought to underestimate risk for black women.[18] This model has also been demonstrated to underestimate the risk for women with atypical hyperplasia.[19]

Table 1
Selected breast cancer risk assessment models: model outputs, included personal and family risk factors, excluded populations

Model	FHAT[11]	BCRAT[13]	Claus Model[20,23]	BRCAPRO[66]	BOADICEA[27,67,68]	Tyrer-Cuzick[69]
Risk evaluation						
Evaluates risk of developing breast cancer	✓	✓	✓	✓	✓	✓
Evaluates risk of having BRCA1 or BRCA2				✓	✓	✓
Personal risk factor inclusion						
Age	✓	✓	✓	✓	✓	✓
Race/ethnicity	✓	✓		✓		✓
BMI						✓
Age at menarche	✓	✓				✓
Age at first live birth	✓	✓				✓
Age at menopause						✓
Hormone replacement therapy use						✓
Breast density						✓
History of prior breast biopsy	✓	✓				✓
History of atypical ductal hyperplasia	✓	✓				✓a
History of lobular carcinoma in situ						✓a
Family history inclusion						
First-degree relatives	✓	✓	✓	✓	✓	✓
Second-degree relatives	✓		✓	✓	✓	✓
Third-degree relatives	✓			✓	✓	

(continued on next page)

Table 1
(continued)

Model	FHAT[11]	BCRAT[13]	Claus Model[20,23]	BRCAPRO[66]	BOADICEA[27,67,68]	Tyrer-Cuzick[69]
Age at onset of breast cancer	✓		✓	✓	✓	✓
Bilateral breast cancer	✓			✓	✓	✓
Ovarian cancer	✓			✓	✓	✓
Male breast cancer				✓	✓	
Excluded populations		• Personal history of breast cancer, DCIS, LCIS • Known BRCA1/2 mutation • Past chest radiation	• Patients without a family history of breast cancer			

Abbreviations: BCRAT, Breast Cancer Risk Assessment Tool; BMI, body mass index; BOADICEA, Breast and Ovarian Analysis of Disease Incidence and Carrier Estimation Algorithm; DCIS, ductal carcinoma in situ; FHAT, Family History Assessment Tool; LCIS, lobular carcinoma in situ.
[a] May overestimate risk in this population and therefore not be appropriate for use.

Claus model

The Claus model was developed using a population-based, case-control study (Cancer and Steroid Hormone Study [CASH]), conducted by the Centers for Disease Control and Prevention.[20,21] This model does not include nonhereditary risk factors in determining lifetime risk of breast cancer and should be used only for women with at least 1 female first- or second-degree relative with breast cancer, based on the assumption that breast cancer is transmitted in an autosomal dominant manner.[12,22] There are 2 versions of the Claus model: risk tables ("Claus tables"), which are based on the model, and the model itself.[23]

MODELS: BREAST CANCER AND GENETIC RISK
BRCAPRO

BRCAPRO predicts a patient's probability of carrying a *BRCA1* or *BRCA2* mutation, the probability of developing invasive breast cancer or ovarian cancer (if not diagnosed with breast cancer), and the probability of developing a contralateral breast cancer (if breast cancer is present).[24,25] The model relies on family history (including relation, age at diagnosis, pathologic markers, race, ethnicity, and treatment), as well as prevalence and penetrance of *BRCA1* and *BRCA2* and baseline breast cancer rates in the population. The model then applies Bayes theorem.

Breast and Ovarian Analysis of Disease Incidence and Carrier Estimation Algorithm

Breast and Ovarian Analysis of Disease Incidence and Carrier Estimation Algorithm (BOADICEA) is intended for women with a family history that may suggest an increased risk of breast or ovarian cancer, to predict the probability of a *BRCA1* or *BRCA2* mutation and risk of developing breast cancer.[26,27] BOADICEA uses family history of breast and ovarian cancer to calculate risk.

Tyrer-Cuzick Model (International Breast Cancer Study)

The Tyrer-Cuzick model estimates a patient's risk of a *BRCA1* or *BRCA2* mutation and risk of developing an invasive or in situ cancer over time by using genetic and hormonal risk factors. Tyrer-Cuzick is particularly useful in populations that are at high risk based on family history where models such as the BCRAT are not as effective.[13] In addition, it predicts the risk of both invasive and in situ cancers rather than just invasive cancers. Importantly, this model has been demonstrated to overestimate invasive cancer risk in women with lobular carcinoma in situ and atypical hyperplasia, and other models may be more accurate for these patient populations.[28,29]

GERMLINE GENETIC TESTING

Genetic testing for breast cancer has grown considerably in recent history. When genetic testing for breast cancer was first available, only limited gene panels, typically evaluating only *BRCA1* and *BRCA2*, were available. However, only up to 30% of *genetically linked* breast cancers are driven by germline *BRCA1/2* mutations.[6] Now, multigene assays evaluating for high-, moderate-, and low-penetrance genes beyond just *BRCA1/2* are available. Therefore, there is a potential group of patients who received limited or single-gene genetic testing before 2014 who may benefit from repeat/expanded testing.[30]

Although expanding the criteria for germline genetic testing is gaining popularity and the NCCN guidelines become more inclusive every year, there remain several obstacles to testing. One of the main concerns is who will perform the genetic counseling and testing. Although there were an estimated 4700 genetic counselors in the United States in 2019, 17 states had 20 or fewer genetic counselors in the entire state, and 4 states had 5 or less.[31] Furthermore, many genetic counselors are not involved in direct patient care, opting instead to work for companies in industry or pharma; and of those seeing patients, many work in noncancer areas, such as prenatal genetics. To combat this problem, some have advocated for physicians to perform their own counseling and testing,[32] which is supported by several organizations in official statements and by providing education.[7,9,32] Beyond those limitations, cost also remains a concern. After identifying the association of *BRCA1* and *BRCA2* with breast cancer in the 1990s,[33,34] 1 company was performing all *BRCA1/2* testing. However, in 2013, the supreme court invalidated the gene patents for that company,[35] thus opening the door for new companies to offer genetic testing related to cancer; this ultimately led to the rapid decline in the cost of genetic testing from more than $4000 for *BRCA1/2* testing alone to now offering multigene panels for $250.[36] Although still not free or feasible for some patients, it is certainly much more attainable for many. It is also worth noting that direct-to-consumer testing is available, but it has not been validated for clinical use, and any "positive" results from these tests should be confirmed in a clinically approved laboratory certified by the Clinical Laboratory Improvement Amendments.[10]

Of the numerous clinically approved testing companies currently offering germline genetic testing, options include both limited and expanded panels. Some favor a more limited approach, testing for only those genes that are most likely to be related to the history presented. However, others prefer to test all genes that may have implications for the patient, even if the risk of harboring such a mutation is low, particularly given the decreasing cost and minimal difference in risk to the patient. Once a test is selected, patient samples can now be provided via multiple methods, such as blood draws and buccal swabs, or even saliva samples, although blood samples tend to be the most reliable (ie, adequate for testing).

When the results from a test return, 5 possible outcomes may be reported for any given variant identified: benign, likely benign, pathogenic, likely pathogenic, or variant of uncertain significance (VUS). As the names imply, benign and likely benign variants are considered "negative," and no further recommendations are typically required. In contrast, pathogenic and likely pathogenic variants are considered "positive" test results, and providers can refer to national guidelines, such as those published by the NCCN, for management recommendations.[10] For VUS findings, it is important to remember that these are actually considered "negative" as well, meaning that no intervention or management decision should be altered based on this finding. Although VUS rates for *BRCA1* and *BRCA2* have steadily declined as more patients have been tested, the expansion of testing to many other genes has yielded a notable increase in overall VUS rates.[37] However, this should similarly decline as again more patients, and particularly more diverse patient populations, are tested.

In addition, racial and ethnic disparities exist in access to and uptake of genetic testing for all cancers and in breast cancer in particular, with previous work demonstrating racial and ethnic disparities in genetic testing for solid tumor malignancies.[38,39] In breast cancer, previous work has shown how contributing factors such as decreased provider referrals, access, and awareness has led to lower rates of genetic testing for black women compared with their white counterparts.[40–44] As genetic testing becomes more and more common, it will be critical to make sure that all patients from diverse ethnic backgrounds have equal access to testing and to ensure the risk models and testing reflect the diversity of potential outcomes and risks based on racial and ethnic origins.

Genetic testing and risk modeling demonstrate the need for interdisciplinary care for the patient at high risk for the development of breast cancer. Although access to a genetic counselor allows for increased genetic testing and timely counseling, not all centers and patients have access.[45,46] In this setting, surgeons can play a critical role in conducting initial risk assessment, identifying patients who may benefit from genetic counseling, and often recommending and ordering genetic testing.[32]

IMAGE-BASED SCREENING FOR BREAST CANCER IN HIGH-RISK POPULATIONS

In addition to the general population screening guidelines, the NCCN has screening guidelines for patients with high- or moderate-risk gene mutations related to breast cancer. According to the 2022 NCCN guidelines, patients with high-risk gene mutations (ie, $\geq$50% absolute lifetime risk of breast cancer [BRCA1, BRCA2, CDH1, PALB2, PTEN, and TP53]) should follow specific screening guidelines. The NCCN recommends that for BRCA1 and BRCA2 mutation carriers, breast awareness should start at age 18 years, with clinical breast examinations every 6 to 12 months starting at age 25 years. Furthermore, breast cancer imaging/screening for women aged 25 to 29 years should include an annual breast MRI with contrast, or if MRI is unavailable, annual mammogram, with consideration of tomosynthesis. Women aged 30 to 75 years should receive an annual mammogram with consideration of tomosynthesis and a breast MRI with contrast; beyond age 75 years, management should be conducted on an individual basis. Notably, these same screening guidelines apply to women with BRCA1/2 mutations even after a breast cancer diagnosis, if they have residual breast tissue (underwent lumpectomy or only a unilateral mastectomy). Patients with a high-risk TP53 mutation have similar recommendations as those patients who are BRCA1/2 mutation carriers except for clinical breast examinations beginning at an even earlier age (ie, age 20 years or at the age of the earliest diagnosed breast cancer in the family if younger than 20 years). The recommendations for those women with CDH1, PALB2, and PTEN mutations consist of an annual mammogram with consideration of tomosynthesis and breast MRI with contrast starting at age 30 years.[47]

The NCCN recommends that those patients with moderate-risk mutations (20% to 50% absolute lifetime risk of developing breast cancer, ie, ATM, BARD1, CDH1, CHEK2, and NF1) undergo annual screening mammography with consideration of tomosynthesis and breast MRI with contrast. The age of starting this screening depends on the gene mutation. For instance, those with CDH1 and NF1 are recommended to begin screening mammography and MRI at age 30 years, whereas women with ATM, CHEK2, and BARD1 mutations are recommended to begin at age 40 years.[47]

Because women with high-risk genes tend to develop breast cancer at a younger age when breast tissue is dense, the sensitivity of mammography alone is lower. In high-risk women, the sensitivity of MRI detecting a breast abnormality ranges from 77% to 100% with a specificity of 81% to 98.9%; this compares to mammography, which has a sensitivity of 12.5% to 40% and specificity of 93% to 100%. Therefore, mammography in association with MRI is the standard screening recommendation in these moderate- to high-risk women.[48] There are certain criteria required for the administration of a high-quality MRI screening, including regional availability, a radiologist with breast MRI imaging experience, the ability to perform biopsy under MRI guidance, and dedicated breast coils specific for breast imaging.[47] In addition to unavailability, reasons for declining MRIs for screening purposes include patient claustrophobia, patient time constraints, financial concerns, referral issues, body habitus, body implants, and frailty.[49]

Screening with whole breast ultrasonography (WBUS) is another imaging tool used for women who cannot or do not wish to undergo MRIs. Overall, this modality is well tolerated, widely available, relatively inexpensive, and does not require intravenous contrast or ionizing radiation. WBUS has been shown to detect cancers not seen on mammography with a greater sensitivity in dense breast. Concerns include the need for a highly experienced technologist and the inability to detect calcifications.[50]

Contrast-enhanced mammography (CEM), which uses modified digital mammography with the addition of an intravenous contrast agent, is another imaging modality that is not standard for breast cancer screening, yet shows promise for the future.[51] In a retrospective study by Sung and colleagues,[51] 904 patients received baseline CEM screenings with 1-year follow-up. Results showed a breast cancer detection rate of 15.5 of 1000, sensitivity increased from 50% with the standard mammography to 87.5% with CEM (p = 0.03), and specificity was 93.7% (95% confidence interval, 91.9%–95.3%).[51] Other imaging modalities, such as thermography, which detects localized skin temperature gradients and produces a heat map of the breast (thermogram), have been theorized to identify developing tumors; yet, there is insufficient evidence to support its use in breast cancer screening.[52]

ROLE OF RISK-REDUCING BREAST SURGERY

According to the NCCN guidelines, bilateral risk-reducing mastectomy (BRRM) may be considered and discussed with all women with a high-risk pathogenic/likely pathogenic germline genetic mutation, which includes BRCA1, BRCA2, CDH1, PALB2, PTEN, and TP53. Discussions should include the degree of protection, reconstruction options, and residual breast cancer risk with age and life expectancy.[47] Surgical risk-reducing mastectomies include simple, total, skin-sparing, or nipple-sparing mastectomies, all of which have been shown to be safe and feasible options for women choosing a risk-reducing surgery. Regardless of the type of mastectomy, the goal is to remove as much of the breast tissue as possible for the obvious reason of reducing the risk of developing breast cancer.[48] In a review of 201 BRCA1/2 carriers, Yao and colleagues demonstrated that nipple-sparing mastectomies have a low rate of complications and locoregional recurrence. Loss of the nipple areolar complex occurred in 1.8% of the patients, flap necrosis in 2.5%, and there were 4 recurrences (none at the nipple areolar complex and 3 in patients with cancer) over a mean follow-up time of 32.6 months.[53] Reconstruction options using implant-based (silicone or saline) prepectoral or postpectoral versus autogenous flap grafts should be part of the discussion with the patient when they are opting for BRRM.[48]

BRRM reduces the risk of developing breast cancer by more than 90%[54]; however, the survival benefit is unclear. According to Heemskerk-Gerritsen and colleagues,[55] who reviewed 2857 BRCA1/2 mutation carriers in the Netherlands, 42% of the BRCA1 and 35% of the BRCA2 mutation carriers received BRRMs. During a mean follow-up of 10 years, breast cancer-specific survival of women at age 65 years with BRCA1 mutations was 93% for patients receiving surveillance versus 99.7% for those who had BRRM, in contrast to patients with a BRCA2 mutation, for which rates were 98% and 100%, respectively. Overall, they concluded that BRRM for BRCA1 mutation carriers was associated with lower mortality, but not necessarily for BRCA2 mutation carriers.[55]

Consideration around unwanted secondary effects such as chronic pain, decreased body image, and decreased sexual satisfaction also needs to be part of the BRRM discussion. A 2018 Cochrane review looked at these psychosocial effects, reporting that generally, patients were satisfied with their decision for BRRM, but their psychological well-being was impacted.[54] In particular, Gahm and colleagues[56] demonstrated in their review of 59 women post-BRRM that 69% reported chronic pain, 71% reported discomfort in their breasts, and 85% had reduced sexual sensations, which all negatively impacted their enjoyment of sex. However, their quality of life and feelings of regret were not a factor.[56] An additional Cochrane review specifically focused on the psychosocial interventions and the effect these had on the quality of life and emotional well-being in female BRCA mutation carriers who underwent BRRM. Unfortunately, only 2 studies with small sample sizes fit the review criteria and no conclusions could be drawn from the data. These findings (or lack thereof) further emphasize the importance of supporting women when they choose this type of elective risk-reducing surgery and the need for further research in this area of long-term outcomes for risk-reducing surgery.[57]

TREATMENT OF BREAST CANCER IN HIGH-RISK PATIENTS

For women with a genetic predisposition to breast cancer who develop breast cancer, survival outcomes may vary. However, a systematic review and meta-analysis of 66 studies of patients with breast cancer and BRCA1/2 mutations noted that the evidence was inconclusive, because some studies suggested worse outcomes, whereas others demonstrated relatively more favorable survival outcomes.[58] Given no clear difference in survival outcomes, patients with BRCA1/2 mutations and breast cancer may still be eligible for breast-conserving therapy (lumpectomy and radiation), similar to those patients with breast cancer and no BRCA1/2 mutation.[59] However, patients with BRCA1/2 mutations do have an increased risk of developing a contralateral (or second primary) breast cancer, potentially as high as greater than 30%, depending on the age at diagnosis of the first breast cancer.[60] As such, many women with BRCA1/2 mutations and breast cancer may opt for bilateral mastectomies (1 therapeutic and 1 prophylactic) to reduce that risk of a second breast cancer.[61]

Beyond surgery, there are now systemic therapy options that are specific to women with a genetic predisposition to breast cancer. For example, the recently published OlympiA trial demonstrated that women with BRCA1/2 mutations and early breast cancer may benefit from 1 year of an adjuvant poly(adenosine diphosphate-ribose) polymerase inhibitor (PARPi).[62] Similar benefits were previously demonstrated for women with BRCA1/2 mutations and metastatic/advanced breast cancer as well.[63,64] In addition to its impact on systemic therapy options, the results of genetic testing may also impact radiation therapy recommendations, because women with TP53 mutations or homozygous ATM mutations are generally advised to avoid therapeutic radiation.[65] As more women with a genetic predisposition to (breast) cancer are identified, more research will undoubtedly reveal additional areas where we can personalize treatment recommendations for our patients.

SUMMARY

Genetic testing plays an important role in assessing breast cancer risk and often the risk of other types of cancers. Accurate risk assessment and stratification represents a critical element of identifying who is best served by increased surveillance and consideration of other prevention or treatment options while also limiting overtreatment and unnecessary testing. Given the implications of these types of genetic test results, the indications for testing will likely continue to expand, and ideally, more women with a genetic predisposition to breast cancer will be identified before they are diagnosed with breast cancer and thus have the option to consider effective screening and prevention management strategies.

CLINICS CARE POINTS

- Women aged 25 years or older should undergo breast cancer risk assessment, particularly those with a family history of cancer.

- Multiple risk models exist to help evaluate a patient's risk of developing breast cancer, and they differ based on the risk factors included and the types of risk calculations provided.
- Not all risk models are appropriate for assessing breast cancer risk for every patient.
- The indications for germline genetic testing are continually expanding.
- Depending on the risk level or known genetic mutation, increased imaging surveillance may be recommended.
- Depending on the risk level or known genetic mutation, BRRM may be considered.

DISCLOSURE

- The authors report no proprietary or commercial interest in any product mentioned or concept.
- Dr J.K. Plichta is a recipient of research funding by the Color Foundation (PI: J.K. Plichta). She serves on the National Comprehensive Cancer Network (NCCN) Breast Cancer Screening Committee.

REFERENCES

1. Breast cancer facts & figures, Am Cancer Soc, 2021, Available at: https://www.cancer.org/content/dam/cancer-org/research/cancer-facts-and-statistics/annual-cancer-facts-and-figures/2020/cancer-facts-and-figures-2020.pdf. Accessed August 4, 2021.
2. Rojas K, Stuckey A. Breast cancer epidemiology and risk factors. Clin Obstet Gynecol 2016;59:651–72.
3. Shiovitz S, Korde LA. Genetics of breast cancer: a topic in evolution. Ann Oncol 2015;26:1291–9.
4. Valencia OM, Samuel SE, Viscusi RK, et al. The role of genetic testing in patients with breast cancer: a review. JAMA Surg 2017;152:589–94.
5. Keeney MG, Couch FJ, Visscher DW, et al. Non-BRCA familial breast cancer: review of reported pathology and molecular findings. Pathology 2017;49:363–70.
6. Economopoulou P, Dimitriadis G, Psyrri A. Beyond BRCA: new hereditary breast cancer susceptibility genes. Cancer Treat Rev 2015;41:1–8.
7. Consensus Guideline on Hereditary Genetic Testing for Patients With and Without Breast Cancer. Available at: https://www.breastsurgeons.org/about/statements/PDF_Statements/BRCA_Testing.pdf. Accessed August/13/2018.
8. Owens DK, Davidson KW, Krist AH, et al. Risk assessment, genetic counseling, and genetic testing for BRCA-related cancer. JAMA 2019;322:652.
9. Rajagopal PS, Nielsen S, Olopade OI. USPSTF recommendations for BRCA1 and BRCA2 testing in the context of a transformative national cancer control plan. JAMA Netw Open 2019;2:e1910142.
10. Daly MB, Pal T, Berry MP, et al. Genetic/familial high-risk assessment: breast, ovarian, and pancreatic, version 2.2021, NCCN clinical practice guidelines in oncology. J Natl Compr Canc Netw 2021;19:77–102.
11. Gilpin C, Carson N, Hunter A. A preliminary validation of a family history assessment form to select women at risk for breast or ovarian cancer for referral to a genetics center. Clin Genet 2000;58:299–308.
12. Cintolo-Gonzalez JA, Braun D, Blackford AL, et al. Breast cancer risk models: a comprehensive overview of existing models, validation, and clinical applications. Breast Cancer Res Treat 2017;164:263–84.
13. https://bcrisktool.cancer.gov/.

14. Gail MH, Brinton LA, Byar DP, et al. Projecting individualized probabilities of developing breast cancer for white females who are being examined annually. J Natl Cancer Inst 1989;81:1879–86.
15. Matsuno RK, Costantino JP, Ziegler RG, et al. Projecting individualized absolute invasive breast cancer risk in asian and pacific islander american women. J Natl Cancer Inst 2011;103:951–61.
16. Gail MH, Costantino JP, Pee D, et al. Projecting individualized absolute invasive breast cancer risk in african american women. J Natl Cancer Inst 2007;99: 1782–92.
17. Banegas MP, John EM, Slattery ML, et al. Projecting Individualized absolute invasive breast cancer risk in US hispanic women. J Natl Cancer Inst 2017;109: djw215.
18. Adams-Campbell LL, Makambi KH, Palmer JR, et al. Diagnostic accuracy of the Gail model in the Black Women's Health Study. Breast J 2007;13:332–6.
19. Pankratz VS, Hartmann LC, Degnim AC, et al. Assessment of the accuracy of the Gail model in women with atypical hyperplasia. J Clin Oncol 2008;26:5374–9.
20. Claus EB, Risch N, Thompson WD. Genetic analysis of breast cancer in the cancer and steroid hormone study. Am J Hum Genet 1991;48:232–42.
21. Evans DGR, Howell A. Breast cancer risk-assessment models. Breast Cancer Res 2007;9:213.
22. Kim G, Bahl M. Assessing risk of breast cancer: a review of risk prediction models. J Breast Imaging 2021;3:144–55.
23. Claus EB, Risch N, Thompson WD. Autosomal dominant inheritance of early-onset breast cancer. Implications for risk prediction. Cancer 1994;73:643–51.
24. Parmigiani G, Berry D, Aguilar O. Determining carrier probabilities for breast cancer-susceptibility genes BRCA1 and BRCA2. Am J Hum Genet 1998;62: 145–58.
25. Mazzola E, Blackford A, Parmigiani G, et al. Recent enhancements to the genetic risk prediction model BRCAPRO. Cancer Inform 2015;14s2:CIN.S17292.
26. Antoniou AC, Pharoah PD, McMullan G, et al. A comprehensive model for familial breast cancer incorporating BRCA1, BRCA2 and other genes. Br J Cancer 2002; 86:76–83.
27. Antoniou AC, Pharoah PP, Smith P, et al. The BOADICEA model of genetic susceptibility to breast and ovarian cancer. Br J Cancer 2004;91:1580–90.
28. Valero MG, Zabor EC, Park A, et al. The tyrer–cuzick model inaccurately predicts invasive breast cancer risk in women with LCIS. Ann Surg Oncol 2020;27:736–40.
29. Boughey JC, Hartmann LC, Anderson SS, et al. Evaluation of the Tyrer-Cuzick (International Breast Cancer Intervention Study) model for breast cancer risk prediction in women with atypical hyperplasia. J Clin Oncol 2010;28:3591–6.
30. Maxwell KN, Wubbenhorst B, D'Andrea K, et al. Prevalence of mutations in a panel of breast cancer susceptibility genes in BRCA1/2-negative patients with early-onset breast cancer. Genet Med 2015;17:630–8.
31. Cosgrove J., Genetic services: information on genetic counselor and medical geneticist workforces, In: Office G.A., Online, 2019, United State Government Accountability Office, 1-45, Available at: https://www.gao.gov/assets/gao-20-593.pdf. Accessed January 4, 2022.
32. Plichta JK, Sebastian ML, Smith LA, et al. Germline genetic testing: what the breast surgeon needs to know. Ann Surg Oncol 2019;26:2184–90.
33. Hall JM, Lee MK, Newman B, et al. Linkage of early-onset familial breast cancer to chromosome 17q21. Science 1990;250:1684–9.

34. Wooster R, Neuhausen SL, Mangion J, et al. Localization of a breast cancer susceptibility gene, BRCA2, to chromosome 13q12-13. Science 1994;265:2088–90.
35. Supreme Court Decision in Association for Molecular Pathology v. Myriad Genetics, Inc. 2013. Available at: https://www.supremecourt.gov/opinions/12pdf/12-398_1b7d.pdf. Accessed September 11, 2016.
36. Plichta JK, Griffin M, Thakuria J, et al. What's new in genetic testing for cancer susceptibility? Oncology (Williston Park) 2016;30:787–99.
37. Welsh JL, Hoskin TL, Day CN, et al. Clinical decision-making in patients with variant of uncertain significance in BRCA1 or BRCA2 genes. Ann Surg Oncol 2017;24:3067–72.
38. Dillon J, Ademuyiwa FO, Barrett M, et al. Disparities in genetic testing for heritable solid-tumor malignancies. Surg Oncol Clin N Am 2022;31:109–26.
39. Ademuyiwa FO, Salyer P, Ma Y, et al. Assessing the effectiveness of the National Comprehensive Cancer Network genetic testing guidelines in identifying African American breast cancer patients with deleterious genetic mutations. Breast Cancer Res Treat 2019;178:151–9.
40. Chapman-Davis E, Zhou ZN, Fields JC, et al. Racial and ethnic disparities in genetic testing at a hereditary breast and ovarian cancer center. J Gen Intern Med 2021;36:35–42.
41. Forman AD, Hall MJ. Influence of race/ethnicity on genetic counseling and testing for hereditary breast and ovarian cancer. Breast J 2009;15(Suppl 1):S56–62.
42. Reid S, Cadiz S, Pal T. Disparities in genetic testing and care among black women with hereditary breast cancer. Curr Breast Cancer Rep 2020;12:125–31.
43. Cragun D, Weidner A, Lewis C, et al. Racial disparities in BRCA testing and cancer risk management across a population-based sample of young breast cancer survivors. Cancer 2017;123:2497–505.
44. Ademuyiwa FO, Salyer P, Tao Y, et al. Genetic counseling and testing in african american patients with breast cancer: a nationwide survey of US breast oncologists. J Clin Oncol 2021;39(36):4020–8.
45. Eichmeyer JN, Zuckerman DS, Beck TM, et al. The value of a genetic counselor for patient identification. J Clin Oncol 2012;30:97.
46. Pederson HJ, Hussain N, Noss R, et al. Impact of an embedded genetic counselor on breast cancer treatment. Breast Cancer Res Treat 2018;169:43–6.
47. Daly M.B., Pal T., Arun B., et al., NCCN Clinical Practice Guidelines in Oncology: Genetic/Familial High-Risk Assessment: Breast, Ovarian, and Pancreatic, Version 2022. Available online at: https://www.nccn.org/professionals/physician_gls/pdf/genetics_bop.pdf. Accessed January 4, 2022.
48. Bland KCE, Klimberg V, Gradishar W. The breast comprehensive management of benign and malignant diseases. 5th ed. Philadelphia, PA: Elsevier; 2018.
49. Vourtsis A, Berg WA. Breast density implications and supplemental screening. Eur Radiol 2019;29:1762–77.
50. Geisel J, Raghu M, Hooley R. The role of ultrasound in breast cancer screening: the case for and against ultrasound. Semin Ultrasound CT MR 2018;39:25–34.
51. Sung JS, Lebron L, Keating D, et al. Performance of dual-energy contrast-enhanced digital mammography for screening women at increased risk of breast cancer. Radiology 2019;293:81–8.
52. Vreugdenburg TD, Willis CD, Mundy L, et al. A systematic review of elastography, electrical impedance scanning, and digital infrared thermography for breast cancer screening and diagnosis. Breast Cancer Res Treat 2013;137:665–76.

53. Yao K, Liederbach E, Tang R, et al. Nipple-sparing mastectomy in BRCA1/2 mutation carriers: an interim analysis and review of the literature. Ann Surg Oncol 2015;22:370–6.

54. Carbine NE, Lostumbo L, Wallace J, et al. Risk-reducing mastectomy for the prevention of primary breast cancer. Cochrane Database Syst Rev 2018;4: Cd002748.

55. Heemskerk-Gerritsen BAM, Jager A, Koppert LB, et al. Survival after bilateral risk-reducing mastectomy in healthy BRCA1 and BRCA2 mutation carriers. Breast Cancer Res Treat 2019;177:723–33.

56. Gahm J, Wickman M, Brandberg Y. Bilateral prophylactic mastectomy in women with inherited risk of breast cancer–prevalence of pain and discomfort, impact on sexuality, quality of life and feelings of regret two years after surgery. Breast 2010; 19:462–9.

57. Jeffers L, Reid J, Fitzsimons D, et al. Interventions to improve psychosocial well-being in female BRCA-mutation carriers following risk-reducing surgery. Cochrane Database Syst Rev 2019;10:Cd012894.

58. van den Broek AJ, Schmidt MK, van 't Veer LJ, et al. Worse breast cancer prognosis of BRCA1/BRCA2 mutation carriers: what's the evidence? A systematic review with meta-analysis. PLoS One 2015;10:e0120189.

59. van den Broek AJ, Schmidt MK, van 't Veer LJ, et al. Prognostic impact of breast-conserving therapy versus mastectomy of BRCA1/2 mutation carriers compared with noncarriers in a consecutive series of young breast cancer patients. Ann Surg 2019;270:364–72.

60. van den Broek AJ, van 't Veer LJ, Hooning MJ, et al. Impact of age at primary breast cancer on contralateral breast cancer risk in BRCA1/2 mutation carriers. J Clin Oncol 2016;34:409–18.

61. Ludwig KK, Neuner J, Butler A, et al. Risk reduction and survival benefit of prophylactic surgery in BRCA mutation carriers, a systematic review. Am J Surg 2016;212:660–9.

62. Tutt ANJ, Garber JE, Kaufman B, et al. Adjuvant olaparib for patients with BRCA1- or BRCA2-mutated breast cancer. N Engl J Med 2017;377(6):523–33.

63. Robson M, Im SA, Senkus E, et al. Olaparib for metastatic breast cancer in patients with a germline BRCA mutation. N Engl J Med 2017;377:523–33.

64. Litton JK, Rugo HS, Ettl J, et al. Talazoparib in patients with advanced breast cancer and a germline BRCA mutation. N Engl J Med 2018;379:753–63.

65. Gradishar WJ, Moran MS, Abraham J, et al. NCCN Guidelines: Breast Cancer (version 1.2022) 2021;1. 2022. Available at: https://www.nccn.org/professionals/physician_gls/pdf/breast.pdf. Accessed December 13, 2021.

66. Berry DA, Iversen ES Jr, Gudbjartsson DF, et al. BRCAPRO validation, sensitivity of genetic testing of BRCA1/BRCA2, and prevalence of other breast cancer susceptibility genes. J Clin Oncol 2002;20:2701–12.

67. Antoniou AC, Cunningham AP, Peto J, et al. The BOADICEA model of genetic susceptibility to breast and ovarian cancers: updates and extensions. Br J Cancer 2008;98:1457–66.

68. https://ccge.medschl.cam.ac.uk/boadicea/boadicea-web-application/. [Accessed 4 January 2022].

69. https://ems-trials.org/riskevaluator/. [Accessed 4 January 2022].

Breast Cancer Pathology in the Era of Genomics

Hannah Y. Wen, MD, PhD[a], Laura C. Collins, MD[b],*

KEYWORDS

- Breast cancer • Germline testing • Special histologic subtype • Multigene assay
- Ki67 • PD-L1 • Mutation profiling • ctDNA

KEY POINTS

- Genomic medicine offers the potential to identify the molecular underpinnings of a patient's breast cancer guiding targeted therapeutic options.
- In early-stage breast cancer, histopathology and tumor biomarker information, supported by multigene assays, for women with ER-positive disease, are fundamental in guiding treatment.
- Genomics in breast pathology is utilized for risk stratification, tumor classification, predictive/prognostic testing, identification of actionable targets, and monitoring for disease progression or treatment resistance.

INTRODUCTION

The era of genomic medicine provides an opportunity for pathologists to offer greater detail about the molecular underpinnings of a patient's cancer and thereby more targeted therapeutic options. For patients with breast cancer, the principal application at this time is in the advanced stage or metastatic setting. In early-stage breast cancer, routine histopathology along with breast tumor biomarker information (estrogen receptor [ER], progesterone receptor [PR], and human epidermal growth factor receptor 2 [HER2]), supported by multigene assays, for women with ER-positive breast cancers, remain fundamental in guiding treatment decisions.

In this review article, the role of genomics in breast cancer pathology, as it pertains to risk management, classification of special tumor types, predictive and prognostic

This article previously appeared in *Hematology/Oncology Clinics* volume 37 issue 1 February 2023.

SOURCE OF FUNDING SUPPORT: H. Wen is supported in part by a National Institutes of Health/National Cancer Institute Cancer Center Support Grant (P30CA008748).

[a] Department of Pathology and Laboratory Medicine, Memorial Sloan Kettering Cancer Center, New York, NY, USA; [b] Department of Pathology, Beth Israel Deaconess Medical Center, Harvard Medical School, Boston, MA, USA
* Corresponding author.
E-mail addresses: weny@mskcc.org (H.Y.W.); lcollins@bidmc.harvard.edu (L.C.C.)

testing, identification of actionable therapeutic targets, and monitoring for disease progression or development of treatment resistance is discussed.

GERMLINE TESTING

About 5% to 10% of breast cancers are hereditary, with *BRCA1* and *BRCA2* germline mutations accounting for most such cases.[1] Other breast cancer susceptibility genes include *PALB2, CHEK2, ATM, CDH1, PTEN, TP53*, and *STK11*, these being associated with lower lifetime risks for breast cancer than *BRCA1* and *BRCA2*.

The advent of multigene panel testing has enabled comprehensive detection of pathologic mutations, which can inform risk-reducing strategies, such as enhanced screening, prophylactic surgery, and chemoprevention. In addition, with the emergence of new treatment options, such as polyadenosine diphosphate-ribose polymerase (PARP) inhibitors, *BRCA* germline testing is not only a strategy for surveillance and prevention but also has become a predictive marker for PARP inhibitor treatment.[2–6] Furthermore, as next-generation sequencing technology is increasingly used in germline analysis, detection of germline variants beyond *BRCA1/2* is readily accomplished. Studies have shown pathogenic or likely pathogenic germline variants in 17% of patients with advanced cancer, including therapeutically actionable germline alterations in 8% of patients.[7,8] Thus, in patients with advanced cancer, germline sequencing analysis could have a complementary role to tumor sequencing analysis for therapy selection.

TUMOR CLASSIFICATION

In patients with newly diagnosed breast carcinoma, accurate categorization of tumor type, grade, and biomarker status, along with tumor size, the presence or absence of lymphovascular invasion, and axillary lymph node metastases, guide management. Most breast carcinomas are invasive carcinomas of no special type (NST, also known as invasive ductal carcinoma). Approximately 10% to 15% of breast carcinomas are invasive lobular carcinomas, with the remaining 5% together comprising the special histologic subtypes, such as tubular, mucinous, invasive cribriform, and invasive micropapillary carcinomas, among others. Almost 70% of breast carcinomas are ER positive; 15% to 20% demonstrate HER2 overexpression/amplification and 10% are ER, PR, and HER2 negative (triple negative). Genomic testing is not necessary for the diagnosis and management of these more frequently occurring carcinomas, and molecular subtyping with assays such as the PAM50 to provide the intrinsic tumor subtype (luminal A or B, HER2 enriched, or basal) are not indicated in routine clinical practice. Broadly speaking, ER-positive, HER2-negative tumors, or luminal-like carcinomas, have a more indolent clinical course than HER2-positive or triple-negative carcinomas (which overlap with basal-like).

As will be discussed in a later section, multigene assays, in conjunction with clinical and pathologic features, are used to guide the need for adjuvant chemotherapy in women with early-stage ER-positive breast cancer; patients with HER2-positive disease or triple-negative carcinomas (NST) receive adjuvant or neoadjuvant chemotherapy regimens. There are, however, some special subtypes of ER-, PR-, and HER2-negative breast cancers that have a more indolent clinical course, and for those patients, chemotherapy is not indicated. It is this small subset of triple-negative tumors for which genomic assays may be helpful to ensure accurate tumor classification so as to avoid overtreatment with chemotherapy. Increasingly, antibodies are being made available to some of the fusion proteins resulting from gene rearrangements present in various cancers auguring in the advent of molecular immunohistochemistry as a more readily accessible and affordable diagnostic tool.[9]

ADENOID CYSTIC CARCINOMA

Adenoid cystic carcinoma is an uncommon breast cancer type comprising less than 1% of all breast carcinomas. In most cases, the histologic pattern of this tumor is readily recognizable, being composed of both epithelial and myoepithelial cells arrayed in a cribriform or trabecular pattern with the production of basement membrane material contained within pseudolumens created by the myoepithelial cells (**Fig. 1**). In addition to these morphologically characteristic patterns, there is a solid, basaloid variant that bears greater resemblance to conventional high-grade triple-negative breast cancer and that may be difficult to distinguish on microscopic examination alone (**Fig. 2**).[10–14]

The molecular alteration characteristic of adenoid cystic carcinoma is translocation and fusion of *MYB* or *MYBL1* with either *NFIB* or other gene partners.[15,16] The resulting gene fusion can be identified through cytogenetic analysis using a dual break-apart probe to MYB or through sequencing analysis. An immunohistochemical assay using an MYB antibody is also available, but although sensitive, this is less specific (see **Fig. 2**).[17,18]

Although most adenoid cystic carcinomas are considered low grade and have an indolent clinical course, the solid basaloid variant often demonstrates high nuclear grade and may have zones of necrosis prompting concern for more aggressive behavior.[12,14] There are insufficient data on the outcome of this particular variant of adenoid cystic carcinoma to inform a specific management recommendation, but accurate diagnostic categorization will help build knowledge on the prognosis of this tumor for future treatment decisions.

SECRETORY CARCINOMA

Secretory carcinoma is another uncommon triple-negative (or low ER-positive) tumor subtype with indolent behavior. It has a particular predisposition for occurring in children, although a broad age range of individuals may be affected. There are characteristic morphologic features that should raise the pathologic differential diagnostic consideration of secretory carcinoma, such as cells with finely vacuolated cytoplasm, the presence of secretions in the ductular lumens, and bland tumor cell nuclei (**Fig. 3**); however, the architectural growth pattern can vary considerably (circumscribed, solid,

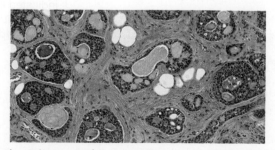

Fig. 1. Adenoid cystic carcinoma. In this conventional adenoid cystic carcinoma, the tumor is readily recognized by its cribriform growth pattern, the presence of a mixed population of epithelial and myoepithelial cells, and the deposition of basement membrane material in "pseudolumens."

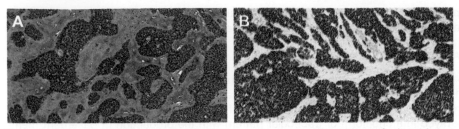

Fig. 2. Solid basaloid variant of adenoid cystic carcinoma. (*A*) This variant of adenoid cystic carcinoma can be more challenging to recognize, given the solid growth pattern, the often higher grade nuclei and the relative absence of obvious basement membrane material (hematoxylin and eosin stain). (*B*) MYB immunostain. Nuclear expression of MYB can be helpful in supporting the diagnosis.

microcystic, infiltrative) and the occasional presence of a central scar or sclerotic area can confound. Again, in adult women, the diagnosis of a triple negative breast cancer without the qualifier of this special histologic subtype may result in overtreatment.

An *ETV6::NTRK3* gene fusion characterizes secretory carcinoma.[19] As with the *MYB::NFIB* gene fusion in adenoid cystic carcinoma, this gene fusion can be identified through cytogenetic analysis with a dual break-apart probe to ETV6 or NTRK3. A pan-TRK immunohistochemical antibody is available and can be used to screen for this tumor subtype (see **Fig. 3**).[20,21] This, in conjunction with confirmation of the *ETV6::NTRK3* gene fusion either with in situ hybridization or sequencing analysis, can be used to support diagnosis and treatment decisions.

Most patients with secretory carcinoma are managed with surgical excision alone. Rare cases of recurrence and late metastases have been reported.[22] Such patients have been demonstrated to benefit from treatment with pan-TRK inhibitors[23] emphasizing the potential role for molecular analysis in therapeutic decision-making.

TALL-CELL CARCINOMA WITH REVERSED POLARITY

Tall-cell carcinoma with reversed polarity is a relatively recently described entity characterized by an *IDH2* mutation (~80% of cases) and *PIK3CA* or *PIK3R1* mutations (up to 60% of cases).[24] These tumors most commonly occur in postmenopausal women and have an indolent clinical course, with lymph node metastases only rarely described. Microscopically, the tumor is composed of solid, papillary tumor cell nests of tall cells with reversed polarity (ie, the nucleus is located at the apical rather than the

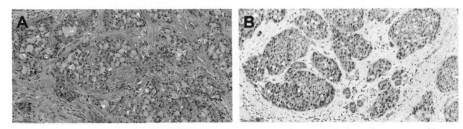

Fig. 3. Secretory carcinoma. (*A*) Secretory carcinoma can be a mimic for other types of breast carcinoma. Here the tumor displays a microcystic or cribriform type growth pattern, with luminal secretions. The tumor cells are relatively bland. (*B*) pan-TRK immunostain. Nuclear positivity is supportive of the diagnosis of secretory carcinoma.

basal aspect of the cell), conferring a striking morphologic appearance (**Fig. 4**). The nuclei are low grade. The tumor is usually ER, PR, and HER2 negative; occasionally low ER positivity is reported.

With greater recognition of this tumor entity, the special histologic subtype should be provided so as to prevent the patient being treated as having a triple-negative breast cancer, NST. Mutation profiling may be used to identify the *IDH2 R172* mutation pathognomonic of this tumor. There is also an IDH2 R172 antibody that can be used for the immunohistochemical evaluation of this tumor (see **Fig. 4**).[25]

The limited data available suggest this tumor may be managed with surgical excision alone.

ADENOMYOEPITHELIOMA/MALIGNANT ADENOMYOEPITHELIOMA

Adenomyoepithelioma is a rare benign epithelial-myoepithelial tumor. Exceptionally, malignant transformation may occur. New data suggest that ER-negative adenomyoepitheliomas are more likely to harbor *HRAS* mutations, and it is these tumors that seem to have the greatest propensity for malignant transformation.[26,27] This observation suggests the possibility of using mutation profiling to identify which patients may be at risk for the development of carcinoma in this setting, thereby dictating a more stringent follow-up protocol. As with MYB and IDH2 R172, there is an antibody to NRAS Q61R that also recognizes HRAS Q61R and KRAS Q61R; however, experience with its use as a diagnostic or prognostic tool is limited at this time.[28]

ER-positive adenomyoepitheliomas are more likely to demonstrate *PIK3CA* mutations and do not seem to have the same risk as their ER-negative counterparts, albeit with limited data.[26]

PROGNOSTIC AND PREDICTIVE TESTING

For early-stage ER-positive/HER2-negative invasive breast carcinoma, the decision whether to give adjuvant chemotherapy hinges on the risk of distant recurrence. Several multigene assays have been developed to estimate this risk, including the 21-gene recurrence score assay (Oncotype Dx),[29] the 70-gene signature (MammaPrint),[30] the 50-gene assay (PAM50, Prosigna),[31] the 12-gene assay (EndoPredict),[32] and the Breast Cancer Index (BCI).[33] All assays are prognostic, providing an estimate of the risk of distant relapse. The 21-gene assay is both prognostic and predictive of chemotherapy benefit. These assays have been endorsed by the National Comprehensive Cancer Network (NCCN),[34] the American Society of Clinical Oncology (ASCO),[35–38] and St Gallen[39–41] guidelines for adjuvant treatment decisions in patients with early-stage, hormone receptor–positive breast cancer. The 21-gene assay is

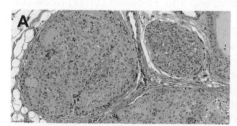
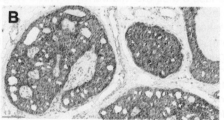

Fig. 4. Tall-cell carcinoma with reversed polarity. (*A*) The characteristic features of this tumor: solid papillary tumor cell nests, with cells of low-grade cytology and reversed polarity. (*B*) If needed, an IDH2 R172 immunostain can confirm the diagnosis.

included in the prognostic staging in the AJCC Cancer Staging 8th Edition.[42] Of these multigene assays, the 21-gene recurrence score assay and the 70-gene signature assay are supported by level I clinical evidence, discussed later in detail.

21-Gene Recurrence Score Assay (Oncotype Dx)

The 21-gene recurrence score assay is a reverse transcriptase polymerase chain reaction (RT-PCR)-based test. The gene panel includes 16 cancer-related genes and 5 reference genes.[29] Derived recurrence scores range from 0 to 100, a higher score indicating a greater risk of recurrence. In the original publication, the cutoff points to classify low-, intermediate-, and high-risk groups were recurrence scores of less than 18, 18 to 30, and greater than or equal to 31, respectively.[29] These scores were later modified to recurrence scores of 0 to 10, 11 to 25, and greater than 25 in the prospective clinical trials.[43–45] The Trial Assigning Individualized Options for Treatment (TAILORx), a prospective randomized trial, found no benefit to chemotherapy in patients with early-stage ER-positive, HER2-negative, node-negative breast cancer with recurrence scores between 0 and 25, with the exception of young patients ($\leq$50 yrs) with recurrence scores of 16 to 25 who were shown to derive some benefit from chemotherapy.[43,44] The RxPONDER (Rx for Positive Node, Endocrine Responsive Breast Cancer) trial further validated the utility of the 21-gene recurrence score in patients with node-positive disease, demonstrating that postmenopausal patients with ER-positive, HER2-negative breast cancer with 1 to 3 positive lymph nodes and recurrence scores between 0 and 25 could be treated with endocrine therapy alone.[45] In contrast, premenopausal patients with 1 to 3 positive lymph nodes derived significant benefit from chemotherapy even in the setting of low recurrence scores.[45] The 21-gene recurrence score assay has had significant impact on adjuvant chemotherapy decisions (see separate article in this issue of the Clinics).

A significant association was also observed between the 21-gene recurrence score and the risk of locoregional recurrence (LRR) in both node-negative and node-positive patients.[46–48] The potential application of the 21-gene recurrence score for locoregional therapy decision-making in patients with early-stage ER-positive, HER2-negative breast cancer is under active investigation.

70-Gene Signature Assay (MammaPrint)

The 70-gene signature assay is a DNA microarray–based assay.[49] Multivariate analysis showed it to be an independent factor in predicting disease outcome in both patients with node-negative and those with node-positive breast cancer in a retrospective cohort.[30] Its clinical utility was validated in a prospective randomized phase 3 trial, the Microarray in Node-Negative and 1 to 3 Positive Lymph Node Disease May Avoid Chemotherapy (EORTC 10041/BIG 3-04 MINDACT).[50] The study assessed both the genomic risk (using the 70-gene signature) and the clinical risk (using a modified version of Adjuvant! Online). Patients with discordant clinical and genomic risks (low clinical risk/high genomic risk or high clinical risk/low genomic risk) were randomized to chemotherapy or no chemotherapy. It was found that patients with high clinical risk and low genomic risk had similar 5-year distant recurrence-free survival with or without adjuvant chemotherapy.[50] In patients with low clinical risk, genomic testing provided no added value as there was no significant benefit from the use of adjuvant chemotherapy regardless of genomic risk.[50] Thus, the 70-gene signature is of greatest value among patients with high clinical risk in whom its use led to a 46% reduction in the administration of adjuvant chemotherapy.[50]

The Integration of Genomic and Clinical Information in Prognostic Estimates

As described earlier for the MINDACT trial, genomic testing is best used in combination with clinicopathologic factors.[50] In fact, secondary analyses of the TAILORx trial found that incorporation of clinical risk stratification based on tumor size and histologic grade added prognostic information to the 21-gene recurrence score.[51] A new tool, RSClin, which integrates the 21-gene recurrence score and selected clinical-pathological features (tumor grade, tumor size, and age), has been shown to provide more accurate prognostic information than recurrence score or clinicopathologic factors alone.[52]

Favorable Histologic Subtypes

Several special histologic subtypes of invasive breast cancer such as tubular carcinoma, cribriform carcinoma, pure mucinous carcinoma, encapsulated papillary carcinoma, and solid papillary carcinoma are associated with favorable prognoses. There are no data addressing whether multigene assays provide additional prognostic and predictive information in patients with these favorable histologic subtypes. Retrospective analysis of such cases has demonstrated the 21-gene recurrence scores to be lower than those of conventional invasive ductal carcinomas, high-risk recurrence scores being less frequently identified, in line with their favorable histology.[53,54] A high-risk recurrence score in any of these special histologic subtypes should prompt a careful pathologic review to confirm the diagnosis and identify tissue factors in the tumor sample that may have influenced the results.

Multigene Assays and Biomarker Assessment

ER, PR, and HER2 are among the 16 cancer-related genes assessed in the 21-gene assay. The 70-gene signature assay and PAM50 report gene expression–based "intrinsic" subtypes (luminal A, luminal B, HER2-enriched, and basal-like). However, these assays are not recommended as primary screening tests for biomarker assessment due to the lack of clinical validation supporting their utility in identifying patients for endocrine or HER2-targeted therapy. Validated immunohistochemistry (IHC) and/or in situ hybridization (ISH) remain the recommended standard tests for ER, PR, and HER2 in breast cancer according to ASCO/CAP guidelines.[55,56] Although a high concordance between standard IHC/ISH and the 21-gene RT-PCR assay for ER and PR status was observed,[57–60] a substantial false-negative rate for HER2 status by RT-PCR has been reported.[59–61] This discordance likely reflects a dilutional effect from contaminating nonneoplastic tissue such as normal breast epithelium, stroma, and tumor infiltrating lymphocytes, an inherent disadvantage of mRNA-based assays compared with IHC/ISH on intact tissue sections.

KI67

Although not genomic in nature, Ki67 assessment is briefly discussed here as a matter of interest.

Ki67 is a marker of cell proliferation. The Ki67 labeling index as assessed by immunohistochemistry is an established prognostic and predictive marker in early-stage breast cancer.[62] However, its clinical utility is limited due to the lack of interobserver and interlaboratory reproducibility and the lack of a standardized cutoff. A Ki67 index cutoff point of 14% was selected to distinguish between luminal A and luminal B breast cancer intrinsic subtype based on analysis of a cohort of breast cancers classified by PAM50.[63] The 14% cutoff was adopted by the 2011 St Gallen International Breast Cancer Consensus Guideline[64]; however, this was changed to 20% in the

2013 Guideline.[65] The 2021 St Gallen Consensus Conference endorsed the recent International Ki67 in Breast Cancer Working Group (IKWG) recommendation using Ki67 less than or equal to 5% (very low) or Ki67 greater than or equal to 30% (very high) to estimate prognosis and guide chemotherapy,[66] but more than one-third of the panel voted "Ki67 threshold not known"[41], highlighting the lack of consensus that complicates use of Ki67 to guide therapy.

The IKWG recommendations set forth preanalytic requirements and a standardized visual scoring method to ensure uniform performance and interpretation of immunohistochemistry for Ki67.[66] Ki67 assessment is recommended only for hormone receptor–positive, HER2-negative early-stage breast cancer with Ki67 cutoffs of less than or equal to 5% or greater than or equal to 30%, as noted above. Even with careful attention to preanalytic issues and standardized scoring methods, there is still substantial interobserver/interlaboratory variability when Ki67 is in the greater than 5% and less than 30% range, limiting clinical applicability.

Recently, Ki67 assessment has been used to select patients for abemaciclib therapy. The Food and Drug Administration (FDA) approved abemaciclib, a CDK4/6 inhibitor, combined with endocrine therapy for hormone receptor-positive, HER2-negative, node-positive, high-risk early breast cancer with Ki67 greater than or equal to 20%. The approval was based on the MonarchE trial[67] but limited to a subset of patients with high recurrence risk and Ki67 greater than or equal to 20%. The FDA also approved the Ki-67 IHC MIB-1 pharmDx (Dako Omnis) assay as a companion diagnostic test for this indication. Updated analysis of the MonarchE study found Ki67 to be prognostic but not predictive.[68] Abemaciclib benefit was observed regardless of Ki67 status. The ASCO-updated recommendations broadened the application to patients with either 4 or more positive axillary lymph nodes or 1 to 3 positive axillary lymph nodes and either grade 3 disease, tumor size greater than or equal to 5 cm, or Ki67 greater then or equal to 20%, in keeping with the MonarchE trial design.[67]

For the aforementioned reasons, there is wide variation in utilization of Ki67 testing in breast cancer among pathology laboratories. Automated scoring by digital image analysis is still investigational but holds the promise of improving agreement and throughput, which is reported to take an average of 9 minutes/case using the IKWG recommended manual scoring method.

TUMOR-INFILTRATING LYMPHOCYTES

The prognostic and predictive value of tumor-infiltrating lymphocytes (TILs) is well established. An increased level of TILs is an independent predictor of response to neoadjuvant chemotherapy in all breast cancer subtypes.[69,70] In triple-negative breast cancer, high-level TILs are associated with better prognosis.[71,72] The presence of TILs is also associated with response to immunotherapy with programmed cell death ligand 1 (PD1/PD-L1) inhibitors. The percentage of stromal TILs is scored as the area of tumor stroma occupied by mononuclear inflammatory cells over total intratumoral stromal area, according to the recommendations by the International TILs Working Group.[73] The percentage of stromal TILs is a continuous variable, ranging from 0% to 100%. Every 10% increment in stromal TILs corresponds to an improved outcome.[69,72] Different studies used different cutoffs of stromal TILs in data analysis. Early studies used cutoffs of 60% or 50% TILs to define lymphocyte-predominant breast cancer.[69,71] Proposed TILs cutoffs of 30%, 20%, 10%, and even 5% have also been used.[74] There are currently no recommendations for a clinically relevant threshold and, therefore, scoring TILs is not implemented in daily practice outside of research or clinical trial settings.

TREATMENT DECISIONS

As noted in the introduction, genomic testing of breast cancers to identify actionable targets, with the exception of the few special histologic subtypes discussed earlier, currently applies to the advanced stage or metastatic settings. Sequencing assays using tumor tissue are required to identify mutations, such as *ESR1*, *PIK3CA*, and *AKT1*. However, early detection evaluating circulating tumor cells may eliminate the need for a biopsy of the metastatic site (see later section and separate article in this issue of the Clinics).

Knowledge bases such as OncoKB that annotate somatic mutations for clinical significance offer the promise of personalized treatment options based on the cancer genome.[75]

IMMUNE CHECKPOINT INHIBITORS AND PD-L1 TESTING

Evaluation of the tumor for susceptibility to immune checkpoint inhibitors, such as pembrolizumab, is often requested in patients with advanced or metastatic triple-negative breast cancer. It is important to know that the drugs are approved for use in patients with tumors demonstrated to express PD-L1 using the appropriate FDA-approved companion diagnostic assay (**Table 1**). Each drug requires a different assay; each assay a specific vendor platform and antibody; and each antibody a different scoring system and different thresholds of positivity. Needless to say, this presents considerable challenges even for larger pathology laboratories in academic medical centers, as validation across platforms is not straightforward, and the relative infrequency of test interpretation makes maintaining proficiency and reproducibility difficult.[76,77] In spite of these hurdles, pathologists are committed to providing the information needed to care for patients with breast cancer, either with an in-house test option or by sending a tissue block to a reference laboratory. It is incumbent on both pathologists and oncologists to understand which test is indicated and to know what assay to order. That said, pembrolizumab was recently approved for high-risk early-stage triple-negative breast cancer in combination with chemotherapy as neoadjuvant treatment regardless of PD-L1 expression.[78]

Additional indicators of susceptibility to immune checkpoint inhibitors include tumor mutational burden, microsatellite instability, and mismatch repair defects. Most breast cancers have a low mutational burden, and microsatellite instability and mismatch

Table 1 Food and Drug Administration–approved companion diagnostic assays for programmed cell death ligand 1 in breast cancer		
	SP142[a]	**22C3 pharmDx**
Immunotherapy	Atezolizumab	Pembrolizumab
Platform	Ventana BenchMark	DAKO
Scoring methods	Immune cells (IC)	Combined positive score (CPS)
Positivity definition	IC ≥ 1%	CPS ≥ 10
Clinical trial	IMpassion 130	KEYNOTE-355
Breast cancer subtype	Locally advanced or metastatic TNBC	Locally advanced or metastatic TNBC
Chemotherapy	Nab-paclitaxel	Taxane or gemcitabine-carboplatin

Abbreviation: TNBC, triple-negative breast cancer.
[a] Indication since withdrawn.

repair defects are uncommon.[79] However, any opportunity to provide treatment benefit in patients with metastatic disease is invariably sought in the appropriate clinical setting. Tumor mutational burden information is provided with sequencing assays along with any specific somatic and/or genomic alterations present.

ESR1 MUTATIONS

The development of endocrine therapy resistance secondary to somatic alterations such as *ESR1* mutations in women with ER-positive metastatic breast cancer is a treatment challenge, particularly among those treated with aromatase inhibitors in this setting[80,81]; this seems to be less of an issue in primary ER-positive breast cancers, but emerging evidence suggests the presence of *ESR1* mutations in women with early-stage disease is associated with poorer disease-free and overall survival.[82] Despite being an established mechanism of endocrine resistance, *ESR1* mutations are not used as a biomarker to guide endocrine therapy, as current practice is to switch to fulvestrant after disease progression on aromatase inhibitors regardless of *ESR1* mutation status. The ASCO guideline does not recommend routine testing for *ESR1* mutations for hormonal receptor-positive, HER2-negative metastatic breast cancer.[83]

HER2 OVEREXPRESSION, AMPLIFICATION, AND MUTATION

HER2 overexpression and/or amplification is determined at the time of primary diagnosis, with approximately 15% to 20% of breast cancers being classified as HER2 "positive" and eligible for HER2-targeted therapies. Until recently, women with tumors lacking HER2 overexpression or amplification were ineligible for these therapeutic agents. However, emerging data demonstrating improved outcomes with the antibody drug conjugate trastuzumab deruxtecan (T-DXd) for patients with HER2 IHC 1+ and HER2 2+, fluorescence in situ hybridization nonamplified tumors have prompted reevaluation of how HER2 IHC-negative tumors are categorized, that is, the need for stricter attention to the separation of 0 and 1+ cases, as there are now treatment implications for this group.[84,85]

Further opportunities for HER2-targeted therapy in patients without demonstrated HER2 overexpression or amplification have been identified among patients with tumors harboring *HER2* mutations.[33] Activating HER2 mutations occur at a frequency of 2% to 3% overall in primary breast cancers with a particular preponderance seen in invasive lobular carcinomas (~8%). The pan-HER inhibitor neratinib has been shown to provide a clinical benefit rate of 31% in a pretreated population of patients with metastatic breast cancer.[33,86]

PIK3CA MUTATIONS FOR PI3K INHIBITOR TREATMENT

In the advanced stage or metastatic setting, identification of patients whose tumors harbor *PIK3CA* mutations offers the opportunity for treatment with the *PIK3CA* inhibitor, alpelisib, in combination with fulvestrant for hormonal receptor–positive/HER2-negative advanced breast cancer in postmenopausal women, or in male patients.[87] *PIK3CA* mutations are identified in up to 45% of patients with ER+, HER2-negative advanced breast cancer[88] and therefore offer a large potential pool of patients who may benefit from this therapy. Furthermore, trials exploring efficacy of alpelisib in patients with *PIK3CA*-mutated *HER2*+ breast cancer are ongoing.[89]

CIRCULATING TUMOR DNA

Circulating tumor DNA (ctDNA) is tumor-derived fragmented DNA present in the bloodstream. The sampling and analysis of ctDNA, also known as "liquid biopsy," offers a minimally invasive approach to genomic profiling and disease monitoring. The FDA approved the liquid biopsy next-generation sequencing (NGS)-based FoundationOne Liquid CDx test as a companion diagnostic device for specific indications, including the identification of *PIK3CA* mutations in breast cancer for treatment with alpelisib.[87]

The plasmaMATCH trial, a prospective trial evaluating the sensitivity of ctDNA to identify actionable mutations in advanced breast cancer, found that the agreement for mutation identification between ctDNA digital PCR and targeted sequencing using tissue biopsies was 96% to 99%.[90] Analytical validation of MSK-ACCESS (Memorial Sloan Kettering—Analysis of Circulating cfDNA to Examine Somatic Status), an institutional NGS platform for detection of somatic alterations in 129 genes in cell-free DNA, demonstrated 92% de novo sensitivity and 99% specificity.[91] Liquid biopsy does not replace tissue biopsy, given the importance of histology diagnosis, but potentially provides a valid alternative sampling strategy, especially when the metastatic site is not amendable for biopsy or a tissue sample obtained is not suitable for molecular analysis.

Multiple studies have demonstrated the potential utility of ctDNA in prognostication and in monitoring treatment response and disease progression in advanced breast cancer.[92–101] However, data are limited to retrospective analyses of prospective trials. In patients with early-stage breast cancer treated with neoadjuvant therapy, detection of ctDNA was associated with poor response and disease recurrence.[102,103] In a prospective multicenter study, detection of ctDNA was associated with relapse in early-stage breast cancer after ostensibly curative therapy, with ctDNA being detected at a median lead time of 10.7 months before clinical relapse.[104] There are no data to demonstrate that clinical intervention following early detection of molecular residual disease translates into improved patient outcome, limiting practical utility at this time. As such, current ASCO and NCCN guidelines do not recommend the use of ctDNA to guide adjuvant therapy in early-stage breast cancer or disease assessment and monitoring in the metastatic setting.[38]

THE UTILITY OF GENOMIC ANALYSIS IN RESOLVING DIAGNOSTIC DILEMMAS

In addition to identifying actionable somatic mutations and predisposing germline variants, genomic analysis can assist in diagnosis when definitive tumor classification cannot be accomplished based on histology and immunohistochemistry. A common clinical dilemma is the determination of primary tumor site in patients presenting with metastatic disease. For patients with a prior history of carcinoma, comparative genomic analysis of paired primary and metastatic tumor samples can determine whether a clonal relationship exists. Genomic comparison can also distinguish local recurrences from new primary carcinomas in patients with prior breast cancer. More challenging are situations in which the patient's history is noncontributory or a primary tumor sample is unavailable for comparison. Certain genomic alterations or combined patterns of mutation are associated with specific tumor types and help to predict tumor origin: examples include *APC* loss-of-function mutations in colorectal cancers, *TMPRSS2::ERG* fusions in prostate cancers, an ultraviolet-associated mutational signature of C > T substitutions in cutaneous melanomas, and the co-occurrence of *TP53* and *CTNNB1* mutations in endometrial cancer.[105] Breast carcinomas, except for certain special histologic subtypes, do not have unique genomic alterations. However, the absence of certain common mutations may be informative. For example, *EGRF* or *KRAS* mutations favor a carcinoma of pulmonary over mammary origin. Penson and colleagues reported a machine learning approach to the prediction of tumor type using genomic data.[105] The correct tumor type was predicted for 73.8% of 7791 patients in the training set and 74.1% of 11,644 patients in an independent cohort.[105] The performance was highest in tumor types with distinctive molecular profiles, such as uveal melanoma, glioma, and colorectal cancer, whereas lowest in esophagogastric, ovarian, and head and neck cancers due to molecular heterogeneity among these tumors and the lack of distinguishing genomic alterations.[105] The algorithm identified carcinomas of mammary type with sensitivity and specificity values of 0.876 and 0.761, respectively, in 1181 patients with breast cancer included in the study cohort.[105]

SUMMARY

It is now well recognized that breast cancer is a heterogeneous disease. Optimal treatment is dictated by tumor biology and a multidisciplinary approach. Advances in genomics have further improved our understanding of breast cancer biology, with robust genomic assays becoming more easily accessible and being increasingly used in daily practice to assist in diagnosis, classification, risk stratification, and the detection of relevant germline mutations and actionable targets. For early-stage breast cancer, treatment is mainly informed by conventional clinicopathologic factors and biomarkers (ER, PR, HER2) using immunohistochemistry and/or in situ hybridization. Systemic therapy is largely driven by histology and receptor subtype. For early-stage hormonal receptor–positive, HER2-negative breast cancer, the use of multigene assays is well established for risk stratification and treatment escalation/deescalation. For advanced breast cancer, transcriptomic, genomic, epigenomic, and proteomic landscapes may inform personalized treatment options. The translation of such data into individualized treatment plans conferring survival benefits is the challenge ahead.

REFERENCES

1. Antoniou A, Pharoah PD, Narod S, et al. Average risks of breast and ovarian cancer associated with BRCA1 or BRCA2 mutations detected in case Series unselected for family history: a combined analysis of 22 studies. Am J Hum Genet 2003;72:1117–30.
2. Robson M, Im SA, Senkus E, et al. Olaparib for Metastatic Breast Cancer in Patients with a Germline BRCA Mutation. N Engl J Med 2017;377:523–33.
3. Robson ME, Tung N, Conte P, et al. OlympiAD final overall survival and tolerability results: Olaparib versus chemotherapy treatment of physician's choice in patients with a germline BRCA mutation and HER2-negative metastatic breast cancer. Ann Oncol 2019;30:558–66.
4. Litton JK, Rugo HS, Ettl J, et al. Talazoparib in Patients with Advanced Breast Cancer and a Germline BRCA Mutation. N Engl J Med 2018;379:753–63.
5. Litton JK, Hurvitz SA, Mina LA, et al. Talazoparib versus chemotherapy in patients with germline BRCA1/2-mutated HER2-negative advanced breast cancer: final overall survival results from the EMBRACA trial. Ann Oncol 2020;31:1526–35.
6. Tutt ANJ, Garber JE, Kaufman B, et al. Adjuvant Olaparib for Patients with BRCA1- or BRCA2-Mutated Breast Cancer. N Engl J Med 2021;384:2394–405.

7. Mandelker D, Zhang L, Kemel Y, et al. Mutation Detection in Patients With Advanced Cancer by Universal Sequencing of Cancer-Related Genes in Tumor and Normal DNA vs Guideline-Based Germline Testing. Jama 2017;318:825–35.
8. Stadler ZK, Maio A, Chakravarty D, et al. Therapeutic Implications of Germline Testing in Patients With Advanced Cancers. J Clin Oncol 2021;39:2698–709.
9. Hornick JL. Replacing Molecular Genetic Testing With Immunohistochemistry Using Antibodies That Recognize the Protein Products of Gene Rearrangements: "Next-generation" Immunohistochemistry. Am J Surg Pathol 2021;45: 584–6.
10. Shin SJ, Rosen PP. Solid variant of mammary adenoid cystic carcinoma with basaloid features: a study of nine cases. Am J Surg Pathol 2002;26:413–20.
11. D'Alfonso TM, Mosquera JM, MacDonald TY, et al. MYB-NFIB gene fusion in adenoid cystic carcinoma of the breast with special focus paid to the solid variant with basaloid features. Hum Pathol 2014;45:2270–80.
12. Slodkowska E, Xu B, Kos Z, et al. Predictors of Outcome in Mammary Adenoid Cystic Carcinoma: A Multi-Institutional Study. Am J Surg Pathol 2020;44:214–23.
13. Massé J, Truntzer C, Boidot R, et al. Solid-type adenoid cystic carcinoma of the breast, a distinct molecular entity enriched in NOTCH and CREBBP mutations. Mod Pathol 2020;33:1041–55.
14. Schwartz CJ, Brogi E, Marra A, et al. The clinical behavior and genomic features of the so-called adenoid cystic carcinomas of the solid variant with basaloid features. Mod Pathol 2022;35:193–201.
15. Persson M, Andrén Y, Mark J, et al. Recurrent fusion of MYB and NFIB transcription factor genes in carcinomas of the breast and head and neck. Proc Natl Acad Sci U S A 2009;106:18740–4.
16. Kim J, Geyer FC, Martelotto LG, et al. MYBL1 rearrangements and MYB amplification in breast adenoid cystic carcinomas lacking the MYB-NFIB fusion gene. J Pathol 2018;244:143–50.
17. West RB, Kong C, Clarke N, et al. MYB expression and translocation in adenoid cystic carcinomas and other salivary gland tumors with clinicopathologic correlation. Am J Surg Pathol 2011;35:92–9.
18. Brill LB 2nd, Kanner WA, Fehr A, et al. Analysis of MYB expression and MYB-NFIB gene fusions in adenoid cystic carcinoma and other salivary neoplasms. Mod Pathol 2011;24:1169–76.
19. Tognon C, Knezevich SR, Huntsman D, et al. Expression of the ETV6-NTRK3 gene fusion as a primary event in human secretory breast carcinoma. Cancer Cell 2002;2:367–76.
20. Hechtman JF, Benayed R, Hyman DM, et al. Pan-Trk Immunohistochemistry Is an Efficient and Reliable Screen for the Detection of NTRK Fusions. Am J Surg Pathol 2017;41:1547–51.
21. Harrison BT, Fowler E, Krings G, et al. Pan-TRK Immunohistochemistry: A Useful Diagnostic Adjunct For Secretory Carcinoma of the Breast. Am J Surg Pathol 2019;43:1693–700.
22. Hoda RS, Brogi E, Pareja F, et al. Secretory carcinoma of the breast: clinicopathologic profile of 14 cases emphasising distant metastatic potential. Histopathology 2019;75:213–24.
23. Shukla N, Roberts SS, Baki MO, et al. Successful Targeted Therapy of Refractory Pediatric ETV6-NTRK3 Fusion-Positive Secretory Breast Carcinoma. JCO Precis Oncol 2017;2017.
24. Chiang S, Weigelt B, Wen HC, et al. IDH2 Mutations Define a Unique Subtype of Breast Cancer with Altered Nuclear Polarity. Cancer Res 2016;76:7118–29.

25. Pareja F, da Silva EM, Frosina D, et al. Immunohistochemical analysis of IDH2 R172 hotspot mutations in breast papillary neoplasms: applications in the diagnosis of tall cell carcinoma with reverse polarity. Mod Pathol 2020;33:1056–64.

26. Geyer FC, Li A, Papanastasiou AD, et al. Recurrent hotspot mutations in HRAS Q61 and PI3K-AKT pathway genes as drivers of breast adenomyoepitheliomas. Nat Commun 2018;9:1816.

27. Watanabe S, Otani T, Iwasa T, et al. A Case of Metastatic Malignant Breast Adenomyoepithelioma With a Codon-61 Mutation of HRAS. Clin Breast Cancer 2019;19:e589–92.

28. Pareja F, Toss MS, Geyer FC, et al. Immunohistochemical assessment of HRAS Q61R mutations in breast adenomyoepitheliomas. Histopathology 2020;76:865–74.

29. Paik S, Shak S, Tang G, et al. A multigene assay to predict recurrence of tamoxifen-treated, node-negative breast cancer. N Engl J Med 2004;351:2817–26.

30. van de Vijver MJ, He YD, van't Veer LJ, et al. A gene-expression signature as a predictor of survival in breast cancer. N Engl J Med 2002;347:1999–2009.

31. Parker JS, Mullins M, Cheang MC, et al. Supervised risk predictor of breast cancer based on intrinsic subtypes. J Clin Oncol 2009;27:1160–7.

32. Filipits M, Rudas M, Jakesz R, et al. A new molecular predictor of distant recurrence in ER-positive, HER2-negative breast cancer adds independent information to conventional clinical risk factors. Clin Cancer Res 2011;17:6012–20.

33. Ma XJ, Salunga R, Dahiya S, et al. A five-gene molecular grade index and HOX-B13:IL17BR are complementary prognostic factors in early stage breast cancer. Clin Cancer Res 2008;14:2601–8.

34. Gradishar WJ, Moran MS, Abraham J et al. Breast Cancer, Version 3.2022, NCCN Clinical Practice Guidelines in Oncology. J Natl Compr Canc Netw. 20, 2022, 691-722; Accessed July 2022.

35. Harris LN, Ismaila N, McShane LM, et al. Use of Biomarkers to Guide Decisions on Adjuvant Systemic Therapy for Women With Early-Stage Invasive Breast Cancer: American Society of Clinical Oncology Clinical Practice Guideline. J Clin Oncol 2016;34:1134–50.

36. Krop I, Ismaila N, Andre F, et al. Use of Biomarkers to Guide Decisions on Adjuvant Systemic Therapy for Women With Early-Stage Invasive Breast Cancer: American Society of Clinical Oncology Clinical Practice Guideline Focused Update. J Clin Oncol 2017;35:2838–47.

37. Andre F, Ismaila N, Henry NL, et al. Use of Biomarkers to Guide Decisions on Adjuvant Systemic Therapy for Women With Early-Stage Invasive Breast Cancer: ASCO Clinical Practice Guideline Update-Integration of Results From TAILORx. J Clin Oncol 2019;37:1956–64.

38. Andre F, Ismaila N, Allison KH, et al. Biomarkers for Adjuvant Endocrine and Chemotherapy in Early-Stage Breast Cancer: ASCO Guideline Update. J Clin Oncol 2022;40:1816–37.

39. Coates AS, Winer EP, Goldhirsch A, et al. Tailoring therapies–improving the management of early breast cancer: St Gallen International Expert Consensus on the Primary Therapy of Early Breast Cancer 2015. Ann Oncol 2015;26:1533–46.

40. Burstein HJ, Curigliano G, Loibl S, et al. Estimating the benefits of therapy for early-stage breast cancer: the St. Gallen International Consensus Guidelines for the primary therapy of early breast cancer 2019. Ann Oncol 2019;30:1541–57.

41. Burstein HJ, Curigliano G, Thürlimann B, et al. Customizing local and systemic therapies for women with early breast cancer: the St. Gallen International Consensus Guidelines for treatment of early breast cancer 2021. Ann Oncol 2021;32:1216–35.

42. Amin MB, Greene FL, Edge SB, et al. The Eighth Edition AJCC Cancer Staging Manual: Continuing to build a bridge from a population-based to a more "personalized" approach to cancer staging. CA Cancer J Clin 2017;67:93–9.

43. Sparano JA, Gray RJ, Makower DF, et al. Prospective Validation of a 21-Gene Expression Assay in Breast Cancer. N Engl J Med 2015;373:2005–14.

44. Sparano JA, Gray RJ, Makower DF, et al. Adjuvant Chemotherapy Guided by a 21-Gene Expression Assay in Breast Cancer. N Engl J Med 2018;379:111–21.

45. Kalinsky K, Barlow WE, Gralow JR, et al. 21-Gene Assay to Inform Chemotherapy Benefit in Node-Positive Breast Cancer. N Engl J Med 2021;385:2336–47.

46. Mamounas EP, Tang G, Fisher B, et al. Association between the 21-gene recurrence score assay and risk of locoregional recurrence in node-negative, estrogen receptor-positive breast cancer: results from NSABP B-14 and NSABP B-20. J Clin Oncol 2010;28:1677–83.

47. Mamounas EP, Liu Q, Paik S, et al. 21-Gene Recurrence Score and Locoregional Recurrence in Node-Positive/ER-Positive Breast Cancer Treated With Chemo-Endocrine Therapy. J Natl Cancer Inst 2017;109.

48. Turashvili G, Chou JF, Brogi E, et al. 21-Gene recurrence score and locoregional recurrence in lymph node-negative, estrogen receptor-positive breast cancer. Breast Cancer Res Treat 2017;166:69–76.

49. van 't Veer LJ, Dai H, van de Vijver MJ, et al. Gene expression profiling predicts clinical outcome of breast cancer. Nature 2002;415:530–6.

50. Cardoso F, van't Veer LJ, Bogaerts J, et al. 70-Gene Signature as an Aid to Treatment Decisions in Early-Stage Breast Cancer. N Engl J Med 2016;375:717–29.

51. Sparano JA, Gray RJ, Ravdin PM, et al. Clinical and Genomic Risk to Guide the Use of Adjuvant Therapy for Breast Cancer. N Engl J Med 2019;380:2395–405.

52. Sparano JA, Crager MR, Tang G, et al. Development and Validation of a Tool Integrating the 21-Gene Recurrence Score and Clinical-Pathological Features to Individualize Prognosis and Prediction of Chemotherapy Benefit in Early Breast Cancer. J Clin Oncol 2021;39:557–64.

53. Turashvili G, Brogi E, Morrow M, et al. The 21-gene recurrence score in special histologic subtypes of breast cancer with favorable prognosis. Breast Cancer Res Treat 2017;165:65–76.

54. Tadros AB, Wen HY, Morrow M. Breast Cancers of Special Histologic Subtypes Are Biologically Diverse. Ann Surg Oncol 2018;25:3158–64.

55. Allison KH, Hammond MEH, Dowsett M, et al. Estrogen and Progesterone Receptor Testing in Breast Cancer: ASCO/CAP Guideline Update. J Clin Oncol 2020;38:1346–66.

56. Wolff AC, Hammond MEH, Allison KH, et al. Human Epidermal Growth Factor Receptor 2 Testing in Breast Cancer: American Society of Clinical Oncology/College of American Pathologists Clinical Practice Guideline Focused Update. J Clin Oncol 2018;36:2105–22.

57. O'Connor SM, Beriwal S, Dabbs DJ, et al. Concordance between semiquantitative immunohistochemical assay and oncotype DX RT-PCR assay for estrogen and progesterone receptors. Appl Immunohistochem Mol Morphol 2010;18:268–72.

58. Kraus JA, Dabbs DJ, Beriwal S, et al. Semi-quantitative immunohistochemical assay versus oncotype DX(®) qRT-PCR assay for estrogen and progesterone receptors: an independent quality assurance study. Mod Pathol 2012;25: 869–76.

59. Park MM, Ebel JJ, Zhao W, et al. ER and PR immunohistochemistry and HER2 FISH versus oncotype DX: implications for breast cancer treatment. Breast J 2014;20:37–45.

60. Neely C, You S, Mendoza PM, et al. Comparing breast biomarker status between routine immunohistochemistry and FISH studies and Oncotype DX testing, a study of 610 cases. Breast J 2018;24:889–93.

61. Dabbs DJ, Klein ME, Mohsin SK, et al. High false-negative rate of HER2 quantitative reverse transcription polymerase chain reaction of the Oncotype DX test: an independent quality assurance study. J Clin Oncol 2011;29:4279–85.

62. Yerushalmi R, Woods R, Ravdin PM, et al. Ki67 in breast cancer: prognostic and predictive potential. Lancet Oncol 2010;11:174–83.

63. Cheang MC, Chia SK, Voduc D, et al. Ki67 index, HER2 status, and prognosis of patients with luminal B breast cancer. J Natl Cancer Inst 2009;101:736–50.

64. Goldhirsch A, Wood WC, Coates AS, et al. Strategies for subtypes–dealing with the diversity of breast cancer: highlights of the St. Gallen International Expert Consensus on the Primary Therapy of Early Breast Cancer 2011. Ann Oncol 2011;22:1736–47.

65. Goldhirsch A, Winer EP, Coates AS, et al. Personalizing the treatment of women with early breast cancer: highlights of the St Gallen International Expert Consensus on the Primary Therapy of Early Breast Cancer 2013. Ann Oncol 2013;24:2206–23.

66. Nielsen TO, Leung SCY, Rimm DL, et al. Assessment of Ki67 in Breast Cancer: Updated Recommendations From the International Ki67 in Breast Cancer Working Group. J Natl Cancer Inst 2021;113:808–19.

67. Johnston SRD, Harbeck N, Hegg R, et al. Abemaciclib Combined With Endocrine Therapy for the Adjuvant Treatment of HR+, HER2-, Node-Positive, High-Risk, Early Breast Cancer (monarchE). J Clin Oncol 2020;38:3987–98.

68. Harbeck N, Rastogi P, Martin M, et al. Adjuvant abemaciclib combined with endocrine therapy for high-risk early breast cancer: updated efficacy and Ki-67 analysis from the monarchE study. Ann Oncol 2021;32:1571–81.

69. Denkert C, Loibl S, Noske A, et al. Tumor-associated lymphocytes as an independent predictor of response to neoadjuvant chemotherapy in breast cancer. J Clin Oncol 2010;28:105–13.

70. Denkert C, von Minckwitz G, Darb-Esfahani S, et al. Tumour-infiltrating lymphocytes and prognosis in different subtypes of breast cancer: a pooled analysis of 3771 patients treated with neoadjuvant therapy. Lancet Oncol 2018;19:40–50.

71. Loi S, Sirtaine N, Piette F, et al. Prognostic and predictive value of tumor-infiltrating lymphocytes in a phase III randomized adjuvant breast cancer trial in node-positive breast cancer comparing the addition of docetaxel to doxorubicin with doxorubicin-based chemotherapy: BIG 02-98. J Clin Oncol 2013; 31:860–7.

72. Loi S, Drubay D, Adams S, et al. Tumor-Infiltrating Lymphocytes and Prognosis: A Pooled Individual Patient Analysis of Early-Stage Triple-Negative Breast Cancers. J Clin Oncol 2019;37:559–69.

73. Salgado R, Denkert C, Demaria S, et al. The evaluation of tumor-infiltrating lymphocytes (TILs) in breast cancer: recommendations by an International TILs Working Group 2014. Ann Oncol 2015;26:259–71.

74. Loi S, Michiels S, Adams S, et al. The journey of tumor-infiltrating lymphocytes as a biomarker in breast cancer: clinical utility in an era of checkpoint inhibition. Ann Oncol 2021;32:1236–44.
75. Chakravarty D, Gao J, Phillips SM, et al. OncoKB: A Precision Oncology Knowledge Base. JCO Precis Oncol 2017;2017.
76. Han G, Schell MJ, Reisenbichler ES, et al. Determination of the number of observers needed to evaluate a subjective test and its application in two PD-L1 studies. Stat Med 2022;41:1361–75.
77. Reisenbichler ES, Han G, Bellizzi A, et al. Prospective multi-institutional evaluation of pathologist assessment of PD-L1 assays for patient selection in triple negative breast cancer. Mod Pathol 2020;33:1746–52.
78. Schmid P, Cortes J, Pusztai L, et al. Pembrolizumab for Early Triple-Negative Breast Cancer. N Engl J Med 2020;382:810–21.
79. Sajjadi E, Venetis K, Piciotti R, et al. Mismatch repair-deficient hormone receptor-positive breast cancers: Biology and pathological characterization. Cancer Cell Int 2021;21:266.
80. Schiavon G, Hrebien S, Garcia-Murillas I, et al. Analysis of ESR1 mutation in circulating tumor DNA demonstrates evolution during therapy for metastatic breast cancer. Sci Transl Med 2015;7:313ra182.
81. Clatot F, Perdrix A, Beaussire L, et al. Risk of early progression according to circulating ESR1 mutation, CA-15.3 and cfDNA increases under first-line anti-aromatase treatment in metastatic breast cancer. Breast Cancer Res 2020; 22:56.
82. Dahlgren M, George AM, Brueffer C, et al. Preexisting Somatic Mutations of Estrogen Receptor Alpha (ESR1) in Early-Stage Primary Breast Cancer. JNCI Cancer Spectr 2021;5.
83. Burstein HJ, Somerfield MR, Barton DL, et al. Endocrine Treatment and Targeted Therapy for Hormone Receptor-Positive, Human Epidermal Growth Factor Receptor 2-Negative Metastatic Breast Cancer: ASCO Guideline Update. J Clin Oncol 2021;39:3959–77.
84. Modi S, Park H, Murthy RK, et al. Antitumor Activity and Safety of Trastuzumab Deruxtecan in Patients With HER2-Low-Expressing Advanced Breast Cancer: Results From a Phase Ib Study. J Clin Oncol 2020;38:1887–96.
85. Modi S, Jacot W, Yamashita T, et al. Trastuzumab Deruxtecan in Previously Treated HER2-Low Advanced Breast Cancer. N Engl J Med 2022;387:9–20.
86. Hyman DM, Piha-Paul SA, Won H, et al. HER kinase inhibition in patients with HER2- and HER3-mutant cancers. Nature 2018;554:189–94.
87. André F, Ciruelos E, Rubovszky G, et al. Alpelisib for PIK3CA-Mutated, Hormone Receptor-Positive Advanced Breast Cancer. N Engl J Med 2019;380:1929–40.
88. Martínez-Sáez O, Chic N, Pascual T, et al. Frequency and spectrum of PIK3CA somatic mutations in breast cancer. Breast Cancer Res 2020;22:45.
89. Pérez-Fidalgo JA, Criscitiello C, Carrasco E, et al. A phase III trial of alpelisib + trastuzumab ± fulvestrant versus trastuzumab + chemotherapy in HER2+ PIK3CA-mutated breast cancer. Future Oncol 2022;18:2339–49.
90. Turner NC, Kingston B, Kilburn LS, et al. Circulating tumour DNA analysis to direct therapy in advanced breast cancer (plasmaMATCH): a multicentre, multi-cohort, phase 2a, platform trial. Lancet Oncol 2020;21:1296–308.
91. Rose Brannon A, Jayakumaran G, Diosdado M, et al. Enhanced specificity of clinical high-sensitivity tumor mutation profiling in cell-free DNA via paired normal sequencing using MSK-ACCESS. Nat Commun 2021;12:3770.

92. Dawson SJ, Tsui DW, Murtaza M, et al. Analysis of circulating tumor DNA to monitor metastatic breast cancer. N Engl J Med 2013;368:1199–209.
93. Fribbens C, Garcia Murillas I, Beaney M, et al. Tracking evolution of aromatase inhibitor resistance with circulating tumour DNA analysis in metastatic breast cancer. Ann Oncol 2018;29:145–53.
94. O'Leary B, Hrebien S, Morden JP, et al. Early circulating tumor DNA dynamics and clonal selection with palbociclib and fulvestrant for breast cancer. Nat Commun 2018;9:896.
95. O'Leary B, Cutts RJ, Liu Y, et al. The Genetic Landscape and Clonal Evolution of Breast Cancer Resistance to Palbociclib plus Fulvestrant in the PALOMA-3 Trial. Cancer Discov 2018;8:1390–403.
96. Paoletti C, Schiavon G, Dolce EM, et al. Circulating Biomarkers and Resistance to Endocrine Therapy in Metastatic Breast Cancers: Correlative Results from AZD9496 Oral SERD Phase I Trial. Clin Cancer Res 2018;24:5860–72.
97. Hrebien S, Citi V, Garcia-Murillas I, et al. Early ctDNA dynamics as a surrogate for progression-free survival in advanced breast cancer in the BEECH trial. Ann Oncol 2019;30:945–52.
98. O'Leary B, Cutts RJ, Huang X, et al. Circulating Tumor DNA Markers for Early Progression on Fulvestrant With or Without Palbociclib in ER+ Advanced Breast Cancer. J Natl Cancer Inst 2021;113:309–17.
99. Kingston B, Cutts RJ, Bye H, et al. Genomic profile of advanced breast cancer in circulating tumour DNA. Nat Commun 2021;12:2423.
100. Bardia A, Su F, Solovieff N, et al. Genomic Profiling of Premenopausal HR+ and HER2- Metastatic Breast Cancer by Circulating Tumor DNA and Association of Genetic Alterations With Therapeutic Response to Endocrine Therapy and Ribociclib. JCO Precis Oncol 2021;5.
101. Tolaney SM, Toi M, Neven P, et al. Clinical Significance of PIK3CA and ESR1 Mutations in Circulating Tumor DNA: Analysis from the MONARCH 2 Study of Abemaciclib plus Fulvestrant. Clin Cancer Res 2022;28:1500–6.
102. Radovich M, Jiang G, Hancock BA, et al. Association of Circulating Tumor DNA and Circulating Tumor Cells After Neoadjuvant Chemotherapy With Disease Recurrence in Patients With Triple-Negative Breast Cancer: Preplanned Secondary Analysis of the BRE12-158 Randomized Clinical Trial. JAMA Oncol 2020;6:1410–5.
103. Magbanua MJM, Swigart LB, Wu HT, et al. Circulating tumor DNA in neoadjuvant-treated breast cancer reflects response and survival. Ann Oncol 2021;32:229–39.
104. Garcia-Murillas I, Chopra N, Comino-Méndez I, et al. Assessment of Molecular Relapse Detection in Early-Stage Breast Cancer. JAMA Oncol 2019;5:1473–8.
105. Penson A, Camacho N, Zheng Y, et al. Development of Genome-Derived Tumor Type Prediction to Inform Clinical Cancer Care. JAMA Oncol 2020;6:84–91.

Breast Cancer Screening Modalities, Recommendations, and Novel Imaging Techniques

Sarah Nielsen, DO[a], Anand K. Narayan, MD, PhD[b],*

KEYWORDS

- Cancer screening guidelines • Health care providers • Mammography • Screening
- Breast neoplasm

KEY POINTS

- Screening mammography reduces breast cancer mortality.
- The American Society of Breast Surgeons recommends that average-risk women undergo breast cancer screening every year starting at age 40.
- Women with risk factors for breast cancer may benefit from earlier, supplemental screening.
- Black, Hispanic, and Asian women are more likely to be diagnosed with breast cancer before the age of 50.

INTRODUCTION

Breast cancer remains the second leading cause of cancer death for women in the United States.[1] In the United States in 2022, the American Cancer Society (ACS) estimates that 290,560 will be diagnosed with breast cancer. Approximately 43,780 Americans will die from this disease.[2] Roughly 1 in 1000 American men (.01%) will develop breast cancer. Owing to the increased availability of screening and treatment, breast cancer mortality has significantly declined in the United States. Mammography remains the only validated screening tool for breast cancer and is the gold standard for breast imaging. The goal of any mammography screening program is the detection of small, node-negative tumors with the least amount of morbidity to the patient and cost to society. However, there are limitations to mammography, one of which is the variable sensitivity based on breast density. Supplemental screening modalities using

This article previously appeared in *Surgical Clinics* volume 103 issue 1 February 2023.

[a] Section Head – Breast Imaging, Department of Radiology, Marshfield Clinic Health System, Marshfield Clinic – Wausau Center, 2727 Plaza Drive, Wausau, WI 54401, USA; [b] Equity, Department of Radiology, University of Wisconsin-Madison, 600 Highland Avenue, F6/178C, Madison, WI 53792-3252, USA
* Corresponding author.
E-mail address: anarayan@uwhealth.org
Twitter: @AnandKNarayan (A.K.N.)

digital breast tomosynthesis (DBT), screening ultrasound (US), breast MRI, and molecular breast imaging (MBI) may be considered based on the patient's risk level and breast density. Higher-risk women should start mammographic screening earlier and may benefit from supplemental screening modalities. This article reviews the fundamentals of mammography screening and current age-based mammography screening recommendations, supplemental breast cancer screening recommendations in women at higher-than-average risk, and novel imaging technologies.

DISCUSSION
Breast Cancer Screening

Mammography
Technique and physics. A mammogram is a radiographic examination of the breast, either displayed on film or on a digital computer monitor. Since 2000, full-field digital mammography (FFDM) has largely replaced film-screen mammography. When a digital mammogram is performed, the patient's breast is placed in compression and X-rays travel through the breast and onto a detector. The detector converts X-rays into electrical signals. The electrical signals are sent to a computer for processing and to the radiologist for interpretation. When looking at a mammogram one will see various shades of gray based on the differential attenuation characteristics of the tissue. Specifically, fat attenuates fewer X-rays than fibroglandular tissue and appears darker gray. Fibroglandular and stromal tissue appear lighter white, as do mineral deposits such as calcifications within a malignant lesion appearing bright white. With the invention of digital mammography came improved contrast resolution. As cancer is radiopaque, good contrast resolution is necessary to be able to discern the subtle differences between a cancer and the normal surrounding fibroglandular tissue. Compression also helps with finding abnormalities by spreading out the tissues and minimizing motion artifacts.

There are two standard views in screening mammography named for the direction of the X-ray beam from the source to the detector: craniocaudal (CC) and mediolateral oblique (MLO) (**Fig. 1**).

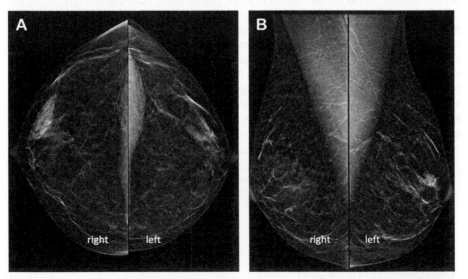

Fig. 1. (*A*) Standard craniocaudal (CC) mammographic views. (*B*) Standard mediolateral oblique (MLO) mammographic views.

For the CC view, the patient's breast is positioned on the image detector with the paddle compressing the breast in the superior to inferior direction. The image should ideally include the cleavage area and some of the pectoralis muscle (seen in roughly 30%). These landmarks help to ensure that an adequate amount of tissue is included and that a portion of tissue harboring a malignancy is not excluded. When looking at a CC view on a monitor, the lateral breast is placed superior to the screen, and the medial breast is inferior.

For the MLO view, the machine is angled generally 40 to 60° to image as much of the pectoralis muscle as possible. A line drawn from the nipple to the chest wall should be within 1 cm of the same line drawn on the CC view to ensure adequate tissue inclusion. Breast cancers may develop within the axillary tail and it is essential to include as much tissue from this region as possible. When looking at an MLO view on a monitor, superior is superior, and inferior is inferior.

The radiation dose is very low in mammography. Compression decreases the radiation dose by decreasing the number of photons needed to penetrate the breast tissue. One screening FFDM is about equivalent to simply living for approximately 7 weeks (background radiation),[3] or flying for roughly 13,000 miles.[4] Combining both FFDM with three-dimensional (tomosynthesis) images increases the dose to ~ 2.5 mGy, which is well below the American College of Radiology's (ACR) 3 mGy per film cutoff. New technology allows the two-dimensional (2D) images to be reconstructed from the 3D images that drop the dose by an estimated 43%.[5] Regardless if your facility performs 2D ± tomosynthesis ± reconstructed 2D views, mammography is a very low dose radiation procedure.

Radiation dose and image quality in mammography are heavily regulated under the Mammography Quality Standards Act (MQSA) Program passed in 1992. All facilities performing mammography in the United States must be certified by the Food and Drug Administration (FDA) or an FDA-approved Certifying State. Certification requires standards to be met in the quality of mammographic equipment, personnel who perform and interpret mammography, and reporting. MQSA requires that all facilities have a procedure in place for following abnormal findings and tracking pathologic results from biopsy procedures. The facility is inspected annually by trained FDA or state inspectors. In addition, the ACR evaluates both phantom and patient images from each machine that performs mammography to ensure minimum quality standards are met. If your facility is an ACR Breast Imaging Center of Excellence it means it has received full accreditation by the ACR in all imaging modalities.

Interpretation of a Mammogram

When interpreting a mammogram, the radiologist uses the Breast Imaging Reporting and Data System (BI-RADS) lexicon.[6] The BI-RADS lexicon is used to describe and classify findings, and each mammogram is given a final BI-RADS assessment category (0–6) (**Fig. 2**) The BI-RADS lexicon serves to standardize reports, and allow for clear communication between the clinicians and radiologists, and what, if anything, needs to be done next. Screening mammograms are performed on the asymptomatic breast. Screening mammograms with potential abnormalities are typically given a BI-RADS category 0 assessment and are subsequently evaluated with a diagnostic mammogram or US at the discretion of the radiologist.

On mammograms, cancers present as masses, asymmetries, calcifications, or architectural distortions. A mass is 3-dimensional and occupies space. It is seen on two different mammographic projections. The shape of a mass is described as oval, round or irregular, whereas the margins are described as circumscribed, obscured, microlobulated, indistinct, and spiculated. The density of a mass can be reported as high, equal,

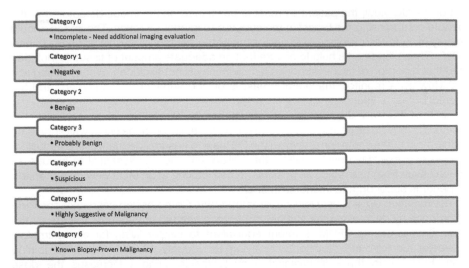

Fig. 2. BI-RADS assessment categories.

low, or fat-containing density. The several different types of asymmetry involve a spectrum of mammographic findings that represent unilateral deposits of fibroglandular tissue not conforming to the definition of a radiodense mass. The asymmetry is visible on only one projection. Focal (involving less than a quadrant), global (involving at least one quadrant), and developing (new, increasing) asymmetries have concave-outward borders, whereas a radiodense mass displays completely or partially convex-outward borders. Architectural distortion, which can occur with our without a central mass, is used to describe speculations radiating from a point and focal retraction at the edge of the parenchyma. In the absence of a history of trauma or surgery, architectural distortion is suspicious of malignancy or radial scar and should be biopsied. Typically benign calcifications are generally larger than those associated with malignancy (coarse, round, rod-like, rim, dystrophic, or "layering" milk of calcium on 90° medial-lateral images). The morphology of calcifications associated with malignancy are usually very small requiring the use of magnification and are described as amorphous, coarse heterogeneous, fine pleomorphic, and fine linear or fine linear branching. The distribution is used to describe the arrangement of calcifications in the breast. Distribution descriptors are diffuse, regional, grouped, linear, and segmental. It should be noted that in evaluating the likelihood of malignancy for calcifications, the distribution is at least as important as the morphology. The radiologists generally report the location of abnormal findings either as a clock position or by quadrant and include the distance from the nipple.

Using the BI-RADS lexicon and assessment system, a quality audit is generated. The current BI-RADS atlas establishes clear definitions for how to determine whether findings in a screening mammogram are true-positive (TP), true-negative (TN), false-positive (FP), or false-negative (FN). From these outcomes, the metrics of sensitivity (TP/TP + FN), specificity (TN/TN + FP), and positive predictive value (PPV) (TP/TP + FN) are calculated.[6] PPV is a measure of how likely it is that a positive test result indicates presence of disease with three subtypes: PPV1, PPV2, and PPV3 (**Fig. 3**). The commonly used performance metrics for screening mammography are recall rate, cancer detection rate (CDR), and PPVs.

The National Mammography Database (NMD) is a component of the ACR National Radiology Data Registry established in 2008. The NMD is a robust automated data

PPV1	PPV2	PPV3
• PPV1 is the percentage of patients recalled from screening for additional imaging who receive a cancer diagnosis. PPV1 is a useful metric for monitoring the success of screening interpretations by incorporating both the cancer detection rate (CDR) and the recall rate in a single metric.	• PPV2 is the percentage of all diagnostic examinations recommended for biopsy or surgical consultation that result in a cancer diagnosis and is a useful metric representing the radiologist's interpretive recommendations.	• PPV3 is the percentage of all known biopsies performed after positive findings of diagnostic evaluations and is useful at the society level because it reflects clinical care actually delivered.

Fig. 3. Positive predictive value definitions.

collection process that accrues screening mammography interpretation and biopsy results in addition to other clinical practice data from over 200 volunteer facilities across 30 states. For quality improvement purposes, the NMD was designed to enable mammographic facilities and radiologists to compare their mammography performance with that of their peers locally, regionally, and nationally. The screening performance metrics (CDR, recall, and PPVs) are calculated for all facilities by use of the standard BI-RADS audit procedures, and provide practice-based screening performance benchmark data.[7]

Benefits of Early Detection Through Mammography Screening

Early detection of breast cancer with screening mammography significantly reduces the risk of death from the disease.[8,9] The strongest evidence is provided by randomized controlled studies (RCTs) and pooled estimates from eight RCTs showing that mammography can reduce breast cancer mortality by at least 20%.[10] Meta-analyses of RCTs have been the primary source of evidence supporting the benefit of screening mammography in guideline development. Observational studies evaluating breast cancer screening must be interpreted with caution because of susceptibility to biases, including selection bias, lead time bias, length bias, and others.[11] However, RCTs were conducted decades ago with obsolete older film screen technology and protocols. With advances in digital mammography technology, the ACS concluded that large, methodologically rigorous observational studies can provide valuable information about the contemporary effectiveness of screening mammography.[10] Numerous observational studies have shown mortality reductions of 40% or greater with organized screening.[12–17]

BREAST CANCER SCREENING RECOMMENDATIONS FOR WOMEN OF AVERAGE RISK

Because screening mammography reduces breast cancer mortality, every major guideline-producing organization in the United States has recommended screening mammography in average-risk women.[18] However, recommendations differ about when women should start screening and how often they should undergo mammographic screening (**Fig. 4**). We describe the varying perspectives used to inform each screening guideline recommendation.

American Society of Breast Surgeons

The American Society of Breast Surgeons (ASBrS) published guidelines in 2019 derived from a literature review conducted by an expert panel. The ASBrS recommended that average-risk women undergo breast cancer screening every year starting at age 40. Although noting that there are disadvantages of starting annual screening mammography at the age of 40, the ASBrS noted that meta-analyses of randomized control trials found that screening mammography reduced breast cancer mortality.

They noted that USPSTF guidelines weighed the results from statistical models generated by the Cancer Intervention and Surveillance Modeling Network (CISNET). Analyses of CISNET models have confirmed that screening strategies starting every year beginning at age 40 yield the largest reductions in breast cancer mortality. The USPSTF opted to base their recommendations on efficiency frontiers evaluating the average gain in life-years per additional mammogram performed per 1000 women. The ASBrS guidelines prioritized mortality reduction benefits over efficiency frontiers.

In addition, they recommended that women with a life expectancy of at least 10 years should continue screening mammography every year. While noting that randomized control trials excluded women older than 74, the ASBrS noted that observational studies have found survival benefits of screening mammography in older women without severe co-morbidities[19] and that false positives would be expected to be lower compared with younger populations.

American Cancer Society

The ACS developed its recommendations using standardized methodologies derived from the Institute of Medicine,[20] supplemented by Breast Cancer Surveillance Consortium (BCSC) data.[21] Compared with premenopausal women who underwent mammographic screening every year, premenopausal women who underwent mammographic screening every 2 years were more likely to be diagnosed with poorer prognosis breast cancers. In contrast, post-menopausal women undergoing

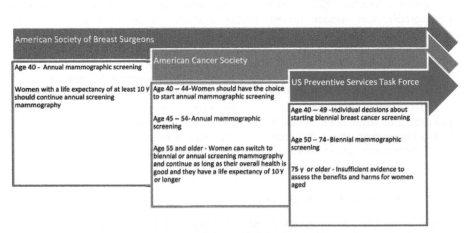

Fig. 4. Summary of breast cancer screening guidelines by Professional societies for average risk women.

screening every 2 years showed no statistically significant increases in advanced-stage breast cancers compared with women undergoing screening every year.

The ACS noted that women between the ages of 40 to 44 showed less morbidity and mortality from breast cancer compared with other 5-year age categories. Consequently, the ACS recommended that average-risk women start annual screening at the age of 45. If women between the ages of 40 to 44 year old chose to initiate breast cancer screening, the ACR recommended that they undergo annual screening. With comparatively fewer benefits of annual screening mammography in women after menopause, the ACS recommended that starting at age 55 (the age at which the majority of women are post-menopausal), average-risk women should transition to biennial screening or continue annual screening.

Beyond the age of 74, the ACS noted that age is one of the most important risk factors for breast cancer. Women between the ages of 75 to 79 show the highest breast cancer incidence rates. 26% of breast cancer deaths are attributable to breast cancer diagnoses after the age of 74. Consequently, the ACS recommended that women continue screening mammography as long as their overall health is good and they have a life expectancy of 10 years or longer.

US Preventive Services Task Force

The US Preventive Services Task Force (USPSTF) is a volunteer panel of 16 nationally recognized experts in primary care, prevention, and evidence-based medicine. Details regarding guideline development methods are described elsewhere.[22] In determining their recommendation, the USPSTF noted that most of the benefits of mammographic screening result from biennial screening during ages 50 to 74 years. While noting that mammographic screening between the ages of 40 to 49 may reduce breast cancer mortality, they noted that comparatively smaller numbers of breast cancer deaths were averted by starting screening at age 40 instead of age 50, whereas the number of FP results and unnecessary biopsies increased by starting screening at age 40.

The USPSTF found that current evidence is insufficient to assess the benefits and harms for women aged 75 years or older, citing a lack of randomized control trial data in women in this age group. However, they cited CISNET modeling studies suggesting that screening women older than 74 year old may be beneficial among women with no or low comorbidity.

Harms Associated with Mammographic Screening, Diagnosis, and Treatment

The USPSTF conducted a systematic review and meta-analysis to estimate potential harms of screening including FPs, overdiagnosed/overtreated breast cancers, anxiety, pain during procedures, and radiation exposure.[23] Of these harms, the USPSTF identified overdiagnosis/overtreatment and FPs as the two major potential harms associated with screening mammography.

Overdiagnosis/Overtreatment

Overdiagnosis/overtreatment refers to the diagnosis and treatment of breast cancers that would not cause harm during a patient's lifetime because these cancers would progress too slowly, not progress at all, or resolve spontaneously. According to the USPSTF, overdiagnosis/overtreatment is the principal harm associated with screening mammography.

The USPSTF systematic review found estimates of overdiagnosis/overtreatment ranging between 0% to 54% of breast cancer cases. A major methodological challenge associated with the quantitative estimation of over-diagnosis is that currently we do not have ways to identify or predict which cancers will progress.[24] Widely ranging estimates about the magnitude and extent of overdiagnosis/overtreatment present challenges for health care providers who are counseling their patients about the potential harms of mammographic screening.

False Positives

The USPSTF systematic review estimated the cumulative probability of FP results based on data from the BCSC[25,26] They found that FP results were highest among women receiving annual mammography, 40 to 49-year-old women, women with extremely dense breast tissue, and/or women using combination hormone therapy.

To evaluate the consequences of FP examinations, USPSTF identified four systematic reviews with varying conclusions about the impacts of FPs. One study was nested within the Digital Mammographic Imaging Screening Trial, a randomized control trial.[27] Tosteson and colleagues found that women with FP results were more likely to experience short-term anxiety however did not experience any differences in anxiety or health-related quality of life 1 year later. In addition, women with FP mammography results were more likely to state that they would undergo screening mammography in the future. Overall, the USPSTF concluded that the absolute magnitude and time course of anxiety experienced by individual women after FPs were difficult to estimate and varied widely.

Maximizing the Benefits and Reducing Potential Harms Associated with Screening Mammography

The ACS emphasized the need to minimize the harms of FP examinations from screening mammography.[28] Screening mammography recalls are common in the United States;[29] however, the vast majority of recalls turn out to be normal.[30] Framing recalls as part of a continuous portion of the screening process in which additional images are occasionally required to complete the imaging evaluation, health care providers can help reduce anxiety associated with recalls. In addition, radiology practices can implement strategies to reduce harm associated with FPs from mammographic screening.[31–33] Emerging technologies like artificial intelligence offer the prospect of reducing variation in mammography performance.[34] By adopting these interventions, radiology practices can maximize the benefits of screening mammography while reducing potential harms.

BREAST CANCER SCREENING RECOMMENDATIONS FOR HIGH-RISK WOMEN

The principal goal of breast cancer screening is to detect small, non-palpable, node-negative breast cancers to allow the least morbid treatments and mortality. Identifying women at the highest risk of disease can direct the use of supplemental screening in addition to screening mammography.

Population Subgroups at Increased Risk

The ASBrS cites the National Comprehensive Cancer Network (NCCN) guidelines for characterizing women as high risk for breast cancer including the following groups **(Fig. 5)**[35,36] In only 5% to 10% of women with breast cancer is a known genetic mutation identified.[37]

Breast Cancer Risk Assessment

Women with risk factors for breast cancer can benefit from earlier, supplemental screening. The ASBrS and NCCN recommend all women undergo a formal risk assessment at 25 year old.[38]

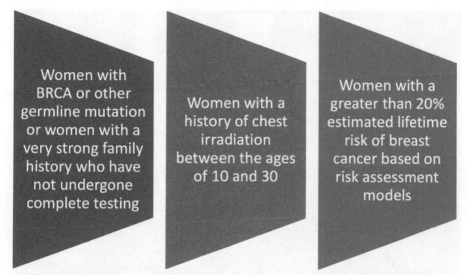

Fig. 5. Women categorized as high risk for breast cancer according to NCCN guidelines.

To determine whether a woman is at average or increased risk, the assessment begins with gathering patient genetic, familial, personal, reproductive, demographic, lifestyle factors, and factors such as the number of biopsies (especially those finding atypical hyperplasia, lobular carcinoma in situ, and flat epithelial atypia). The family history should be assessed for first-degree, second-degree, and third-degree relatives on both the maternal and paternal sides of the family.

Many statistical models have been developed to estimate the risk of developing breast cancer and the risk of carrying a heritable genetic mutation. Common models include Gail model, Claus, BRCAPRO, BOADICEA, and Tyrer-Cuzick. Each model incorporates and weighs different sets of risk factors. Hence, the models can give different estimates for the same woman. To improve discriminatory accuracy, a few models also include modifiable lifestyle risk factors such as body mass index, alcohol use, exercise, and non-modifiable mammographic breast density (MBD). The modified Tyrer-Cuzick 8 risk-assessment model includes MBD, which is an important risk factor. The Tyrer-Cuzick model is the most comprehensive but is also the most time intensive.[39] To determine eligibility for MRI screening, the ACS and NCCN recommend using models that are largely dependent on family history (eg, Claus, BRCAPRO and Tyrer-Cuzick) and recommend against using models with limited family history (eg, Gail or modified Gail).[40]

Implications of Breast Density

Breast density is a mammographic assessment of the ratio of fibroglandular tissue (white) to fat (gray) in the breast. The ACR BI-RADS atlas[6] requires reporting of breast density in every mammogram report as fatty (A), scattered (B), heterogeneously dense (C), or extremely dense (D). The fatty and scattered categories (A and B) are considered non-dense, whereas the heterogeneously and extremely dense (C and D) are considered dense (**Fig. 6**). Nearly 43% of women aged 40 to 74 year old have dense breasts.[41]

Mammographic density is one of the strongest risk factors for breast cancer. Women with extremely dense mammographic patterns show four to six times higher

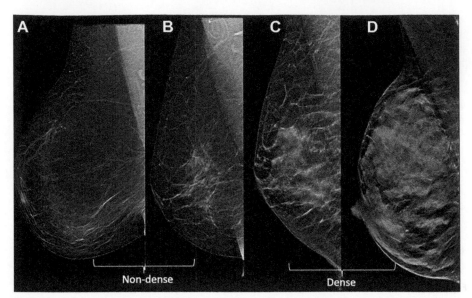

Fig. 6. BI-RADS Breast Density Categories: (*A*) Fatty (*B*) Scattered fibroglandular (*C*) Heterogeneously Dense (*D*) Extremely dense.

risk of developing breast cancer compared with those with fatty breasts[41,42] Another implication of dense breasts is the masking effect, or reduced sensitivity of mammography in detecting noncalcified cancers in women with dense breasts. The sensitivity of mammography in the detection of breast cancer is close to 90% for fatty breasts and drops to 60% for women with extremely dense breasts.[43] This masking effect can cause a delay in diagnosis, potentially resulting in an interval, clinically palpable tumor. An interval cancer is one that manifests within 1 year of a normal mammogram. Interval cancers typically have a worse prognosis than cancers detected by radiologic screening, and interval cancer rates increase with increasing breast density.[44]

The definition of "dense" is subjective by the radiologist and therefore inter-observer variability can be significant among radiologists. Improving the consistency of screening recommendations based on density assessments has led to the growth of automated software programs for reliable and reproducible quantitative and volumetric breast density assessment. Application of deep learning (DL) methods for density assessment is an emerging area of research.

In the United States, currently at least 38 states require patients to be notified about their breast density and what it means to have dense breasts.[43] Because of the limitations of mammography, supplemental screening has been advocated for women with dense breast tissue. In 2019, the FDA proposed a rule to the MQSA Act that would make it a national requirement that all mammography centers in all states communicate information about dense breast tissue to their patients. As of this date, this proposed rule is under review.

SUPPLEMENTAL SCREENING MODALITIES

As risk assessments become more comprehensive with the incorporation of breast density, more women are being notified of their lifetime risk for breast cancer. For women deemed high risk, the screening guidelines are relatively well-defined. For women with intermediate-risk and/or increased breast density, supplemental screening modalities should be discussed with these women. Available options include anatomic screening with DBT and whole-breast ultrasound (WBUS), and functional screening with breast MRI, contrast-enhanced digital mammography (CEDM), MBI, and fluorodeoxyglucose-PET dedicated breast imaging. The American College of Radiology Appropriateness Criteria are evidence-based guidelines for specific clinical conditions that are reviewed annually by a multidisciplinary expert panel. The ACR Appropriateness Criteria reviewed the evidence regarding supplemental Breast Cancer Screening based on Breast Density and lifetime risk.[45] (Table 1).

Digital Breast Tomosynthesis

DBT, approved by the FDA in 2011, is an X-ray mammography technique in which tomographic images of the breast are reconstructed from multiple low-dose projections acquired by moving the X-ray tube in an arc over a limited angular range (Fig. 7). DBT technique reduces the impact of overlapping breast tissue which ultimately increases the conspicuity of lesions while reducing FPs due to summation. The FDA has approved software for the reconstruction of 2D synthetic views from 3D acquired data, which allows the radiation dose to remain comparable to that of conventional FFDM and has permitted DBT with synthetic reconstruction to replace FFDM.[46]

The use of DBT is widespread and currently many facilities in the United States offer DBT as their primary screening modality. Two prospective European screening trials[44,47] showed an incremental CDR of 2.3 and 2.7 per 1000 screening examinations with DBT as compared with digital mammography alone. Friedwald and colleagues,[48] using a multi-institutional retrospective analysis, showed an incremental CDR of 1.2 cancers per 1000 screening examination with DBT. However, for extremely dense breasts, there was no improvement in cancer detection for DBT over DM.[49] Additional benefits of adding DBT to 2D mammography is the reduction in recall rate, with a meta-analysis showing an absolute reduction in recall rate of 0.8% to 3.6%.[50] The ACR Appropriateness criteria suggest that DBT is appropriate for all women regardless of breast density and risk status.[45]

Whole-Breast Ultrasound

Multiple studies confirm the incremental cancer detection capabilities of WBUS in women with higher risk. ACRIN 6666 was a prospective, multicenter trial, randomized to the sequence of mammography and US, designed to evaluate the performance of screening US in conjunction with mammography in high-risk women.[51] Screening US was associated with the detection of an additional 4.2 cancers per 1000 women screened. However, these additional cancers were balanced by a large increase in FP findings and reduce PPVs. In the Japan Strategic Anti-cancer Randomized Trial (J-START), asymptomatic women between the ages of 40 to 49 were randomized to undergo mammography and ultrasonography versus mammography alone twice in 2 years.[52] Women undergoing supplemental screening US had more cancers detected than those undergoing mammography alone; however, specificity was lower. With increased experience with screening-breast US and technological advances, some of the limitations associated with screening-breast US may diminish.[53]

Contrast Enhanced Breast MRI

The ASBrS notes that contrast-enhanced breast MRI is more sensitive than either mammography and/or US.[54] In addition, cancers detected on breast MRI were more likely to be invasive carcinomas, whereas cancers detected on mammography

Table 1
Summary of ACR recommendations for supplemental screening based on cancer risk and breast density

Modality	Average Risk		Intermediate Risk		High Risk	
	Non-dense	Dense	Non-dense	Dense	Non-dense	Dense
Digital breast tomosynthesis	Usually appropriate	Usually appropriate	Usually appropriate	Usually appropriate	Usually appropriate	Usually appropriate
Whole-breast ultrasound	Usually not appropriate	May be appropriate	Usually not appropriate	May be appropriate	May be appropriate	Usually appropriate
Breast MRI	Usually not appropriate	May be appropriate	May be appropriate	May be appropriate	Usually appropriate	Usually appropriate
Abbreviated breast MRI	Usually not appropriate	May be appropriate	May be appropriate	May be appropriate	May be appropriate	Usually appropriate
Molecular breast imaging	Usually not appropriate	Usually not appropriate	Usually not appropriate	Usually not appropriate	Usually not appropriate	Usually not appropriate
Contrast-enhanced mammography	Usually not appropriate	May be appropriate	Usually not appropriate	May be appropriate	May be appropriate	May be appropriate

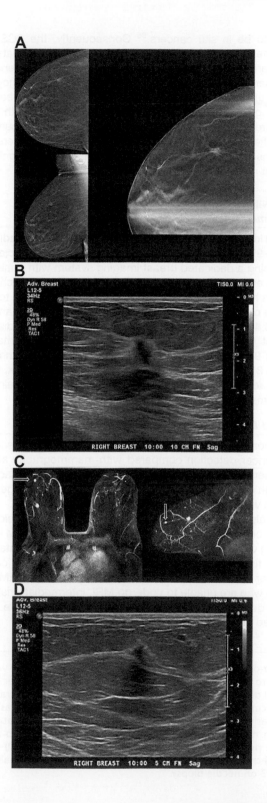

were more likely to be in situ cancers.[55] Consequently, the ACS advocates MRI screening for women with an approximately 20% to 25% or greater lifetime risk of breast cancer, regardless of breast density.[40] The ASBrS recommends that these patients should be offered MR screening starting at age 25 and mammography at age 30, or 10 years before the first-degree relative was diagnosed, but no earlier than age 25. Emerging data suggest that MRI may be beneficial in women with extremely dense breast tissue, regardless of underlying breast cancer risk. A multicenter, randomized, controlled trial in the Netherlands found that supplemental MRI screening in women with extremely dense breast tissue resulted in the diagnosis of significantly fewer interval cancers than mammography alone.[56]

EMERGING SCREENING TECHNOLOGIES
Molecular Breast Imaging

MBI is a functional imaging technique involving the injection of a radiopharmaceutical agent (technetium-99m sestamibi) and obtaining CC and MLO projections (similar to mammography) using a dedicated breast imaging system with dual-head solid-state detectors. Studies evaluating MBI as a supplemental screening technique for women with dense breasts have shown an incremental CDR between 7.5 to 8 per 1000. The median tumor size of cancer detected by MBI only is 1 cm, with an additional recall rate of 5.9% to 8.4%[57–59] As Tc-99 sestamibi is systemically distributed, tissues outside the breast receive the largest radiation dose. The estimated whole-body dose for 8 mi of Tc-99 sestamibi is 2.1 to 2.6 mSv which is below annual natural background levels of $\sim$3 mSv.[60] Concerns regarding MBI radiation risk, though disputed, have led to it slow adoption in clinical practice. However, MBI remains a sensitive tool for supplemental imaging and further studies are needed.

Contrast-Enhanced Digital Mammography

By enhancing tumor vascularity, contrast-enhanced breast MRI screening substantially increases cancer detection compared with mammography and/or breast US. However, the dissemination of breast MRI has been limited by lack of widespread availability and high costs. CEDM uses CEDM platforms to leveraged enhanced cancer detection from vascular imaging.

Initial studies evaluating CEDM as a screening modality have yielded promising results.[61] Sung and colleagues[62] evaluated the performance of CEDM in 904 women undergoing screening CEDM for a variety of indications (dense breasts, family history of breast cancer in a first-degree relative, personal history of breast cancer) and found high CDRs (15.5 per 1000 women) and high sensitivity (87.5%). CEM may be an alternative for patients who are unable to undergo MRI, intermediate-risk patient populations who do not qualify for MRI screening, and as an alternative to breast MRI in settings with limited access to breast MRI.

Fig. 7. (A) A 63-year-old woman presenting for screening mammogram with tomosynthesis. Patient was found to have a focal asymmetry in the right upper outer breast, which persisted on additional diagnostic spot compression views. (B) Focused ultrasound of the right breast found a 0.9-cm mass at 10:00, 10 cm from the nipple, which was subsequently biopsied revealing invasive lobular carcinoma, grade 2/3. (C) A pre-operative MRI evaluation showed the known malignancy in the right breast at 10:00, but also revealed a second smaller mass in the right breast at 10:00 at anterior depth (arrow). (D) MR-directed ultrasound showed a 0.6-cm mass at 10:00, 5 cm from the nipple, which revealed invasive lobular carcinoma grade 2/3 on needle biopsy.

Abbreviated Breast MRI

Abbreviated breast MRI examinations reduce image acquisition and interpretation times to increase access and decrease costs associated with breast MRIs. Chen and colleagues[63] found no statistically significant differences in sensitivity comparing full breast MRI protocols with abbreviated breast MRI protoools. The ECOG-ACRIN Cancer Research Group conducted a prospective, multicenter, study in the United States and Germany.[64] Among women with dense breasts undergoing screening, abbreviated breast MRI was associated with a higher rate of invasive breast cancer detection (incremental cancer detection increase of 7 cancers per 1000 women).

Generalizability of Screening Recommendations

A major limitation of the existing literature is that randomized control trials used for meta-analyses incorporated study populations with limited numbers of racial/ethnic minorities. As a result, observational studies and statistical models have been used to address gaps in randomized control trial data.

Using SEER population registries, Banegas and colleagues[65] found that Hispanic and Black women had a 10% to 50% greater risk of breast cancer-specific mortality compared with non-Hispanic white women. Stapleton and Oseni and colleagues[66] found that Black, Hispanic, and Asian women were more likely to be diagnosed with breast cancer before the age of 50. In part, due to the potential harms of delayed onset of screening mammography in racial/ethnic minority women, the ASBrS recommends annual screening mammography starting at age 40 in average-risk women.

For transgender patients who are at average risk, ACR recommendations for breast cancer screening were based on expert opinion derived from limited data.[67] For average-risk transgender patients, the ACR recommends annual screening starting at age 40 for male-to-female transgender patients who have used hormones for 5 years as well as female-to-male transgender patients who have not undergone mastectomy [99]. Individuals who identify as lesbian, gay, bisexual, or queer are less likely to present for cancer screening, emphasizing the importance of creating and fostering inclusive environments.[68]

SUMMARY

In summary, breast cancer is the second leading cause of cancer death among women in the United States. Mammography screening in average-risk women reduces breast cancer mortality. Black, Hispanic, and Asian women are more likely to be diagnosed with breast cancer before the age of 50. To reduce disparities and prevent the maximum number of breast cancer deaths, the ASBrS recommends that average-risk women undergo breast cancer screening every year starting at age 40. Women with risk factors for breast cancer can benefit from earlier, supplemental screening. Emerging technologies such as contrast-enhanced mammography and abbreviated breast MRI may facilitate early detection and improve patient outcomes in the appropriate clinical settings.

CLINICS CARE POINTS

- Screening mammography reduces breast cancer mortality
- The American Society of Breast Surgeons recommends that average-risk women undergo breast cancer screening every year starting at age 40

- Women with risk factors for breast cancer can benefit from earlier, supplemental screening
- Black, Hispanic, and Asian women are more likely to be diagnosed with breast cancer before the age of 50
- The American College of Radiology recommends annual screening starting at age 40 for male-to-female transgender patients who have used hormones for 5 years as well as female-to-male transgender patients who have not undergone mastectomy

DISCLOSURE

The authors have nothing to disclose.

REFERENCES

1. Smith RA, Andrews KS, Brooks D, et al. Cancer screening in the United States, 2019: A review of current American Cancer Society guidelines and current issues in cancer screening. CA Cancer J Clin 2019;69(3):184–210.
2. Siegel RL, Miller KD, Fuchs HE, et al. Cancer statistics, 2022. CA Cancer J Clin 2022;72(1):7–33.
3. Radiation Dose to Adults from Common Imaging Examinations. ACR Available at: https://www.acr.org/-/media/ACR/Files/Radiology-Safety/Radiation-Safety/Dose-Reference-Card.pdf Google Scholar.
4. Calculate Your Radiation Dose. EPA Available at: https://www.epa.gov/radiation/calculate-your-radiation-dose Google Scholar.
5. Garayoa J, Hernandez-Giron I, Castillo M, et al. In: Fujita H, Hara T, Muramatsu C, editors. Digital breast tomosynthesis: image quality and dose Saving of the Synthesized image. Breast imaging. IWDM 2014. Lecture notes in computer Science, 8539. Cham: Springer; 2014. https://doi.org/10.1007/978-3-319-07887-8_22.
6. Sickles EA, D'Orsi CJ. ACR BI-RADS Follow-up and Outcome Monitoring. In: D'Orsi CJ, Sickles EA, Mendelson EB, et al, editors. ACR BI-RADS atlas, breast imaging reporting and data system. Reston, VA: American College of Radiology; 2013 [Google Scholar].
7. Lee CS, Moy L, Friedewald SM, et al. Harmonizing Breast Cancer Screening Recommendations: Metrics and Accountability. AJR Am J Roentgenol 2018;210(2):241–5.
8. Smith RA, Duffy SW, Gabe R, et al. The randomized trials of breast cancer screening: what have we learned? Radiol Clin North Am 2004;42(5):793-v.
9. Tabár L, Yen AM, Wu WY, et al. Insights from the breast cancer screening trials: how screening affects the natural history of breast cancer and implications for evaluating service screening programs. Breast J 2015;21(1):13–20.
10. Oeffinger KC, Fontham ET, Etzioni R, et al. Breast Cancer Screening for Women at Average Risk: 2015 Guideline Update From the American Cancer Society [published correction appears in JAMA. JAMA 2015;314(15):1599–1614, 1406.
11. Narayan AK, Lee CI, Lehman CD. Screening for Breast Cancer. Med Clin North Am 2020;104(6):1007–21.
12. Broeders M, Moss S, Nyström L, et al. The impact of mammographic screening on breast cancer mortality in Europe: a review of observational studies. J Med Screen 2012;19(Suppl 1):14–25.
13. Coldman A, Phillips N, Wilson C, et al. Pan-Canadian study of mammography screening and mortality from breast cancer [published correction appears in. J Natl Cancer Inst 2015;107(1):dju404.

14. Pocobelli G, Weiss NS. Breast cancer mortality in relation to receipt of screening mammography: a case-control study in Saskatchewan, Canada. Cancer Causes Control 2015;26(2):231–7.

15. Yen AM, Tsau HS, Fann JC, et al. Population-Based Breast Cancer Screening With Risk-Based and Universal Mammography Screening Compared With Clinical Breast Examination: A Propensity Score Analysis of 1 429 890 Taiwanese Women. JAMA Oncol 2016;2(7):915–21.

16. Morrell S, Taylor R, Roder D, et al. Mammography service screening and breast cancer mortality in New Zealand: a National Cohort Study 1999-2011. Br J Cancer 2017;116(6):828–39.

17. Moss SM, Nyström L, Jonsson H, et al. The impact of mammographic screening on breast cancer mortality in Europe: a review of trend studies. J Med Screen 2012;19(Suppl 1):26–32.

18. Narayan AK, Lehman CD. Mammography Screening Guideline Controversies: Opportunities to Improve Patient Engagement in Screening. J Am Coll Radiol 2020;17(5):633–6.

19. Badgwell BD, Giordano SH, Duan ZZ, et al. Mammography before diagnosis among women age 80 years and older with breast cancer. J Clin Oncol 2008; 26(15):2482–8.

20. Brawley O, Byers T, Chen A, et al. New American Cancer Society process for creating trustworthy cancer screening guidelines. JAMA 2011;306(22):2495–9.

21. Miglioretti DL, Zhu W, Kerlikowske K, et al. Breast Tumor Prognostic Characteristics and Biennial vs Annual Mammography, Age, and Menopausal Status. JAMA Oncol 2015;1(8):1069–77.

22. Harris RP, Helfand M, Woolf SH, et al. Current methods of the US Preventive Services Task Force: a review of the process. Am J Prev Med 2001;20(3 Suppl): 21–35.

23. Nelson HD, Pappas M, Cantor A, et al. Harms of Breast Cancer Screening: Systematic Review to Update the 2009 U.S. Preventive Services Task Force Recommendation. Ann Intern Med 2016;164(4):256–67 [published correction appears in Ann Intern Med. 2018 Nov 20;169(10):740].

24. Puliti D, Duffy SW, Miccinesi G, et al. Overdiagnosis in mammographic screening for breast cancer in Europe: a literature review. J Med Screen 2012;19(Suppl 1): 42–56.

25. Breast Cancer Surveillance Consortium. Breast Cancer Surveillance Consortium. Available at URL: https://www.bcsc-research.org/. Accessed July 09, 2020.

26. Hubbard RA, Kerlikowske K, Flowers CI, et al. Cumulative probability of false-positive recall or biopsy recommendation after 10 years of screening mammography: a cohort study. Ann Intern Med 2011;155(8):481–92 [published correction appears in Ann Intern Med. 2014 May 6;160(9):658].

27. Tosteson AN, Fryback DG, Hammond CS, et al. Consequences of false-positive screening mammograms. JAMA Intern Med 2014;174(6):954–61.

28. Lehman CD, Arao RF, Sprague BL, et al. National Performance Benchmarks for Modern Screening Digital Mammography: Update from the Breast Cancer Surveillance Consortium. Radiology 2017;283(1):49–58.

29. Nelson HD, O'Meara ES, Kerlikowske K, et al. Factors Associated With Rates of False-Positive and False-Negative Results From Digital Mammography Screening: An Analysis of Registry Data. Ann Intern Med 2016;164(4): 226–35.

30. Berg WA. Benefits of screening mammography. JAMA 2010;303(2):168–9.

31. Burnside ES, Park JM, Fine JP, et al. The use of batch reading to improve the performance of screening mammography. AJR Am J Roentgenol 2005;185(3):790–6.
32. Froicu M, Mani KL, Coughlin B. Satisfaction With Same-Day-Read Baseline Mammography. J Am Coll Radiol 2019;16(3):321–6.
33. Dontchos BN, Narayan AK, Seidler M, et al. Impact of a Same-Day Breast Biopsy Program on Disparities in Time to Biopsy. J Am Coll Radiol 2019;16(11):1554–60.
34. Lehman CD, Yala A, Schuster T, et al. Mammographic Breast Density Assessment Using Deep Learning: Clinical Implementation. Radiology 2019; 290(1):52–8.
35. NCCN Guidelines Version 1.2021 Breast Cancer Screening and Diagnosis.
36. NCCN Guidelines Version 1.2022 Breast Cancer Risk Reduction.
37. Claus EB, Schildkraut JM, Thompson WD, et al. The genetic attributable risk of breast and ovarian cancer. Cancer 1996;77(11):2318–24.
38. The American Society of Breast Surgeons website. Position statement on screening mammography. Available at: www.breastsurgeons.org/docs/statements/PositionStatement-on-Screening-Mammography.pdf.
39. Monticciolo DL, Newell MS, Moy L, et al. Breast Cancer Screening in Women at Higher-Than-Average Risk: Recommendations From the ACR. J Am Coll Radiol 2018;15(3 Pt A):408–14.
40. Saslow D, Boetes C, Burke W, et al. American Cancer Society guidelines for breast screening with MRI as an adjunct to mammography. CA Cancer J Clin 2007;57(2):75–89 [published correction appears in CA Cancer J Clin. 2007 May--Jun;57(3):185].
41. McCormack VA, dos Santos Silva I. Breast density and parenchymal patterns as markers of breast cancer risk: a meta-analysis. Cancer Epidemiol Biomarkers Prev 2006;15(6):1159–69.
42. Yaghjyan L, Colditz GA, Rosner B, et al. Mammographic breast density and breast cancer risk: interactions of percent density, absolute dense, and non-dense areas with breast cancer risk factors. Breast Cancer Res Treat 2015; 150(1):181–9.
43. DenseBreast-Info. Legislation and regulation. 2015. Available at. https://densebreast-info.org/legislation.aspx. Google Scholar.
44. Ciatto S, Houssami N, Bernardi D, et al. Integration of 3D digital mammography with tomosynthesis for population breast-cancer screening (STORM): a prospective comparison study. Lancet Oncol 2013;14(7):583–9.
45. Expert Panel on Breast Imaging, Weinstein SP, Slanetz PJ, et al. ACR Appropriateness Criteria® Supplemental Breast Cancer Screening Based on Breast Density. J Am Coll Radiol 2021;18(11S):S456–73.
46. Svahn TM, Houssami N, Sechopoulos I, et al. Review of radiation dose estimates in digital breast tomosynthesis relative to those in two-view full-field digital mammography. Breast 2015;24(2):93–9.
47. Skaane P, Bandos AI, Gullien R, et al. Comparison of digital mammography alone and digital mammography plus tomosynthesis in a population-based screening program. Radiology 2013;267(1):47–56.
48. Friedewald SM, Rafferty EA, Rose SL, et al. Breast cancer screening using tomosynthesis in combination with digital mammography. JAMA 2014;311(24):2499–507.
49. Rafferty EA, Durand MA, Conant EF, et al. Breast Cancer Screening Using Tomosynthesis and Digital Mammography in Dense and Nondense Breasts. JAMA 2016;315(16):1784–6.

50. Houssami N. Digital breast tomosynthesis (3D-mammography) screening: data and implications for population screening. Expert Rev Med Devices 2015; 12(4):377–9.

51. Berg WA, Blume JD, Cormack JB, et al. Combined screening with ultrasound and mammography vs mammography alone in women at elevated risk of breast cancer. JAMA 2008;299(18):2151–2163 [published correction appears in JAMA. 2010 Apr 21;303(15):1482].

52. Ohuchi N, Suzuki A, Sobue T, et al. Sensitivity and specificity of mammography and adjunctive ultrasonography to screen for breast cancer in the Japan Strategic Anti-cancer Randomized Trial (J-START): a randomised controlled trial. Lancet 2016;387(10016):341–8.

53. Weigert J, Steenbergen S. The connecticut experiments second year: ultrasound in the screening of women with dense breasts. Breast J 2015;21(2):175–80.

54. Kuhl CK, Schrading S, Leutner CC, et al. Mammography, breast ultrasound, and magnetic resonance imaging for surveillance of women at high familial risk for breast cancer. J Clin Oncol 2005;23(33):8469–76.

55. Sung JS, Stamler S, Brooks J, et al. Breast Cancers Detected at Screening MR Imaging and Mammography in Patients at High Risk: Method of Detection Reflects Tumor Histopathologic Results. Radiology 2016;280(3):716–22.

56. Bakker MF, de Lange SV, Pijnappel RM, et al. Supplemental MRI Screening for Women with Extremely Dense Breast Tissue. N Engl J Med 2019;381(22): 2091–102.

57. Rhodes DJ, Hruska CB, Phillips SW, et al. Dedicated dual-head gamma imaging for breast cancer screening in women with mammographically dense breasts. Radiology 2011;258(1):106–18.

58. Rhodes DJ, Hruska CB, Conners AL, et al. Journal club: molecular breast imaging at reduced radiation dose for supplemental screening in mammographically dense breasts. AJR Am J Roentgenol 2015;204(2):241–51.

59. Shermis RB, Wilson KD, Doyle MT, et al. Supplemental Breast Cancer Screening With Molecular Breast Imaging for Women With Dense Breast Tissue. AJR Am J Roentgenol 2016;207(2):450–7.

60. Hruska CB. Let's Get Real about Molecular Breast Imaging and Radiation Risk. Radiol Imaging Cancer 2019;1(1):e190070. Published 2019 Sep 27.

61. Jochelson MS, Lobbes MBI. Contrast-enhanced Mammography: State of the Art. Radiology 2021;299(1):36–48. https://doi.org/10.1148/radiol.2021201948.

62. Sung JS, Lebron L, Keating D, et al. Performance of Dual-Energy Contrast-enhanced Digital Mammography for Screening Women at Increased Risk of Breast Cancer. Radiology 2019;293(1):81–8.

63. Chen SQ, Huang M, Shen YY, et al. Application of Abbreviated Protocol of Magnetic Resonance Imaging for Breast Cancer Screening in Dense Breast Tissue. Acad Radiol 2017;24(3):316–20.

64. Comstock CE, Gatsonis C, Newstead GM, et al. Comparison of Abbreviated Breast MRI vs Digital Breast Tomosynthesis for Breast Cancer Detection Among Women With Dense Breasts Undergoing Screening. JAMA 2020;323(8):746–56 [published correction appears in JAMA. 2020 Mar 24;323(12):1194].

65. Banegas MP, Li CI. Breast cancer characteristics and outcomes among Hispanic Black and Hispanic White women. Breast Cancer Res Treat 2012;134(3): 1297–304.

66. Stapleton SM, Oseni TO, Bababekov YJ, et al. Race/Ethnicity and Age Distribution of Breast Cancer Diagnosis in the United States. JAMA Surg 2018;153(6): 594–5.

67. Monticciolo DL, Malak SF, Friedewald SM, et al. Breast Cancer Screening Recommendations Inclusive of All Women at Average Risk: Update from the ACR and Society of Breast Imaging. J Am Coll Radiol 2021;18(9):1280–8.
68. Perry H, Fang AJ, Tsai EM, et al. Imaging Health and Radiology Care of Transgender Patients: A Call to Build Evidence-Based Best Practices. J Am Coll Radiol 2021;18(3 Pt B):475–80.

Testing for Inherited Susceptibility to Breast Cancer

Mark Robson, MD

KEYWORDS

- Genetic susceptibility • Genetic testing • Genetic risk

KEY POINTS

- Early approaches to genetic testing for breast cancer risk were based on certain assumptions about the nature of that predisposition.
- With the passage of time, the therapeutic relevance of inherited risk has become clearer and centered the sensitivity of testing.
- The importance of sensitivity has led to calls for universal testing of all breast cancer patients.
- A combination of age-based and guideline-based testing offers extremely high sensitivity and a negative predictive value.
- Broad (universal) testing using large multigene panels introduces the risk of misinterpretation and mismanagement of genetic alterations that are less familiar to nongenetics clinicians.

INTRODUCTION

Although 1 in 8 (12.9%) US women will develop breast cancer in their lifetime,[1] not everyone is at the same risk for the disease. Individual women are at higher or lower degrees of risk based on well-known factors such as age at menarche and menopause, age at first live birth, parity, and mammographic density. Environmental factors such as obesity and alcohol may also play a role. Family history, of course, has long been known to be one of the major contributors to the variation in individual breast cancer risk.[2] Shared genetic factors largely mediate this influence of family history. Based on a Nordic twin study, 31% (95% confidence interval [CI] 11%–51%) of the variation in breast cancer risk can be attributed to heredity.[3]

Over the last 40 years, a huge scientific effort has identified the genetic underpinnings of much (but not all) of this hereditability. These genetic factors are

This article previously appeared in Hematology/Oncology Clinics volume 37 issue 1 February 2023.

Breast Medicine Service, Department of Medicine, Memorial Hospital for Treatment of Cancer and Allied Disease, Memorial Sloan Kettering Cancer Center, Weill Cornell Medical College, 300 East 66th Street, Room 813, New York, NY 10065, USA
E-mail address: robsonm@mskcc.org
Twitter: @MarkRobsonMD (M.R.)

conventionally divided into 3 broad categories: (1) rare high-penetrance genetic variants (present in <1% of the population with relative risks of 5 or higher), (2) rare moderate penetrance variants (<1% prevalence, relative risks of generally 2–5), and (3) common variants (also known as single-nucleotide polymorphisms [SNPs], present in >1% of the population, sometimes nearly 50%, and associated with relative risks of <1.5, more commonly <1.2). What follows is a brief discussion of these categories.

RARE, HIGH-PENETRANCE VARIANTS

Rare, high-penetrance variants are responsible for familial cancer syndromes that were first suspected because of pedigree analysis. Familial cancer syndromes, including those that involve breast cancer, nearly always manifest an autosomal dominant pattern of predisposition. Traditionally, these syndromes were recognized by (1) the apparent transmission of the predisposition by both males and females, with a 50% chance of a parent passing the predisposing genetic variant to each child; (2) onset of disease at a younger age than in the general population; (3) increased risk of bilateral cancers in paired organs, such as the breasts; and (4) often increased risks at more than one organ site. Before the era of routine genetic testing, the penetrance (risk of cancer) associated with these rare variants appeared to be very high, often over 90%.

The first familial cancer syndromes described were linked to rare cancers, such as retinoblastoma (Hereditary retinoblastoma, described in twins by Benedict in 1929) and childhood sarcoma (Li-Fraumeni syndrome, first described in 1969).[4,5] Interestingly, the first description of Li-Fraumeni syndrome, eventually shown to be due to pathogenic variants in TP53, noted the association of childhood sarcoma with very early-onset breast cancer. These syndromes were very rare, and it was not until Henry Lynch described autosomal dominant colon/endometrial and breast/ovary cancer families that consideration was given to the potential role of rare variants in the causation of common malignancies.[6,7] Newman and King compiled the statistical evidence for a rare "breast cancer gene" in 1988 and, using the techniques available at that time, localized the position of this gene, which came to be known as BRCA1, to 17q21.[8,9] The gene itself was cloned in 1994, with a second gene, BRCA2, identified shortly thereafter.[10,11]

Although pathogenic variants in BRCA1 and BRCA2 cause the hereditary breast and ovarian cancer syndrome (HBOC), breast cancer is seen in several other familial cancer syndromes. Li-Fraumeni (TP53) was mentioned earlier. Breast cancer is also a component tumor of Cowden syndrome (PTEN), hereditary diffuse gastric cancer (CDH1), and the Peutz-Jeghers syndrome (STK11).[12–14] Fortunately, these syndromes are quite rare, unlike HBOC.

RARE, MODERATE PENETRANCE VARIANTS

The high-penetrance genes associated with autosomal dominant cancer syndromes were mainly identified through positional cloning techniques. This approach was feasible due to the ability to easily "track" the gene through pedigrees and seek recombination events. Other risk genes were identified through candidate gene approaches, often in women who were not part of families with clear autosomal dominant transmission. For example, breast cancer risk was noted to be increased in women from families in which children had been diagnosed with ataxia-telangiectasia, a recessive disorder of childhood that was found to be associated with alterations in the ATM gene.[15] CHEK2 was initially identified as a possible cause of Li-Fraumeni syndrome.[16] The presence of a common CHEK2 founder variant in

Northern Europe (c.1100delC) facilitated the establishment of this gene as a less-penetrant susceptibility gene.[17] Other genes became candidates because of a growing understanding of the components of DNA damage repair pathways and the ability to conduct large case-control studies using next-generation sequencing technology, including studies comparing the entire exomes of women with or without cancer.

It has been challenging to come to a consensus on a list of breast cancer susceptibility genes. In general, moderate penetrance variants do not cause a recognizable autosomal dominant pedigree pattern, and the associated risks are similar to those associated with having an affected first-degree relative (relative risk of 1.8–1.9).[18,19] This presents 2 issues. First, large studies are needed to establish whether a particular gene has a statistically significant association with risk. This is further complicated by the observation that some genes may have subtype-specific predispositions (eg, for estrogen receptor-negative disease but not for the more common estrogen receptor-positive disease). Second, because pathogenic variants in individual genes are rare, defining the exact degree of associated risk has been complicated by statistical variation within relatively wide CIs. Two large recent population-based case-control studies have gone far toward consolidating a list of accepted susceptibility genes. The Breast Cancer Association Consortium (BCAC) published an analysis of 34 suspected susceptibility genes in 60,466 women with breast cancer and 53,461 controls.[20] Hu and colleagues reported an analysis of 28 genes in 32,247 women with breast cancer and 32,544 controls from the CARRIERS Consortium.[21] The results of these studies are summarized in **Table 1**.

Genes associated with significantly increased risks in both studies were *ATM*, *CHEK2*, *BRCA1*, *BRCA2*, and *PALB2*. Genes associated with risk in the larger BCAC analysis but not the CARRIERS analysis were *BARD1*, *MSH6*, *RAD51 C*, and *RAD51D*. Although the associations did not reach statistical significance in the CARRIERS study, this may have been a result of the difference in sample size, since the prevalence of alterations in these genes was similar between the 2 studies, with similar odds ratios. Certain known associations (eg, *CDH1*, *NF1*, *PTEN*, *STK11*, *TP53*) were not clearly identified in these population-based studies. This may be because many of these syndromes present at a young age with clinical features (*PTEN*, *NF1*, *STK11*) or with malignancy (*TP53*). These individuals would not be included in a population-based ascertainment of breast cancer cases (who would be excluded if a mutation were known) and controls (who would be excluded if they manifested clinical features of a predisposition syndrome). It is important to note that breast cancer associations were *not* confirmed for several genes that are often included on commercial multigene panels, including *BRIP1*, *NBN*, and *RAD50*.

In both reports, *ATM* and *CHEK2* variants were associated with greater risks of estrogen receptor (ER)-positive disease than of ER-negative. For *BARD1*, *BRCA1*, *BRCA2*, *PALB2*, *RAD51C*, and *RAD51D*, risks of an ER-negative disease were greater. In the BCAC analysis, there were also age effects, with odds ratios declining significantly with age for *BRCA1*, *BRCA2*, *CHEK2*, *PALB2*, *PTEN*, and *TP53*.

Taken together, these studies clearly establish *ATM*, *CHEK2*, and *PALB2* as breast cancer susceptibility genes. *ATM* and *CHEK2* would be considered of moderate penetrance, while the risk associated with *PALB2* variants is similar to that resulting from *BRCA2* variants, and *PALB2* could therefore be considered a high-penetrance gene. There are also indications that *BARD1*, *RAD51C*, and *RAD51D* variants are linked to an increased risk of ER-negative breast cancer although the risk of breast cancer overall is only marginally increased. Another important outcome of these studies is the estimate of pathogenic variant prevalence in the general population

Table 1
Statistically significant associations with all breast cancer genes in either population-based study[20,21]

Gene	BCAC (48,826 Cases, 50,703 Controls)			CARRIERS (32,247 Cases, 32,544 Controls)		
	N (%) Cases	N (%) Controls	OR (95% CI)	N (%) Cases	N (%) Controls	OR (95% CI)
ATM	294 (0.6%)	150 (0.3%)	2.10 (1.71–2.57)	253 (0.78%)	134 (0.41%)	1.82 (1.46–2.27)
BARD1	62 (0.12%)	32 (0.06%)	2.09 (1.35–3.23)	49 (0.15%)	35 (0.11%)	1.37 (0.87–2.16)
BRCA1	515 (1.05%)	58 (0.11%)	10.57 (8.02–13.93)	275 (0.87%)	37 (0.11%)	7.62 (5.33–11.27)
BRCA2	754 (1.54%)	135 (0.27%)	5.85 (4.85–7.06)	417 (1.29%)	78 (0.24%)	5.23 (4.07–6.77)
CHEK2	704 (1.44%)	315 (0.625)	2.54 (2.21–2.91)	349 (1.08%)	138 (0.42%)	2.47 (2.02–3.05)
MSH6	39 (0.08%)	23 (0.05%)	1.96 (1.15–3.33)	39 (0.12%)	32 (0.10%)	1.13 (0.70–1.83)
PALB2	274 (0.56%)	55 (0.11%)	5.02 (3.73–6.76)	148 (0.46%)	38 (0.12%)	3.83 (2.68–5.63)
RAD51C	54 (0.11%)	26 (0.05%)	1.93 (1.20–3.11)	41 (0.13%)	35 (0.11%)	1.20 (0.75–1.93)
RAD51D	51 (0.10%)	25 (0.05%)	1.80 (1.11–2.93)	26 (0.08%)	14 (0.04%)	1.72 (0.88–3.51)

Abbreviations: CI, confidence interval; OR, odds ratio.

| Table 2 | | |
| Prevalence of pathogenic variants in relevant genes in 83,247 combined controls[20,21] | | |
Gene	N	%
ATM	284	0.34%
BARD1	67	0.08%
BRCA1	95	0.11%
BRCA2	213	0.26%
CHEK2	453	0.54%
PALB2	93	0.11%
RAD51 C	61	0.07%
RAD51D	39	0.05%

(Table 2). These results suggest that approximately 0.37% (1 in 270) of control women carry a pathogenic variant in BRCA1 or BRCA2, and 0.99% (1 in 100) carry a variant in ATM, CHEK2, or PALB2 (assuming that the number of women carrying variants in 2 or more genes is small).

COMMON VARIATION AND BREAST CANCER RISK

Although variants in high- or moderate-penetrance genes are more common than initially suspected, they are still quite rare and cannot account for a substantial portion of the heritability of breast cancer. Therefore, more heritability must result from common variation.

The invention of massively parallel, "next-generation" sequencing facilitated large-scale whole-genome sequencing that allowed an appreciation of the staggering amount of normal variation in the human population.[22] The 1000 Genomes project assessed the whole genomes of over 2500 individuals from around the world and cataloged 84.7 million SNPs, 3.6 million short insertion/deletions, and 60,000 structural variants. Early on, researchers realized that this variation could, in theory, be used to identify genomic regions associated with breast cancer susceptibility.[23] A series of genome-wide association studies (GWAS) were conducted, comparing the prevalence of individual SNPs in cases and controls to identify specific loci associated with case status (reviewed in the paper by Lilyquist and colleagues[24]). These studies identified over 180 individual SNPs associated with breast cancer with high degrees of statistical significance (called "genome-wide significance," generally requiring $P < 10^{-5}$ or greater, in order to adjust for extreme multiple testing).

Each SNP is associated with a very small increase in risk (odds ratios >1.4 and most with OR of 1.10 or less), limiting the value as individual predictors. However, knowledge of genotypes (and associated risks) at multiple SNPs allows the construction of polygenic risk scores (PRS), which can be more meaningful. As an example, Mavaddat and colleagues reported on the construction and validation of a breast cancer PRS using 313 SNPs from a prior GWAS.[25] Each standard deviation of the PRS was associated with an increase in hazard ratio of 1.61 (95% CI 1.57–1.65), and women with the highest PRS have an estimated lifetime risk of 32.6% (compared to 2% for those with the lowest). PRS also modify contralateral breast cancer risk as well as risks in women with pathogenic variants in BRCA1 or BRCA2 or moderate-penetrance genes.[26–30] PRS is largely independent of traditional risk factors although PRS obviously does make some contribution to familial risk.[31] After appropriate adjustment for this shared component of risk, PRS can be combined with existing risk-assessment models to generate a comprehensive risk assessment for women without identified genetic susceptibility and for women with alterations in moderate-penetrance genes.[28,32–36] Clinical deployment of these comprehensive models is underway although there are still many aspects of the clinical use of PRS that remain to be standardized.[37]

INTRODUCTION OF GENETIC TESTING FOR BREAST CANCER SUSCEPTIBILITY

In the early 1990s, while researchers were seeking to identify BRCA1 (and BRCA2), parallel conversations began about how to offer genetic testing to the families participating in the discovery studies, particularly the unaffected relatives. As moderate-penetrance genes were not yet identified, discussions were exclusively about testing for BRCA1/2 variants. The conversations were shaped by several assumptions, many of which have since been shown to be incorrect.

The first assumption was that pathogenic variants in these genes would be rare, even though the segregation analysis of Newman and King predicted an allele frequency of 0.0006 (which corresponds to a heterozygote prevalence of 0.11%, exactly what was observed for BRCA1 in the BCAC controls described above).[9] The second assumption was that women with pathogenic variants would be at extremely high risk of breast cancer (80% or greater by age 70), along with a substantially increased risk of ovarian cancer.[38,39] Along with this pessimistic understanding of risk, there was also uncertainty about the effectiveness of preventive interventions like mastectomy and salpingo-oophorectomy.[40,41] Breast MRI was not yet available. There were no immediately obvious therapeutic implications for women who had cancer. And, lastly, there was substantial concern about the possibility of adverse psychological response to the finding of a pathogenic variant as well as negative social consequences such as discrimination and stigmatization.[42] Despite these limitations, there was significant (but not universal) interest in testing among women who had participated in the research ascertainments.[43] And, in the United States, there was rapid commercialization and promotion of testing, particularly since the group that identified BRCA1 was tightly linked to a commercial enterprise that established an exclusive patent position on the gene sequence and uses thereof.

Because of the complexities surrounding germline genetic testing and because testing was at first exclusively for personal utility (with no clearly effective clinical interventions), a rigorous paradigm was deployed for pretest counseling, documented informed consent, and posttest counseling to ensure understanding both before and after testing, as well as to provide support in the event of adverse psychological responses.[44–47] Germline genetic testing was to be handled differently than other tests used for asymptomatic individuals because of the perceived exceptional nature of this information. The closest paradigm was Huntington's disease rather than hypercholesterolemia. Not all agreed with this concept of "genetic exceptionalism,"[48] but the principle of pretest genetic counseling became established and, in many places, a prerequisite to testing.

CHALLENGES TO THE STANDARD MODEL

Since 1996, when BRCA testing began to become widely available (at least in the United States), the utility and necessity of the standard model for genetic testing in breast cancer have been questioned. Many of the assumptions that underlay the genetic counseling model have turned out to be incorrect. The breast and ovarian cancer risks associated with pathogenic variants in BRCA1 and BRCA2 are significantly higher than those of the general population but not as high as those calculated from the study of the early high-risk families.[49] Severe psychological distress in reaction to test results has not been limiting although some individuals do experience adverse responses to genetic information.[50] Systemic discrimination and stigmatization have not materialized. And preventive interventions such as risk-reducing mastectomy, risk-reducing salpingo-oophorectomy, and enhanced surveillance with breast MRI are all clearly effective (although not completely so).[51–59] All these factors argued for the potential *clinical* utility of testing for unaffected women, which eventually led to the endorsement of testing for appropriate unaffected women by the U.S. Preventive Services Task Force.[60,61]

While various lines of evidence were establishing the potential benefit in unaffected women, the *therapeutic* importance of testing women with breast cancer also became clear. Among families who participated in the efforts to clone *BRCA1* and *BRCA2*, there was a clear increased incidence of bilateral cancer, as would be expected from a high-penetrance single-gene predisposition. Once the genes were identified, the absolute risks of metachronous contralateral disease were found to be high in women with breast cancer and pathogenic variants. In 1 large analysis, the risk of contralateral cancer in women with *BRCA1* pathogenic variants was 40% in the 20 years after the index diagnosis.[49] For women with *BRCA2* variants, the risk was 26%. In response to this risk, a significant number of women with pathogenic variants opt for bilateral mastectomy at the time of initial surgery, even if they are otherwise candidates for breast conservation. While this approach clearly reduces the risk of second breast cancer, the impact on survival is controversial. Some reports have suggested an overall survival benefit; however, these studies are not definitive, and the conclusions probably do not apply to all patients.[62,63] Age at diagnosis, risk of mortality from index cancer diagnosis, and whether the pathogenic variant is in *BRCA1* or *BRCA2* are all likely to impact any potential survival benefit. Hence, breast conservation is not contraindicated in *BRCA* carriers.[64] Nonetheless, knowledge of BRCA status at diagnosis can be extremely important in guiding women and their surgeons in choice of local therapy.

Knowledge of *BRCA* status is also important in guiding the selection of systemic therapy. In the metastatic setting, platinum-based chemotherapy treatment appears to be more effective than taxanes in patients with *BRCA*-associated triple-negative breast cancer.[65] In addition, treatment of *BRCA* carriers with metastatic disease using inhibitors of poly-ADP-ribose polymerase (PARP inhibitors, eg, olaparib, talazoparib) provides an advantage in progression-free (but not overall) survival compared to physician's choice of nonplatinum chemotherapies.[66–68] Recently, the OlympiA study demonstrated that the addition of a PARP inhibitor to a standard adjuvant therapy improved survival.[69]

Knowledge of *BRCA* status has been important to decisions about local treatment since the early 1990s and is now important to treatment selection in both late and early-stage disease. For this reason, some have recommended that genetic testing be offered to all women with breast cancer.[70] It would not be possible to deploy this model using the standard testing approach of pretest and posttest counseling by trained genetics professionals, as there simply are not enough genetic counselors and the workforce is not evenly geographically distributed. There is, however, significant literature on "mainstreaming" genetic testing, also known as clinician-directed testing, illustrating that it is safe and acceptable to both patients and providers.[71–76] One could therefore envision a "2-track" system whereby affected women who need genetic information rapidly for treatment decision-making could receive clinician-directed testing after pretest education while unaffected women seeking risk assessment (or women with a past diagnosis for who the information is not immediately therapeutically relevant) could receive standard pretest counseling. Apart from efficiency, 1 additional advantage to a cascade approach (testing affected women and then extending testing to family members of those found to carry pathogenic variants) is that all *BRCA* carriers in the population could, in theory, be identified much more quickly than by unselected population screening.[77]

CONSIDERATIONS REGARDING UNIVERSAL TESTING

Genetic testing of all women with breast cancer at the time of diagnosis would have several potential benefits. If such testing became a part of standard care, it would substantially reduce the chance that a *BRCA* carrier would be "missed." It could also reduce existing racial and geographic disparities in genetic testing related to access to pretest counseling. As mentioned, it could accelerate the identification of most if not all carriers in the population if cascade testing were effective. And early modeling studies suggest that the approach could be cost-effective compared to family history-based testing although these were based on European cost assumptions which may not be appropriate for all health systems.[78,79]

The question then becomes, why not use universal testing? The first question is whether testing *all* women with breast cancer is necessary to achieve the stated goals, or whether strict adherence to guideline criteria-based testing would be sufficient.[80] Guidelines vary from country to country, and even among health systems within a country. In the United States, the National Comprehensive Cancer Network (NCCN) guidelines are the most widely accepted (**Table 3**). These guidelines are quite permissive and very nonspecific. In a large analysis of unselected women with breast cancer seen at the Mayo Clinic between 2000 and 2016, Yadav and colleagues reported that 1872 of 3907 women (47.9%) met the 2019 NCCN criteria.[81] These criteria limited testing of women with triple-negative breast cancer to those aged 60 years or younger, so the proportion of women meeting the 2022 criteria (with no age limit on triple-negative disease) is likely to be slightly higher. The sensitivity of the older NCCN criteria was 86.9% (93/107) for *BRCA1* or *BRCA2* alterations and 82.6% (100/122) for *BRCA1*, *BRCA2*, or *PALB2* alterations. It is likely that the more recent criteria (testing all women with triple-negative cancer) are more sensitive, as another recent analysis indicated that approximately 3% of such women carried a *BRCA1*,

Table 3	
NCCN criteria for genetic testing (version 2.2022)	
Age	**Additional Criteria**
≤45	No other criteria needed
46–50	Multiple synchronous or metachronous primaries ≥1 Close relative with breast, ovary, prostate, pancreas cancer Unknown or limited family history
≥51	≥1 Close relative with breast cancer ≤ 50, male breast, ovarian, pancreas, metastatic prostate ≥2 Close relatives with breast and/or prostate cancer (at any age) ≥3 Diagnoses of breast cancer (total, including bilateral/metachronous) in patient and relatives
Any	Triple-negative breast cancer Lobular breast cancer with family history of diffuse gastric cancer Male breast cancer ≥1 Relative with male breast cancer Ashkenazi Jewish ancestry

BRCA2, or *PALB2* pathogenic variant if they were older than 65 years.[82] The sensitivity of the NCCN criteria for moderate-penetrance genes such as *CHEK2* and *ATM* was lower (67/110, 60.9%),[81] which is not unexpected as the criteria are designed to identify strong predispositions.

While the sensitivity analyses suggest that the NCCN criteria are insufficient, it is important to remember that the prevalence of pathogenic variants is quite low overall. Therefore, the negative predictive value (NPV) of the NCCN criteria (even without expanding to all triple-negative disease) is very high. Of the 2035 women not meeting the NCCN criteria, 2021 did not have *BRCA1* or *BRCA2* alterations (NPV 99.3%), and 2013 did not have *BRCA1*, *BRCA2*, or *PALB2* alterations (NPV 98.9%). If onetests all women aged 60 years or younger and those older than 60 years who meet the NCCN criteria, the NPV of these combined criteria for *BRCA1* or *BRCA2* would be 99.6%.

Taken together, these data suggest that women who are older than 60 years and do not otherwise meet the NCCN criteria are very unlikely to carry a *BRCA1*, *BRCA2*, or *PALB2* alteration that would have immediate clinical relevance (either for surgical treatment or for treatment with a PARP inhibitor).[83] Testing all women 60 or younger would increase the number of women tested by about 20% (from the approximately 50% who meet the NCCN criteria to approximately 70% of all patients). This approach would still have a slightly lower NPV for non-BRCA predisposition genes (97.8%). However, alterations in genes other than *BRCA1*, *BRCA2*, and *PALB2* do not have immediate therapeutic relevance. Contralateral cancer risks are undefined, and thus, finding pathogenic variants does not support routine preventive mastectomy,[84] especially since a meaningful proportion of women carrying moderate-risk variants are not even at elevated cancer risk due to modification by polygenic risk and traditional risk factors.[28,33,36] Universal testing will therefore substantially increase the number of women who need to be tested (and thus societal cost) and, since nearly all testing is now done through multigene panels, will increase the chance that a woman will be found to carry either a variant of uncertain significance or a pathogenic alteration in a gene that is not therapeutically actionable and may be of uncertain relevance to her family members.[85]

SUMMARY

There has been enormous progress since the discovery of *BRCA1* and *BRCA2* in the mid-1990s. Germline variation has clear relevance with decisions for women with breast cancer and their families regarding surgical prevention, cancer surveillance, and treatment of established early- and late-stage disease. Because of this clear clinical utility (at least for *BRCA1* and *BRCA2*), the traditional referral/genetic counseling model presents a potential barrier to getting women the information they need in a timely manner. For time-sensitive treatment decision-making, newer clinician-directed testing approaches should be promoted. At the same time, the involvement of genetic counselors and other clinical cancer genetics professionals is critical for result interpretation, especially for variants of uncertain significance and pathogenic variants in genes other than *BRCA1* or *BRCA2*. This involvement is crucial to avoid misinterpretation and mismanagement while also ensuring appropriate family engagement for cascade testing when appropriate. Older women with breast cancer (older than 60 years) who do not meet the current NCCN criteria are extremely unlikely to carry a pathogenic variant in *BRCA1*, *BRCA2*, and probably *PALB2*. Multigene panel testing may identify non-*BRCA* variants in this setting although the NPV of the NCCN criteria is high even for these genes. If multigene panel testing is performed, whether in women meeting NCCN criteria or not, engagement of genetics professionals in the posttest setting is even more crucial as the interpretation of non-*BRCA* variants and determination of associated risks is a dynamic field. This is particularly the case if a panel is chosen that includes several genes that are not typically associated with breast cancer.

CLINICS CARE POINTS

- NCCN criteria have a high, but less than 100%, sensitivity for the detection of pathogenic variants in *BRCA1* and *BRCA2* and an even lower sensitivity for the detection of pathogenic variants in "moderate-penetrance" genes.
- Including an age threshold (eg, testing women younger than 60 years without regard to criteria and using risk-based testing above that age) will improve sensitivity marginally.
- Broader testing will identify more pathogenic variants in genes other than *BRCA1* and *BRCA2*. These variants do not have treatment implications (apart from *PALB2*), and the risks to unaffected women are highly modified by polygenic risk and by traditional risk factors. This modification is such that a significant proportion of women with pathogenic variants in moderate-penetrance genes are not at significantly increased risk of breast cancer.
- If broad testing is to be undertaken without pretest counseling, it is essential that a cancer genetics professional be engaged to assist interpretation and management of variants that are unfamiliar to the ordering clinician.

DISCLOSURE

Dr M. Robson reports personal fees from Research to Practice, Intellisphere, myMedEd, Change Healthcare, and Physician's Education Resources; consulting for Artios Pharma (uncompensated), AstraZeneca (uncompensated), Daiichi-Sankyo (uncompensated), Epic Sciences (uncompensated), Merck (uncompensated), Pfizer (uncompensated), Tempus Labs (uncompensated), and Zenith Pharma (uncompensated); grants from AstraZeneca (institution, clinical trials), Merck (institution, clinical trial), Pfizer (institution, clinical trial); and other support from AstraZeneca (editorial services) and Pfizer (editorial services), all outside the submitted work. Dr M. Robson is supported by the Breast Cancer Research Foundation and the NIH/NCI Cancer Center Support Grant P30 CA008748.

REFERENCES

1. Siegel RL, Miller KD, Fuchs HE, et al. Cancer statistics, 2022. CA Cancer J Clin 2022;72(1):7–33.
2. Pharoah PD, Antoniou AC, Easton DF, et al. Polygenes, risk prediction, and targeted prevention of breast cancer. N Engl J Med 2008;358(26):2796–803.
3. Mucci LA, Hjelmborg JB, Harris JR, et al. Familial Risk and Heritability of Cancer Among Twins in Nordic Countries. JAMA 2016;315(1):68–76.
4. Benedict WL. Homologous Retinoblastoma in Identical Twins. Trans Am Ophthalmol Soc 1929;27:173–6.
5. Li FP, Fraumeni JF Jr. Soft-tissue sarcomas, breast cancer, and other neoplasms. A familial syndrome? Ann Intern Med 1969;71(4):747–52.
6. Lynch HT, Krush AJ. Carcinoma of the breast and ovary in three families. Surg Gynecol Obstet 1971;133(4):644–8.
7. Lynch HT, Krush AJ, Larsen AL. Heredity and multiple primary malignant neoplasms: six cancer families. Am J Med Sci 1967;254(3):322–9.

8. Hall JM, Lee MK, Newman B, et al. Linkage of early-onset familial breast cancer to chromosome 17q21. Science 1990;250(4988):1684–9.
9. Newman B, Austin MA, Lee M, et al. Inheritance of human breast cancer: evidence for autosomal dominant transmission in high-risk families. Proc Natl Acad Sci U S A 1988;85(9):3044–8.
10. Miki Y, Swensen J, Shattuck-Eidens D, et al. A strong candidate for the breast and ovarian cancer susceptibility gene BRCA1. Science 1994;266(5182):66–71.
11. Wooster R, Bignell G, Lancaster J, et al. Identification of the breast cancer susceptibility gene BRCA2. Nature 1995;378(6559):789–92.
12. Hansford S, Kaurah P, Li-Chang H, et al. Hereditary Diffuse Gastric Cancer Syndrome: CDH1 Mutations and Beyond. JAMA Oncol 2015;1(1):23–32.
13. Hearle N, Schumacher V, Menko FH, et al. Frequency and spectrum of cancers in the Peutz-Jeghers syndrome. Clin Cancer Res 2006;12(10):3209–15.
14. Hendricks LAJ, Hoogerbrugge N, Schuurs-Hoeijmakers JHM, et al. A review on age-related cancer risks in PTEN hamartoma tumor syndrome. Clin Genet 2021;99(2):219–25.
15. Swift M, Reitnauer PJ, Morrell D, et al. Breast and other cancers in families with ataxia-telangiectasia. N Engl J Med 1987;316(21):1289–94.
16. Bell DW, Varley JM, Szydlo TE, et al. Heterozygous germ line hCHK2 mutations in Li-Fraumeni syndrome. Science 1999;286(5449):2528–31.
17. Meijers-Heijboer H, van den Ouweland A, Klijn J, et al. Low-penetrance susceptibility to breast cancer due to CHEK2(*)1100delC in noncarriers of BRCA1 or BRCA2 mutations. Nat Genet 2002;31(1):55–9.
18. Collaborative Group on Hormonal Factors in Breast C. Familial breast cancer: collaborative reanalysis of individual data from 52 epidemiological studies including 58,209 women with breast cancer and 101,986 women without the disease. Lancet 2001;358(9291):1389–99.
19. Pharoah PD, Day NE, Duffy S, et al. Family history and the risk of breast cancer: a systematic review and meta-analysis. Int J Cancer 1997;71(5):800–9.
20. Breast Cancer Association C, Dorling L, Carvalho S, et al. Breast Cancer Risk Genes - Association Analysis in More than 113,000 Women. N Engl J Med 2021;384(5):428–39.
21. Hu C, Hart SN, Gnanaolivu R, et al. A Population-Based Study of Genes Previously Implicated in Breast Cancer. N Engl J Med 2021;384(5):440–51.
22. Genomes Project C, Auton A, Brooks LD, et al. A global reference for human genetic variation. Nature 2015;526(7571):68–74.
23. Uffelmann E, Huang QQ, Munung NS, et al. Genome-wide association studies. Nat Rev Methods Primers 2021;1(1):59.
24. Lilyquist J, Ruddy KJ, Vachon CM, et al. Common Genetic Variation and Breast Cancer Risk-Past, Present, and Future. Cancer Epidemiol Biomarkers Prev 2018;27(4):380–94.
25. Mavaddat N, Michailidou K, Dennis J, et al. Polygenic Risk Scores for Prediction of Breast Cancer and Breast Cancer Subtypes. Am J Hum Genet 2019;104(1): 21–34.
26. Lakeman IMM, van den Broek AJ, Vos JAM, et al. The predictive ability of the 313 variant-based polygenic risk score for contralateral breast cancer risk prediction in women of European ancestry with a heterozygous BRCA1 or BRCA2 pathogenic variant. Genet Med 2021;23(9):1726–37.
27. Kuchenbaecker KB, McGuffog L, Barrowdale D, et al. Evaluation of Polygenic Risk Scores for Breast and Ovarian Cancer Risk Prediction in BRCA1 and BRCA2 Mutation Carriers. J Natl Cancer Inst 2017;109(7).

28. Gao C, Polley EC, Hart SN, et al. Risk of Breast Cancer Among Carriers of Pathogenic Variants in Breast Cancer Predisposition Genes Varies by Polygenic Risk Score. J Clin Oncol 2021;39(23):2564–73.

29. Binkley TK, Binkley C. Porcelain-fused-to-metal crowns as replacements for denture teeth in removable partial denture construction. J Prosthet Dent 1987; 58(1):53–6.

30. Barnes DR, Rookus MA, McGuffog L, et al. Polygenic risk scores and breast and epithelial ovarian cancer risks for carriers of BRCA1 and BRCA2 pathogenic variants. Genet Med 2020;22(10):1653–66.

31. Kapoor PM, Mavaddat N, Choudhury PP, et al. Combined Associations of a Polygenic Risk Score and Classical Risk Factors With Breast Cancer Risk. J Natl Cancer Inst 2021;113(3):329–37.

32. Carver T, Hartley S, Lee A, et al. CanRisk Tool-A Web Interface for the Prediction of Breast and Ovarian Cancer Risk and the Likelihood of Carrying Genetic Pathogenic Variants. Cancer Epidemiol Biomarkers Prev 2021;30(3):469–73.

33. Gallagher S, Hughes E, Kurian AW, et al. Comprehensive Breast Cancer Risk Assessment for CHEK2 and ATM Pathogenic Variant Carriers Incorporating a Polygenic Risk Score and the Tyrer-Cuzick Model. JCO Precis Oncol 2021;5.

34. Hughes E, Tshiaba P, Wagner S, et al. Integrating Clinical and Polygenic Factors to Predict Breast Cancer Risk in Women Undergoing Genetic Testing. JCO Precis Oncol 2021;5.

35. Hurson AN, Pal Choudhury P, Gao C, et al. Prospective evaluation of a breast-cancer risk model integrating classical risk factors and polygenic risk in 15 cohorts from six countries. Int J Epidemiol 2022;50(6):1897–911.

36. Lee A, Mavaddat N, Wilcox AN, et al. BOADICEA: a comprehensive breast cancer risk prediction model incorporating genetic and nongenetic risk factors. Genet Med 2019;21(8):1708–18.

37. Polygenic Risk Score Task Force of the International Common Disease A. Responsible use of polygenic risk scores in the clinic: potential benefits, risks and gaps. Nat Med 2021;27(11):1876–84.

38. Easton DF, Ford D, Bishop DT. Breast and ovarian cancer incidence in BRCA1-mutation carriers. Breast Cancer Linkage Consortium. Am J Hum Genet 1995; 56(1):265–71.

39. Easton DF, Steele L, Fields P, et al. Cancer risks in two large breast cancer families linked to BRCA2 on chromosome 13q12-13. Am J Hum Genet 1997;61(1): 120–8.

40. Stefanek ME. Bilateral prophylactic mastectomy: issues and concerns. J Natl Cancer Inst Monogr 1995;(17):37–42.

41. Struewing JP, Watson P, Easton DF, et al. Prophylactic oophorectomy in inherited breast/ovarian cancer families. J Natl Cancer Inst Monogr 1995;(17):33–5.

42. Burke W, Kahn MJ, Garber JE, et al. First do no harm" also applies to cancer susceptibility testing. Cancer J Sci Am 1996;2(5):250–2.

43. Lerman C, Narod S, Schulman K, et al. BRCA1 testing in families with hereditary breast-ovarian cancer. A prospective study of patient decision making and outcomes. JAMA 1996;275(24):1885–92.

44. Wilfond BS, Rothenberg KH, Thomson EJ, et al. Cancer genetic susceptibility testing: ethical and policy implications for future research and clinical practice. Cancer Genetic Studies Consortium, National Institutes of Health. J Law Med Ethics 1997;25(4):243–51, 230.

45. Geller G, Botkin JR, Green MJ, et al. Genetic testing for susceptibility to adult-onset cancer. The process and content of informed consent. JAMA 1997; 277(18):1467–74.

46. Biesecker BB, Boehnke M, Calzone K, et al. Genetic counseling for families with inherited susceptibility to breast and ovarian cancer. JAMA 1993;269(15):1970–4.

47. Statement of the American Society of Human Genetics on genetic testing for breast and ovarian cancer predisposition. Am J Hum Genet 1994;55(5):i–iv.

48. Green MJ, Botkin JR. Genetic exceptionalism" in medicine: clarifying the differences between genetic and nongenetic tests. Ann Intern Med 2003;138(7): 571–5.

49. Kuchenbaecker KB, Hopper JL, Barnes DR, et al. Risks of Breast, Ovarian, and Contralateral Breast Cancer for BRCA1 and BRCA2 Mutation Carriers. JAMA 2017;317(23):2402–16.

50. Schwartz MD, Peshkin BN, Hughes C, et al. Impact of BRCA1/BRCA2 mutation testing on psychologic distress in a clinic-based sample. J Clin Oncol 2002; 20(2):514–20.

51. Warner E. Impact of MRI surveillance and breast cancer detection in young women with BRCA mutations. Ann Oncol 2011;22(Suppl 1):i44–9.

52. Rebbeck TR, Lynch HT, Neuhausen SL, et al. Prophylactic oophorectomy in carriers of BRCA1 or BRCA2 mutations. N Engl J Med 2002;346(21):1616–22.

53. Rebbeck TR, Friebel T, Lynch HT, et al. Bilateral prophylactic mastectomy reduces breast cancer risk in BRCA1 and BRCA2 mutation carriers: the PROSE Study Group. J Clin Oncol 2004;22(6):1055–62.

54. Passaperuma K, Warner E, Causer PA, et al. Long-term results of screening with magnetic resonance imaging in women with BRCA mutations. Br J Cancer 2012; 107(1):24–30.

55. Meijers-Heijboer H, van Geel B, van Putten WL, et al. Breast cancer after prophylactic bilateral mastectomy in women with a BRCA1 or BRCA2 mutation. N Engl J Med 2001;345(3):159–64.

56. Li X, You R, Wang X, et al. Effectiveness of Prophylactic Surgeries in BRCA1 or BRCA2 Mutation Carriers: A Meta-analysis and Systematic Review. Clin Cancer Res 2016;22(15):3971–81.

57. Kauff ND, Satagopan JM, Robson ME, et al. Risk-reducing salpingo-oophorectomy in women with a BRCA1 or BRCA2 mutation. N Engl J Med 2002;346(21):1609–15.

58. Hartmann LC, Sellers TA, Schaid DJ, et al. Efficacy of bilateral prophylactic mastectomy in BRCA1 and BRCA2 gene mutation carriers. J Natl Cancer Inst 2001; 93(21):1633–7.

59. Chiarelli AM, Prummel MV, Muradali D, et al. Effectiveness of screening with annual magnetic resonance imaging and mammography: results of the initial screen from the ontario high risk breast screening program. J Clin Oncol 2014; 32(21):2224–30.

60. Force USPST, Owens DK, Davidson KW, et al. Risk Assessment, Genetic Counseling, and Genetic Testing for BRCA-Related Cancer: US Preventive Services Task Force Recommendation Statement. JAMA 2019;322(7):652–65.

61. Force USPST. Genetic risk assessment and BRCA mutation testing for breast and ovarian cancer susceptibility: recommendation statement. Ann Intern Med 2005; 143(5):355–61.

62. Heemskerk-Gerritsen BA, Rookus MA, Aalfs CM, et al. Improved overall survival after contralateral risk-reducing mastectomy in BRCA1/2 mutation carriers with a

history of unilateral breast cancer: a prospective analysis. Int J Cancer 2015; 136(3):668–77.

63. Evans DG, Ingham SL, Baildam A, et al. Contralateral mastectomy improves survival in women with *BRCA1/2*-associated breast cancer. Breast Cancer Res Treat 2013;140(1):135–42.

64. Trombetta MG, Dragun A, Mayr NA, et al. ASTRO Radiation Therapy Summary of the ASCO-ASTRO-SSO Guideline on Management of Hereditary Breast Cancer. Pract Radiat Oncol 2020;10(4):235–42.

65. Tutt A, Tovey H, Cheang MCU, et al. Carboplatin in *BRCA1/2*-mutated and triple-negative breast cancer BRCAness subgroups: the TNT Trial. Nat Med 2018; 24(5):628–37.

66. Robson M, Im SA, Senkus E, et al. Olaparib for Metastatic Breast Cancer in Patients with a Germline BRCA Mutation. N Engl J Med 2017;377(6):523–33.

67. Litton JK, Rugo HS, Ettl J, et al. Talazoparib in Patients with Advanced Breast Cancer and a Germline BRCA Mutation. N Engl J Med 2018;379(8):753–63.

68. Gelmon KA, Fasching PA, Couch FJ, et al. Clinical effectiveness of olaparib monotherapy in germline BRCA-mutated, HER2-negative metastatic breast cancer in a real-world setting: phase IIIb LUCY interim analysis. Eur J Cancer 2021; 152:68–77.

69. Tutt ANJ, Garber JE, Kaufman B, et al. Adjuvant Olaparib for Patients with *BRCA1*- or *BRCA2*-Mutated Breast Cancer. N Engl J Med 2021;384(25): 2394–405.

70. Manahan ER, Kuerer HM, Sebastian M, et al. Consensus Guidelines on Genetic' Testing for Hereditary Breast Cancer from the American Society of Breast Surgeons. Ann Surg Oncol 2019;26(10):3025–31.

71. Yoon SY, Wong SW, Lim J, et al. Oncologist-led BRCA counselling improves access to cancer genetic testing in middle-income Asian country, with no significant impact on psychosocial outcomes. J Med Genet 2022;59(3):220–9.

72. Stromsvik N, Olsson P, Gravdehaug B, et al. It was an important part of my treAT-Ment": a qualitative study of Norwegian breast Cancer patients' experiences with mainstreamed genetic testing. Hered Cancer Clin Pract 2022;20(1):6.

73. Ramsey ML, Tomlinson J, Pearlman R, et al. Mainstreaming germline genetic testing for patients with pancreatic cancer increases uptake. Fam Cancer 2022;17:1–7.

74. Hamilton JG, Symecko H, Spielman K, et al. Uptake and acceptability of a mainstreaming model of hereditary cancer multigene panel testing among patients with ovarian, pancreatic, and prostate cancer. Genet Med 2021;23(11):2105–13.

75. Bokkers K, Zweemer RP, Koudijs MJ, et al. Positive experiences of healthcare professionals with a mainstreaming approach of germline genetic testing for women with ovarian cancer. Fam Cancer 2022;21(3):295–304.

76. Bokkers K, Vlaming M, Engelhardt EG, et al. The Feasibility of Implementing Mainstream Germline Genetic Testing in Routine Cancer Care-A Systematic Review. Cancers (Basel) 2022;14(4).

77. Offit K, Tkachuk KA, Stadler ZK, et al. Cascading After Peridiagnostic Cancer Genetic Testing: An Alternative to Population-Based Screening. J Clin Oncol 2020; 38(13):1398–408.

78. Sun L, Brentnall A, Patel S, et al. A Cost-effectiveness Analysis of Multigene Testing for All Patients With Breast Cancer. JAMA Oncol 2019;5(12):1718–30. https://doi.org/10.1001/jamaoncol.2019.3323.

79. Norum J, Grindedal EM, Heramb C, et al. BRCA mutation carrier detection. A model-based cost-effectiveness analysis comparing the traditional family history

approach and the testing of all patients with breast cancer. ESMO Open 2018; 3(3):e000328.

80. Beitsch PD, Whitworth PW, Hughes K, et al. Underdiagnosis of Hereditary Breast Cancer: Are Genetic Testing Guidelines a Tool or an Obstacle? J Clin Oncol 2019; 37(6):453–60.

81. Yadav S, Hu C, Hart SN, et al. Evaluation of Germline Genetic Testing Criteria in a Hospital-Based Series of Women With Breast Cancer. J Clin Oncol 2020;38(13): 1409–18.

82. Boddicker NJ, Hu C, Weitzel JN, et al. Risk of Late-Onset Breast Cancer in Genetically Predisposed Women. J Clin Oncol 2021;39(31):3430–40.

83. Desai NV, Yadav S, Batalini F, et al. Germline genetic testing in breast cancer: Rationale for the testing of all women diagnosed by the age of 60 years and for risk-based testing of those older than 60 years. Cancer 2021;127(6):828–33.

84. Tung NM, Boughey JC, Pierce LJ, et al. Management of Hereditary Breast Cancer: American Society of Clinical Oncology, American Society for Radiation Oncology, and Society of Surgical Oncology Guideline. J Clin Oncol 2020; 38(18):2080–106.

85. Robson M. Management of Women With Breast Cancer and Pathogenic Variants in Genes Other Than *BRCA1* or *BRCA2*. J Clin Oncol 2021;39(23):2528–34.

A New Landscape of Testing and Therapeutics in Metastatic Breast Cancer

Geetha Jagannathan, MBBS[1], Marissa J. White, MD[1],
Rena R. Xian, MD[1,2], Leisha A. Emens, MD, PhD[3],
Ashley Cimino-Mathews, MD[1,2,*]

KEYWORDS

- Biomarkers • Metastasis • Breast cancer • PD-L1 • Tumor mutation burden
- Companion diagnostic

KEY POINTS

- Biomarker testing on metastatic breast carcinoma enables selection of targeted therapies, and companion diagnostics are required assays coupled to an associated therapy.
- The National Comprehensive Cancer Network (NCCN) recommends biomarker assessment of hormone receptor status, HER2, and *BRCA1/2* on all metastatic breast carcinomas, and suggests second-line biomarker assessment of *PIK3CA* on metastatic hormone receptor positive, HER2 negative carcinomas.
- The NCCN recommends biomarker assessment of PD-L1 on metastatic triple negative carcinomas, with assessment of tumor mutation burden, mismatch repair protein status/microsatellite instability, and *NTRK* status in select circumstances.

OVERVIEW

Metastatic breast cancer remains an incurable disease, with significantly lower 5-year survival (28%) compared with localized cancer (99%) and cancers with nodal involvement (86%).[1] The therapeutic options for patients with metastatic breast cancer were historically limited; however, research has generated new and promising targeted therapies for patients with metastatic breast cancer. Targeted therapies typically

This article previously appeared in Clinics in Laboratory Medicine volume 43 issue 2 June 2023.
This article originally appeared in *Surgical Pathology Clinics* Volume 15 Issue 1, March 2022.
[1] Department of Pathology, The Johns Hopkins University School of Medicine, 401 N Broadway, Weinberg 2242, Baltimore, MD 21287, USA; [2] Department of Oncology, The Johns Hopkins University School of Medicine, 401 N Broadway, Weinberg 2242, Baltimore, MD 21287, USA; [3] Department of Oncology, UPMC Hillman Cancer Center/Magee Women's Hospital, 5117 Centre Avenue, Room 1.46e, Pittsburgh, PA 15213, USA
* Corresponding author. 401 N Broadway, Weinberg 2242, Baltimore, MD 21287.
E-mail address: acimino1@jhmi.edu

require unique biomarker testing to determine eligibility for treatment, many of which must be performed with one particular assay.

The National Comprehensive Cancer Network (NCCN) clinical practice guidelines recommend assessment of the following biomarkers in metastatic breast cancer: hormone receptors, human epidermal growth factor receptor-2 (HER2), programmed death-ligand 1 (PD-L1) (in triple negative), and germline *BRCA1* and *BRCA2* status, with the option to test for *PIK3CA* as a second line in estrogen receptor (ER)-positive, HER2-negative cancers, and in select circumstances to test for mismatch repair protein status and tumor mutational burden and/or *NTRK* (**Tables 1–3**).[2] Recommended testing methods include immunohistochemistry (IHC), chromogenic in situ hybridization (CISH), fluorescent in situ hybridization (FISH), targeted gene sequencing, and large-panel next-generation sequencing. Many of these biomarkers must be determined using an assay that is designated by the US Food and Drug Administration (FDA) as a companion diagnostic for its associated targeted therapeutic agent.[3–5] In this review, we cover the recommended biomarker assessment, testing methods, and companion diagnostics for metastatic breast cancer.

Summary Box 1: Recommended biomarker assessment in metastatic breast cancer

1. Hormone receptors: ER and PR (all newly metastatic)

2. HER2 (all newly metastatic)

3. PD-L1 by 22C3 in triple-negative metastatic breast carcinomas

4. MSI or dMMR[a]

5. TMB[a]

6. *BRCA1* and *BRCA2* (germline testing on all newly metastatic patients)

7. *PIK3CA* (as a second-line option in ER-positive, HER2-negative metastatic cancer)

8. *NTRK*[a]

dMMR, mismatch repair protein deficiency; MSI, microsatellite instability; PD-L1, programmed death-ligand 1; PR, progesterone receptor; TMB, tumor mutation burden.

[a]In select circumstances.

HORMONE RECEPTOR AND HUMAN EPIDERMAL GROWTH FACTOR RECEPTOR-2 TESTING
Clinical Relevance

ER, progesterone receptor (PR), and HER2 testing are the prototype of predictive and prognostic biomarker testing in breast cancer. Retesting ER, PR, and HER2 on metastatic breast cancers at first occurrence, each recurrence, and on different sites of disease are standard of care. Based on their expression, breast cancers fall into 3 distinct prognostic and predictive groups: (1) hormone receptor positive and HER2 negative, (2) HER2 positive with or without hormone receptor expression, and (3) triple negative for both hormone receptors and HER2. Most often, metastatic disease has the same hormone receptor and HER2 expression profile as the primary tumor. However, a small but significant subset of the metastatic disease shows discordance in expression of these markers, which can significantly impact treatment decisions. In addition, tumoral heterogeneity and divergent clonal evolution can result in the presence of different hormone receptor or HER2 status in different tumor sites or in regions within one tumor (**Fig. 1**).[6,7]

Table 1
Biomarker characteristics for estrogen receptor, progesterone receptor, and human epidermal growth factor receptor-2

Marker	Breast Cancer Subtype Tested	Test Method	Sample Type	Scoring	Companion Diagnostics[5]	Manufacturer	FDA-Approved Drugs
ER and PR	Any	IHC	FFPE	Score intensity and percentage of tumor cells labeling: <1%: Negative ≥1%: Positive 1%–10% ER expression: Low positive	Any FDA-approved antibody platform. No formally designated companion diagnostic		Aromatase inhibitors; tamoxifen; CDK4/6 inhibitors with aromatase inhibitors or fulvestrant
HER2	Any	IHC	FFPE	Score intensity, completeness of membranous labeling and percentage of tumor cells labeling[14]: Negative (score 0 or 1+) Equivocal (2+) Positive (3+)	InSite Her-2/neu KIT	Biogenex Laboratories, Inc	Trastuzumab
					Bond Oracle HER2 IHC System	Leica Biosystems	Trastuzumab
					HercepTest	Dako Denmark A/S	Trastuzumab; pertuzumab; T-DM1
					PATHWAY anti-Her2/neu (4B5) Rabbit Monoclonal Primary Antibody	Ventana Medical Systems, Inc	Trastuzumab; T-DM1
		FISH		Score average HER2 copy number and ratio of HER2 to CEP17 in tumor cells[15]	INFORM HER2 Dual ISH DNA Probe Cocktail	Ventana Medical Systems, Inc	Trastuzumab; T-DM1
					INFORM HER-2/neu	Ventana Medical Systems, Inc	Trastuzumab
					HER2 FISH pharmDx Kit	Dako Denmark A/S	Trastuzumab; Pertuzumab; T-DM1

(continued on next page)

Table 1
(continued)

Marker	Breast Cancer Subtype Tested	Test Method	Sample Type	Scoring	Companion Diagnostics[5]	Manufacturer	FDA-Approved Drugs
					VENTANA HER2 Dual ISH DNA Probe Cocktail	Ventana Medical Systems, Inc	Trastuzumab
					PathVysion HER-2 DNA Probe Kit	Abbott Molecular Inc	Trastuzumab
		CISH		Score average HER2 copy number in tumor cells	SPOT-Light HER2 CISH Kit	Life Technologies Corporation	Trastuzumab
					HER2 CISH pharmDx Kit	Dako Denmark A/S	Trastuzumab
		NGS			FoundationOne CDx	Foundation Medicine, Inc	Trastuzumab; pertuzumab; T-DM1

Abbreviations: CEP17, chromosome enumeration probe 17; CISH, chromogenic in situ hybridization; FFPE, formalin-fixed paraffin-embedded; FISH, fluorescence in situ hybridization; IHC, immunohistochemistry; NGS, next-generation sequencing; T-DM1, ado-trastuzumab emtansine.

Table 2

Biomarker characteristics for immunotherapy: programmed death-ligand 1, tumor mutation burden, and microsatellite instability/mismatch repair protein deficiency

Marker	Breast Cancer Subtype Tested	Test Method	Sample Type	Scoring	Companion Diagnostics	Manufacturer	FDA-Approved Drugs
PD-L1	Advanced HR-negative, HER2-negative	IHC	FFPE	CPS = number of PD-L1⁺ tumor cells plus the number of PD-L1⁺ immune cells (lymphocytes and macrophages only), divided by the total number of tumor cells, multiplied by 100	PD-L1 IHC 22C3 Pharm Dx	Dako North America, Inc	Adjuvant pembrolizumab with chemotherapy (nab-paclitaxel, or paclitaxel, or gemcitabine plus carboplatin)
MSI/d-MMR	Any	IHC/PCR	FFPE	MSI testing evaluates for the presence of additional peaks in microsatellites of tumor in comparison to nonneoplastic tissue dMMR is	Any FDA-approved antibody platform. No companion diagnostic is available at present		Pembrolizumab

(continued on next page)

Table 2
(continued)

Marker	Breast Cancer Subtype Tested	Test Method	Sample Type	Scoring	Companion Diagnostics	Manufacturer	FDA-Approved Drugs
				determined by loss of IHC labeling for MMR proteins, MLH1, PMS2, MSH2, MSH6			
TMB	Any	NGS	FFPE	High TMB is > 10 mutations/ megabase of genome tested	FoundationOne CDx	Foundation Medicine, Inc	Pembrolizumab

Abbreviations: CPS, combined positive score; dMMR, mismatch repair protein deficiency; FFPE, formalin-fixed paraffin-embedded; HR, hormone receptor; MSI, microsatellite instability; NGS, next-generation sequencing; PCR, polymerase chain reaction; PD-L1, programmed death-ligand 1; TMB, tumor mutation burden.

Table 3
Biomarker characteristics for single-gene alterations

Marker	Breast Cancer Subtype Tested	Test Method	Sample Type	Companion Diagnostics	Manufacturer	FDA-Approved Drugs
PIK3CA mutations	HR-positive, HER2-negative	PCR	Blood for circulating tumor DNA or FFPE	therascreen PIK3CA RGQ PCR Kit	QIAGEN GmbH	Alpelisib
		NGS	Blood for circulating tumor DNA	FoundationOne Liquid CDx	Foundation Medicine, Inc	
		NGS for somatic and germline detection	FFPE	FoundationOne CDx	Foundation Medicine, Inc	Alpelisib
BRCA1/BRCA2 germline and somatic mutations	Any	Germline testing by PCR and Sanger sequencing	Blood	BRACAnalysis CDx	Myriad Genetic Laboratories, Inc	Olaprib Talazoparib
NTRK fusions	Secretory carcinomas	NGS	FFPE	FoundationOne CDx	Foundation Medicine, Inc	Larotrectinib

Abbreviations: FFPE, formalin-fixed paraffin-embedded; HR, hormone receptor; NGS, next-generation sequencing; PCR, polymerase chain reaction.

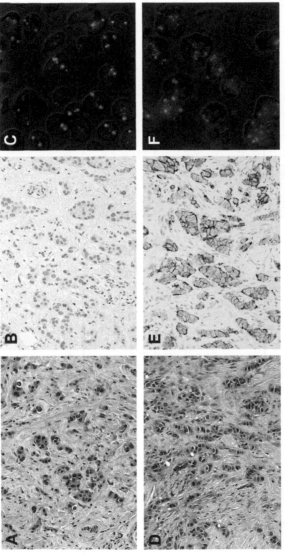

Fig. 1. Tumoral HER2 heterogeneity within a pleomorphic lobular carcinoma. Most of this primary invasive lobular carcinoma displays classic morphology with uniform cells arranged singly and in nests. (*A*, hematoxylin-eosin [H&E], original magnification ×200). This classic component is negative for HER2 protein overexpression by IHC (*B*, original magnification ×200) and is negative for *HER2* amplification by FISH, with a *HER2:CEP17* ratio of 1.6 and a *HER2* copy number of 2.3 signals per cell (*C*; green = *CEP17*, red = *HER2* locus). However, a subset of this tumor is pleomorphic, with enlarged and variably sized nuclei (*D*, H&E, original magnification ×200). This pleomorphic component is equivocal (IHC 2+) for HER2 overexpression by IHC (*E*, ×200) and is positive for *HER2* amplification by FISH, with a *HER2:CEP17* ratio of 4.4 and a *HER2* copy number of 8.7 signals/cell (*F*; green = *CEP17*, red = *HER2* locus). Tumoral HER2 heterogeneity could result in disparate biomarker profiles in different metastatic sites, or clonal expansion and predominance of biomarker profile.

Two notable independent prospective studies, the Breast Recurrence In Tissues Study (BRITS) and DESTINY studies, evaluated the changes in ER, PR, and HER2 expression in the primary tumor and any subsequent recurrences, both locoregional and distant metastases. A pooled analysis of the 2 studies' data by Amir and colleagues[8] showed that the overall discordance rates for the 3 markers were 12.6%, 31.2%, and 5.5%, respectively. Among the 3 markers, expression of PR was more often discordant than ER and HER2. The trend in the PR expression discordance was often a conversion from a positive to a negative result. This decrease or loss of PR is relevant (**Fig. 2**), because it can signal poorer response to antihormonal therapy.[9]

The discordance is explained by a wide variety of factors, including tumor biology (eg, tumor heterogeneity, clonal evolution), preanalytical variables (eg, tissue fixation, method of staining), and analytical variables (eg, subjectivity of scoring, interobserver variability). The current NCCN and American Society of Clinical Oncology (ASCO) guidelines recommend retesting all new metastatic breast cancers for ER, PR, and HER2 status. Retesting is especially important when the markers were previously unknown, initially negative, or not overexpressed. The conversion of hormone receptors and HER2 from negative to positive expression is the most clinically significant. In the analysis of Amir and colleagues,[8] 13% of hormone receptor-negative and 5% of HER2-negative primary tumors gained expression of the biomarkers in their respective metastatic tumor foci. Biomarker discordances contributed to change in therapy in approximately 14% of the patients enrolled in the 2 studies.[8] Retesting offers a subset of patients an additional treatment option with endocrine therapy, CDK 4/6 inhibitors, and/or trastuzumab.[10] Patients with discordant ER and HER2 results due to biomarker conversion tend to have worse survival than those with concordant biomarker results.[11]

Testing Techniques

ASCO and College of American Pathologists (CAP) jointly developed guidelines for the interpretation and reporting of ER, PR, and HER2 in breast cancer. As of this writing, the most recent updates to the guidelines for ER/PR and HER testing occurred in 2020 and 2018, respectively.[12,13] ER and PR testing are routinely performed by IHC. The latest guidelines recommend classifying tumors with an ER labeling of 1% to 10% as "ER low positive." These tumors more closely resemble basallike breast cancers in histology, molecular profile, and response to neoadjuvant chemotherapy than ER-positive breast cancers. The data on the benefit of endocrine therapy in this group are limited and potentially low. However, these patients are still eligible to receive endocrine therapy.[12] Cases with less than 10% ER labeling and those close to the threshold require a laboratory-specific standard operating procedure such as a second pathologist to review the score to ensure reproducibility.

HER2 assessment can be performed by IHC, FISH, CISH, or silver in situ hybridization (SISH). Although IHC is commonly used as first line for its quick turnaround time and cost-effectiveness, any approved method of testing may be used for first-line testing. An equivocal result is reflexed to a different testing method to provide a definitive result. The algorithms for the interpretation of hormone receptor and HER2 expression in metastatic tumors are the same as those for primary tumors, and guidelines are available for free online from the CAP.[14,15]

Challenges and Practical Considerations

Although specific IHC assays for ER and PR are not formally designated as FDA-approved companion diagnostic tests, in practice they function as companion

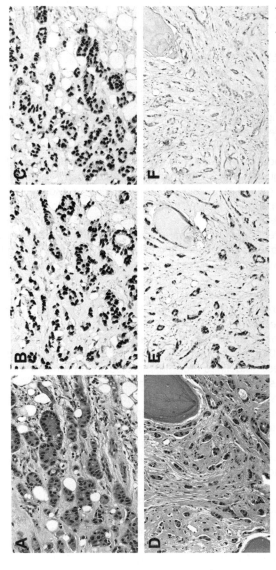

Fig. 2. PR discordance between a primary and metastatic tumor to bone in a decalcified specimen. This primary invasive ductal carcinoma (*A*, H&E, original magnification ×200) is diffusely and strongly positive for estrogen receptor (ER) (*B*, original magnification ×200) and PR (*C*, original magnification ×200). However, although biomarker testing on the patient's metastatic tumor in the iliac crest bone (*D*, H&E, original magnification ×200) shows concordant ER expression (*E*, original magnification ×200), the PR is discordant with negative (0%) labeling (*F*, original magnification ×200). Absence of biomarker labeling in a decalcified specimen could reflect true discordance, or a false-negative result due to the decalcification process.

diagnostics to deem patients as candidates for endocrine therapy. On the other hand, there are specific FDA companion diagnostic tests for HER2, as detailed in **Table 1**.

The most common distant site of breast cancer metastasis is the bone.[16] Biomarker expression testing in this setting is particularly challenging due to the confounding effects of decalcification on antigenicity and DNA integrity in bone specimens. Rapidly acting, strong acid buffers such as hydrochloric acid lower the antigenicity of the tumor cells and frequently produce false-negative results in hormone receptor and HER2 expression results by IHC (see **Fig. 2**), as well as false-negative amplification of *HER2* by FISH.[17] Weaker acid buffers containing acetic acid and formic acid and chelating agents such as EDTA[18] are currently more widely used. Although they are slow acting, their use improves antigen preservation and stability. Bone fragments should be separated out from soft tissue in these specimens to minimize the amount of tissue subjected to decalcification. Biomarker testing can also be performed on cytology specimens, which have results comparable to core biopsies.[19]

Key points Box 1: Estrogen receptor, progesterone receptor, and human epidermal growth factor receptor-2 testing in metastatic breast cancer

1. ER, PR, and HER2 should be retested on all new metastases due to the possibility of discordance and potential management changes.

2. ER-low positive is a new category of tumors with 1% to 10% ER labeling; patients are eligible for endocrine therapy but are less likely to benefit from it.

3. Decalcification with strong acid buffers can cause false-negative results for ER, PR, and HER2 expression; this is mitigated but not eliminated with agents containing EDTA and weaker acids.

4. When sampling and grossing metastatic tumors in bone, the soft tissue fragments should be separated out to avoid decalcification of the entire tumor and to improve biomarker assessment.

PROGRAMMED DEATH-LIGAND 1 TESTING FOR IMMUNOTHERAPY
Clinical Relevance

Immunotherapy has shown a long-lasting, durable treatment response in various tumor types. Triple-negative breast carcinoma (TNBC) and HER2-positive carcinoma often display brisk tumor-infiltrating lymphocytes (TILs), reflecting a host antitumor immune response.[20] The checkpoint inhibitor pembrolizumab targeting the programmed death 1 (PD-1) receptor recently gained regular FDA approval for both high-risk early (regardless of programmed death-ligand 1 [PD-L1] status) and locally advanced unresectable or metastatic TNBC (for PD-L1+ disease); this reflects a major advance for an aggressive breast tumor subtype for which few targeted therapies are available. For advanced PD-L1+ TNBC, pembrolizumab in combination with several chemotherapeutic options (nab-paclitaxel, or paclitaxel, or gemcitabine plus carboplatin) is endorsed by the FDA.[21] Notably, the use of atezolizumab in combination with nab-paclitaxel demonstrated clinical activity in randomized phase 3 clinical trials of advanced TNBC[22]; however, the accelerated approval for its use in this setting was voluntarily withdrawn by the sponsor in 2021. Of note, the FDA also granted full approval for the addition of pembrolizumab to standard neoadjuvant chemotherapy, followed by pembrolizumab monotherapy, for high-risk early-stage TNBC regardless of PD-L1 expression.[23]

Testing Techniques

IHC for PD-L1 is used to identify patients with metastatic TNBC who are eligible for checkpoint inhibition with pembrolizumab. As of this writing, there is one FDA-approved companion diagnostic assay for the use of pembrolizumab in TNBC (see **Table 2**). To guide the use of pembrolizumab in the advanced disease setting, the PD-L1 status of a tumor is determined by the combined positive score (CPS), which is the number of PD-L1$^+$ tumor cells plus the number of PD-L1$^+$ immune cells (lymphocytes and macrophages only), divided by the total number of tumor cells, multiplied by 100. A tumor is considered PD-L1 positive, and the patient eligible for pembrolizumab, when the CPS score is 10 or more (**Fig. 3**). The only FDA-approved PD-L1 companion diagnostic that uses the CPS scoring system is the PD-L1 IHC 22C3 pharmDx assay ("22C3 assay"). For high-risk early-stage TNBC, the addition of pembrolizumab to standard neoadjuvant chemotherapy is a treatment option regardless of PD-L1 status, so PD-L1 testing to determine eligibility for neoadjuvant immunotherapy is not recommended.[23]

For the clinical trials and during the accelerated approval period for atezolizumab with nab-paclitaxel, the PD-L1 status of a breast tumor was determined by the immune cell (IC) score, which is the percentage of the tumor area occupied by PD-L1$^+$ immune cells (TILs, plasma cells, neutrophils, eosinophils, and macrophages). A tumor was considered PD-L1 positive, and the patient eligible for atezolizumab, when the IC score was 1% or greater (see **Fig. 3**). The PD-L1 companion diagnostic that used the IC scoring system was the Ventana PD-L1 (SP142) assay ("SP142 assay"). The indication for atezolizumab in advanced TNBC was voluntarily withdrawn by the sponsor in 2021.

Challenges and Practical Considerations

PD-L1 testing currently should only be performed on tumor samples from patients with locally advanced or metastatic TNBC, and only upon request from the oncologist. The PD-L1 22C3 IHC assay can be performed on both newly obtained metastatic tumor samples and archival primary tumors. Exploratory biomarker analyses from patients on clinical trials with atezolizumab showed that the likelihood of a positive PD-L1 result does vary between the primary and metastatic tumor, as well as between different metastasis niche sites. In general, metastases tend to have fewer TILs than primary tumors, decreasing the chances of having immune cells present to express PD-L1. In addition, metastases to the liver and brain tend to have fewer TILs than metastases to other sites such as the lung.[24] It is not known if this extends to PD-L1 expression as determined by the 22C3 assay. Given the totality of the data, it is preferable to avoid PD-L1 testing on liver samples if possible. Of note, the PD-L1 IHC assays are not validated for decalcified bone specimens, cytology cell blocks or smears, or circulating tumor cells.

Unlike chemotherapy, which causes well-recognized cytotoxic side effects, immunotherapy causes a spectrum of immune-related adverse events (irAEs), affecting various organ systems. Pathologists need to be aware of and recognize the histopathology of irAEs across organ types, including dermatitis, thyroiditis, hepatitis, colitis, and potentially fatal pneumonitis.[25]

Key Points Box 2: Programmed death-ligand 1 testing in metastatic breast cancer

1. PD-L1 testing is currently indicated for patients with locally advanced or metastatic TNBC

2. The 22C3 assay uses the CPS scoring system to determine patient eligibility for pembrolizumab plus chemotherapy for advanced TNBC

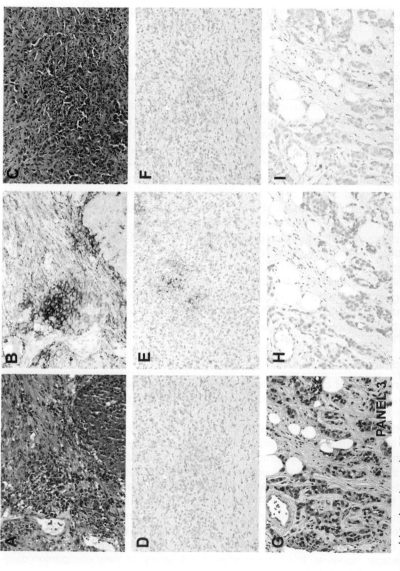

Fig. 3. PD-L1 immunohistochemistry: the PD-L1 IHC 22C3 pharmDx assay. PANEL 1: A locally advanced, primary TNBC (*A*, H&E, original magnification ×200) is PD-L1 positive by the 22C3 assay, with a CPS of 10 or more (*B*, original magnification ×200). This patient is eligible for pembrolizumab plus approved chemotherapy. PANEL 2: The archival primary tumor of a patient with metastatic TNBC (*C*, H&E, original magnification ×200) is PD-L1 negative by the 22C3 assay, with a CPS less than 10 (*F*, original magnification ×200). This patient is not eligible for pembrolizumab.

3. The CPS score is the total number of PD-L1$^+$ cells (tumor cells plus mononuclear immune cells), divided by the total number of tumor cells, multiplied by 100, with a positivity cutoff in breast cancer of 10 or more.

4. PD-L1 testing can be performed on either new metastatic tumor biopsies or archival primary tumor samples.

MISMATCH REPAIR PROTEIN DEFICIENCY, MICROSATELLITE INSTABILITY, AND TUMOR MUTATION BURDEN TESTING

Clinical Relevance

Some tumor types have higher tumor mutation burden (TMB) than others. Mutations accumulate in tumors by various mechanisms, including mutations (germline or somatic) in genes involved in repair of DNA base pair mismatches (mismatch protein [MMR] proteins) or double-strand DNA breaks (BRCA1/2). As mutations accumulate, tumor cells express new antigens on the cell surface and can become highly immunogenic and susceptible to immunotherapy.[26]

The prevalence of mismatch repair protein deficiency (dMMR) in breast cancer ($\sim$2%) is significantly lower than that in cancers of the colon ($\sim$15–20%) and endometrium ($\sim$20–30%). dMMR testing and microsatellite instability (MSI) testing have become standard of care in colon and endometrial carcinomas, whereas their use in breast cancers is limited. dMMR breast cancers are frequently high grade, associated with high TILs, and often negative for PR expression.[27] A high TMB is seen in about 5% of breast cancers, which predominantly includes TNBC and metastatic tumors. Among metastatic tumors, high TMB is more frequently seen in metastatic lobular carcinoma than metastatic ductal carcinoma. These tumors are also associated with high TILs and BRCA1/2 germline mutations (**Fig. 4**).[28]

Single-agent pembrolizumab is now approved for any advanced solid tumor with MSI-high status, dMMR, or high TMB. Pembrolizumab is the first drug to be ever approved based on biomarkers across all tumor types (ie, a "tumor agnostic" approval).[29]

Testing Techniques

MMR testing in breast cancer is based on techniques that have been widely used in colorectal and endometrial cancers. The most commonly used testing methods are IHC or polymerase chain reaction (PCR). IHC assays for MMR proteins, namely MLH1, PMS1, MSH2, and MSH6, evaluate for loss of nuclear expression in the tumor cells. MSI is formally assessed by PCR to look for the presence of additional peaks in microsatellites in the tumor compared with normal nonneoplastic tissue. The tumors that are microsatellite unstable are further classified based on the number of unstable markers as MSI low (1 marker) and MSI high ($\geq$2 markers). In April 2021, the FDA approved the MMR IHC assay VENTANA MMR RxDx (Roche) as companion diagnostic for selecting endometrial cancers for dostarlimab-gxly immunotherapy.[30] At present, there are no MMR or MSI companion diagnostics for breast cancer. Any FDA-cleared assay may be used to determine eligibility for immunotherapy; however, this may change in the future, as new companion diagnostics are developed.[30,31]

TMB is determined either by whole-genome or whole-exome sequencing, or by sequencing targeted regions of the genome. TMB is defined as the total number of somatic mutations in a megabase of the genomic sequence analyzed. Tumors with 10 or more mutations per megabase of the genome are generally accepted as having high TMB. Unlike MSI and MMR testing, TMB testing has a companion diagnostic assay,

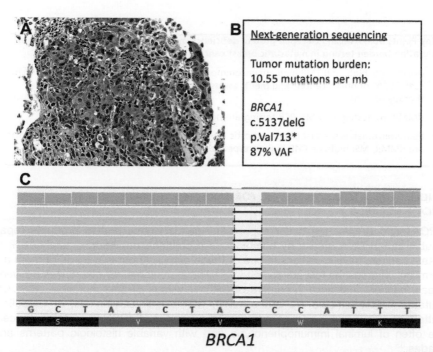

BRCA1

Fig. 4. BRCA1 mutation in a TNBC with high tumor mutation burden. This TNBC metastatic to the brain (*A*, H&E, original magnification ×200) underwent next-generation sequencing (NGS). NGS revealed a high tumor mutation burden of 10.55 mutations per megabase (Mb) (where high TMB is ≥ 10 mutations per Mb) and a pathogenic *BRCA1* mutation (*B, C*). The *BRCA1* mutation was previously identified as a germline change. In the tumor, this mutation has a variant allele frequency (VAF) of 87%, which is consistent with loss of heterozygosity (LOH), and biallelic inactivation of *BRCA1* in the tumor. High TMB makes the patient eligible for single-agent pembrolizumab, and the germline *BRCA1* mutation (with LOH in the tumor) makes the patient eligible for PARP inhibitors.

the FoundationOneCDx assay (Foundation Medicine, Inc) (see **Table 2**), which is often required to determine patient eligibility for single-agent pembrolizumab.

Challenges and Practical Considerations

Studies on dMMR and MSI in breast cancer have shown some major drawbacks to MMR IHC in breast cancer: (1) IHC for MMR proteins shows significant heterogeneity within the tumors, which can be particularly problematic in small biopsies, and (2) loss of MMR proteins by IHC does not correlate well with MSI testing by PCR in breast cancer. Thus, the 2 testing methods (IHC and PCR) cannot be used interchangeably in breast cancer, unlike what is done in colon or endometrial cancer. Loss of MMR proteins by IHC is more frequent than MSI.[32] At present, there are no breast cancer-specific testing guidelines for dMMR and MSI testing.

Assessment of TMB can be particularly useful in metastatic TNBC. Testing is largely driven by the oncologist in circumstances in which there are no other satisfactory treatment options available. However, because MSI and TMB are included in most next-generation sequencing assays performed for actionable mutations, this information will be available for any tumor subjected to broad sequencing.

> **Key Points Box 3: Mismatch repair protein deficiency, microsatellite instability, and tumor mutation burden testing in metastatic breast cancer**
>
> 1. dMMR, MSI high, and TMB high are uncommon findings in breast cancers; however, TMB is seen in 5% of breast cancers and merits assessment on metastatic tumors with limited therapy options.
> 2. dMMR IHC testing and MSI PCR testing are not interchangeable in breast cancer.
> 3. Pembrolizumab is the first tumor-agnostic PD-L1 inhibitor for use in advanced tumors that are dMMR, MSI-high, or TMB-high, irrespective of tumor type.

SINGLE-GENE ALTERATION TESTING FOR TARGETED THERAPY
BRCA 1 and BRCA 2

BRCA1 and *BRCA2* are tumor suppressor genes whose protein products repair double-strand DNA breaks by homologous recombination. Approximately 10% of breast cancers have mutations in one of these genes. About two-thirds of them are germline, whereas the rest are somatic.[33,34] There are some key differences between breast cancers that arise in carriers of *BRCA1* versus *BRCA2* mutations. *BRCA1*-mutated breast cancers are often TNBC, metaplastic carcinomas, or medullary pattern and have high nuclear grade and TILs (see **Fig. 4**). *BRCA2*-mutated cancers are often of luminal immunophenotype and with variable histologic patterns and grades.[35]

Poly(adenosine diphosphate-ribose) polymerase (PARP) inhibitors (olaparib and talazoparib) and platinum-based chemotherapies are effective in patients with *BRCA1/2*-mutated breast cancers. In breast cancer, PARP inhibitors are currently approved only for patients with metastatic breast cancer and *germline* mutation in either gene.[36] In contrast, PARP inhibitors are approved for use in patients with ovarian carcinoma and either *germline or somatic BRCA1/2* mutations. Recent trials have shown that PARP inhibitors are also effective in patients with breast cancer and somatic *BRCA1/2* mutations, which, if approved, would expand the population of eligible patients.[37] *BRCA* testing not only offers a targeted therapeutic option to patients but also helps identify family members who may be at risk, and *BRCA* testing is initiated by the treating oncologist. The companion diagnostic assay is BRACAnalysisCDx (Myriad Genetic Laboratories, Inc), which uses Sanger sequencing and multiplex PCR to detect various *BRCA* mutations (see **Table 3**). This assay is currently only intended to detect germline mutations.

PIK3CA

Most (70%) breast cancers are hormone receptor positive and HER2 negative. The first line of treatment of these cancers, whether primary or metastatic, is endocrine therapy to suppress the tumor's estrogen-dependent growth. In the metastatic setting, CDK4/6 inhibitors are also considered first line in ER-positive, HER2-negative cancers (no additional testing except ER positivity required). However, about half of these patients will eventually develop resistance to endocrine therapy. One strategy to overcome the resistance is by inhibiting the PI3K/AKT/mTOR pathway components, which regulate cell functions such as growth, division, and survival. About 40% of hormone receptor-positive and HER2-negative tumors harbor activating mutations in *PIK3CA* (**Fig. 5**). At present, *PIK3CA* inhibitor alpelisib, in combination with selective estrogen receptor downregulator fulvestrant, is a second-line therapy in patients with metastatic breast cancer who have progressed on endocrine therapy with

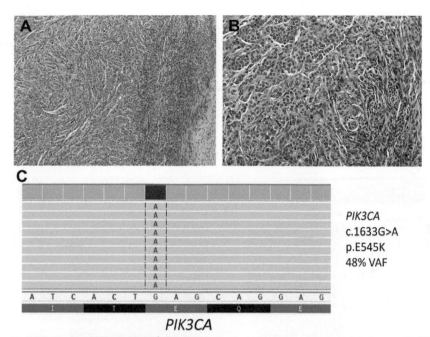

Fig. 5. *PIK3CA* mutation in an ER⁺ breast carcinoma. Sections of an ovarian tumor (*A*, H&E, original magnification ×100) reveal nests of uniform cells (*B*, H&E, X200) that are diffusely ER⁺ (not shown), consistent with a metastasis from the patient's known breast primary. Next-generation sequencing revealed a pathogenic *PIK3CA* mutation (*C*) with 48% variant allele frequency (VAF). The p.E545K mutation is one of the most common activating mutations in *PIK3CA* commonly detected in breast carcinoma. This *PIK3CA* mutation makes the patient eligible for *PIK3CA*-targeted therapy.

or without CDK4/6 inhibitors.[38] The treating oncologist initiates *PIK3CA* testing. There are 3 companion diagnostic assays available to detect *PIK3CA* mutations: therascreen *PIK3CA* RGQ PCR Kit (PCR test), FoundationOne Liquid CDx assay (NGS test), and FoundationOne CDx assay (NGS test) (see **Table 3**).[39] The first 2 assays can be performed on patients' blood samples using circulating tumor DNA. *PIK3CA* is the only biomarker in breast cancer that has been approved for detection in the blood through circulating tumor DNA.[40–42]

NTRK Testing

NTRK inhibitors (larotrectinib and entrectinib) are newly developed targeted therapies for solid tumors with fusions involving genes of the *NTRK* family, independent of tumor histology.[43,44] In the breast, secretory carcinomas are a rare tumor type accounting for less than 0.15% of all invasive breast cancers. These tumors are characterized by unique histology with intracellular and extracellular eosinophilic secretions, typically TNBC phenotype, and a pathognomonic *ETV6-NTRK3* gene fusion (**Fig. 6**). These tumors are identical to their counterparts in the salivary gland, thyroid, and skin.[45] Most of these tumors are indolent, whereas a small subset is aggressive with late recurrences and may benefit from *NTRK* inhibitors.

NTRK testing is unique because it is triggered by the pathologist upon histologic diagnosis of secretory carcinoma rather than by the treating clinician. Until recently, *NTRK* fusions were detected by molecular methods such as FISH and NGS. Now, a

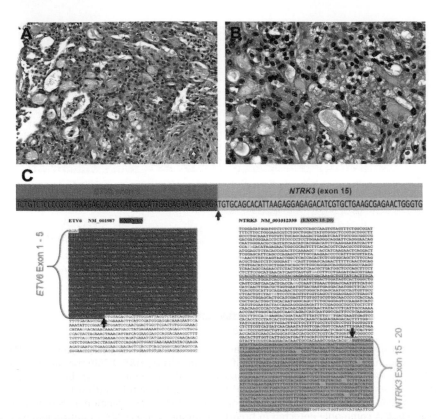

Fig. 6. NTRK-ETV6 translocation in primary secretory carcinoma of the breast. This primary breast carcinoma displays cribriform architecture (*A*, H&E, original magnification ×200), uniform nuclei, and eosinophilic luminal secretions (*B*, H&E, original magnification ×400), suggesting secretory carcinoma. Targeted gene sequencing confirms the presence of a translocation between *ETV6* exons 1 to 5 and *NTRK* exons 15 to 20 (*C*), confirming the diagnosis of secretory carcinoma. If the patient were to develop metastatic disease, the presence of the *NTRK-ETV6* translocation would make the patient eligible for *NTRK*-targeted therapy.

pan-*NTRK* IHC stain is available, and the *ETV6-NTRK* fusion causes a nuclear localization of the fusion protein and nuclear labeling with IHC. Diffuse and/or at least focally strong nuclear labeling with IHC has good sensitivity (83%) and specificity (100%) in detecting the *ETV6-NTRK3* fusion in secretory carcinomas of the breast.[46] IHC may be a valuable and cost-effective screening tool for secretory carcinomas, but it is not an approved companion diagnostic and molecular testing is required to confirm gene rearrangements in tumors in which *NTRK* inhibitors are being considered. The approved companion diagnostic for *NTRK* analysis is the next-generation sequencing platform FoundationOne CDx assay (see **Table 3**).[47] *NTRK* analysis is typically part of large next-generation sequencing platforms and will be assessed in all breast cancer subtypes submitted for sequencing. However, the vast majority of breast cancers known to have *NTRK* alterations are secretory carcinomas.[48]

Key Points Box 4: Single mutation testing in metastatic breast cancer

1. Patients with germline *BRCA1/2* mutations and metastatic breast cancer are eligible for therapy with PARP inhibitors

2. Patients with somatic *PIK3CA* mutations in ER-positive, HER2-negative metastatic breast cancer are eligible for targeted therapy with alpelisib

3. Patients with *NTRK* rearrangement metastatic breast secretory carcinomas are eligible for targeted therapy with larotrectinib and entrectinib

4. Although *NTRK* assessment can be performed on any breast cancer subtype, there is no utility in testing nonsecretory carcinomas.

5. IHC to detect NTRK protein is an effective screening and diagnostic tool in secretory carcinomas, but molecular confirmation is required for treatment with NTRK inhibitors.

FUTURE DIRECTIONS
Novel Assays

Liquid biopsies of blood for circulating tumor DNA (ctDNA) is a time- and cost-effective, noninvasive method for obtaining tumor material for testing. Liquid biopsies have a unique advantage of capturing tumor heterogeneity within a single tumor site and across multiple metastases. ctDNA testing can be used to detect new actionable genetic alterations in tumors that progress, to measure tumor burden, and to monitor tumor relapse or metastasis.[49] Two of the most common single-gene alterations detected by testing ctDNA are *PIK3CA* and *ESR1,* both relevant therapeutically.[50] At present, the only FDA-approved companion diagnostic assay that uses ctDNA in breast cancer is for detecting *PIK3CA* for treatment with alpelisib. All other uses of ctDNA in breast cancer remain experimental at present.

Emerging Biomarkers

The presence of TILs is both a prognostic and predictive biomarker in breast cancer.[51,52] Society-level guidelines for scoring and reporting TILs and clinical guidelines for meaningful use of this information will be required before TILs can be incorporated into clinical practice.

Another big challenge in the interpretation of biomarkers is interobserver and intraobserver variability. Image digitization and image analysis technologies may provide reproducible, objective, and accurate assessment of biomarkers, as platforms are validated and approved for clinical use.[53] Finally, novel anti-HER2 therapeutic agents such as antibody drug conjugates have shown beneficial responses even in HER2 nonamplified breast cancers in clinical trials, leading to a proposed new category of breast tumors, "HER2-low."[54] Future testing algorithms may see inclusion of this category to identify tumors that respond well to emerging anti-HER2 agents.

SUMMARY

Metastatic breast cancers remain a challenge to treat. However, the landscape of testing and therapeutics in these cancers is evolving rapidly. As new targeted therapeutics are developed, corresponding companion diagnostic assays are also being developed to determine which patients will benefit from these therapies Sequencing platforms are a cost-effective tool to comprehensively gather genomic information on multiple biomarkers simultaneously to guide therapy. It is important for the practicing pathologist to be aware of biomarker recommendations and testing platforms to effectively participate in and guide the multidisciplinary care of patients with metastatic breast cancer.

DISCLOSURE

G. Jagannathan: None; M.J. White: None; R.R. Xian: None; L.A. Emens: honoraria from AbbVie, Amgen, Celgene, Chugai, GCPR, Gilead, Gritstone, MedImmune, Peregrine, Shionogi, and Syndax; honoraria and travel support from AstraZeneca, Bayer, MacroGenics, Replimune, and Vaccinex; travel support from Bristol Myers Squibb, Genentech/Roche, and Novartis; potential future stock from Molecuvax; institutional support from AbbVie, Aduro Biotech, AstraZeneca, the Breast Cancer Research Foundation, Bristol Myers Squibb, Bolt Therapeutics, Compugen, Corvus, CyTomX, the US Department of Defense, EMD Serono, Genentech, Maxcyte, Merck, the National Cancer Institute, the NSABP Foundation, SU2C, Silverback, Roche, the Translational Breast Cancer Research Consortium, Takeda, Tempest, and HeritX; royalties from Aduro Biotech; A. Cimino-Mathews: Research grants to institution from Bristol-Myers Squibb; consultancy/honoraria to self from Bristol-Myers Squibb and Roche.

REFERENCES

1. Female breast cancer — cancer stat facts. Available at: https://seer.cancer.gov/statfacts/html/breast.html. Accessed January 2, 2021.
2. NCCN Clinical Practice Guidelines in Oncology (NCCN Guidelines): Breast Cancer. NCCN.org. 2021. Available at: https://www.nccn.org/guidelines/category_1. Accessed April 26, 2021.
3. Jørgensen JT, Hersom M. Companion diagnostics-a tool to improve pharmacotherapy. Ann Transl Med 2016;4(24). https://doi.org/10.21037/atm.2016.12.26.
4. U.S. FDA. Developing and labeling in vitro companion diagnostic devices for a specific group of oncology therapeutic products guidance for industry. FDA guidance documents. 2020. Available at: https://www.fda.gov/vaccines-blood-biologics/guidance-compliance-regulatory-information-biologics/biologics-guidances. Accessed April 25, 2021.
5. U.S. FDA. List of Cleared or Approved Companion Diagnostic Devices (In Vitro and Imaging Tools). 2021. Available at: https://www.fda.gov/medical-devices/in-vitro-diagnostics/list-cleared-or-approved-companion-diagnostic-devices-in-vitro-and-imaging-tools. Accessed April 28, 2021.
6. Allott EH, Geradts J, Sun X, et al. Intratumoral heterogeneity as a source of discordance in breast cancer biomarker classification. Breast Cancer Res 2016;18(1):1–11.
7. Jabbour MN, Massad CY, Boulos FI. Variability in hormone and growth factor receptor expression in primary versus recurrent, metastatic, and post-neoadjuvant breast carcinoma. Breast Cancer Res Treat 2012;135(1):29–37.
8. Amir E, Clemons M, Purdie CA, et al. Tissue confirmation of disease recurrence in breast cancer patients: pooled analysis of multi-centre, multi-disciplinary prospective studies. Cancer Treat Rev 2012;38(6):708–14.
9. Bardou VJ, Arpino G, Elledge RM, et al. Progesterone receptor status significantly improves outcome prediction over estrogen receptor status alone for adjuvant endocrine therapy in two large breast cancer databases. J Clin Oncol 2003;21(10):1973–9.
10. Van Poznak C, Somerfield MR, Bast RC, et al. Use of biomarkers to guide decisions on systemic therapy for women with metastatic breast cancer: American Society of Clinical Oncology clinical practice guideline. J Clin Oncol 2015;33(24):2695–704.

11. Hoefnagel LDC, Moelans CB, Meijer SL, et al. Prognostic value of estrogen receptor α and progesterone receptor conversion in distant breast cancer metastases. Cancer 2012;118(20):4929–35.

12. Allison KH, Hammond MEH, Dowsett M, et al. Estrogen and progesterone receptor testing in breast cancer: ASCO/CAP guideline update. J Clin Oncol 2020; 38(12):1346–66.

13. Wolff AC, Elizabeth Hale Hammond M, Allison KH, et al. Human epidermal growth factor receptor 2 testing in breast cancer: American society of clinical oncology/ college of American pathologists clinical practice guideline focused update. J Clin Oncol 2018;36(20):2105–22.

14. Estrogen and progesterone receptor testing in breast cancer guideline update. American Society of Clinical Oncology/College of American Pathologists; 2020. Available at: https://www.cap.org/protocols-and-guidelines/cap-guidelines/ current-cap-guidelines/guideline-recommendations-for-immunohistochemical- testing-of-estrogen-and-progesterone-receptors-in-breast-cancer. Accessed April 19, 2021.

15. HER2 testing in breast cancer. American Society of Clinical Oncology/College of American Pathologists; 2018. Available at: https://www.cap.org/protocols-and- guidelines/cap-guidelines/current-cap-guidelines/recommendations-for-human- epidermal-growth-factor-2-testing-in-breast-cancer. Accessed April 26, 2021.

16. Chen MT, Sun HF, Zhao Y, et al. Comparison of patterns and prognosis among distant metastatic breast cancer patients by age groups: a SEER population- based analysis. Sci Rep 2017;7(1):1–8.

17. Clark BZ, Yoest JM, Onisko A, et al. Effects of hydrochloric acid and formic acid decalcification on breast tumor biomarkers and HER2 fluorescence in situ hybrid- ization. Appl Immunohistochem Mol Morphol 2019;27(3):223–30.

18. van Es SC, van der Vegt B, Bensch F, et al. Decalcification of breast cancer bone metastases With EDTA does not affect ER, PR, and HER2 results. Am J Surg Pathol 2019;43(10):1355–60.

19. Pareja F, Murray MP, Jean RD, et al. Cytologic assessment of estrogen receptor, progesterone receptor, and HER2 status in metastatic breast carcinoma. J Am Soc Cytopathol 2017;6(1):33–40.

20. Cimino-Mathews A. Tumor-in filtrating lymphocytes and PD-L1 in breast cancer (and, what happened to medullary carcinoma?). Diagn Histopathol 2021;1–7.

21. Cortes J, Cescon DW, Rugo HS, et al. Pembrolizumab plus chemotherapy versus placebo plus chemotherapy for previously untreated locally recurrent inoperable or metastatic triple-negative breast cancer (KEYNOTE-355): a randomised, placebo-controlled, double-blind, phase 3 clinical trial. Lancet 2020; 396(10265):1817–28.

22. Schmid P, Adams S, Rugo HS, et al. Atezolizumab and Nab-paclitaxel in advanced triple-negative breast cancer. N Engl J Med 2018;379(22):2108–21.

23. Schmid P, Cortes J, Pusztai L, et al. Pembrolizumab for early triple-negative breast cancer. N Engl J Med 2020;382(9):810–21.

24. Cimino-Mathews A, Ye X, Meeker A, et al. Metastatic triple-negative breast can- cers at first relapse have fewer tumor-infiltrating lymphocytes than their matched primary breast tumors: a pilot study. Hum Pathol 2013;44(10):2055–63.

25. Michot JM, Bigenwald C, Champiat S, et al. Immune-related adverse events with immune checkpoint blockade: a comprehensive review. Eur J Cancer 2016;54: 139–48.

26. Fusco MJ, West HJ, Walko CM. Tumor mutation burden and cancer treatment. JAMA Oncol 2021;7(2):316.

27. Cheng AS, Leung SCY, Gao D, et al. Mismatch repair protein loss in breast cancer: clinicopathological associations in a large British Columbia cohort. Breast Cancer Res Treat 2020;179(1):3–10.

28. Barroso-Sousa R, Jain E, Cohen O, et al. Prevalence and mutational determinants of high tumor mutation burden in breast cancer. Ann Oncol 2020;31(3):387–94.

29. Marabelle A, Fakih M, Lopez J, et al. Association of tumour mutational burden with outcomes in patients with advanced solid tumours treated with pembrolizumab: prospective biomarker analysis of the multicohort, open-label, phase 2 KEYNOTE-158 study. Lancet Oncol 2020;21(10):1353–65.

30. U.S. FDA. FDA grants accelerated approval to dostarlimab-gxly for dMMR endometrial cancer. Drug approvals and databases. Available at: https://www.fda.gov/drugs/drug-approvals-and-databases/fda-grants-accelerated-approval-dostarlimab-gxly-dmmr-endometrial-cancer. Accessed April 26, 2021.

31. Venetis K, Sajjadi E, Haricharan S, et al. Mismatch repair testing in breast cancer: The path to tumor-specific immuno-oncology biomarkers. Transl Cancer Res 2020;9(7):4060–4.

32. Fusco N, Lopez G, Corti C, et al. Mismatch repair protein loss as a prognostic and predictive biomarker in breast cancers regardless of microsatellite instability. JNCI Cancer Spectr 2018;2(4). https://doi.org/10.1093/jncics/pky056.

33. Winter C, Nilsson MP, Olsson E, et al. Targeted sequencing of BRCA1 and BRCA2 across a large unselected breast cancer cohort suggests that one-third of mutations are somatic. Ann Oncol 2016;27(8):1532–8.

34. Nik-Zainal S, Davies H, Staaf J, et al. Landscape of somatic mutations in 560 breast cancer whole-genome sequences. Nature 2016;534(7605):47–54.

35. Sønderstrup IMH, Jensen MBR, Ejlertsen B, et al. Subtypes in BRCA-mutated breast cancer. Hum Pathol 2019;84:192–201.

36. Robson M, Im S-A, Senkus E, et al. Olaparib for metastatic breast cancer in patients with a Germline BRCA mutation. N Engl J Med 2017;377(6):523–33.

37. Tung NM, Robson ME, Ventz S, et al. TBCRC 048: phase II study of olaparib for metastatic breast cancer and mutations in homologous recombination-related genes. J Clin Oncol 2020;38(36):4274–82.

38. André F, Ciruelos E, Rubovszky G, et al. Alpelisib for PIK3CA-mutated, hormone receptor–positive advanced breast cancer. N Engl J Med 2019;380(20):1929–40.

39. Martínez-Saéz O, Chic N, Pascual T, et al. Frequency and spectrum of PIK3CA somatic mutations in breast cancer. Breast Cancer Res 2020;22(1):1–9.

40. U.S. FDA. FDA approves first PI3K inhibitor for breast cancer. Available at: https://www.fda.gov/news-events/press-announcements/fda-approves-first-pi3k-inhibitor-breast-cancer. Accessed April 26, 2021.

41. U.S. FDA. FDA approves liquid biopsy NGS companion diagnostic test for multiple cancers and biomarkers. Available at: https://www.fda.gov/drugs/fda-approves-liquid-biopsy-ngs-companion-diagnostic-test-multiple-cancers-and-biomarkers. Accessed April 26, 2021.

42. U.S. FDA. FDA approves alpelisib for metastatic breast cancer. Available at: https://www.fda.gov/drugs/resources-information-approved-drugs/fda-approves-alpelisib-metastatic-breast-cancer. Accessed April 26, 2021.

43. Scott LJ. Larotrectinib: first global approval. Drugs 2019;79(2):201–6.

44. Al-Salama ZT, Keam SJ. Entrectinib: first global approval. Drugs 2019;79(13):1477–83.

45. Diallo R, Schaefer KL, Bankfalvi A, et al. Secretory carcinoma of the breast: a distinct variant of invasive ductal carcinoma assessed by comparative genomic hybridization and immunohistochemistry. Hum Pathol 2003;34(12):1299–305.

46. Harrison BT, Fowler E, Krings G, et al. Pan-TRK immunohistochemistry. Am J Surg Pathol 2019;43(12):1693–700.
47. U.S. FDA. FDA approves companion diagnostic to identify NTRK fusions in solid tumors for Vitrakvi. Available at: https://www.fda.gov/drugs/fda-approves-companion-diagnostic-identify-ntrk-fusions-solid-tumors-vitrakvi. Accessed April 25, 2021.
48. Remoué A, Conan-Charlet V, Bourhis A, et al. Non-secretory breast carcinomas lack NTRK rearrangements and TRK protein expression. Pathol Int 2019; 69(2):94–6.
49. Canzoniero JVL, Park BH. Use of cell free DNA in breast oncology. Biochim Biophys Acta 2016;1865(2):266–74.
50. Buono G, Gerratana L, Bulfoni M, et al. Circulating tumor DNA analysis in breast cancer: Is it ready for prime-time? Cancer Treat Rev 2019;73:73–83.
51. Tan PH, Ellis I, Allison K, et al. The 2019 World Health Organization classification of tumours of the breast. Histopathology 2020;77(2):181–5.
52. Tan PH, Ellis I, Allison K, et al. World Health Organization Classification of Tumours: breast tumors. 5th editionVol 2. Lyon, France: IARC Press; 2019.
53. Dermawan JK, Mukhopadhyay S, Shah AA. Frequency and extent of cytokeratin expression in paraganglioma: an immunohistochemical study of 60 cases from 5 anatomic sites and review of the literature. Hum Pathol 2019;93:16–22.
54. Tarantino P, Hamilton E, Tolaney SM, et al. HER2-low breast cancer: pathological and clinical landscape. J Clin Oncol 2020;38(17):1951–62.

Primary Care

Primary Care

Individualizing Breast Cancer Risk Assessment in Clinical Practice

Amy E. Cyr, MD[a],*, Kaitlyn Kennard, MD[b]

KEYWORDS

- Breast cancer risk • High risk • Risk assessment • Risk models • Risk factors
- Risk reduction • Screening

KEY POINTS

- Multiple tools exist to assess future breast cancer risk for individual patients.
- A risk calculator may depend heavily on family history, the risk of a genetic mutation, prior biopsy results, breast density, lifestyle, and hormonal factors.
- Choice of risk model depends on which risk factors apply to a patient.
- Risk calculations inform both screening and risk-reduction options.
- Although many risk factors are nonmodifiable, patients can reduce their risk to some extent with lifestyle modifications.

INTRODUCTION

Breast cancer (BC) is the most common malignancy in American women.*,[1] Mortality has declined, in part because screening detects cancers at an early stage.[2] For most women, screening means annual mammography, starting at 40 years of age. Mammography improves survival, with the caveat that some women undergo procedures for benign findings or treatment for clinically insignificant cancers.[2,3] For women whose BC risk is above average, the addition of annual breast magnetic resonance imaging (MRI) to mammography is superior to mammography alone.[4] Women identified as high risk (HR) are also eligible for risk-reducing endocrine therapy or surgery.

This chapter discusses BC risk factors, tools used to identify HR patients, and how to use this information to reduce BC-related morbidity and mortality.

This article previously appeared in *Surgical Oncology Clinics* volume 32 issue 4 October 2023
[a] Department of Medicine, Washington University, Box 8056, 660 South Euclid Avenue, Saint Louis, MO 63110, USA; [b] Department of Surgery, Washington University, Box 8051, 660 South Euclid Avenue, Saint louis, MO 63110, USA
* Corresponding author.
E-mail address: amycyr@wustl.edu

Clinics Collections 14 (2024) 93–107
https://doi.org/10.1016/j.ccol.2024.02.012
2352-7986/24/© 2024 Elsevier Inc. All rights reserved.

DISCUSSION
Nonmodifiable Risk Factors

Age and race

White women have the highest BC rate, followed by Black women, although this gap has narrowed. Hispanic, American Indian, and Pacific Islander women have the lowest incidence. Aging increases risk, but the incidence has increased for women aged 20 to 49 years, while remaining stable or declining for older women.[5]

Although all young women are more likely to have higher stage and more aggressive disease, at all ages, these poor prognostic indicators disproportionately affect Black women. In addition, stage-for-stage, young Black women are twice as likely to die from BC as White women.[6]

Thoracic radiation

For children and young adults treated with thoracic radiation, the incidence of BC by the age of 55 years is as high as 29%.[7] Radiation increases the risk for both estrogen receptor positive (ER+) and negative (ER−) disease. Patient age during therapy, radiation dose, use of alkylating agents, and therapy-related suppression of ovarian function impact the degree of risk attributable to radiation.[7–9] Thoracic radiation is not a variable in any risk model but is a stand-alone indication for HR screening and risk-reducing therapy.[4]

Breast density

Increased breast density is an independent risk factor for BC.[10,11] Women with the highest level of density have a 4-fold increase in risk compared with women with minimal density. Density is, in part, heritable (Asian women, for instance, have the highest breast density), but higher alcohol intake and the use of hormone replacement therapy (HRT) also increase density.[11] Many patients taking endocrine therapy see a decrease in breast density; some studies suggest that this mammographic change is prognostic and predictive.[10]

Pathologies

Benign breast disease comprises nonproliferative lesions, proliferative lesions without atypia, atypical hyperplasia, and lobular carcinoma in situ (LCIS). Nonproliferative pathologies increase risk minimally and only for women with a family history (FHx). Proliferative change without atypia doubles risk, atypical hyperplasia increases risk 4-fold, and LCIS increases risk 8- to 10-fold.[12,13] A younger age at diagnosis of benign disease further increases risk, and for women of any age, the increased risk persists for 2 decades. Although the risk affects both breasts, the ipsilateral breast is twice as likely as the contralateral breast to develop a cancer within the first 5 years after biopsy (within the first 10 years for women with atypia).[12,14]

BC predisposition genes

The widespread use of multigene panel testing identifies cancer-predisposing variants. These pathogenic variants are overall rare, but the incidence of ATM and CHEK2 mutations is 1% to 2% in White Europeans or European descendants, while the incidence of BRCA mutations is about 2.5% in the Ashkenazi Jewish population.[15,16]

High-penetrance genes like BRCA1, BRCA2, and TP53 increase lifetime BC risk to at least 50%, while moderate penetrance genes like ATM, BARD1, CDH1, CHEK2, RAD51 C, RAD51D, and STK11 increase lifetime risk to 20% to 50%; the gene, specific variant, and FHx modify the risk. While most pathogenic ATM variants increase lifetime BC risk to under 30%, lifetime risk with the missense variant c.7271 T > G approaches that of BRCA2. Lifetime BC risk with PALB2, often classified as moderately penetrant, and with PTEN may exceed 50%.[15–17] Risk with moderately penetrant variants can be further refined with polygenic risk scores (PRSs).[15]

Pathogenic ATM and CHEK2 variants primarily increase the risk of ER+ disease, suggesting a possible role for endocrine prophylaxis. In contrast, *BARD1*, *RAD51 C*, and *RAD51D* increase ER cancer risk.[15,17]

Risk Models

Risk models incorporate nonmodifiable and modifiable variables to estimate BC risk. Model choice depends on (1) why a patient may be HR and (2) how the information will drive management.

Breast cancer risk assessment tool

Gail and colleagues used data from Caucasian women aged 35 to 74 years to develop a model to calculate invasive and noninvasive BC risk. Their model included age of menarche and first parity, number of biopsies, presence of atypia, and number of affected female first-degree relatives (FDRs).[18]

Other investigators refined the model and limited its prediction to an invasive disease. This modified Gail model, or National Cancer Institute Breast Cancer Risk Assessment Tool (BCRAT), calculates risk over the next 5 years and by the age of 90 years (**Box 1**).[19,20]

The BCRAT performs well at the population level, measured by the expected-to-observed (E/O) event ratio, but this varies by subpopulation: Although modifications to the BCRAT incorporated data from African American, Asian, Pacific Islander, and Hispanic women, BCRAT performance is poorer in non-White populations.[21–23]

The model underestimates risk in general. In one study evaluating model performance in women with atypia, investigators expected 34.9 cancers but observed 58 (E/O 0.6). For individual women, the concordance statistic (or area under the curve [AUC]) was 0.50 (95% confidence interval [CI] 0.44–0.55), no better than the flip of a coin.[24] A meta-analysis showed that the BCRAT performs poorly at the individual level for women without atypia as well.[25] In addition, female FDRs are the only included FHx, so the model underestimates risk for patients with an extended or paternal FHx or affected male relatives.

The BCRAT is more likely to underestimate, rather than overestimate, lifetime risk, so it is best used to determine eligibility for endocrine therapy (as it was used in chemoprevention trials), but not for screening MRI.

Breast Cancer Surveillance Consortium

Tice and colleagues assessed density alone to predict BC risk and calculated an AUC of 0.67 (95% CI 0.66–0.70), equivalent to the AUC calculated using BCRAT variables.

Box 1
BCRAT (Gail model)

- Available online at https://bcrisktool.cancer.gov/
- Calculates risk at 5 years and by the age of 90 years
- Cannot be used for patients younger than 35 years or with a BRCA mutation or LCIS
- Underestimates lifetime risk for patients with atypia and those with extended or paternal family history
- Better used to determine endocrine therapy eligibility rather than to direct screening recommendations

Adding density to BCRAT variables modestly improved the AUC.[26] They further refined and validated their risk model using data from the Breast Cancer Surveillance Consortium (BCSC) registries, limiting FHx of affected FDR to yes/no, and adding categories of benign disease (nonproliferative, proliferative without atypia, proliferative with atypia, and LCIS) (**Box 2**).[27]

The final model underestimates the risk for young women, those with fatty density, Asian and Hispanic women, and Black women, while overpredicting risk overall (E/O 1.04, 95% CI 1.03–1.06); AUC was 0.665. Only 3% of women had a 5-year risk over 3%, and about 7% had a 10-year risk over 5%. For women with proliferative disease, the addition of that pathology to the risk calculation identifies 3 times as many as HR.[28,29]

Because BCSC provides 5- and 10-year risk but not lifetime BC risk, it is best used to determine eligibility for endocrine prophylaxis.[30]

International Breast Cancer Intervention Study model
Developed with the data from the International Breast Cancer Intervention Study (IBIS), the Tyrer-Cuzick, or IBIS model (**Box 3**), calculates the likelihood of having a BRCA-related cancer and refines that calculation with risk attributable to personal factors. The software is downloadable, and there is an online platform. Although not a default setting with the most recent software (version 8), IBIS creators recommend inclusion of competing mortality.[31–33]

Unlike BCRAT, IBIS incorporates diverse risk factors, including hormonal history, BRCA status, and breast density. Body mass index (BMI) refines the risk attributable to density. An elevated BMI independently adds risk for postmenopausal women; the protective effect of increased BMI in premenopausal women is not addressed in the model.[32,33]

FHx includes bilateral breast, ovarian, and male BCs. Unaffected relatives and their current age (or age at death) further refine results.[32,33]

Biopsy history includes benign/nonproliferative disease, hyperplasia, atypia, and LCIS. Pathologies such as adenosis, apocrine change, and mild usual ductal hyperplasia (UDH) are considered nonproliferative. Proliferative disease includes moderate or florid UDH, sclerosing adenosis, and papillomas. Atypia includes atypical ductal and lobular hyperplasia, but not flat epithelial atypia. The calculated relative risk attributed to atypia is 4-fold, while that for LCIS is 8-fold.[31,32]

IBIS overestimates risk for women with LCIS and atypia, however.[34–36] In one study, the AUC for women with LCIS was only 0.493.[29] Another reported an E/O ratio of 1.48 in patients with LCIS and an AUC of 0.54 (95% CI 0.48–0.62).[36]

IBIS performs well across ethnic populations but may overestimate the risk for Hispanic women while underestimating that for African Americans. It also overestimates

---

Box 2
BCSC Risk Model

- Available online at https://tools.bscs-scc.org/BC5yearRisk/calculator.htm
- Calculates invasive breast cancer risk at 5 and 10 years
- Incorporates personal risk factors, including breast density, biopsy history, and limited family history but is not validated in women with implants
- Underestimates risk in younger women, non-Caucasian women, and women with minimal breast density
- Can be used to determine eligibility for endocrine prophylaxis

---

Box 3
IBIS (Tyrer-Cuzick model)

- Available online at https://ibis.ikonopedia.com or at https://www.ems-trials.org/riskevaluator/

- Calculates breast cancer risk at 5 or 10 years and by the age of 85 years and calculates the likelihood of carrying a BRCA mutation

- Incorporates personal risk factors, including breast density, biopsy history, and extensive family history

- Overestimates lifetime risk with extended follow-up and for patients with atypia or LCIS

- Can be used to determine eligibility for high-risk screening or for endocrine prophylaxis

---

the risk for women with the highest risk, for BRCA carriers, and with longer follow-up.[37,38] PRS data can be added and improve model performance.[39]

CanRisk

CanRisk (**Box 4**), previously known as Breast and Ovarian Analysis of Disease Incidence and Carrier Estimation Algorithm, was developed using a cohort of women diagnosed with BC before the age of 55 years.[40]

It incorporates diverse variables, such as hormonal and lifestyle risk factors, breast density, personal cancer history, and risk-reducing surgery, but not biopsy history. Relevant FHx includes breast, ovarian, male breast, and pancreatic cancers, along with BC receptor information.[40–42] Like IBIS, a PRS can be included.[43]

CanRisk is time-consuming but valuable in some situations. *BRCA1*, *BRCA2*, *ATM*, *PALB2*, *CHEK2*, *RAD51 C*, *RAD51D*, *BARD1*, and *BRIP1* mutations are included, so it is helpful for calculating risk with moderately penetrant genes and for women who do not have a familial moderate penetrance gene. CanRisk provides 5- or 10-year and lifetime BC risk, ovarian cancer risk, and contralateral BC risk for patients with a personal history of cancer.[44]

CanRisk, available online,[44] is frequently updated and performs better than other models at both population and individual levels. In one study, E/O ratios ranged from 0.88 to 1.12, depending on the thoroughness of the variable input, with AUCs ranging from 0.61 to 0.70.[45]

Claus

Claus and colleagues assumed a dominant allele could explain hereditary cancer and proposed a model using data from Caucasian BC patients (age 20–54 years) and matched controls (**Box 5**). Input includes up to 2 relatives (FDR and second-degree

---

Box 4
CanRisk

- Available online at https://canrisk.org

- Calculates breast, ovarian, and contralateral breast cancer risk at 5 or 10 years and by the age of 80 years

- Incorporates personal risk factors, including breast density, extensive family history, and various cancer predisposition genes

- Frequently updated and able to refine risk due to moderately penetrant genes

- Results determine eligibility for high-risk screening

Box 5
Claus

- Determines breast cancer risk using published risk tables
- Calculates breast cancer risk in 10-year increments, up to the age of 79 years
- Incorporates up to 2 first- or second-degree relatives with breast or ovarian cancer
- Less robustly validated and may underestimate breast cancer risk
- Results determine eligibility for high-risk screening

---

relatives with BC and FDRs with ovarian cancer) and age at diagnosis. Risk estimates are available in table form or online.[46]

In one cohort, Claus underpredicted cancers (E/O ratio 1.69, 95% CI 1.48–1.87), and the AUC was lower than that for other models evaluated in the same study (AUC 0.59, 95% CI 0.56–0.62).[47]

BRCAPRO

BRCAPRO (**Box 6**) shares many features with IBIS and CanRisk. It incorporates unaffected FDR and second-degree relatives and those with bilateral breast and ovarian cancer. Cancer receptors, race, ethnicity, and risk-reducing surgery can be included. Like IBIS, it determines cancer risk based on the likelihood of having a *BRCA* gene. It provides an estimated risk of breast, ovarian, or contralateral BC.[48,49] Unlike IBIS, BRCAPRO does not include competing mortality, and there is no free online tool.

At the population level, BRCAPRO overestimates risk for older women and those without a significant FHx, while underestimating risk overall, especially for younger women and for those with a more extensive FHx. Discrimination at the individual level is similar, but somewhat inferior, to that of IBIS and BCRAT.[37,47]

Ask2Me

Although several of these risk calculators incorporate germline mutations, management guidelines, including those provided by testing companies and the National Comprehensive Cancer Network (NCCN), report broad lifetime cancer risks.[16] The online All Syndromes Known to Man Evaluator (Ask2Me) provides an age-adjusted estimate of cancer risk associated with any of almost 3-dozen genes. It also provides risk in 5-year intervals, which can guide the timing of risk-reducing interventions.[50,51]

The website is updated less frequently than others, including CanRisk and NCCN. For instance, NCCN currently recommends consideration of HR screening for women with BARD1 and reports no increase in ovarian cancer risk, while Ask2Me continues to show an increased ovarian cancer risk. Ask2Me references NCCN and other professional society guidelines, but as of the date of this writing, that information is outdated.[49,50]

Box 6
BRCAPRO

- Available with a commercial software package
- Calculates breast, ovarian, and contralateral breast cancer risk
- Incorporates a complex family history of breast or ovarian cancer
- May underestimate breast cancer risk, especially for young patients
- Results determine eligibility for high-risk screening

Artificial intelligence

Deep learning–based convolutional neural networks improve cancer detection and refine mammographic breast density classification. These and other artificial intelligence tools also use mammographic images to provide risk stratification. The AUCs reported with deep learning are equivalent or superior to those of the tools discussed in this chapter. However, minority women are underrepresented in many data sets used to develop this technology, and tools need to be validated in diverse screening populations.[52]

Polygenic risk scores

While some BCs are attributable to highly or moderately penetrant genes, most result from common alleles. Individually these minimally affect risk. For patients with many HR alleles, though, the increase in BC risk may be significant and is reflected in a PRS.

PRS data are applicable to non-White populations, help predict contralateral BC risk, and refine risk with moderately penetrant genes.[53–55] Addition of PRS to standard risk factors improves model performance over that with either PRS or standard risk factors alone. Such refinements to risk calculations may in the future not only identify women as HR but identify those with low risk who may not need yearly mammography. PRS may even determine risk for certain types of BC (for instance ER+ disease), informing management.[54,56] Outside of their inclusion in models like IBIS and CanRisk; however, PRS are not yet routinely used to make clinical decisions.

Choosing a model

Table 1 summarizes the variables included in these frequently used models, which represent only a proportion of available models. As with those discussed here, others were developed and validated using different sets of data and incorporate variable risk factors. Model performance, therefore, varies by patient subpopulation (age, risk factors, ethnicity, etc).[37]

Investigators have compared the population-level calibration and individual-level discrimination of these models. Discrimination is best for CanRisk and IBIS. All models, with the exception of CanRisk, underestimate risk in patients with the lowest risk and overestimate in patients with the highest risk.[57] IBIS identifies the highest proportion of HR women.[58] Most models predict risk better for luminal than for nonluminal cancers.[59]

Based on performance, ease of use, accessibility, and utility for directing management, we recommend BCRAT, BCSC, or IBIS for identifying patients eligible for endocrine prophylaxis and the FHx-based models (especially IBIS and CanRisk) to determine eligibility for HR screening.[60–62]

Modifiable Risk Factors

Modifiable risk factors impact BC risk to a lesser degree than most nonmodifiable factors but remain important. Addressing these empowers patients while lowering their risk for diseases beyond BC.

Physical activity

Increasing physical activity lowers BC risk. Regular exercise may delay the onset of menarche, increase the length of the menstrual cycle, and increase the number of anovulatory cycles, decreasing exposure to sex hormones. Studies, though, show the benefit of exercise in the absence of menstrual cycle changes.[63] Aerobic exercise may also induce changes in insulin sensitivity, antioxidant defense, epigenetic mechanisms, and intracellular signaling pathways.[64]

Table 1
Variables included in selected risk models

Risk Factor	BCRAT	IBIS	CanRisk	BRCAPRO	Claus	BCSC
Age	•	•	•	•	•	•
Race/ethnicity	•			•		•
Ashkenazi Jewish		•	•	•		
Menarche	•	•	•	•		
First parity	•	•	•	•		
Menopause		•	•			
Atypia	•	•				•
LCIS	NA	•				•
Prior biopsy	•	•				•
Breast density		•	•			•
PRS		•	•			
BRCA status	NA	•	•	•		
Other genes			•			
History of breast cancer	NA	NA	•	•		
BMI		•	•			
Family history variables						
Affected FDR	•	•	•	•	•	•
Non–FDR		•	•	•	•	
Male relatives		•	•	•		
Bilateral cancers	NA	•	•	•		
Cancer receptors	NA		•	•		
Ovarian cancer		•	•	•	•	
Other cancers		•				

Abbreviations: BCRAT, Breast Cancer Risk Assessment Tool; BCSC, breast cancer surveillance consortium; BMI, body mass index; FDR, first-degree relative; IBIS, breast cancer intervention study; LCIS, lobular carcinoma in situ; NA, not applicable (the model is not applicable to patients with this factor); PRS, polygenic risk score.

Moderate to vigorous activity reduces risk by an average of 25% in premenopausal and postmenopausal women, both lean and obese. There is a dose-dependent relationship, but the optimal level of physical activity for risk reduction remains unclear.[65]

Hormonal
Women using estrogen plus progestin have a higher risk of both ER+ and ER− disease. Combination HRT also interferes with mammographic sensitivity. The risk is most pronounced with longer HRT use and with current or recent use.[66,67]

Data on estrogen replacement therapy (ERT) are less clear. While some observational studies reported higher BC incidence and mortality, randomized trials showed that ERT lowered incidence and mortality compared with placebo, with the greatest reduction in ER+ cancers. ERT did not appear to interfere with cancer detection by mammography.[66–69] Given these high-level data, ERT appears to be safe, even for HR women.

Diet and alcohol
The Mediterranean diet (excluding alcohol) is protective, especially for postmenopausal women, independent of body weight and BMI.[70] Conversely, a diet high in

refined sugar and fat increases BC risk, which may result from inflammatory processes.[71]

Despite the concern about the pro-estrogen effect of soy, studies consistently show its protective effects. Phytoestrogens are structurally similar to estradiol and bind to ER-alpha in the breast and uterus and ER-beta in the cardiovascular system, urogenital tract, and bone. Soy binds to ER more weakly than does estradiol and has a higher affinity for ER-beta. Soy may therefore act as a selective ER modulator, lowering the risk of an ER+ disease and reducing recurrence risk in women with a personal history of cancer.[72,73]

Dairy products may lower BC risk. Breast tissue has receptors for vitamin D, which moderates cell proliferation, malignant cell differentiation, apoptosis, and angiogenesis. The impact of dairy depends, however, on the dairy product, its fat content, and a patient's menopausal status.[74]

Alcohol use contributes to a significant proportion of BCs, especially ER+ tumors. It increases risk in a dose-dependent fashion, likely though ER-dependent pathways. This seems to be independent of alcohol type. The most susceptible period for carcinogenesis is likely the period after menarche and before first pregnancy.[75,76]

Weight

A higher BMI in early adulthood lowers BC risk.[77] However, weight gain and postmenopausal obesity increase BC risk: Each 5-kg/m^2 increase in BMI may increase risk by 12%. The increase in risk is most pronounced for nonusers of HRT. Even a 2-kg weight loss, though, reduces the risk of postmenopausal BC.[77–79] The benefit extends beyond BC risk reduction: Even a modest weight loss reduces the risk of other chronic diseases. Importantly, women who are aware of the link between elevated BMI and BC risk are more likely to participate in weight loss interventions.[80]

The Impact of Risk Assessment on Management Options

Endocrine prophylaxis reduces the risk of ER+ disease by 50% to 86%. It also reduces the risk of benign disease and biopsy frequency. Endocrine therapies, however, have side effects and adverse events. The American Society of Clinical Oncology and the United States Preventive Services Task Force note that the women most likely to benefit are those with a 5-year risk of at least 3%, usually calculated with the BCRAT, or a 10-year risk of at least 5% using IBIS.[62,81] Patient uptake of endocrine prophylaxis is low, but women who are aware of their risk status are more likely to opt in.[82]

These risk calculations also drive screening, which reduces mortality and morbidity. Those with a lifetime risk of 20% or higher, for instance benefit from the addition of breast MRI to annual mammography. The FHx-dependent calculators, especially IBIS, BRCAPRO, and CanRisk, are excellent tools for identifying women eligible for HR screening.[4,83,84]

CHALLENGES AND OPPORTUNITIES

We need to identify HR women before they should start screening, to optimize early detection and utilize the opportunity for risk-reducing therapy. Some women, including Ashkenazi Jews who (have a 1 in 40 chance of carrying a BRCA mutation) and Black women (who are significantly more likely to be diagnosed with BC before the age of 40 years), need risk assessment well before the age of 40 years.[4]

While it is beyond the scope of this chapter to discuss barriers to enhanced screening and risk-reducing therapies, a few points deserve mention. People of color are more likely to present with advanced disease, less likely to participate in screening, less likely to be offered genetic assessment, and more likely to die from cancer. Beyond race, other factors related to disparities include geography, socioeconomic status, insurance status, and gender identity. Unfortunately, HR screening may be out of financial reach for patients with substantial out-of-pocket costs or those limited by barriers like transportation needs. Nonbinary individuals may not be offered assigned sex-appropriate screening or may be unwelcome in those environments.[3,85,86]

SUMMARY

Patients can only benefit from HR screening and management if they are aware of their risk status and their options and can access those options. We have excellent tools for identifying HR patients, but we need to reach traditionally underserved populations and ensure their access to these services.

*We recognize that gender identity may differ from sex assigned at birth. For the purposes of this chapter, "women" refers to individuals assigned female sex at birth.

CLINICS CARE POINTS

- Women with a lifetime breast cancer risk of ≥20% are considered "high risk" and benefit from the addition of screening breast MRI to annual mammography. Family history-based tools like IBIS, BRCAPRO, and CanRisk are the best risk models to assess a patient's eligibility for high-risk screening.
- Women with a 5-year breast cancer risk of ≥1.7% are eligible for endocrine prophylaxis; those with a 5-year risk of ≥3% or a 10-year risk ≥5% are most likely to benefit. Based on professional society guidelines and their use in clinical trials, BCRAT, BCSC, and IBIS are the best risk models to assess a patient's eligibility for endocrine prophylaxis.
- Patient awareness of high-risk status improves their adherence to screening recommendations.
- Women can lower their breast cancer risk by maintaining a healthy BMI, being physically active, eating a healthy diet, and limiting alcohol use.

DISCLOSURE

The authors have nothing to disclose.

REFERENCES

1. NCI. National Cancer Institute: Cancer Statistics. Available at: https://www.cancer.gov/about-cancer/understanding/statistics#:~:text=The%20most%20common%20cancers%20(listed,endometrial%20cancer%2C%20leukemia%2C%20pancreatic%20cancer. Accessed January 29, 2023.
2. Duffy SW, Tabár L, Yen AM, et al. Mammography screening reduces rates of advanced and fatal breast cancers: Results in 549,091 women. Cancer 2020; 126(13):2971–9.
3. Monticciolo DL, Malak SF, Friedewald SM, et al. Breast cancer screening recommendations inclusive of all women at average risk: update from the ACR and Society of Breast Imaging. J Am Coll Radiol 2021;18(9):1280–8.
4. Monticciolo DL, Newell MS, Moy L, et al. Breast cancer screening in women at higher-than-average risk: recommendations from the ACR. J Am Coll Radiol 2018;15(3 Pt A):408–14.

5. Ellington TD, Miller JW, Henley SJ, et al. Trends in breast cancer incidence, by race, ethnicity, and age among women aged ≥20 years - United States, 1999-2018. MMWR Morb Mortal Wkly Rep 2022;71(2):43–7.

6. Baquet CR, Mishra SI, Commiskey P, et al. Breast cancer epidemiology in blacks and whites: disparities in incidence, mortality, survival rates and histology. J Natl Med Assoc 2008;100(5):480–8.

7. Travis LB, Hill D, Dores GM, et al. Cumulative absolute breast cancer risk for young women treated for Hodgkin lymphoma. J Natl Cancer Inst 2005;97(19): 1428–37.

8. Inskip PD, Sigurdson AJ, Veiga L, et al. Radiation-related new primary solid cancers in the childhood cancer survivor study: comparative radiation dose response and modification of treatment effects. Int J Radiat Oncol Biol Phys 2016;94(4):800–7.

9. Veiga LH, Curtis RE, Morton LM, et al. Association of breast cancer risk after childhood cancer with radiation dose to the breast and anthracycline use: a report from the Childhood Cancer Survivor Study. JAMA Pediatr 2019;173(12): 1171–9.

10. Atakpa EC, Thorat MA, Cuzick J, et al. Mammographic density, endocrine therapy and breast cancer risk: a prognostic and predictive biomarker review. Cochrane Database Syst Rev 2021;10(10):CD013091.

11. Cuzick J, Warwick J, Pinney E, et al. Tamoxifen-induced reduction in mammographic density and breast cancer risk reduction: a nested case-control study. J Natl Cancer Inst 2011;103(9):744–52.

12. Hartmann LC, Sellers TA, Frost MH, et al. Benign breast disease and the risk of breast cancer. N Engl J Med 2005;353(3):229–37.

13. Wen HY, Brogi E. Lobular Carcinoma in situ. Surg Pathol Clin 2018;11(1):123–45.

14. London SJ, Connolly JL, Schnitt SJ, et al. A prospective study of benign breast disease and the risk of breast cancer. JAMA 1992;267(7):941–4.

15. Graffeo R, Rana HQ, Conforti F, et al. Moderate penetrance genes complicate genetic testing for breast cancer diagnosis: ATM, CHEK2, BARD1 and RAD51D. Breast 2022;65:32–40.

16. National Comprehensive Cancer Network Clinical Practice Guidelines in Oncology: Genetic/Familial High-Risk Assessment: Breast, Ovarian, and Pancreatic Version 2.2023. Available at: https://www.nccn.org/professionals/physician_gls/pdf/genetics_bop.pdf. Accessed January 29, 2023.

17. Lowry KP, Geuzinge HA, Stout NK, et al. Breast cancer screening strategies for women with ATM, CHEK2, and PALB2 pathogenic variants: a comparative modeling analysis. JAMA Oncol 2022;8(4):587–96.

18. Gail MH, Brinton LA, Byar DP, et al. Projecting individualized probabilities of developing breast cancer for white females who are being examined annually. J Natl Cancer Inst 1989;81(24):1879–86.

19. Costantino JP, Gail MH, Pee D, et al. Validation studies for models projecting the risk of invasive and total breast cancer incidence. J Natl Cancer Inst 1999;91(18): 1541–8.

20. National Cancer Institute: Breast Cancer Risk Assessment Tool. Available at: https://bcrisktool.cancer.gov/. Accessed January 29, 2023.

21. Banegas MP, John EM, Slattery ML, et al. Projecting individualized absolute invasive breast cancer risk in US Hispanic Women. J Natl Cancer Inst 2017;109(2). https://doi.org/10.1093/jnci/djw215.

22. Gail MH, Costantino JP, Pee D, et al. Projecting individualized absolute invasive breast cancer risk in African American women. J Natl Cancer Inst 2007;99(23):

1782–92 [published correction appears in J Natl Cancer Inst. 2008 Aug 6;100(15):1118] [published correction appears in J Natl Cancer Inst. 2008 Mar 5;100(5):373].

23. Matsuno RK, Costantino JP, Ziegler RG, et al. Projecting individualized absolute invasive breast cancer risk in Asian and Pacific Islander American women. J Natl Cancer Inst 2011;103(12):951–61.

24. Pankratz VS, Hartmann LC, Degnim AC, et al. Assessment of the accuracy of the Gail model in women with atypical hyperplasia. J Clin Oncol 2008;26(33):5374–9.

25. Wang X, Huang Y, Li L, et al. Assessment of performance of the Gail model for predicting breast cancer risk: a systematic review and meta-analysis with trial sequential analysis. Breast Cancer Res 2018;20(1):18.

26. Tice JA, Cummings SR, Ziv E, et al. Mammographic breast density and the Gail model for breast cancer risk prediction in a screening population. Breast Cancer Res Treat 2005;94(2):115–22.

27. Tice JA, Cummings SR, Smith-Bindman R, et al. Using clinical factors and mammographic breast density to estimate breast cancer risk: development and validation of a new predictive model. Ann Intern Med 2008;148(5):337–47.

28. Tice JA, Miglioretti DL, Li CS, et al. Breast Density and Benign Breast Disease: Risk Assessment to Identify Women at High Risk of Breast Cancer. J Clin Oncol 2015;33(28):3137–43.

29. Tice JA, Bissell MCS, Miglioretti DL, et al. Validation of the breast cancer surveillance consortium model of breast cancer risk. Breast Cancer Res Treat 2019; 175(2):519–23.

30. Breast Cancer Surveillance Consotium Risk Calculator. Available at: https://tools. bcsc-scc.org/BC5yearRisk/calculator.htm. Accessed May 20, 2023.

31. Tyrer J, Duffy SW, Cuzick J. A breast cancer prediction model incorporating familial and personal risk factors. Stat Med 2004;23(7):1111–30. https://doi.org/10. 1002/sim.1668.

32. IBIS Breast Cancer Risk Evaluation Tool, Available at: https://ems-trials.org/ riskevaluator/. Accessed January 29, 2023.

33. Brentnall AR, Cuzick J. Risk models for breast cancer and their validation. Stat Sci 2020;35(1):14–30.

34. Boughey JC, Hartmann LC, Anderson SS, et al. Evaluation of the Tyrer-Cuzick (International Breast Cancer Intervention Study) model for breast cancer risk prediction in women with atypical hyperplasia. J Clin Oncol 2010;28(22):3591–6.

35. Valero MG, Zabor EC, Park A, et al. The Tyrer-Cuzick model inaccurately predicts invasive breast cancer risk in women with LCIS. Ann Surg Oncol 2020;27(3): 736–40.

36. Lo LL, Milne RL, Liao Y, et al. Validation of the IBIS breast cancer risk evaluator for women with lobular carcinoma in-situ. Br J Cancer 2018;119(1):36–9.

37. Cintolo-Gonzalez JA, Braun D, Blackford AL, et al. Breast cancer risk models: a comprehensive overview of existing models, validation, and clinical applications. Breast Cancer Res Treat 2017;164(2):263–84.

38. Kurian AW, Hughes E, Simmons T, et al. Performance of the IBIS/Tyrer-Cuzick model of breast cancer risk by race and ethnicity in the Women's Health Initiative. Cancer 2021;127(20):3742–50.

39. Maas P, Barrdahl M, Joshi AD, et al. Breast cancer risk from modifiable and nonmodifiable risk factors among white women in the United States. JAMA Oncol 2016;2(10):1295–302.

40. Antoniou AC, Pharoah PD, McMullan G, et al. A comprehensive model for familial breast cancer incorporating BRCA1, BRCA2 and other genes. Br J Cancer 2002; 86(1):76–83.
41. Antoniou AC, Cunningham AP, Peto J, et al. The BOADICEA model of genetic susceptibility to breast and ovarian cancers: updates and extensions. Br J Cancer 2008;98(8):1457–66.
42. Lee AJ, Cunningham AP, Tischkowitz M, et al. Incorporating truncating variants in PALB2, CHEK2, and ATM into the BOADICEA breast cancer risk model. Genet Med 2016;18(12):1190–8.
43. Mavaddat N, Ficorella L, Carver T, et al. Incorporating alternative Polygenic Risk Scores into the BOADICEA breast cancer risk prediction model. Cancer Epidemiol Biomarkers Prev 2023. https://doi.org/10.1158/1055-9965.EPI-22-0756.
44. CanRisk. Available at: https://www.canrisk.org/. Accessed February 10, 2023.
45. Yang X, Eriksson M, Czene K, et al. Prospective validation of the BOADICEA multifactorial breast cancer risk prediction model in a large prospective cohort study. J Med Genet 2022;59(12):1196–205. https://doi.org/10.1136/jmg-2022-108806.
46. Claus EB, Schildkraut JM, Thompson WD, et al. The genetic attributable risk of breast and ovarian cancer. Cancer 1996;77(11):2318–24.
47. McCarthy AM, Guan Z, Welch M, et al. Performance of breast cancer risk-assessment models in a large mammography cohort. J Natl Cancer Inst 2020; 112(5):489–97. https://doi.org/10.1093/jnci/djz177.
48. Parmigiani G, Berry D, Aguilar O. Determining carrier probabilities for breast cancer-susceptibility genes BRCA1 and BRCA2. Am J Hum Genet 1998;62(1): 145–58. https://doi.org/10.1086/301670.
49. Mazzola E, Blackford A, Parmigiani G, et al. Recent enhancements to the genetic risk prediction model BRCAPRO. Cancer Inform 2015;14(Suppl 2):147–57. https://doi.org/10.4137/CIN.S17292.
50. Ask2Me: The All Syndromes Known to Man Evaluator, 2023. Available at: https:// ask2me.org/. Accessed January 29, 2023.
51. Braun D, Yang J, Griffin M, et al. A Clinical decision support tool to predict cancer risk for commonly tested cancer-related germline mutations. J Genet Couns 2018;27(5):1187–99. https://doi.org/10.1007/s10897-018-0238-4.
52. Gastounioti A, Desai S, Ahluwalia VS, et al. Artificial intelligence in mammographic phenotyping of breast cancer risk: a narrative review. Breast Cancer Re 2022;24(1):14. https://doi.org/10.1186/s13058-022-01509-z.
53. Ho WK, Tai MC, Dennis J, et al. Polygenic risk scores for prediction of breast cancer risk in Asian populations. Genet Med 2022;24(3):586–600. https://doi.org/10. 1016/j.gim.2021.11.008.
54. Gao G, Zhao F, Ahearn TU, et al. Polygenic risk scores for prediction of breast cancer risk in women of African ancestry: a cross-ancestry approach. Hum Mol Genet 2022;31(18):3133–43. https://doi.org/10.1093/hmg/ddac102.
55. Kramer I, Hooning MJ, Mavaddat N, et al. Breast cancer polygenic risk score and contralateral breast cancer risk. Am J Hum Genet 2020;107(5):837–48. https:// doi.org/10.1016/j.ajhg.2020.09.001.
56. Mavaddat N, Michailidou K, Dennis J, et al. Polygenic risk scores for prediction of breast cancer and breast cancer subtypes. Am J Hum Genet 2019;104(1):21–34. https://doi.org/10.1016/j.ajhg.2018.11.002.
57. Li SX, Milne RL, Nguyen-Dumont T, et al. Prospective evaluation over 15 years of six breast cancer risk models. Cancers 2021;13(20). https://doi.org/10.3390/cancers13205194.

58. Coopey SB, Acar A, Griffin M, et al. The impact of patient age on breast cancer risk prediction models. Breast J 2018;24(4):592–8.
59. McCarthy AM, Liu Y, Ehsan S, et al. Validation of breast cancer risk models by race/ethnicity, family history and molecular subtypes. Cancers 2021;14(1). https://doi.org/10.3390/cancers14010045.
60. National Comprehensive Cancer Network Clinical Practice Guidelines in Oncology: Breast Cancer Screening and Diagnosis version 1.2022. Available at: https://www.nccn.org/professionals/physician_gls/pdf/breast-screening.pdf. Accessed January 29, 2023.
61. National Comprehensive Cancer Network Clinical Practice Guidelines in Oncology: Breast Cancer Risk Reduction Version 1.2023. Available at: https://www.nccn.org/professionals/physician_gls/pdf/breast_risk.pdf. Accessed January 29, 2023.
62. Visvanathan K, Fabian CJ, Bantug E, et al. Use of endocrine therapy for breast cancer risk reduction: ASCO clinical practice guideline update. J Clin Oncol 2019;37(33):3152–65.
63. Howell A, Anderson AS, Clarke RB, et al. Risk determination and prevention of breast cancer. Breast Cancer Res 2014;16(5):446.
64. Korn AR, Reedy J, Brockton NT, et al. The 2018 World Cancer Research Fund/American Institute for Cancer Research Score and Cancer Risk: a longitudinal analysis in the NIH-AARP Diet and Health Study. Cancer Epidemiol Biomarkers Prev 2022;31(10):1983–92.
65. Lynch BM, Neilson HK, Friedenreich CM. Physical activity and breast cancer prevention. Recent Results Cancer Res 2011;186:13–42.
66. Collaborative Group on Hormonal Factors in Breast Cancer. Type and timing of menopausal hormone therapy and breast cancer risk: individual participant meta-analysis of the worldwide epidemiological evidence. Lancet 2019; 394(10204):1159–68.
67. Chen CL, Weiss NS, Newcomb P, et al. Hormone replacement therapy in relation to breast cancer. JAMA 2002;287(6):734–41.
68. Chlebowski RT, Anderson GL, Aragaki AK, et al. Association of menopausal hormone therapy with breast cancer incidence and mortality during long-term follow-up of the Women's Health Initiative randomized clinical trials. JAMA 2020;324(4): 369–80.
69. Million Women Study Collaborators. Breast cancer and hormone-replacement therapy in the Million Women Study. Lancet 2003;362(9382):419–27 [published correction appears in Lancet. 2003 Oct 4;362(9390):1160].
70. Buja A, Pierbon M, Lago L, et al. Breast cancer primary prevention and diet: an umbrella review. Int J Environ Res Public Health 2020;17(13). https://doi.org/10.3390/ijerph17134731.
71. Albuquerque RC, Baltar VT, Marchioni DM. Breast cancer and dietary patterns: a systematic review. Nutr Rev 2014;72(1):1–17.
72. Wei Y, Lv J, Guo Y, et al. Soy intake and breast cancer risk: a prospective study of 300,000 Chinese women and a dose-response meta-analysis. Eur J Epidemiol 2020;35(6):567–78.
73. Messina MJ, Wood CE. Soy isoflavones, estrogen therapy, and breast cancer risk: analysis and commentary. Nutr J 2008;7:17.
74. Dong JY, Zhang L, He K, et al. Dairy consumption and risk of breast cancer: a meta-analysis of prospective cohort studies. Breast Cancer Res Treat 2011; 127(1):23–31.
75. Starek-Świechowicz B, Budziszewska B, Starek A. Alcohol and breast cancer. Pharmacol Rep 2023;75(1):69–84.

76. Chen WY, Rosner B, Hankinson SE, et al. Moderate alcohol consumption during adult life, drinking patterns, and breast cancer risk. JAMA 2011;306(17):1884–90.
77. Suzuki R, Iwasaki M, Inoue M, et al. Body weight at age 20 years, subsequent weight change and breast cancer risk defined by estrogen and progesterone receptor status–the Japan public health center-based prospective study. Int J Cancer 2011;129(5):1214–24.
78. Renehan AG, Pegington M, Harvie MN, et al. Young adulthood body mass index, adult weight gain and breast cancer risk: the PROCAS Study (United Kingdom). Br J Cancer 2020;122(10):1552–61.
79. Teras LR, Patel AV, Wang M, et al. Sustained weight loss and risk of breast cancer in women 50 years and older: a pooled analysis of prospective data. J Natl Cancer Inst 2020;112(9):929–37.
80. Burkbauer L, Goldbach M, Huang C, et al. Awareness of link between obesity and breast cancer risk is associated with willingness to participate in weight loss intervention. Breast Cancer Res Treat 2022;194(3):541–50.
81. Owens DK, Davidson KW, Krist AH, et al. Medication use to reduce risk of breast cancer: US Preventive Services Task Force Recommendation Statement. JAMA 2019;322(9):857–67.
82. Huilgol YS, Keane H, Shieh Y, et al. Elevated risk thresholds predict endocrine risk-reducing medication use in the Athena screening registry. NPJ Breast Cancer 2021;7(1):102.
83. US Preventative Services Task Force. Breast Cancer: Screening, Available at: https://www.uspreventiveservicestaskforce.org/uspstf/recommendation/breast-cancer-screening. Accessed January 29, 2023.
84. American Cancer Society Recommendations for the Early Detection of Breast Cancer. Available at: https://www.cancer.org/cancer/breast-cancer/screening-tests-and-early-detection/american-cancer-society-recommendations-for-the-early-detection-of-breast-cancer.html. Accessed January 29, 2023.
85. Stringer-Reasor EM, Elkhanany A, Khoury K, et al. Disparities in breast cancer associated with African American identity. Am Soc Clin Oncol Educ Book 2021;41:e29–46.
86. Khan A, Rogers CR, Kennedy CD, et al. Genetic evaluation for hereditary cancer syndromes among African Americans: a critical review. Oncol 2022;27(4):285–91.

Psychological Aspects of Breast Cancer

Jennifer Kim Penberthy, PhD[a],*, Anne Louise Stewart, MD[a],
Caroline F. Centeno, BS[a], David R. Penberthy, MD, MBA[b]

KEYWORDS

- Breast cancer • Distress • Depression • Anxiety • Psychotherapy

KEY POINTS

- Anxiety, depression, cognitive impairment, adjustment disorders, sleep disturbance and associated fatigue, posttraumatic stress, body image issues, and sexual dysfunction are the most frequently described psychological symptoms and disorders in women with breast cancer.
- Distress screening and psychological assessment is used to identify patients with breast cancer requiring therapeutic support and intervention throughout the treatment course.
- Psychotherapeutic approaches have proved effective in managing psychological symptoms and disorders in patients diagnosed with breast cancer.
- Addressing psychological symptoms can help improve compliance with treatment, outcomes, psychological symptoms, and quality of life.
- Patients diagnosed with breast cancer should be supported with these techniques during the entire oncological trajectory.

INTRODUCTION
Prevalence of Breast Cancer

Breast cancer is a complex and heterogeneous group of diseases in terms of occurrence, impact, therapeutic response, and clinical outcomes. It is the most commonly occurring cancer in women and the most common cancer overall. More than 2.26 million new cases of breast cancer were reported in women globally in 2020 alone. At the end of that same year, there were 7.8 million women alive diagnosed with breast cancer in the past 5 years. In the United States, breast cancer is the most common malignancy diagnosed in women, with an estimated 290,560 cases diagnosed in

This article previously appeared in Psychiatric Clinics volume 46 issue 3 September 2023.
[a] Department of Psychiatry & Neurobehavioral Sciences, UVA Cancer Center, University of Virginia School of Medicine & Health System, PO Box 800623, Charlottesville, VA 22908, USA;
[b] Department of Radiation Oncology, Penn State Cancer Institute, Penn State Health Milton S. Hershey College of Medicine, Hershey, PA, USA
* Corresponding author.
E-mail address: jkp2n@UVAHealth.org

Clinics Collections 14 (2024) 109–128
https://doi.org/10.1016/j.ccol.2024.02.011
2352-7986/24/© 2024 Elsevier Inc. All rights reserved.

2022 and 43,780 deaths from the disease in the same year.[1] One in eight women will develop breast cancer in her lifetime.

Breast cancer occurs worldwide and can occur at any age after puberty and with increasing rates in later life.[2] Breast cancer represents the number two oncological cause of death and 25% of all new cancer diagnoses in women, with the highest incidence in the age range from 55 to 64 years.[2] Breast cancer is a rare malignancy in men, accounting for less than 1% of all cases of cancer.[3] Rates of breast cancer in the United States vary by race and ethnicity. Non-Hispanic white women (137.6 per 100,000) and non-Hispanic Black women (129.6 per 100,000) have the highest incidence of breast cancer (rate of new breast cancer cases) overall. Hispanic women have the lowest incidence (99.9 per 100,000). Incidence rates for non-Hispanic Asian and Pacific Islanders and non-Hispanic American Indian/Alaska Natives are in the middle at 106.9 and 111.3 per 100,000 cases, respectively.[4]

Despite the growing and aging global population, and the increasing number of new breast cancer diagnoses, survival rates have improved due to advancements in early detection and treatment.[5] Women with a history of breast cancer are the largest group of cancer survivors in high-income countries, and as of January 2022, there were more than 3.8 million women with a history of breast cancer in the United States, which include women currently being treated and women who have finished treatment.[6] Thus, this growing population of women warrants our attention and our efforts to better understand their stressors and mental health needs.

Most women diagnosed with breast cancer experience at least some psychosocial distress during the course of their breast cancer diagnosis and treatment. The level of distress varies from woman to woman and over the course of diagnosis and treatment. Cancer-related distress can be expected to dissipate with time for most of the women diagnosed with cancer. For others, however, such distress may interfere substantially with their psychological well-being, quality of life, physical comfort, and the ability to make appropriate treatment decisions and adhere to treatment.[7] Psychosocial distress can be related to physical problems such as illness or disability, psychological problems, family issues, and social concerns such as those related to employment, insurance, and supportive care access. In this chapter, the authors focus on the *psychological impact* of the diagnosis and treatment of breast cancer in women specifically, including psychological symptoms and disorders. They also explore research regarding effective treatments.

Definitions

Breast cancer arises in the lining cells of the ducts or lobules in the glandular tissue of the breast. Initially, the cancerous growth is confined to the duct or lobule ("in situ") where it generally causes no symptoms and has minimal potential for spread. Over time, these in situ cancers may progress and invade the surrounding breast tissue, spreading to the nearby lymph nodes or other organs in the body. If a woman dies of breast cancer, it is typically because of widespread metastasis.[8]

Breast cancer is not a transmissible or infectious disease. Unlike some cancers that have infection-related causes, such as human papillomavirus infection and cervical cancer, there are no known viral or bacterial infections linked to the development of breast cancer. In fact, about half of breast cancers develop in women who have no identifiable breast cancer risk factor other than gender (female) and age (over 40 years). Certain factors increase the risk of breast cancer, including increasing age, obesity, harmful use of alcohol, family history of breast cancer, history of radiation exposure, reproductive history (such as age that menstrual periods began and age at first pregnancy), tobacco use, and unopposed estrogen over time, including postmenopausal hormone therapy.[9] Pregnancy may lower risk due to the interruption of the stimulatory effects of estrogen. Patients with breast cancer who know that they are at increased risk of having hereditary breast cancer may experience heightened levels of psychological distress.[10]

Modern breast cancer treatments are varied and highly effective, especially when the disease is identified early and the patient is adherent to treatment. Typical treatment of breast cancer consists of a combination of surgical removal, radiation therapy, and medication such as hormonal therapy, chemotherapy, or targeted biological therapy. These treatments target the microscopic cancer that has spread from the breast tumor through the blood. The combination of treatments prevents cancer growth and saves lives and can be physically and psychologically stressful to endure. Psychological and physical symptoms can interfere with well-being and treatment compliance[11] and are therefore very important to address.

BACKGROUND
Psychological Impact

Breast cancer diagnosis and treatments are often associated with significant psychological distress. This distress negatively affects psychosocial adjustment to the disease process and health outcomes.[12] Importantly, increased distress in patients with breast cancer has been associated with poorer physical and mental health during treatment.[11]

Being given the diagnosis of breast cancer is often overwhelmingly distressing in and of itself and can create an enormous stress for the patient who now has to deal with new and challenging issues of treatment choices.[13] Undergoing testing, receiving the diagnosis, understanding the prognosis, undergoing treatments, handling side effects, managing possible relapses, and facing an uncertain future are all stages of a stressful process that can cause psychological distress and negatively affect psychological health and well-being, including quality of life, treatment compliance, and outcome.

This heightened stress can lead to or worsen existing anxiety, depression, or other psychological symptoms. Many patients experience multiple concurrent psychological issues during their cancer care trajectory. The most prevalent psychological symptoms in patients with breast cancer include anxiety, depression, impaired cognitive function, as well as physical symptoms such as pain, sleep disturbances, sexual dysfunction, and fatigue, which can trigger fear of death or recurrence, altered body image, and diminished well-being.[14-18]

Patients who receive the diagnosis of breast cancer may progress through stages of coping with the news. These stages include difficulty accepting the diagnosis, failing to acknowledge the seriousness of the situation, and feeling angry or becoming tearful and distraught. Eventually these phases of shock, denial, and emotional reaction typically give way to efforts to adjust, a desire to seek treatment, and hope for health. It is important for providers to understand these stages in their patients and not assume that a patient's emotional response is fixed or even necessarily unhealthy. Allowing time for the patient to process the news of their diagnosis and evaluate treatment options is an important and ongoing part of effective treatment and support.[18]

Different psychological issues arise in different phases of treatment. These phases coincide with aspects of the clinical course of the illness and related treatments. Studies show highest distress at transition points in treatment: at the time of diagnosis, awaiting treatment, during and on completion of treatment, at follow-up visits, at time of recurrence, and at time of treatment failure.[19] In addition, multiple variables affect distress over the course of diagnosis and treatment. These variables include age, sex, personality, and variables related to the impact of treatment such as side effects, social support, and socioeconomic status.[19] Overall, approximately 30% of women show significant distress at some point during the illness, and the number is greater in women with recurrent disease whose family members are also distressed.[20]

Cancer treatment approach can affect symptom presentation. In patients who undergo surgical procedures for breast cancer, the rate of significant psychological dysfunction ranges from 30% to 47%, without any significant difference between those who undergo breast-conserving surgery versus a modified radical mastectomy. Significantly, 20% to 45% continue to meet criteria for their psychiatric disorder 1 year postsurgery, and 10% endorse ongoing disorders 6 years after their operation.[21] Research indicates that 40% of patients with breast cancer report anxiety while undergoing radiotherapy, and this percentage remains stable throughout the course of radiation.[22] Chemotherapy is one of the most stressful aspects of a breast cancer diagnosis, with up to 90% of patients reporting some level of distress during their course of chemotherapy.[23] Chemotherapies can lead to poor functioning, fatigue, depression, anger, and mood disturbance posttreatment.[24] Much of the distress surrounding chemotherapy stems from the anticipation and experiences of unpleasant physical side effects,[25] which are related to specific chemotherapy agents used.

Why Identifying Psychological Symptoms Is Important

The link between psychological and physical health in patients with breast cancer is well documented. Anxiety can manifest as physical symptoms such as muscle tension or sleep disturbance, which may increase the risk of depression.[26] For patients with breast cancer diagnosed with depressive symptoms, mortality rates were found to be nearly 26 times higher and 39 times higher in patients diagnosed with major depression. Importantly, a decrease in depression symptoms was associated with longer survival.[27,28] Diagnosis and treatment of psychological symptoms and disorders improves patients' adherence to therapy and quality of life.[29] Adherence to treatment is important because the effectiveness of breast cancer therapies depends on receiving the full course of treatment. Partial treatment is less likely to lead to a positive outcome.[30]

Distress Screening and Psychological Assessment

It is important to identify psychological stressors in order to plan a proper treatment approach. A full discussion of all psychological assessment tools is beyond the scope of this chapter. A comprehensive literature review published in *Seminars in Oncology Nursing* concluded that psychological health in patients with cancer was determined by a balance between the stress and burden posed by the cancer experience and the resources available for coping.[31] For all of these reasons, screening, assessing, and treating psychological symptoms and disorders is of utmost importance in this patient population.

The Institute of Medicine's 2008 report, Cancer Care for the Whole Patient: Meeting Psychosocial Health Needs, called attention to the importance of addressing the psychological problems associated with cancer and noted that leaving these needs unmet could result in decreased well-being and reduced treatment adherence and threaten patients' return to health.[32] Recognizing this, the National Comprehensive Cancer Network issued a consensus statement recommending distress screening and management as a standard of care within oncology health services delivery. In 2012, the American College of Surgeons Commission on Cancer (CoC) added distress screening to its accreditation standards for cancer programs; this requires development and implementation of a process to integrate and monitor on-site psychosocial distress screening and referral for the provision of psychosocial care.[32]

Distress, defined as the overburden or the inability to cope with negative affect–eliciting events, exists along a continuum, ranging from feelings of vulnerability, sadness, and fears to problems that can become disabling. Distress may be experienced as a reaction to the disease and its treatment and also as a result of the consequences of the disease on social functioning.[33] Many of the instruments used to assess patients with breast cancer attempt to measure what is referred to as health-related quality of life (HRQOL).[34,35] HRQOL assessments are self-rated subjective evaluations of health and well-being generally in at least 4 areas: psychological functioning, physical functioning, social functioning, and symptoms and side effects. In this chapter the authors focus on the areas of psychological functioning.

An instrument commonly used to assess psychological distress is the Distress Thermometer and Problem List from the National Comprehensive Cancer Network. The Distress Thermometer itself is a one-item, 11-point Likert scale represented on a visual graphic of a thermometer that ranges from 0 (no distress) to 10 (extreme distress), with which patients indicate their level of distress over the course of the prior week.[36] Specific problems encountered can also be endorsed.

Specific symptoms can be assessed by more specialized assessments including the Hospital Anxiety and Depression scale,[37] the Short Form-36 of the Medical Outcomes Study,[38] Brief Symptom Inventory,[39] Cancer Rehabilitation Evaluation System tool,[40] the Functional Assessment of Cancer Therapy-Breast,[41] and the Quality of Life Breast Cancer Instrument.[42] Distress screening followed by targeted assessment of relevant symptoms with standardized, valid, and reliable psychological assessment tools is recommended in order to create an appropriate and effective treatment intervention.

Inconsistency in research methodology, including use of various assessment tools, some of which are not validated or reliable, has led to differing reports of symptoms and their impact. Distress and psychological assessment in patients with breast cancer has made progress, but caution is recommended in evaluating the research.[43]

DISCUSSION
Common Psychological Symptoms

Although research demonstrates common psychological symptoms that occur in patients with breast cancer, it is important to remember the wide variability across individual women. The psychosocial impact of breast cancer must be understood in the context of multiple issues that affect women's coping, quality of life, and well-being, including socioeconomic and cultural factors, social support, access to health care, and the presence of other chronic illness or life crises. In addition, there are differing psychological challenges that coincide with clinical course of the illness and related treatments. With these caveats in mind, the authors briefly review the research regarding common psychological symptoms (**Table 1**).

Adjustment Disorders

Problems in adjusting to a breast cancer diagnosis or treatment may lead to significant distress beyond what is normally seen in response to such stressor and lead to functional impairment, resulting in a diagnosis of adjustment disorder. Adjustment disorders can be defined as with depression or anxiety or both. Recent research found that 38.6% of patients with breast cancer met criteria for adjustment disorder with depression.[44] Another 2020 study found that 37.5% of patients with breast cancer

Table 1
Common psychological symptoms and estimates of prevalence in breast cancer

Symptom	Prevalence (%)
PTSD	0–32
Anxiety	10–30
Depression	10–30
Cognitive impairment	12–82
Sexual dysfunction	43–83
Sleep disturbances	50–90
Body image disturbances	75–92

met criteria for adjustment disorder symptoms during the course of treatment and up to 5 years posttreatment.[45] Onset of an adjustment disorder can occur at any time during the cancer continuum but is most likely, as are many symptoms, to present during transition points, where new stressors ensue. Making a diagnosis of adjustment disorder can be challenging, as it is can seem similar to other depressive and anxiety disorders.

Anxiety and Depression

Research shows that about one-third of patients with breast cancer display symptoms of anxiety and depression,[46] and these numbers were found to be even higher during COVID, with one study reporting more than half of patients with breast cancer suffered from depression (51.2%), anxiety (62.8%), sleep problems (51.2%), and posttraumatic stress disorder (PTSD) symptoms (35.3%).[47] Clinically relevant symptoms of anxiety and depression are common at the initial diagnosis and during active treatment, when treatment side effects may have more of a negative impact.[48] High prevalence of depressive symptoms and anxiety have also been observed in survivorship,[49] with one study finding depressive symptoms persisting for at least 2 years after diagnosis in 20% of women.[50]

Anxiety is common in patients with breast cancer,[13] with rates ranging from 10% to 30%. Anxiety may be related to anticipation of negative outcomes and the uncertainty about the future. Anxiety is also frequently related to concern over recurrence and the worry of treatment side effects during and after treatments.[51] Recent findings suggest that anxiety is more prevalent than depression, although other studies report comparable rates of between 10% and 30%.[46]

The rate of depression in patients with breast cancer is estimated to be between 10% and 30%, depending on the study population, study design, and choice of depression measure.[13] Depressive symptoms have been shown to negatively affect compliance with treatment regime, reduce patient quality of life and self-care, and decrease immunity and chances of survival.[52] Diagnosing depression can be challenging in patients with cancer because symptoms of depression overlap with physical symptoms related to treatment. Chronic fatigue and decreased social interactions are also common responses to breast cancer that can affect depressive symptoms.[53] Research indicates that women with a primary breast cancer diagnosis remain vulnerable to psychological disorders for many years,[54] highlighting the significant psychological impact of this medical condition.

Cancer-Related Cognitive Impairment

Cognitive difficulties in patients with breast cancer began to appear in the literature in the 1990s,[55] associated with the increasing use of postoperative adjuvant chemotherapy. Because symptoms were more frequently reported in women who received very high-dose chemotherapy, the concern was that cognitive impairment might become a dose-limiting treatment toxicity. Fortunately, over the past 20 years, there has been a deescalation of both the intensity and generalized use of adjuvant chemotherapy in patients with breast cancer. Because of this initial association of cognitive impairment with chemotherapy treatment, early research focused on what was referred to as "chemobrain."

The reported prevalence of cognitive impairment following treatment of breast cancer is somewhat variable. There was preliminary evidence of measurable neurocognitive effects among patients with breast cancer who were exposed to chemotherapy. Subsequent studies have documented cognitive changes before any cancer-directed therapies, as well as in association with other common breast cancer treatments (eg, radiation, endocrine therapy). According to one survey, 77% of patients who received chemotherapy with and without endocrine therapy and 45% who received only endocrine therapy reported cognitive symptoms during or soon after treatment.[56]

A commonly cited range suggests that 12% to 82% of women will experience cognitive impairment as a result of their cancer treatment.[57] This variability may be attributable to a range of patient factors such as age, menopausal status, and education level.[58] Research also demonstrates that cognitive impairment is often present before the start of chemotherapy,[59] potentially arising as a result of cancer itself. The evolving body of research has led to a renaming of the condition as *cancer-related cognitive impairment*. Although symptoms are most commonly reported in close proximity to initial breast cancer treatments, for some patients, symptoms of cognitive impairment can persist for years after treatment completion.[60]

Sleep Disturbances

Similar to other symptoms, the incidence of sleep disturbance, including insomnia, varies across studies depending on the study design and assessment methods, but most studies report that 60% to 90% of patients with breast cancer endorse significant sleep disturbances.[61] This is much higher than in the healthy population. The prevalence of sleep disorders is higher among patients with breast cancer compared with other cancers, possibly due to the impact of menopausal symptoms triggered by this therapy.[62] Insomnia in patients with breast cancer can be associated with various factors such as psychological distress arising from the cancer diagnosis or adverse effects of cancer therapy. Patients who receive adjuvant endocrine therapy remain at increased risk for insomnia because of the occurrence of menopause.[63] Research exploring the prevalence of patients with breast cancer meeting criteria for an insomnia syndrome report rates of 18.6% to 19%.[64]

Body Image Disturbances and Sexual Dysfunction

A woman's body image is conceptualized as the mental representation of her social and psychological experiences and is shaped by her impression and sense of her physical appearance.[65] Breast cancer treatments typically involve significant changes to a woman's body, potentially including disfiguring surgeries, hair loss, and the emotional and physical impact of hormonal changes resulting from the treatments. A recent study reports that 92% of patients with breast cancer after modified radical mastectomy endorsed body image disturbances.[66] Another study examining patients with breast cancer posttreatment reported a prevalence of body image dissatisfaction of 74.8% confidence interval (CI) (65%–82%).[67]

Psychologically, body image disturbance has demonstrated a direct relationship with low self-confidence, weak social relationships, depression, and problems in sexual functioning.[68,69] Sexual dysfunction in patients with breast cancer is commonly reported, with prevalence rates across the globe between 43% and 75%, and average prevalence rates of 66% to 68%, depending on age.[70] These symptoms have been found to exist during treatment and after treatment. Recent research on young women breast cancer survivors showed an incidence rate as high as 83%.[71] Other recent studies showed that 50% to 75% of breast cancer survivors reported persistent sexual dysfunction.[72] In patients with breast cancer with body image disturbance, 73.4% endorse sexual dysfunctions, suggesting that these women constitute a high-risk group.[73] Body image disturbance and sexual dysfunction are a significant problem for most of the patients with breast cancer and must be addressed in order to facilitate improved quality of life.

Acute Stress Disorder and Posttraumatic Stress Disorder

Acute stress disorder (ASD) and PTSD occur in response to a perceived life-threatening trauma and subsequent related symptoms including recurrent and intrusive thoughts of the experiences associated with cancer, feelings of detachment and emotional numbness, increased arousal, sudden outbursts of anger, avoidance of cancer and treatment-related stimuli, and an exaggerated startle response. These symptoms frequently occur in patients with breast cancer, especially posttreatment. Patients may describe constant concerns, nightmares about the treatment, and worries about recurrence of cancer. Acute stress is differentiated from PTSD by the duration of symptoms, which are limited to 1 month. Most of the research conducted are on PTSD.

Subthreshold symptoms are different than meeting full diagnostic criteria for ASD or PTSD, and some of the challenges in the research literature result from a lack of clarity in assessment, treatment phase, and diagnosis of symptoms or disorder. For example, a 2019 study found that greater than 90% of patients with breast cancer experienced posttraumatic stress symptoms after diagnosis, with no significant improvement until 2 years after hospital discharge.[74] However, in a study that examined full criteria for PTSD, researchers found only 2% of patients breast cancer met criteria 1 year after diagnosis.[75] Another study[76] found the prevalence of breast cancer–related PTSD diagnosis to be 8.1%, and a 2016 meta-analysis reported 9.6% of patients with breast cancer in their sample diagnosed with PTSD.[77] In a recent meta-analysis researchers reported PTSD in 10% of women and endorsed that depending on the methods and inclusion criteria of the studies, the incidence of a PTSD diagnosis after the diagnosis of breast cancer varied widely, with some studies reporting up to 32.3%.[78] Additional research report clinically significant levels of PTSD symptoms from 7.3% to 13.8% depending on the assessment and scoring criteria used.[79] In a study from 2013 on a diverse breast cancer population, researchers found that 23% reported symptoms consistent with a diagnosis of PTSD at baseline, 16.5% at first follow-up, and 12.6% at the second follow-up. Persistent PTSD was observed among 12.1% participants. Among participants without PTSD at baseline, 6.6% developed PTSD at the first follow-up interview. Younger age at diagnosis, being black, and being Asian were associated with PTSD.[80]

PSYCHOTHERAPEUTIC APPROACHES

Increased psychological screening and assessment has heightened the need for effective psychological intervention in patients with breast cancer. Women may present with multiple psychological symptoms that can be addressed at the same time. Some specialized interventions have also been developed and studied to address specific symptoms. It is important to recognize that treating one symptom, such as insomnia, may positively affect other symptoms, such as depression or anxiety. Thus, even targeted treatment approaches may impact other symptoms. Ideally, treatment is provided in an integrated system of care. Supportive services are crucial in a comprehensive cancer center and help ensure care is patient-centered and holistic.

With the growing number and types of interventions for breast cancer survivors, it can be difficult to determine which interventions are appropriate for patients. Rather than using diagnostic or medical treatment status as a guide for psychosocial treatment selection, practitioners can be guided by the patient's psychological needs, such as addressing anxiety or coping with adjusting to their bodily changes. These psychological needs can then be mapped onto relevant evidence-based psychological treatments. Interventions can be offered at any point during the course of diagnosis, treatment, and survivorship. The authors briefly review commonly used empirically based psychotherapeutic interventions with recommendations for use when appropriate (**Table 2**).

Psychoeducation

Psychological and emotional support is often given in conjunction with providing education about breast cancer, its diagnosis, treatment, and other aspects of the cancer experience. This support provides comfort, instills confidence, and reduces the stress of illness and of having to think through and decide on treatment options.[81] Given the complexity of breast cancer care, physicians often do not have the time to extensively discuss treatment options and concerns regarding those options. Psychologists and other mental health care professionals can provide additional information, directly address psychosocial concerns, and aid in the shared decision-making process. Psychoeducation is also often a component in supportive and cognitive–behavioral interventions.

Psychoeducational therapy (PET) is an interdisciplinary approach, including an educational program and a psychological intervention.[82] Research supports the efficacy of psychoeducation in improving adaptive coping strategies and quality of life,

Table 2	
Psychological interventions used in patient populations with breast cancer	
Psychological Intervention	**Definition**
Psychoeducational	Focus on providing information about illness in a social and supportive interaction
Cognitive behavioral psychotherapy	Focus on self-monitoring, behavior change, and cognitive restructuring of maladaptive thoughts and beliefs
Mindfulness-based therapy	Focus on self-regulation, present moment awareness, and acceptance of experience without judgment
Supportive-expressive therapy	Focus on social support, especially in the context of encouraging expression of emotion
Meaning-centered psychotherapy	Focus on sense of self and meaning making
Acceptance and commitment therapy	Focus on increasing psychological flexibility and acceptance

reducing depression and anxiety, and increasing treatment compliance and self-efficacy in women with breast cancer.[83]

Cognitive Behavioral Therapy

Cognitive behavioral therapy (CBT) is a widely used evidence-based practice and is focused on improving coping skills and affect. It is based on a combination of the basic principles of behavioral and cognitive psychology and typically has 3 components: self-monitoring, behavior change, and cognitive restructuring of maladaptive thoughts and beliefs.

In a 2016 review, CBT approaches were shown to be effective for treatment of mood, anxiety, sleep, disorders, PTSD, sexual dysfunction and adjustment disorders, as well as treatment-related side effects in patients with breast cancer.[84] In a more recent meta-analyses, CBT was found to be effective in restructuring negative automatic cognitive schemas,[85] and increasing optimism and positive thought, which help to improve the quality of life of patients with breast cancer.[86]

CBT has been found to be effective in managing anxiety and depression,[87] insomnia,[88] fatigue,[89] and menopausal symptoms[90] and improve quality of life and self-esteem.[91] CBT has been also shown to be effective in managing physical symptoms such as pain, headache, irritable bowel syndrome, nausea, and vomiting[92] and thus may help patients with breast cancer suffering from treatment side effects.

Cognitive and Behavioral Cancer Stress Management (CBCSM) is a structured intervention focused on cancer-related stress management that has demonstrated mixed results in outcome studies with patients with breast cancer. In a recent meta-analysis, CBCSM was found to significantly increase relaxation scores, positive affect, decrease serum cortisol, anxiety, depression, thought avoidance, thought intrusion, and negative mood. However, there was no significant impact on reducing stress or mood disturbances.[93]

Mindfulness-Based Therapy

Mindfulness-based approaches focus on helping patients achieve self-regulation, present moment awareness, and acceptance of experience without judgment. These approaches are particularly appropriate for coping with loss of control, general loss, and grief. Research on such interventions shows benefits including decreased distress, improved sleep, reduced fatigue, improved mood, and reduced anxiety.[94,95] Compared with usual care, mindfulness approaches were found superior in decreasing depression and anxiety in patients with breast cancer.[96]

Mindfulness-based cancer recovery (MBCR) is a cancer-specific modification of mindfulness-based stress reduction.[97] Several MBCR clinical trials have shown efficacy in improving mood, quality of life, and reducing stress.[98,99] Recent meta-analyses provide further support for the effectiveness of mindfulness-based interventions in cancer with moderate to large effect sizes. The investigators reported significant reductions in anxiety and depression in patients receiving mindfulness-based therapy versus control treatment.[100]

Supportive-Expressive Therapy

Supportive-expressive therapy (SET) promotes social support among peers and encourages patients to express disease-related emotions and existential concerns, with a focus on facing and grieving losses.[101] The goals of the therapy include increasing support, enhancing openness and emotional expressiveness, integrating a changed self and body image into the view of self, improving coping skills and interpersonal relationships, and detoxifying feelings around death and dying. SET is based on the idea that participants learn to better cope with their cancer and feel less distressed by expressing emotions and increasing the experience of social support. Clinical trials have examined the effects of SET on potential working mechanisms, finding a decrease in suppression of negative affect and improvements in social functioning. SET has been shown to reduce stress symptoms and improve quality of life in patients with breast cancer.[102]

Meaning-Centered Psychotherapy

Meaning-centered psychotherapy (MCP) emerged from SET and is tailored to patients with advanced cancer. Components include exploring the patient's cancer story, eliciting sense of self, impact of cancer, and exploring sources of meaning. MCP targets psychological, existential, and spiritual distress of patients with breast cancer, with demonstrated significant beneficial effects on quality of life, depression, and hopelessness.[103]

Acceptance and Commitment Therapy

Acceptance and commitment therapy (ACT) has fairly recently been studied in patients with breast cancer. It includes strategies to modify a patient's relationship with their thoughts and feelings so that they can experience them without being dominated by them. Basic ACT strategies include value clarification, commitment to engaging in value-consistent activities, and use of acceptance strategies to cope. These strategies are used to increase psychological flexibility and adaptability, which may increase acceptance of relapse and reduce fears related to breast cancer. In a 2021 study, patients with breast cancer showed significant improvement in subjective cognitive impairment, depression, anxiety, and psychological inflexibility after the ACT intervention.[104] In a recent review and meta-analysis, ACT was found to have significantly improved anxiety, depression, stress, and increased hope in patients with breast cancer.[105]

Diversity Considerations

Although evidence suggests that psychosocial interventions are beneficial for patients with breast cancer at all phases of treatment, historically, most studies have lacked diversity; thus less is known about the effectiveness in these underrepresented populations. Certain populations face unique stressors such as lack of health information, poor patient–provider communication, fearful perceptions of treatment, and distrust of the health care system. Black women are more likely to report lack of social support, greater cancer-related stigma, and poorer breast cancer–related quality of life than White women.[106] Significantly, Black women are 41% more likely to die from breast cancer than White women[106] despite a lower incidence rate. Limited research demonstrates that Black women's coping skills are improved through cognitive reframing and increased knowledge.[107] In addition, a CBT decision-making intervention showed significantly improved self-efficacy, thus enabling Black women to more comfortably engage with their health care team on treatment decisions such as chemotherapy.[107] Overall, effective interventions for diverse populations may have the greatest success when they are culturally informed, but more research is needed.

Psychopharmacologic Drugs and Breast Cancer

Psychiatric treatment holds an important place in the treatment of psychological symptoms in patients with breast cancer. Medications are commonly prescribed in the oncology setting to treat psychiatric disorders frequently exacerbated by cancer. Psychiatric disorders are serious medical conditions that can alter the course and

Table 3
Psychopharmacologic interventions used in patient populations with breast cancer[a]

Pharmacologic Drug	Targeted Symptoms
Mirtazapine	Insomnia, low appetite, nausea[b,c]
Olanzapine	Nausea/vomiting[d]
Lorazepam	Specific procedures or phobias[e]
Bupropion	Fatigue,[f] smoking cessation[g]
Duloxetine	Neuropathic pain[h]
Venlafaxine	Hot flashes[i]
Stimulants	Fatigue[j]

[a] Adapted from Elsevier.[108]
[b] Adapted from Investigational New Drugs.[109]
[c] Adapted from Psychiatry Clin Neurosci.[110]
[d] Adapted from Cochrane Database of Syst Rev.[111]
[e] Adapted from Journal of Clinical Oncology.[112]
[f] Adapted from BMC Cancer.[113]
[g] Adapted from Cancer Causes & Control.[114]
[h] Adapted from Clin J Pain.[115]
[i] Adapted from Breast Cancer Research and Treatment.[116]
[j] Adapted from Cochrane Database Syst Rev.[117]

treatment of cancer and often require psychopharmacologic interventions. These medications can also be a useful tool in treating psychiatric symptoms secondary to the cancer itself and secondary to the cancer treatment. Psychiatrists trained to prescribe to the oncology patient are preferred, as they can tailor medications to the patient, the cancer, and any current or future cancer treatments to avoid drug-drug interactions. A detailed description of appropriate medications is beyond the scope of this chapter, but in addition to treatment of any underlying psychiatric illness, some general thoughts specific to pharmacologic treatment in oncology patients are provided in **Table 3**.

SUMMARY

Breast cancer is the most common cancer in women, with about 1 in 8 women developing breast cancer in their lifetime. Many women diagnosed with breast cancer will experience some distress during their diagnosis or course of treatment or in survival. Cancer-related distress can be expected to dissipate with time for most of the women diagnosed, but in others distress may lead to significant symptoms that interfere with their psychological well-being. Such symptoms include anxiety, depression, sleep and sex disturbances, as well as cognitive disruptions and posttraumatic symptoms. Left untreated, these symptoms can lead to poor quality of life and negatively affect treatment compliance and ultimately, treatment outcome. Thus, distress and related psychological symptoms must be routinely assessed in patients with breast cancer and used to inform care. Various psychotherapeutic interventions have been demonstrated to be effective in addressing symptoms of patients with breast cancer. It is recommended that the patient's psychological needs are used to guide treatment, with specific issues or symptoms mapped onto relevant evidence-based treatments. Psychoeducation and CBT may be most helpful for reducing stress, depression, and anxiety and improving overall coping skills. Mindfulness-based therapies are particularly helpful in coping with loss of control, loss, and grief and can also reduce symptoms of depression and anxiety and improve cognitive functioning. Supportive emotional therapies and meaning-centered therapy focus on connecting with others and enhancing openness and may be most effective for improving social functioning, reducing negative affect, improving quality of life, and reducing hopelessness. ACT focuses on increasing psychological flexibility and acceptance and has promise in reducing stress, anxiety, fears, and depression. Less research has been conducted on patients of color who face unique stressors. Limited research supports the need to implement tailored culturally informed assessments and treatments to these populations. Psychiatric medications also play an important role in addressing the symptoms of this patient population and should be used in conjunction with psychosocial interactions as appropriate.

CLINICS CARE POINTS

- Patients diagnosed with breast cancer have an increased risk for depression, anxiety, cognitive impairments, sleep disruptions, and sexual dysfunction.

- Patients may go through stages of adjusting to the breast cancer diagnosis and treatments. It is important to understand that patients may display a range of emotions and behaviors over time. Do not assume that a patient's emotional response is fixed or even necessarily unhealthy.

- Transition times during diagnosis and treatment (such as diagnosis, treatment implementation, survivorship) are periods of higher risk for patients with breast cancer to experience psychological symptoms.

- Research demonstrates that addressing psychology symptoms can improve compliance with treatment and improve psychological symptoms and quality of life.

- Effective psychotherapeutic interventions are best used to match the patient's presenting symptoms and can be varied over time to address patient needs.

- Psychotropic medications are frequently helpful in addressing symptoms not helped by psychotherapy and are an important aspect of treatment.

DISCLOSURE

The authors have no financial disclosures to make and have no funding sources that supported writing this chapter.

REFERENCES

1. Siegel RL, Miller KD, Fuchs HE, et al. Cancer statistics, 2022. CA Cancer J Clin 2022;72(1):7–33.
2. Stewart BW, Wild CP, Weiderpass E, editors. World cancer report: cancer research for cancer prevention. Lyon: IARC Press; 2020. Available at: https://www.iccp-portal.org/system/files/resources/IARC%20World%20Cancer%20Report%202020.pdf.
3. Rojas K, Stuckey A. Breast cancer epidemiology and risk factors. Clin Obstet Gynecol 2016;59(4):651–72.
4. Cancer stat facts: Female breast cancer. SEER. Available at: https://seer.cancer.gov/statfacts/html/breast.html. Accessed 8 November, 2022.
5. DeSantis C, Ma J, Bryan L, et al. Breast cancer statistics, 2013. CA Cancer J Clin 2014;64(1):52–62.

6. Miller KD, Nogueira L, Devasia T, et al. Cancer treatment and survivorship statistics, 2022. CA Cancer J Clin 2022;72(5):409–36.

7. Zaker MR, Safaripour A, Sabegh SRZ, et al. Supportive intervention challenges for patients with breast cancer: A systematic review. Asian Pacific Journal of Environment and Cancer 2021;4(1). https://doi.org/10.31557/APJEC.2021.4.1.19-24.

8. Mutebi M, Anderson BO, Duggan C, et al. Breast cancer treatment: A phased approach to implementation. Cancer 2020;126(Suppl 10):2365–78.

9. Feng Y, Spezia M, Huang S, et al. Breast cancer development and progression: Risk factors, cancer stem cells, signaling pathways, genomics, and molecular pathogenesis. Genes Dis 2018;5(2):77–106.

10. Chiriac VF, Baban A, Dumitrascu DL. Psychological stress and breast cancer incidence: a systematic review. Clujul Med 2018;91(1):18–26.

11. Dinapoli L, Colloca G, Di Capua B, et al. Psychological aspects to consider in breast cancer diagnosis and treatment. Curr Oncol Rep 2021;23(3):1–7.

12. Montgomery M, McCrone SH. Psychological distress associated with the diagnostic phase for suspected breast cancer: systematic review. J Adv Nurs 2010;66(11):2372–90.

13. Ng CG, Mohamed S, Kaur K, et al. Perceived distress and its association with depression and anxiety in breast cancer patients. PLoS One 2017;12(3):e0172975.

14. Bower JE. Cancer-related fatigue: mechanisms, risk factors, and treatments. Nat Rev Clin Oncol 2014;11(10):597–609.

15. Nowicki A, Krzemkowska E, Rhone P. Acceptance of illness after surgery in patients with breast cancer in the early postoperative period. Pol Przegl Chir 2015;87(11):539–50.

16. Hall DL, Antoni MH, Lattie EG, et al. Perceived fatigue interference and depressed mood: comparison of chronic fatigue syndrome/Myalgic encephalomyelitis patients with fatigued breast cancer survivors. Fatigue 2015;3(3):142–55.

17. Schmid-Büchi S, Halfens RJG, Dassen T, et al. A review of psychosocial needs of breast-cancer patients and their relatives. J Clin Nurs 2008;17:2895–909.

18. Ganz PA. Psychological and social aspects of breast cancer. Oncology (Williston Park) 2008;22(6):642–53.

19. Andrykowski MA, Manne SL. Are psychological interventions effective and accepted by cancer patients? I. Standards and levels of evidence. Ann Behav Med 2006;32(2):93–7.

20. Institute of Medicine (US) and National Research Council (US) National Cancer Policy Board. In: Hewitt M, Herdman R, Holland J, editors. Meeting psychosocial needs of women with breast cancer. Washington (DC): National Academies Press (US); 2004.

21. Moyer A. Psychosocial outcomes of breast-conserving surgery versus mastectomy: a meta-analytic review [published correction appears in Health Psychol 1997 Sep;16(5):442]. Health Psychol 1997;16(3):284–98.

22. Izawa H, Karasawa K, Kawase E, et al. The assessment of anxiety about radiotherapy in patient with early breast cancer receiving breast irradiation. Int J Radiat Oncol Biol Phys 2007;69(3):S589–90.

23. Costanzo ES, Lutgendorf SK, Mattes ML, et al. Adjusting to life after treatment: distress and quality of life following treatment for breast cancer. Br J Cancer 2007;97(12):1625–31.

24. Hack TF, Pickles T, Ruether JD, et al. Predictors of distress and quality of life in patients undergoing cancer therapy: impact of treatment type and decisional role. Psycho Oncol 2010;19(6):606–16.

25. Gibbons A, Groarke A. Coping with chemotherapy for breast cancer: Asking women what works. Eur J Oncol Nurs 2018;35:85–91.

26. Smith HR. Depression in cancer patients: Pathogenesis, implications and treatment (Review). Oncol Lett 2015;9(4):1509–14.

27. Satin JR, Linden W, Phillips MJ. Depression as a predictor of disease progression and mortality in cancer patients: a meta-analysis. Cancer 2009;115(22): 5349–61.

28. Giese-Davis J, Collie K, Rancourt KM, et al. Decrease in depression symptoms is associated with longer survival in patients with metastatic breast cancer: a secondary analysis. J Clin Oncol 2011;29(4):413–20.

29. Hardman A, Maguire P, Crowther D. The recognition of psychiatric morbidity on a medical oncology ward. J Psychosom Res 1989;33(2):235–9.

30. Blaschke TF, Osterberg L, Vrijens B, et al. Adherence to medications: insights arising from studies on the unreliable link between prescribed and actual drug dosing histories. Annu Rev Pharmacol Toxicol 2012;52:275–301.

31. Andrykowski MA, Lykins E, Floyd A. Psychological health in cancer survivors. Semin Oncol Nurs 2008;24(3):193–201.

32. Adler NE, Page AEK, Institute of Medicine (US), Committee on Psychosocial Services to Cancer Patients/Families in a Community Setting. Cancer care for the Whole patient: meeting psychosocial health needs. Washington (DC): National Academies Press (US); 2008.

33. McEvoy MD, McCorkle R. Quality of life issues in patients with disseminated breast cancer. Cancer 1990;66(6 Suppl):1416–21.

34. Cella DF, Bonomi AE, Lloyd SR, et al. Reliability and validity of the Functional Assessment of Cancer Therapy-Lung (FACT-L) quality of life instrument. Lung Cancer 1995;12(3):199–220.

35. Mandelblatt JS, Eisenberg JM. Historical and methodological perspectives on cancer outcomes research. Oncology (Williston Park) 1995;9(11 Suppl):23–32.

36. Ownby KK. Use of the distress thermometer in clinical practice. J Adv Pract Oncol 2019;10(2):175–9.

37. Stern AF. The hospital anxiety and depression scale. Occup Med (Lond) 2014; 64(5):393–4.

38. Zhou K, Li M, Wang W, et al. Reliability, validity, and sensitivity of the Chinese Short-Form 36 Health Survey version 2 (SF-36v2) in women with breast cancer. J Eval Clin Pract 2019;25(5):864–72.

39. Calderon C, Ferrando PJ, Lorenzo-Seva U, et al. Factor structure and measurement invariance of the Brief Symptom Inventory (BSI-18) in cancer patients. Int J Clin Health Psychol 2020;20(1):71–80.

40. Schag CA, Ganz PA, Heinrich RL. CAncer Rehabilitation Evaluation System– short form (CARES-SF). A cancer specific rehabilitation and quality of life instrument. Cancer 1991;68(6):1406–13.

41. Brady MJ, Cella DF, Mo F, et al. Reliability and validity of the Functional Assessment of Cancer Therapy-Breast quality-of-life instrument. J Clin Oncol 1997; 15(3):974–86.

42. Levine MN, Guyatt GH, Gent M, et al. Quality of life in stage II breast cancer: an instrument for clinical trials. J Clin Oncol 1988;6(12):1798–810.

43. Adeyemi OJ, Gill TL, Paul R, et al. Evaluating the association of self-reported psychological distress and self-rated health on survival times among women with breast cancer in the U.S. PLoS One 2021;16(12):e0260481.

44. Tang HY, Xiong HH, Deng LC, et al. Adjustment Disorder in Female Breast Cancer Patients: Prevalence and Its Accessory Symptoms. Curr Med Sci 2020; 40(3):510–7.

45. Wijnhoven LMA, Custers JAE, Kwakkenbos L, et al. Trajectories of adjustment disorder symptoms in post-treatment breast cancer survivors. Support Care Cancer 2022;30(4):3521–30.

46. Saboonchi F, Petersson LM, Wennman-Larsen A, et al. Changes in caseness of anxiety and depression in breast cancer patients during the first year following surgery: patterns of transiency and severity of the distress response. Eur J Oncol Nurs 2014;18(6):598–604.

47. Cui Q, Cai Z, Li J, et al. The Psychological Pressures of Breast Cancer Patients During the COVID-19 Outbreak in China-A Comparison With Frontline Female Nurses. Front Psychiatry 2020;11:559701.

48. Burgess C, Cornelius V, Love S, et al. Depression and anxiety in women with early breast cancer: five year observational cohort study. BMJ 2005; 330(7493):702.

49. Maass SW, Roorda C, Berendsen AJ, et al. The prevalence of long-term symptoms of depression and anxiety after breast cancer treatment: A systematic review. Maturitas 2015;82(1):100–8.

50. Avis NE, Levine BJ, Case LD, et al. Trajectories of depressive symptoms following breast cancer diagnosis. Cancer Epidemiol Biomarkers Prev 2015; 24(11):1789–95.

51. Walker LG, Heys SD, Walker MB, et al. Psychological factors can predict the response to primary chemotherapy in patients with locally advanced breast cancer. Eur J Cancer 1999;35(13):1783–8.

52. Boing L, Pereira GS, Araújo CDCR, et al. Factors associated with depression symptoms in women after breast cancer. Rev Saude Publica 2019;53:30.

53. Denieffe S, Gooney M. A meta-synthesis of women's symptoms experience and breast cancer. Eur J Cancer Care 2011;20(4):424–35.

54. Cohee AA, Adams RN, Fife BL, et al. Relationship Between Depressive Symptoms and Social Cognitive Processing in Partners of Long-Term Breast Cancer Survivors. Oncol Nurs Forum 2017;44(1):44–51.

55. Van Dyk K, Ganz PA. Cancer-Related Cognitive Impairment in Patients With a History of Breast Cancer. JAMA 2021;326(17):1736–7.

56. Buchanan ND, Dasari S, Rodriguez JL, et al. Post-treatment Neurocognition and Psychosocial Care Among Breast Cancer Survivors. Am J Prev Med 2015;49(6 Suppl 5):S498–508.

57. Janelsins MC, Heckler CE, Peppone LJ, et al. Cognitive complaints in survivors of breast cancer after chemotherapy compared with age-matched controls: An analysis from a nationwide, multicenter, prospective longitudinal study. J Clin Oncol 2017;35(5):506–14.

58. Vardy J. Cognitive function in breast cancer survivors. Cancer Treat Res 2009; 151:387–419.

59. Lange M, Giffard B, Noal S, et al. Baseline cognitive functions among elderly patients with localised breast cancer. Eur J Cancer 2014;50(13):2181–9.

60. Hurria A, Somlo G, Ahles T. Renaming "chemobrain. Cancer Invest 2007;25(6): 373–7.

61. Weng YP, Hong RM, Chen VC, et al. Sleep quality and related factors in patients with breast cancer: A cross-sectional study in Taiwan. Cancer Manag Res 2021; 13:4725–33.

62. Simeit R, Deck R, Conta-Marx B. Sleep management training for cancer patients with insomnia. Support Care Cancer 2004;12(3):176–83.

63. Bardwell WA, Profant J, Casden DR, et al. The relative importance of specific risk factors for insomnia in women treated for early-stage breast cancer. Psycho Oncol 2008;17(1):9–18.

64. Savard J, Simard S, Blanchet J, et al. Prevalence, clinical characteristics, and risk factors for insomnia in the context of breast cancer. Sleep 2001;24(5): 583–90.

65. Esplen MJ, Wong J, Warner E, et al. Restoring body image after cancer (ReBIC): Results of a randomized controlled trial. J Clin Oncol 2018;36(8):749–56.

66. Thakur M, Sharma R, Mishra AK, et al. Psychological distress and body image disturbances after modified radical mastectomy among breast cancer survivors: A cross-sectional study from a tertiary care centre in North India. Lancet Regional Health-Southeast Asia 2022;7(100077). https://doi.org/10.1016/j.lansea.2022.100077.

67. Guedes TSR, Dantas de Oliveira NP, Holanda AM, et al. Body image of women submitted to breast cancer treatment. Asian Pac J Cancer Prev 2018;19(6): 1487–93.

68. Fobair P, Stewart SL, Chang S, et al. Body image and sexual problems in young women with breast cancer. Psycho Oncol 2006;15(7):579–94.

69. Fang SY, Lin YC, Chen TC, et al. Impact of marital coping on the relationship between body image and sexuality among breast cancer survivors. Support Care Cancer 2015;23(9):2551–9.

70. Esmat Hosseini S, Ilkhani M, Rohani C, et al. Prevalence of sexual dysfunction in women with cancer: A systematic review and meta-analysis. Int J Reprod Biomed 2022;20(1):1–12.

71. Qi A, Li Y, Sun H, et al. Incidence and risk factors of sexual dysfunction in young breast cancer survivors. Ann Palliat Med 2021;10(4):4428–34.

72. Ljungman L, Ahlgren J, Petersson LM, et al. Sexual dysfunction and reproductive concerns in young women with breast cancer: Type, prevalence, and predictors of problems. Psycho Oncol 2018;27(12):2770–7.

73. Jing L, Zhang C, Li W, et al. Incidence and severity of sexual dysfunction among women with breast cancer: a meta-analysis based on female sexual function index. Support Care Cancer 2019;27(4):1171–80.

74. Oliveri S, Arnaboldi P, Pizzoli SFM, et al. PTSD symptom clusters associated with short- and long-term adjustment in early diagnosed breast cancer patients. Ecancermedicalscience 2019;13:917.

75. Swartzman S, Booth JN, Munro A, et al. Posttraumatic stress disorder after cancer diagnosis in adults: A meta-analysis. Depress Anxiety 2017;34(4):327–39.

76. Carletto S, Porcaro C, Settanta C, et al. Neurobiological features and response to eye movement desensitization and reprocessing treatment of posttraumatic stress disorder in patients with breast cancer. Eur J Psychotraumatol 2019; 10(1):1600832.

77. Wu X, Wang J, Cofie R, et al. Prevalence of posttraumatic stress disorder among breast cancer patients: A meta-analysis. Iran J Public Health 2016;45(12): 1533–44.

78. Brown LC, Murphy AR, Lalonde CS, et al. Posttraumatic stress disorder and breast cancer: Risk factors and the role of inflammation and endocrine function. Cancer 2020;126(14):3181–91.
79. Bulotiene G, Matuiziene M. Posttraumatic stress in breast cancer patients. Acta Med Litu 2014;21(2):43–50.
80. Vin-Raviv N, Hillyer GC, Hershman DL, et al. Racial disparities in posttraumatic stress after diagnosis of localized breast cancer: the BQUAL study. J Natl Cancer Inst 2013;105(8):563–72.
81. Fawzy FI, Fawzy NW, Arndt LA, et al. Critical review of psychosocial interventions in cancer care. Arch Gen Psychiatry 1995;52(2):100–13.
82. Cipolletta S, Simonato C, Faccio E. The effectiveness of psychoeducational support groups for women with breast cancer and their caregivers: A mixed methods study. Front Psychol 2019;10:288.
83. Dolbeault S, Cayrou S, Brédart A, et al. The effectiveness of a psychoeducational group after early-stage breast cancer treatment: results of a randomized French study. Psycho Oncol 2009;18(6):647–56.
84. Zhang J, Xu R, Wang B, et al. Effects of mindfulness-based therapy for patients with breast cancer: A systematic review and meta-analysis. Complement Ther Med 2016;26:1–10.
85. Getu MA, Chen C, Panpan W, et al. The effect of cognitive behavioral therapy on the quality of life of breast cancer patients: a systematic review and meta-analysis of randomized controlled trials [published correction appears in Qual Life Res. 2022 Oct;31(10):3089]. Qual Life Res 2021;30(2):367–84.
86. Stagl JM, Bouchard LC, Lechner SC, et al. Long-term psychological benefits of cognitive-behavioral stress management for women with breast cancer: 11-year follow-up of a randomized controlled trial. Cancer 2015;121(11):1873–81.
87. Ren W, Qiu H, Yang Y, et al. Randomized controlled trial of cognitive behavioural therapy for depressive and anxiety symptoms in Chinese women with breast cancer. Psychiatry Res 2019;271:52–9.
88. Aricò D, Raggi A, Ferri R. Cognitive behavioral therapy for insomnia in breast cancer survivors: A review of the literature. Front Psychol 2016;7:1162.
89. Abrahams HJG, Gielissen MFM, Donders RRT, et al. The efficacy of Internet-based cognitive behavioral therapy for severely fatigued survivors of breast cancer compared with care as usual: A randomized controlled trial. Cancer 2017;123(19):3825–34.
90. Hunter MS, Coventry S, Hamed H, et al. Evaluation of a group cognitive behavioural intervention for women suffering from menopausal symptoms following breast cancer treatment. Psycho Oncol 2009;18(5):560–3.
91. Wojtyna E, Jolanta Ż, Patrycja S. The influence of cognitive-behaviour therapy on quality of life and self-esteem in women suffering from breast cancer. Rep Practical Oncol Radiother 2007;12(2):109–17.
92. Gielissen MF, Verhagen S, Witjes F, et al. Effects of cognitive behavior therapy in severely fatigued disease-free cancer patients compared with patients waiting for cognitive behavior therapy: a randomized controlled trial. J Clin Oncol 2006;24(30):4882–7.
93. Tang M, Liu X, Wu Q, et al. The effects of cognitive-behavioral stress management for breast cancer patients: A systematic review and meta-analysis of randomized controlled trials. Cancer Nurs 2020;43(3):222–37.
94. Cillessen L, Johannsen M, Speckens AEM, et al. Mindfulness-based interventions for psychological and physical health outcomes in cancer patients and

survivors: A systematic review and meta-analysis of randomized controlled trials. Psycho Oncol 2019;28(12):2257–69.
95. Xunlin NG, Lau Y, Klainin-Yobas P. The effectiveness of mindfulness-based interventions among cancer patients and survivors: a systematic review and meta-analysis. Support Care Cancer 2020;28(4):1563–78.
96. Cramer H, Lauche R, Paul A, et al. Mindfulness-based stress reduction for breast cancer-a systematic review and meta-analysis. Curr Oncol 2012;19(5): e343–52.
97. Carlson LE, Speca M. Mindfulness-based cancer Recovery: a Step-by-Step MBSR approach to help you cope with treatment and reclaim your life. New Harbinger, Oakland, CA; 2010.
98. Johannsen M, O'Connor M, O'Toole MS, et al. Efficacy of mindfulness-based cognitive therapy on late post-treatment pain in women treated for primary breast cancer: A randomized controlled trial. J Clin Oncol 2016;34(28):3390–9.
99. Lengacher CA, Reich RR, Paterson CL, et al. Examination of broad symptom improvement resulting from mindfulness-based stress reduction in breast cancer survivors: A randomized controlled trial. J Clin Oncol 2016;34(24):2827–34.
100. Zhang MF, Wen YS, Liu WY, et al. Effectiveness of mindfulness-based therapy for reducing anxiety and depression in patients with cancer: A meta-analysis. Medicine (Baltim) 2015;94(45):e0897.
101. Classen CC, Kraemer HC, Blasey C, et al. Supportive-expressive group therapy for primary breast cancer patients: a randomized prospective multicenter trial. Psycho Oncol 2008;17(5):438–47.
102. Kissane DW, Grabsch B, Clarke DM, et al. Supportive-expressive group therapy for women with metastatic breast cancer: survival and psychosocial outcome from a randomized controlled trial. Psycho Oncol 2007;16(4):277–86.
103. Lichtenthal WG, Roberts KE, Pessin H, et al. Meaning-Centered Psychotherapy and cancer: Finding meaning in the face of suffering. Psychiatr Times 2020; 37(8):23–5.
104. Shari NI, Zainal NZ, Ng CG. Effects of brief acceptance and commitment therapy (ACT) on subjective cognitive impairment in breast cancer patients undergoing chemotherapy. J Psychosoc Oncol 2021;39(6):695–714.
105. Li H, Wu J, Ni Q, et al. Systematic review and meta-analysis of effectiveness of acceptance and commitment therapy in patients with breast cancer. Nurs Res 2021;70(4):E152–60.
106. Whitehead NE, Hearn LE. Psychosocial interventions addressing the needs of Black women diagnosed with breast cancer: a review of the current landscape. Psycho Oncol 2015;24(5):497–507.
107. Sheppard VB, Wallington SF, Willey SC, et al. A peer-led decision support intervention improves decision outcomes in black women with breast cancer. J Cancer Educ 2013;28(2):262–9.
108. Stern TA, Rosenbaum JF, Fricchione GL, et al. Massachusetts general hospital handbook of general hospital Psychiatry. 7th edition. Philadelphia: Elsevier; 2018.
109. Cao J, Ouyang Q, Wang S, et al. Mirtazapine, a dopamine receptor inhibitor, as a secondary prophylactic for delayed nausea and vomiting following highly emetogenic chemotherapy: An open label, randomized, Multicenter Phase III trial. Invest N Drugs 2020;38(2):507–14.
110. Kim SW, Shin IS, Kim JM, et al. Effectiveness of mirtazapine for nausea and insomnia in cancer patients with depression. Psychiatry Clin Neurosci 2008; 62(1):75–83.

111. Sutherland A, Naessens K, Plugge E, et al. Olanzapine for the prevention and treatment of cancer-related nausea and vomiting in adults. Cochrane Database Syst Rev 2018;2018(9). https://doi.org/10.1002/14651858.cd012555.pub2.
112. Traeger L, Greer JA, Fernandez-Robles C, et al. Evidence-based treatment of anxiety in patients with cancer. J Clin Oncol 2012;30(11):1197–205.
113. Salehifar E, Azimi S, Janbabai G, et al. Efficacy and safety of bupropion in cancer-related fatigue, a randomized double blind placebo controlled clinical trial. BMC Cancer 2020;20(1). https://doi.org/10.1186/s12885-020-6618-9.
114. Schnoll RA, Martinez E, Tatum KL, et al. A bupropion smoking cessation clinical trial for cancer patients. Cancer Causes & Control 2010;21(6):811–20.
115. Guan J, Tanaka S, Kawakami K. Anticonvulsants or antidepressants in combination pharmacotherapy for treatment of neuropathic pain in cancer patients: a systematic review and meta-analysis. Clin J Pain 2016;32(8):719–25.
116. Ramaswami R, Villarreal MD, Pitta DM, et al. Venlafaxine in management of hot flashes in women with breast cancer: A systematic review and meta-analysis. Breast Cancer Res Treat 2015;152(2):231237.
117. Minton O, Richardson A, Sharpe M, et al. Drug therapy for the management of cancer related fatigue. Cochrane Database Syst Rev 2010;7:CD006704.

Disparities in Breast Cancer Outcomes and How to Resolve Them

Otis W. Brawley, MD, MACP, FRCP(L)[a,b,*],
Dina George Lansey, MSN, RN[a]

KEYWORDS

- Breast cancer • Disparities in outcome • Race • Area of geographic origin
- Quality of care

KEY POINTS

- Disparities or differences in outcome exist by race, socioeconomic status, and area of residence.
- Disparities in outcome are largely due to differences in quality of care (risk reduction, screening, diagnosis, and treatment).
- The key to overcoming disparities is getting all women high quality care to include prevention/risk reduction, appropriate screening, appropriate diagnosis, and high quality treatment.

BREAST CANCER OUTCOMES

In the western world, breast cancer is the most common lethal cancer in women and the second leading cause of cancer death behind lung cancer.[1] The American Cancer Society estimates that 281,550 women were diagnosed with invasive breast cancer in the United States in 2021 and approximately 43,600 women died from it.[2] The median age at breast cancer diagnosis for American women is 61; 19% were younger than 50 years. In the United States, the lifetime risk of diagnosis of invasive breast cancer is about 13% (1 in 8), and lifetime risk of death is about 3% (1 in 33). It is estimated that nearly 4 million breast cancer survivors live in the United States.

This article previously appeared in Hematology/Oncology Clinics volume 37, issue 1 February 2023

Funding: This work was supported by the National Institutes of Health (P30 CA 0069783 and 1U10CA180820) and Bloomberg Philanthropies.

[a] Department of Oncology, Johns Hopkins School of Medicine, Baltimore, MD, USA;
[b] Department of Epidemiology, Johns Hopkins Bloomberg School of Public Health, Baltimore, MD, USA
* Corresponding author. Johns Hopkins University, 1550 Orleans Street Suite 1m16, Baltimore, MD 21231-2410.
E-mail address: Otis.Brawley@JHU.edu

The diagnosis of noninvasive ductal carcinoma or ductal carcinoma in sutu (DCIS) was rare before the advent of widespread mammography screening. It has increased dramatically over the past 40 years. It is estimated that 50,000 American women were diagnosed in 2021.[3]

The age-adjusted breast cancer mortality rate declined in the United States by more than 40% from 33.2 per 100,000 in 1988 to 19.9 in 2017. Analysis of population data shows that more than 50% of the decline in death rate is attributed to improvements in treatment. Hormonal, chemical, surgical, and radiation therapy of breast cancer have improved dramatically over the past 5 decades.[4] Improvements in and increasing availability of screening as well as increased awareness of breast cancer and the empowerment of women to seek care after appreciating symptoms are also important factors contributing to the decline.[5,6]

DEFINING THE DISPARITIES

While a 40% decline in mortality is significant, review of population data shows that not all populations have enjoyed the progress equally. For example, **Table 1** shows the annualized breast cancer mortality using National Cancer Institute Surveillance, Epidemiology, and End Results (NCI SEER) from 2013 to 2017 with race and ethnicity as used in US Government databases. Much of the discussion in health disparities focuses on the Black disparity because the Black mortality rate is the highest of any race/ethnicity. It is of note that non Hispanic (NH) White women have a mortality disparity when compared to the other races/ethnicities.

The academic discipline of health disparities is the study of differences in outcome. The National Cancer Institute defines cancer health disparities as population differences in cancer measures such as incidence, prevalence, mortality, survival, survivorship, and stage at diagnosis.[7] While most studies focus on differences in outcomes by race, there are also differences when populations are defined by and caused by area of geographic origin, ethnicity, socioeconomic status, and geographic area of residence.

Race is a sociopolitical categorization. It is not a biological categorization. The US Office of Management and Budget defines the racial and ethnic categories for all government databases.[8] According to US Office of Management and Budget (OMB), these definitions are sociopolitical and not based on biology. A complicating factor; race especially in the United States, very commonly correlates with social determinants that can influence disease causation and disease outcome.

Breast cancer mortality rates vary by socioeconomic status irrespective of race. Wealth and culture can influence dietary patterns, weight gain, and birthing habits,

---

Table 1
Annualized age-adjusted US breast cancer incidence and mortality (using 2013–2017 SEER data)

	Incidence	Mortality
All races	128.5	19.9
NH White	137.3	20.3
NH Black	124.8	27.6
API	102.9	11.4
AI/AN	79.5	11.5
Hispanic	99.1	14.1

NH White, Non-Hispanic White, NH Black, Non-Hispanic Black; API, Asian Pacific Islander; AI/AN, American Indian/Alaskan Native.

all of which are correlated with risk of breast cancer. A higher proportion of the socially deprived also receive poorer quality care (from screening, to diagnosis, to treatment). Important to US breast cancer mortality statistics by race is the fact that 21.2% of Black Americans live in poverty compared to 9.0% of White Americans.[9]

Area of geographic origin is a population categorization often confused with race. People originating in Europe are generally considered Caucasian or White race. Europe is an area of at least 840 areas of geographic origins.[10] There can be biologic differences by area of geographic origin. Glucose 6 phosphate dehydrogenase (G6PD) deficiency is an example of a disease that varies by area of geographic origin. There are several known G6PD deficiencies.[11] Each is well described at a molecular level and is associated with a specific geographic area such as the Mediterranean, India, or Sub-Saharan Africa.

Another issue to be considered when looking at population statistics is genetic admixture. Most individuals are not from a homogenous monolithic group. Most humans are a mixture of several areas of geographic origin. Indeed, most American Black persons have inherited traits from several African and several European areas of geographic origin. Again, the point is race is a sociopolitical categorization and not a categorization based on biology.

DIFFERENCES IN STAGE AT DIAGNOSIS

The US SEER database published breast stage distribution for Black and White women using local, regional, and distant as staging descriptors. Data from the period 2010 to 2016 are provided in **Table 2**.

Of the 4 million breast cancer survivors living in the United States today, about 150,000 are living with metastatic disease. Of those living with metastatic disease, three-fourths were originally diagnosed with local or regional stage disease.[9]

Population incidence rates are very much correlated with mammography rates. Increased use of mammography screening is associated with a dramatic rise in the incidence of localized disease at diagnosis. Interestingly, there has not been a decline in distant disease over time. CDC National Center for Health Statistics data suggest that the prevalence of screening in Black and White American women over the past decade is very similar. While there is parity in proportions screened by race, data demonstrating equity in quality of screening are lacking. It is suggested that Black women as a group are more likely to encounter lower quality screening as well as greater delays in diagnostic workup and definitive treatment.[12,13]

Table 2
Stage Distribution and Relative Survival by Race

	All	White	Black
Stage distribution by race (percent), SEER data from 2010 to 2016			
Localized	63	64	55
Regional	30	29	35
Distant	6	6	9
Unstaged	2	1	2
5-y Relative survival by stage and race (percent), SEER data from 2010 to 2016			
Localized	98.9	99.2	96.1
Regional	65.7	86.8	77.7
Distant	28.1	29.4	19.4
Unstaged	55.1	52.7	50.3

Within race/ethnicity, lower socioeconomic status meaning lower income, less education, lack of health insurance, or poor-quality health insurance is also associated with higher mortality rates and lower 5-year survival after diagnosis.

MOLECULAR SUBTYPES BY RACE

Breast cancer is not one disease. There are at least 4 molecular subtypes of breast cancer (**Table 3**). Each has different levels of drug sensitivity or resistance, and each has a different biological behavior.

Luminal A is the most common type of breast cancer. It is less aggressive, slower growing, sensitive to hormonal therapy, and has the best prognosis.

Luminal B cancers tend to be of higher grade than luminal A. They are associated with poorer outcomes.

HER-2 enriched tumors respond to HER-2 blocking agents such as trastuzumab. It is an aggressive form of breast cancer, but success with HER-2 blocking agents have substantially improved outcomes.

Basal-like or triple-negative breast cancer is often referred to as triple-negative breast cancer because it lacks the estrogen receptor, progesterone receptor, and the HER-2 receptor. Hormonal treatments and HER-2 blocking agents are ineffective. Today, triple-negative breast cancer has the poorest prognosis of all 4 subtypes. Basal-like tumors are more common in premenopausal women and women with BRCA1 mutations (**Table 3**).

SURVIVAL AND OUTCOMES

Five-year survival differs by breast cancer subtype within stage.[14] For example, irrespective of race, the proportion alive at 5 years after diagnosis is 92% among women diagnosed with luminal A (hormone receptor positive, HER-2 negative) disease and 77% for all those diagnosed with basal-like (triple negative) disease.[15]

The distribution of breast cancer subtypes among Black and White women is shown in **Fig. 1**.[16] It is of note that approximately 19% of Black women with breast cancer have triple-negative disease compared to about 9% of White women.[17] Women of other races and ethnicities have distributions similar to White Americans. There are no significant differences in the prevalence of progesterone receptor or HER-2 status among the population groups.[18] The significant difference is in the higher incidence rate of estrogen receptor positive (ER +) disease in White women and the substantially lower incidence of ER + disease in Black women.[19] It is the lower proportion of Black patients with disease expressing the estrogen receptor that accounts for the higher proportion of Black women with basal-like, triple-negative disease.

Table 3
Classifying subtypes by receptor status

Molecular Subtype	ER Status	PR Status	HER-2 Status
Luminal A	+	+/−	- ($\leq$14% Ki-67)
Luminal B	+	+/−	+ (or − with >14% Ki-67)
HER-2 overexpressing	-	-	+
Triple negative (basal like)	-	-	-

ER, estrogen receptor; PR, progesterone receptor.

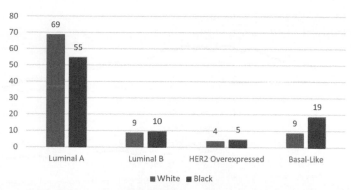

Fig. 1. Breast cancer subtype by race/ethnicity.

There is very little racial/ethnic variation in the prevalence of these markers with the exception of a lower proportion of Black women having disease expressing ER and higher proportion of White women having disease expressing ER.

INCIDENCE AND MORTALITY

Studying trends in breast cancer incidence and mortality in various populations can provide clues relating to breast cancer cause and prevention. It can also help focus screening, diagnostic, and therapeutic efforts such that they are more effective.

From the beginning of the NCI SEER registry in the early 1970s, the White population had a higher incidence rate than the Black population. In recent years, White and Black American women have similar incidence rates (**Fig. 2**). The exception to this pattern is the incidence rate for Black women younger than 45 years has consistently been higher than that of White women, and incidence rates are strikingly higher in White as opposed to Black patients.[17]

Trends in Black and White mortality are available from the SEER registry from the early 1970s (**Fig. 3**). Data for Hispanics, Native Americans/Alaskan Natives, and Asians became available in 1992. It is of note that Black and White women had similar death rates in the 1970s, and the Black-White disparity began several years after effective screening and treatment became widely available. The Black-White mortality disparity for the United States as a whole is greater today than it has ever been.

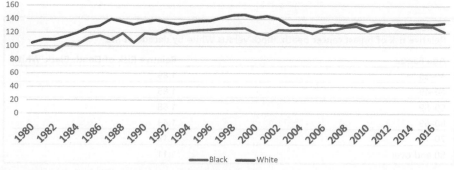

Fig. 2. Breast cancer incidence by race 1980 to 2018.

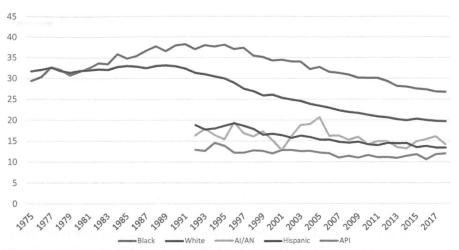

Fig. 3. Breast cancer death rate by race/ethnicity in 1975 to 2018.

When assessing differences in mortality by area of residence, one finds tremendous difference in mortality by state. For example, the annualized death rate is 23.2 per 100,000 among residents of Mississippi and 17.3 per 100,000 among residents of Massachusetts during the period 2014 to 2018. There are 6 states (all with very low death rates) where there are small differences in mortality between Black and White women. Alternatively, there are 12 states where White women have a mortality rate greater than that of Black women, including Massachusetts.

As noted above, Hispanic, American Indian/Alaskan Native (AI/AN), and Asian Pacific islander (API) women have strikingly lower mortality rates than non-Hispanic White and Black American women. Recent Asian immigrants to the United States show lower rates of breast cancer than those who have lived in the United States for many years. Indeed, third- and fourth-generation Asian American women have breast cancer risk similar to White American women.[17] This observation supports the theory that cultural acclamation influences breast cancer risk.

Today, Black women are more likely to die from breast cancer than White women at every age[17] (**Table 4**). The relative risk of death is greater for younger Black women. This likely reflects a higher risk of both diagnosis and a higher risk of more aggressive disease at younger age, especially basal-like or triple-negative disease. Determining the reasons for this pattern is a very active area of research. Identification of these external influences is the key to developing interventions to reduce breast cancer risk.

Table 4
Relative risk of breast cancer death, Black versus White by decade of life

Age Range	Relative Risk of Death Black/White
30–39	1.89
40–49	1.85
50–59	1.68
60–69	1.43
70–79	1.19
80 and over	1.11

Source: NCI SEER.

REASONS FOR THE DISPARITIES

The differences in incidence within populations suggest that there are varying external influences leading to varying incidence and mortality rates. There are some sociocultural reasons for differences in breast cancer incidence and the distribution of breast cancer markers. The rise in incidence since the 1970s is thought to be partlally linked to increasing prevalence of obesity and to declines in the average number of births per female.[20]

ENERGY IMBALANCE

Long-term cohort studies have shown a correlation between high caloric intake, limited or no exercise, and energy storage (overweight or obesity) with the risk of several cancers.[21] The connection between energy imbalance and breast cancer risk is complicated. Women who gain weight as an adult appear to be at greater risk (especially of postmenopausal breast cancer) than those who have been overweight since childhood. How much of the Black-White difference in risk of breast cancer death is due to energy imbalance is unknown.

Over the past 5 decades, there has been a significant rise in the proportion of the population suffering from obesity. In 1970, 15% of Black and White women were obese.[22,23] The prevalence of obesity by race/ethnicity in 2017 and 2018 is provided in **Fig. 4**.

BIRTHING HABITS

Socioeconomically deprived women are more likely to have children at an earlier age. For cultural and economic reasons, they are also less likely to breast feed. Higher parity without breast feeding is associated with increased risk of basal-like breast cancers and reduced risk of luminal A and luminal B breast cancers, especially for cancers diagnosed in premenopausal women. Breastfeeding is more common among White Americans than among Black Americans and is correlated with a lower risk of basal-like or triple-negative breast cancer in later life.[24]

A higher proportion of middle class, college-educated women do not have children or delay childbirth until after the age of 30. This is correlated with an increase in risk of ER + breast cancer.[25]

Another risk factor for ER + breast cancer is the use of postmenopausal hormone therapy.[26] This practice is more common in upper middle class White women than among other minorities. It is not just that poor and Black women have habits that

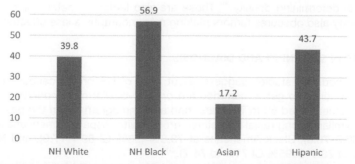

Fig. 4. Prevalence of obesity among adults by race/ethnicity in 2017/2018 (percent). (*Data from* NCHS, National Health and Nutrition Examination survey, 2017-2018.)

increase the risk of poor-prognosis triple-negative disease. More educated White women have habits that increase the risk of better prognosis of ER + disease.

OTHER RISK FACTORS FOR BREAST CANCER

It is estimated that 5% to 10% of breast cancers present in individuals with familial inheritance of susceptibility.[27] Most are autosomal dominant and highly penetrant.[28] Patients with these mutations are often younger at diagnosis and have a higher grade, more aggressive disease. A genetic study has not been thoroughly conducted in African American breast cancer patients.[29] There is some evidence of specific mutations of certain African areas of origin.[30,31] In at least 1 study assessing a diverse group of women with breast cancer, African Americans had a higher rate of polymorphisms and variants of unknown significance than the non-Hispanic, non-Jewish White population.[32]

Area of geographic origin (as opposed to race) may also contribute to the variance in genomic markers.[31] Jemal and colleagues[33] have studied genomic markers by area of geographic origin in Africa and compared them to US-born Black women. US born Black women are commonly an admixture of several of more than 100 recognized areas of geographic origin in Africa and the more than 840 recognized European areas of geographic origin. Compared to US-born Black women, the prevalence rate ratio of triple-negative breast cancer was 0.92 (95% confidence interval [CI] 0.81–1.04) among Western-African-born women with breast cancer, 0.87 (95% CI 0.78–0.98) among Caribbean-born, and 0.53 (95% CI 0.37–0.77) among Eastern-African-born Black women.[34] Again, area of geographic origin is the categorization that should be studied as it can correlate with genetic differences, but the areas used in this study are still quite vast.[35]

The mechanism for increased risk in those with energy imbalance may also be epigenetic.[36] There are metabolic influences on genomics. For example, alterations of glycolysis or hypoxia can reduce transcription of tumor suppressor genes. Hypermethylation of the tumor suppressor genes in the RAS family leads to a higher risk of relapse and worse survival. One of the few surveys comparing epigenetics in Black versus White populations found a higher frequency of hypermethylation in *FASSF1A* among Black participants than among White participants.[37,38]

It is established that women with higher breast density have higher risk of breast cancer. Older studies suggested that Black women had a higher prevalence of dense breasts than White women, and it itself was a risk factor for breast cancer. Mammographic breast density differences across racial groups by itself do not explain differences in breast cancer risk. Age, obesity, reproductive history, and other factors are important in determining density.[39] These are also factors in determining risk. High breast density also obscures tumors making mammography a less effective tool.

DISPARITIES IN SCREENING AND DIAGNOSIS

Population modeling studies suggest about 10% of US breast cancer deaths are attributed to failure to get a mammogram or poor-quality mammography. In 2018, 72.8% of women, aged 50 to 74 years, had a mammogram within the past 2 years. Rates are similar among racial and ethnic groups with Hispanic Americans at 71.5% (95% CI 66.5–76.0), Black Americans at 73.8% (95% CI 69.1–77.9), and NH White Americans at 73.1% (95% CI 71.4 to 74.7).[40]

While the there is little racial variation among Americans receiving "a mammogram," studies however do suggest that poor and minority women are more likely to have

- Screening performed in a nonaccredited clinic with older or poorly maintained imaging equipment;[41]
- Screening in multiple clinics, such that older images are not available for comparison;
- Their image read by a radiologist who does not specialize in mammography;
- Incomplete tracking and follow-up for abnormal screening tests[42];
- The workup of abnormal results often takes longer for poor women than for the middle class White population.[43]

Obesity, which is more common in Black women, may also affect the efficacy of breast cancer screening and treatment. Indeed, obese women have a 20% increased risk of false positives.[44–46]

DISPARITIES IN TREATMENT

Population modeling suggests that 20%–27% of breast cancer deaths are due to receipt of poor-quality treatment. Poor quality of care can manifest itself in numerous ways. Once diagnosed, poor or Black women are also more likely to have delayed treatment than the White population. Lund and colleagues found that 7% of Black women diagnosed with a low-stage potential curable breast cancer in metropolitan Atlanta did not start treatment within 1 year of diagnosis compared to 2% of White women.[47,48]

Numerous studies show that African American women are less likely to receive treatment consistent with National Comprehensive Cancer Network practice guidelines.[49–51] Common indicators of poor care include a higher proportion of patients with positive margins after surgery or no assessment of pathology for ER, PR, and HER-2 status, or even no assessment of lymph nodes for presence of cancer.[51,52] The omission or underdosing of chemotherapy is also common.[53] Obesity can be a reason for underdosing of chemotherapy.

Poor care can sometimes be due to the patient's refusal to accept it.[54] This can be caused by a lack of information or fear and distrust. Partridge and colleagues found that Black patients were much less likely to take prescribed tamoxifen and aromatase inhibitor therapies.[54] The poor insurance status does account for some poor adherence to oral therapies.[55–57] This latter finding is especially important as the greatest documented disparity in treatment is among Black and White women with ER + disease.[58]

Again, we note that women of all races can receive less than optimal therapy. These women are more often poor and disenfranchised.[59–61] They suffer from access issues such as inability to afford care, inability to get paid leave to get care, or lack of transportation to obtain care. The poor are also more likely to suffer from obesity, diabetes, hypertension, cardiovascular disease, respiratory diseases, and other comorbidities that complicate the provision of aggressive treatment.

While Black Americans are less likely to receive high-quality breast cancer care (screening, diagnosis, and treatment) than White Americans, a larger number of White American women get poor-quality care.[55] This is because the US White population is much larger than the Black population (62.8% of the US population compared to 9.3%).[55,62] The absolute number of White Americans living in poverty is twice that of NH Black Americans living in poverty.

The Affordable Care Act (ACA) increased access to care for a large number of Americans beginning in 2014.[63] The ACA has not been in place long enough to effect cancer mortality statistics, but one would predict that it will prevent deaths. The ACA has been associated with increased early detection of breast, colon, and several other cancers.[64,65] Unfortunately, Medicaid expansion under the ACA has occurred in some states and not in others. This portends to greater state-by-state breast cancer disparities.

The provision of quality care matters. In lung cancer, colon cancer, lymphoma, leukemia, and myeloma clinical trials, stage-by-stage, equal treatment consistently yields equal access, and race is not a factor in outcome.[66,67] In some breast cancer studies, there are minor differences in outcome by race. The reasons are unclear but may be differences in biology that are caused or influenced by social determinants of health.

Among breast cancer patients seen in an equal-access facility with high volumes of African American patients, (the Henry Ford Health System) Lehrberg and colleagues[68] found that equal treatment yields equal outcomes among Black and White early-stage, node-negative patients. In an assessment of women with stage 1 to 3 triple-negative breast cancer, Roseland and colleagues[69] found no mortality disparity after adjustment for clinical factors such as age, stage, and Charleston Comorbidity Score (hazard ratio [HR] 1.51, CI 1.10–2.08). Indeed, they found that comorbidity, especially diabetes and hypertension, explained nearly half of the Black-White survival disparity. Black patients were overwhelmingly more obese than White patients (72% compared to 49.7%). Only after adjusting for social deprivation was race no longer significant (HR 1.26, CI 0.84–1.87).

In an analysis by race of women in early stage breast cancer treatment trials, there was near comparable benefit for adjuvant chemotherapy.[70] There were some small mortality differences among African Americans with lymph node-negative disease, but most was attributed to noncancer issues. In Southwest Oncology Group clinical trials evaluating adjuvant therapies, Hirschman and colleagues found that African American women had worse disease-free survival and overall survival than White women (HR 1.95, 95% CI 1.36–2.78).[71] The study found that African American women were more likely to experience discontinuation or delay of treatment than White patients. It is speculated that this was due to economic barriers and transportation issues. It is known that these delays were not due to toxicities.

THE SOLUTION: BRINGING ABOUT HEALTH EQUITY

If we are to have treatments for all, we must study all populations. We need large studies in well-defined populations that are diverse with as many criteria as possible to provide estimates of the burden of mutations in underserved and previously understudied populations.[72] Study of treatment outcomes while carefully defining populations should also continue.[18]

The variation in death rates among the racial groups by state is highly suggestive that something can be done to reduce breast cancer deaths. It also suggests that Black women are not the only women to suffer disparities. We have significant data to show that significant improvement in outcomes can be brought about by providing all Americans with adequate high-quality care.[73] Adequate high-quality care includes prevention, screening, diagnosis, and treatment. Too often, adequate care is interpreted simply as access to treatment. Even then, the utilization of that care and the quality of that care are rarely mentioned.

Utilization of care requires a way of paying for it and accessing it. Elements of a program to reduce disparities in breast cancer require some form of payment or insurance as well as the ability to use that insurance.[74,75] Navigation programs and other efforts to identify patient needs (education, economic as well as logistic) and keep them in the system can be quite useful. Other issues that need to be addressed include transportation and education regarding how to obtain health care.[76]

There are examples of success such as that at the Henry Ford Health System mentioned earlier. At a population level, the Metropolitan Chicago Breast Cancer Task Force sponsored culturally sensitive breast health education and successfully lobbied for passage of the Illinois Reducing Breast Cancer Disparities Act of 2009. This act improved access to high-quality routine mammography screening. The result was a decrease of 13.87% in mortality rates for Black women, the largest decrease in mortality among the 10 US cities with large African American populations.[77]

Cancer research has clearly demonstrated the existence of disparities. Furthermore, it has shown us that a significant reason for disparities in health is people who could benefit from the known science and simply are not getting it. A substantial number of breast cancer deaths could be prevented simply by providing the known science to all.[22,78] In a civilized society, the provision of adequate care is a moral imperative.

CLINICS CARE POINTS

- Disparities in quality of breast care often begins with women getting mammography without the advantage of previous images being compared.
- Disparities often include delays in assessment of abnormal screening tests and delays in treatment when compared to those getting quality care.
- Disparities also include underdosing of chemotherapy or radiation from older lower energy radiation therapy machines.

DISCLOSURE

O.W. Brawley has consulting interests in Genentech, Grail, Agilent, Incyte, PDS Bio, and Lyell Immunopharma. D.G. Lansey reports no conflict of interest.

REFERENCES

1. Sung H, Ferlay J, Siegel RL, et al. Global cancer statistics 2020: GLOBOCAN estimates of incidence and mortality worldwide for 36 cancers in 185 countries. CA Cancer J Clin 2021;71(3):209–49.
2. Siegel RL, Miller KD, Fuchs HE, et al. Cancer Statistics, 2021. CA Cancer J Clin 2021;71(1):7–33.
3. Ward EM, DeSantis CE, Lin CC, et al. Cancer statistics: Breast cancer in situ. CA Cancer J Clin 2015;65(6):481–95.
4. Crew KD, Albain KS, Hershman DL, et al. How do we increase uptake of tamoxifen and other anti-estrogens for breast cancer prevention? NPJ Breast Cancer 2017;3:20.
5. Stedman MR, Feuer EJ, Mariotto AB. Current estimates of the cure fraction: a feasibility study of statistical cure for breast and colorectal cancer. J Natl Cancer Inst Monogr 2014;2014(49):244–54.
6. Plevritis SK, Munoz D, Kurian AW, et al. Association of Screening and Treatment With Breast Cancer Mortality by Molecular Subtype in US Women, 2000-2012. Jama 2018;319(2):154–64.
7. Brawley OW. Health disparities in breast cancer. Obstet Gynecol Clin North Am 2013;40(3):513–23.

8. Friedman DJ, Cohen BB, Averbach AR, et al. Race/ethnicity and OMB Directive 15: implications for state public health practice. Am J Public Health 2000;90(11): 1714–9.
9. Siegel RL, Miller KD, Fuchs HE, et al. Cancer statistics, 2022. CA Cancer J Clin 2022;72(1):7–33.
10. Elhaik E, Tatarinova T, Chebotarev D, et al. Geographic population structure analysis of worldwide human populations infers their biogeographical origins. Nat Commun 2014;5:3513.
11. Koromina M, Pandi MT, van der Spek PJ, et al. The ethnogeographic variability of genetic factors underlying G6PD deficiency. Pharmacol Res 2021;173:105904.
12. Nyante SJ, Abraham L, Aiello Bowles EJ, et al. Diagnostic Mammography Performance across Racial and Ethnic Groups in a National Network of Community-Based Breast Imaging Facilities. Cancer Epidemiol Biomarkers Prev 2022; 31(7):1324–33.
13. Lawson MB, Bissell MCS, Miglioretti DL, et al. Multilevel Factors Associated With Time to Biopsy After Abnormal Screening Mammography Results by Race and Ethnicity. JAMA Oncol 2022. https://doi.org/10.1001/jamaoncol.2022.1990.
14. Howlader NNA, Krapcho M, Miller D, et al. SEER Cancer Statistics Review, 1975-2017. 2020. 2021. Available at: https://seer.cancer.gov/csr/1975_2017/. Accessed October 23, 2022.
15. DeSantis CE, Miller KD, Goding Sauer A, et al. Cancer statistics for African Americans, 2019. CA Cancer J Clin 2019;69(3):211–33.
16. Kong X, Liu Z, Cheng R, et al. Variation in Breast Cancer Subtype Incidence and Distribution by Race/Ethnicity in the United States From 2010 to 2015. JAMA Netw Open 2020;3(10):e2020303.
17. DeSantis CE, Ma J, Gaudet MM, et al. Breast cancer statistics, 2019. CA Cancer J Clin 2019;69(6):438–51.
18. Howard FM, Olopade OI. Epidemiology of Triple-Negative Breast Cancer: A Review. Cancer J 2021;27(1):8–16.
19. Sung H, DeSantis C, Jemal A. Subtype-Specific Breast Cancer Incidence Rates in Black versus White Men in the United States. JNCI Cancer Spectr 2020;4(1): pkz091.
20. Islami F, Goding Sauer A, Miller KD, et al. Proportion and number of cancer cases and deaths attributable to potentially modifiable risk factors in the United States. CA Cancer J Clin 2018;68(1):31–54.
21. Calle EE, Rodriguez C, Walker-Thurmond K, et al. Overweight, obesity, and mortality from cancer in a prospectively studied cohort of U.S. adults. N Engl J Med 2003;348(17):1625–38.
22. Islami F, Siegel RL, Jemal A. The changing landscape of cancer in the USA - opportunities for advancing prevention and treatment. Nat Rev Clin Oncol 2020; 17(10):631–49.
23. Ogden CL, Fryar CD, Martin CB, et al. Trends in Obesity Prevalence by Race and Hispanic Origin-1999-2000 to 2017-2018. Jama 2020;324(12):1208–10.
24. Ambrosone CB, Zirpoli G, Ruszczyk M, et al. Parity and breastfeeding among African-American women: differential effects on breast cancer risk by estrogen receptor status in the Women's Circle of Health Study. Cancer Causes Control 2014;25(2):259–65.
25. Lambertini M, Santoro L, Del Mastro L, et al. Reproductive behaviors and risk of developing breast cancer according to tumor subtype: A systematic review and meta-analysis of epidemiological studies. Cancer Treat Rev 2016;49:65–76.

26. Ravdin PM, Cronin KA, Howlader N, et al. The decrease in breast-cancer incidence in 2003 in the United States. N Engl J Med 2007;356(16):1670–4.
27. Pal T, Bonner D, Cragun D, et al. A high frequency of BRCA mutations in young black women with breast cancer residing in Florida. Cancer 2015;121(23): 4173–80.
28. Offit K, Gilewski T, McGuire P, et al. Germline BRCA1 185delAG mutations in Jewish women with breast cancer. Lancet 1996;347(9016):1643–5.
29. Cragun D, Weidner A, Lewis C, et al. Racial disparities in BRCA testing and cancer risk management across a population-based sample of young breast cancer survivors. Cancer 2017;123(13):2497–505.
30. Friebel TM, Andrulis IL, Balmaña J, et al. BRCA1 and BRCA2 pathogenic sequence variants in women of African origin or ancestry. Hum Mutat 2019; 40(10):1781–96.
31. Ndiaye R, Diop JPD, Bourdon-Huguenin V, et al. Evidence for an ancient BRCA1 pathogenic variant in inherited breast cancer patients from Senegal. NPJ Genom Med 2020;5:8.
32. Nanda R, Schumm LP, Cummings S, et al. Genetic testing in an ethnically diverse cohort of high-risk women: a comparative analysis of BRCA1 and BRCA2 mutations in American families of European and African ancestry. Jama 2005;294(15): 1925–33.
33. Jemal A, Fedewa SA. Is the prevalence of ER-negative breast cancer in the US higher among Africa-born than US-born black women? Breast Cancer Res Treat 2012;135(3):867–73.
34. Sung H, DeSantis CE, Fedewa SA, et al. Breast cancer subtypes among Eastern-African-born black women and other black women in the United States. Cancer 2019;125(19):3401–11.
35. Pinheiro PS, Medina H, Callahan KE, et al. Cancer mortality among US blacks: Variability between African Americans, Afro-Caribbeans, and Africans. Cancer Epidemiol 2020;66:101709.
36. Lara OD, Wang Y, Asare A, et al. Pan-cancer clinical and molecular analysis of racial disparities. Cancer 2020;126(4):800–7.
37. Jiang Y, Cui L, Chen WD, et al. The prognostic role of RASSF1A promoter methylation in breast cancer: a meta-analysis of published data. PLoS One 2012;7(5): e36780.
38. Mehrotra J, Ganpat MM, Kanaan Y, et al. Estrogen receptor/progesterone receptor-negative breast cancers of young African-American women have a higher frequency of methylation of multiple genes than those of Caucasian women. Clin Cancer Res 2004;10(6):2052–7.
39. del Carmen MG, Halpern EF, Kopans DB, et al. Mammographic breast density and race. AJR Am J Roentgenol 2007;188(4):1147–50.
40. Goding Sauer A, Siegel RL, Jemal A, et al. Current Prevalence of Major Cancer Risk Factors and Screening Test Use in the United States: Disparities by Education and Race/Ethnicity. Cancer Epidemiol Biomarkers Prev 2019;28(4):629–42.
41. Betancourt JR, Tan-McGrory A, Flores E, et al. Racial and Ethnic Disparities in Radiology: A Call to Action. J Am Coll Radiol 2019;16(4 Pt B):547–53.
42. Rauscher GH, Murphy AM, Orsi JM, et al. Beyond the mammography quality standards act: measuring the quality of breast cancer screening programs. AJR Am J Roentgenol 2014;202(1):145–51.
43. Ansell D, Grabler P, Whitman S, et al. A community effort to reduce the black/white breast cancer mortality disparity in Chicago. Cancer Causes Control 2009;20(9):1681–8.

44. Griggs JJ, Sorbero ME, Lyman GH. Undertreatment of obese women receiving breast cancer chemotherapy. Arch Intern Med 2005;165(11):1267–73.
45. Cohen SS, Palmieri RT, Nyante SJ, et al. Obesity and screening for breast, cervical, and colorectal cancer in women: a review. Cancer 2008;112(9):1892–904.
46. Elmore JG, Carney PA, Abraham LA, et al. The association between obesity and screening mammography accuracy. Arch Intern Med 2004;164(10):1140–7.
47. Lund MJ, Brawley OP, Ward KC, et al. Parity and disparity in first course treatment of invasive breast cancer. Breast Cancer Res Treat 2008;109(3):545–57.
48. Silber JH, Rosenbaum PR, Clark AS, et al. Characteristics associated with differences in survival among black and white women with breast cancer. Jama 2013; 310(4):389–97.
49. Freedman RA, He Y, Winer EP, et al. Racial/Ethnic differences in receipt of timely adjuvant therapy for older women with breast cancer: are delays influenced by the hospitals where patients obtain surgical care? Health Serv Res 2013;48(5): 1669–83.
50. Griggs JJ, Sorbero ME, Stark AT, et al. Racial disparity in the dose and dose intensity of breast cancer adjuvant chemotherapy. Breast Cancer Res Treat 2003; 81(1):21–31.
51. Obeng-Gyasi S, Asad S, Fisher JL, et al. Socioeconomic and Surgical Disparities are Associated with Rapid Relapse in Patients with Triple-Negative Breast Cancer. Ann Surg Oncol 2021;28(11):6500–9.
52. Breslin TM, Morris AM, Gu N, et al. Hospital factors and racial disparities in mortality after surgery for breast and colon cancer. J Clin Oncol 2009;27(24): 3945–50.
53. Bickell NA, Wang JJ, Oluwole S, et al. Missed opportunities: racial disparities in adjuvant breast cancer treatment. J Clin Oncol 2006;24(9):1357–62.
54. Partridge AH, Wang PS, Winer EP, et al. Nonadherence to adjuvant tamoxifen therapy in women with primary breast cancer. J Clin Oncol 2003;21(4):602–6.
55. Wu XC, Lund MJ, Kimmick GG, et al. Influence of race, insurance, socioeconomic status, and hospital type on receipt of guideline-concordant adjuvant systemic therapy for locoregional breast cancers. J Clin Oncol 2012;30(2):142–50.
56. Huiart L, Ferdynus C, Giorgi R. A meta-regression analysis of the available data on adherence to adjuvant hormonal therapy in breast cancer: summarizing the data for clinicians. Breast Cancer Res Treat 2013;138(1):325–8.
57. Lannin DR, Mathews HF, Mitchell J, et al. Influence of socioeconomic and cultural factors on racial differences in late-stage presentation of breast cancer. Jama 1998;279(22):1801–7.
58. Warner ET, Tamimi RM, Hughes ME, et al. Racial and Ethnic Differences in Breast Cancer Survival: Mediating Effect of Tumor Characteristics and Sociodemographic and Treatment Factors. J Clin Oncol 2015;33(20):2254–61.
59. Griggs JJ, Culakova E, Sorbero ME, et al. Social and racial differences in selection of breast cancer adjuvant chemotherapy regimens. J Clin Oncol 2007;25(18): 2522–7.
60. Griggs JJ, Culakova E, Sorbero ME, et al. Effect of patient socioeconomic status and body mass index on the quality of breast cancer adjuvant chemotherapy. J Clin Oncol 2007;25(3):277–84.
61. Li CI, Beaber EF, Tang MT, et al. Reproductive factors and risk of estrogen receptor positive, triple-negative, and HER2-neu overexpressing breast cancer among women 20-44 years of age. Breast Cancer Res Treat 2013;137(2):579–87.

62. Siegel R, Ward E, Brawley O, et al. Cancer statistics, 2011: the impact of eliminating socioeconomic and racial disparities on premature cancer deaths. CA Cancer J Clin 2011;61(4):212–36.
63. Zhao J, Mao Z, Fedewa SA, et al. The Affordable Care Act and access to care across the cancer control continuum: A review at 10 years. CA Cancer J Clin 2020;70(3):165–81.
64. Le Blanc JM, Heller DR, Friedrich A, et al. Association of Medicaid Expansion Under the Affordable Care Act With Breast Cancer Stage at Diagnosis. JAMA Surg 2020;155(8):1–7.
65. Fedewa SA, Yabroff KR, Smith RA, et al. Changes in Breast and Colorectal Cancer Screening After Medicaid Expansion Under the Affordable Care Act. Am J Prev Med 2019;57(1):3–12.
66. Albain KS, Unger JM, Crowley JJ, et al. Racial disparities in cancer survival among randomized clinical trials patients of the Southwest Oncology Group. J Natl Cancer Inst 2009;101(14):984–92.
67. Dess RT, Hartman HE, Mahal BA, et al. Association of Black Race With Prostate Cancer-Specific and Other-Cause Mortality. JAMA Oncol 2019;5(7):975–83.
68. Lehrberg A, Davis MB, Baidoun F, et al. Outcome of African-American compared to White-American patients with early-stage breast cancer, stratified by phenotype. Breast J 2021;27(7):573–80.
69. Roseland ME, Schwartz K, Ruterbusch JJ, et al. Influence of clinical, societal, and treatment variables on racial differences in ER-/PR- breast cancer survival. Breast Cancer Res Treat 2017;165(1):163–8.
70. Dignam JJ. Re: Racial disparities in cancer survival among randomized clinical trials of the Southwest Oncology Group. J Natl Cancer Inst 2010;102(4):279–80 [author reply: 280–2].
71. Hershman DL, Unger JM, Barlow WE, et al. Treatment quality and outcomes of African American versus white breast cancer patients: retrospective analysis of Southwest Oncology studies S8814/S8897. J Clin Oncol 2009;27(13):2157–62.
72. Omilian AR, Wei L, Hong CC, et al. Somatic mutations of triple-negative breast cancer: a comparison between Black and White women. Breast Cancer Res Treat 2020;182(2):503–9.
73. Siegel RL, Jemal A, Wender RC, et al. An assessment of progress in cancer control. CA Cancer J Clin 2018;68(5):329–39.
74. Gabram SG, Lund MJ, Gardner J, et al. Effects of an outreach and internal navigation program on breast cancer diagnosis in an urban cancer center with a large African-American population. Cancer 2008;113(3):602–7.
75. Natale-Pereira A, Enard KR, Nevarez L, et al. The role of patient navigators in eliminating health disparities. Cancer 2011;117(15 Suppl):3543–52.
76. Starbird LE, DiMaina C, Sun CA, et al. A Systematic Review of Interventions to Minimize Transportation Barriers Among People with Chronic Diseases. J Community Health 2019;44(2):400–11.
77. Polite BN, Gluck AR, Brawley OW. Ensuring Equity and Justice in the Care and Outcomes of Patients With Cancer. Jama 2019;321(17):1663–4.
78. Ma J, Jemal A, Fedewa SA, et al. The American Cancer Society 2035 challenge goal on cancer mortality reduction. CA Cancer J Clin 2019;69(5):351–62.

Diagnosis

Breast Cancer
Risk Assessment, Screening, and Primary Prevention

Elena Michaels, MD, Rebeca Ortiz Worthington, MD, MS, Jennifer Rusiecki, MD, MS*

KEYWORDS

- Breast cancer • Breast cancer risk • Mammogram • Breast MRI
- Chemoprophylaxis • SERM • Aromatase inhibitors • Prophylactic surgery

KEY POINTS

- All women should be assessed by history for breast cancer risk starting at age 18 years and counseled on breast awareness and lifestyle modifications such as weight loss, physical activity, reduced alcohol consumption, and smoking cessation.
- Women with above-average risk for breast cancer include those with a personal or family history of breast cancer, known genetic mutation, history of chest radiation before age 30, history of high-risk lesions, or dense breast tissue on mammography.
- Risk calculators should be used to identify high-risk patients who would benefit from yearly breast MRI screening and risk-reducing medications.
- High-risk individuals should be referred to breast cancer prevention specialists including an oncologist and genetic counselor who can assist in co-managing screening and prevention.

INTRODUCTION

Approximately one in eight women will be diagnosed with breast cancer in their lifetime. Breast cancer risk increases as women age with the highest rate of new diagnoses at ages 70 to 74 years. It is also a leading cause of death for women in their 40s and is the second most common cause of cancer deaths in women.[1,2] Although non-Hispanic white women have the highest annual average breast cancer incidence rate, hormone receptor-negative cancer is more common among black women, and breast cancer death rates are highest in black patients despite lower incidence rates.[3] This is

This article previously appeared in *Medical Clinics* volume 107 issue 2 March 2023.
Department of Medicine, University of Chicago, 5841 South Maryland Avenue, MC 3051, Chicago, IL 60637, USA
* Corresponding author.
E-mail address: jrusiecki@medicine.bsd.uchicago.edu

https://doi.org/10.1016/j.ccol.2024.02.009
2352-7986/24/© 2024 Elsevier Inc. All rights reserved.

thought to be due in large part to socioeconomic factors as well as later-stage diagnosis of disease.[4]

Breast cancer incidence is rising by approximately 0.5% per year.[2] Studies suggest that over half of all breast cancer diagnoses could be prevented through lifestyle changes and the use of risk-reducing medications and surgery.[5] The use of targeted interventions such as genetic counseling, MRI, chemoprophylaxis, and prophylactic surgery for high-risk patients are notably underutilized.[6] This is likely multi-factorial and due to a combination of insufficient provider training, time constraints, and patient preference.

This review provides an outline of performing a breast cancer risk assessment, how to apply a risk-based approach to screening, and recommendations for breast cancer prevention both for average and high-risk groups. It is our goal that this review will give providers an evidence-based review and the skills needed to use an individualized, risk-based approach to breast cancer screening and prevention.

Risk Assessment

Assessment of an individual patient's risk of developing breast cancer is the first step in developing a personalized prevention and screening strategy. A risk assessment should be performed for patients as young as 18 years old and revisited every 5 years. Key items to elicit during a patient's history include the following: (a) personal or family history of breast or ovarian cancer, breast cancer-associated genetic mutation, or family history of genetic breast cancer syndrome; (b) personal history of chest radiation < 30 years old; (c) personal history of a high-risk breast lesion, breast biopsy, or dense breasts on mammography.[7–9] **Fig. 1** shows a model for approaching risk assessment via history. Based on a risk factor review and, if needed, a risk calculation, providers can assign patients to a risk group (**Table 1**).

Risk Factor Review and Counseling

An individual's risk for developing breast cancer is based on modifiable and nonmodifiable risk factors (**Table 2**). Approximately 40% of breast cancers are due to hormonal or reproductive factors, 40% are attributable to modifiable risk factors, and about 10% are due to known genetic mutations.[10] The degree of conferred risk varies substantially by each factor (see **Table 2**).

Nonmodifiable Risk Factors

Past Medical History: Chest Radiation and Proliferative Breast Lesions.

A history of chest radiation as a child or young adult leads to a 40% lifetime risk of developing breast cancer.[11] These patients should be co-managed with a breast specialist.

All patients with a history of biopsy-proven atypical ductal hyperplasia (ADH), atypical lobular hyperplasia (ALH), or lobular carcinoma in situ (LCIS) are at an increased risk of breast cancer.[5] These lesions should be removed. Ductal carcinoma in situ (DCIS), unlike other proliferative breast lesions, is managed and treated as a noninvasive breast cancer. Non-proliferative lesions such as fibroadenoma, epithelial hyperplasia, intraductal papilloma, and phyllodes tumors do not carry an increased risk of breast cancer.[12]

Genetic Factors and Family History of Cancer

A strong family history of cancer is defined as a first or second-degree family member with:

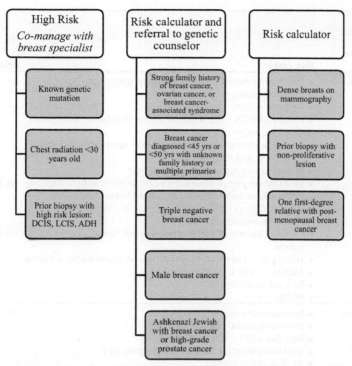

Fig. 1. Risk assessment algorithm. Patients with any of the conditions listed under the "High Risk" box should be comanaged with a breast specialist. Prevention strategies for this group may include prophylactic surgeries, medications, and advanced imaging. Patients with conditions under the "Risk calculation and referral to genetic counselor" box should be offered genetic counseling and based on the results of genetic testing a risk calculation should be performed. For patients that refuse genetic testing, a risk calculation should be performed. For patients with conditions under the "Risk Calculation" box, a risk calculation should be performed. For patients that do not fit into any of these three groupings, a risk calculation is not necessary.

- A known genetic mutation
- Bilateral breast cancer or two or more breast cancer primaries
- Premenopausal breast cancer (<50 years old)
- Ovarian cancer

Table 1		
Risk group		
High	**Moderate**	**Average**
>20% lifetime calculated risk	15% to 19% lifetime calculated risk	<15% lifetime calculated risk
• Chest radiation	• First-degree family member postmenopausal breast cancer	• 0 to 3 hormonal/lifestyle risk factors
• Atypical hyperplasia, DCIS or LCIS	• Dense breast	
• Genetic syndrome	• 3+ hormonal/lifestyle risk factors	
• Significant family history[a]		

[a] ≥2 first-degree relatives with breast cancer, or ≥1 relative with premenopausal breast cancer, or male breast cancer.

Table 2 Risk factors		
Risk Factor Category	**Risk Factor**	**Relative Risk**
Non-modifiable	• Personal or family history of known genetic mutation	RR >4.0
	• Personal history of breast cancer	
	• Personal history of ovarian cancer	
	• History of DCIS, LCIS, atypical ductal or lobular hyperplasia	
	• Chest radiation <30 y of age	
	• Hereditary breast and ovarian cancer syndromes (eg, BRCA 1, BRCA 2, and PALB2)	
	• Strong family history of breast cancer	
	• One first-degree relative with postmenopausal breast cancer	RR 2.1 to 4.0
	• Extremely or heterogeneously dense breast tissue	
	• Genetic factors (CHEK2 mutation carrier, Lynch syndrome, Ataxia telangiectasia)	
	• Personal history of melanoma, thyroid cancer, endometrial cancer	RR 1.1 to 2.0
	• History of ≥1 breast biopsies or breast lesion without atypia	
	• Menarche <12 y, menopause >55 y	
	• DES use or exposure	
	• PCOS	
Modifiable	• Hormone therapy within past 5 y	RR 1.1 to 2.0
	• Postmenopausal obesity, inactivity	
	• First live birth ≥30 y, nulliparity	
	• Oral contraceptive use within the past 10 y	
	• Alcohol consumption	
	• Current smoking	

- Two or more people with breast cancer on the same side of the family
- Male breast cancer, metastatic prostate cancer, or pancreatic cancer

These individuals should be referred to a genetic counselor. Anyone with a personal history of ovarian or pancreatic cancer or 3 or more family members diagnosed with any combination of cancers including breast, pancreatic, or prostate cancer, melanoma, sarcoma, adrenocortical carcinoma, brain tumor, leukemia, gastric, colon, endometrial, thyroid, or kidney cancer, or hamartomatous polyps in the gastrointestinal tract should also be referred per National Comprehensive Cancer Network (NCCN) guidelines.[7,8]

In addition to the above criteria, referral to a genetic counselor is recommended for all women diagnosed with breast cancer under age 45, women diagnosed under 50 years old with an unknown family history or multiple breast primaries, triple-negative breast cancer, male breast cancer, and those of Ashkenazi Jewish heritage diagnosed with breast cancer or high-grade prostate cancer.[7]

Genetic factors that increase a patient's risk for developing breast cancer are genetic mutations and hereditary breast and ovarian cancer syndromes. These include BRCA1, BRCA2, PALB2, CHEK2, Peutz-Jeghers syndrome, Li-Fraumeni syndrome, PTEN hamartoma syndrome, neurofibromatosis 1, and Lynch syndrome.[8]

Modifiable Risk Factors—Lifestyle Counseling

Weight control and physical activity

Postmenopausal overweight or obesity status is associated with an increased risk of breast cancer of 1.03 per 2 kg/m^2 point increase in body mass index (BMI) in postmenopausal women (95% confidence interval [CI] 1.01 to 1.04).[13] In addition, women who experience postmenopausal weight gain can reduce the risk of breast cancer by 8% with every 5 kg/m^2 decrease in BMI.[13]

Several studies have shown that physical activity can reduce cancer risk in postmenopausal women. Any level of physical activity is protective, although a significant reduction in breast cancer risk by 20% was seen in women, regardless of BMI, who performed more than 6.7 metabolic equivalents (MET)-h/wk of physical activity (odds ratio [OR] 0.82, CI 0.7 to 0.92).[14] This is equivalent to a 30-min walk, 4 times a week.

Alcohol
Alcohol consumption of up to 1 to 2 drinks per day is associated with an increased risk of breast cancer. Two cohort studies showed that for every 10 g of alcohol consumed per day, breast cancer risk increased by 10%.[15] Consensus is to limit alcohol use to one drink per day or less and to avoid daily alcohol use.

Modifiable Risk Factors: Hormone and Reproductive Factors

Hormone therapy
The use of hormone therapy (HT) for the treatment of vasomotor symptoms related to menopause has been complicated by the concern about an increased risk of breast cancer. Much of this concern originates from the Women's Health Initiative (WHI), a randomized control trial studying the use of HT in postmenopausal women. The study was terminated early after finding that women who received both estrogen and progestin had a 26% increased incidence of breast cancer (hazard ratio [HR] 1.26; 95% CI, 1.00 to 1.59).[16] This finding partially contributed to changing current prescribing guidelines for postmenopausal HT.

Since the WHI study was published, several prospective, observational studies have shown that estrogen-only HT affects breast cancer risk differently. Most notably, the Nurses' Health Study showed an increase in breast cancer risk for women taking estrogen-only HT starting after 5 years of use and becoming statistically significant after "long-term" use of 20 years or longer (Risk Ratio [RR] 1.42, 95% CI, 1.13 to 1.77).[17] Therefore, NCCN practice guidelines do not recommend against the use of short-term postmenopausal HT of fewer than 5 years duration.[8] However, women and their providers should be aware that there is a small increased breast cancer risk that is more pronounced with progesterone-containing regimens.

Hormone contraceptives
Several studies have shown a small, increased risk of breast cancer from oral contraceptive use. A meta-analysis shows a small but significant increase in breast cancer risk with oral contraceptives (OR 1.15, 95% CI: 1.01 to 1.31, $P = .036$).[18] Conversely, oral contraceptives also have a protective benefit against ovarian and endometrial cancer. The breast cancer risk seen with oral contraception is small and this option should not be withheld from patients based on this risk alone. It is recommended that for women who are concerned specifically about breast cancer risk that providers counsel to limit oral contraceptive use to 5 to 10 years and consider alternative forms of contraception after the age of 40.

Pregnancy and breastfeeding
Counseling on the role of pregnancy in breast cancer risk is complicated. Past pregnancy is not a modifiable risk factor and there are many other factors aside from cancer risk that are considered when planning a pregnancy. Pregnancy under the age of 25 is protective against future breast cancer, whereas women who give birth at or after 30-year-old are at an increased risk of breast cancer. However, nulliparous women have a 2.0 relative risk of breast cancer compared with women who have given birth.[14]

In general, it is recommended that women with an elevated risk of breast cancer who wish to become a pregnant plan for pregnancy at a younger age if possible.

For women who give birth, breastfeeding has a protective benefit against breast cancer. A longer duration of breastfeeding is associated with greater risk reduction, although a benefit has been shown within 5 months.[14] Similar to pregnancy, a myriad of factors can affect a woman's ability to breastfeed but it is recommended that providers counsel on the benefits of breastfeeding.

Risk calculation

After reviewing risk factors a calculator should be used for those with a significant family history, personal history of a breast lesion or biopsy, or dense breasts. Risk calculators account for various personal, genetic, family, and hormonal/reproductive factors to estimate an individual's 5-year, 10-year, or lifetime risk for developing breast cancer (**Table 3**). Elevated 5-year risk is used to determine if an individual qualifies for risk reduction medications. Lifetime risk is used to determine whether to offer MRI in addition to mammography for annual screening.[19–22]

Risk-based screening

Screening and early detection of breast cancer is an important tool in improving breast cancer mortality. Mammography remains the preferred option for screening but the timing and duration of screening are less clear with multiple competing guidelines (**Table 4**). Screening decisions should be based on the patient's risk of breast cancer and providers must engage in shared decision-making to determine the appropriate screening plan (**Fig. 2**).

Average risk

The age to initiate screening varies by guideline but there is a consensus that mammogram screening should be initiated by age 50 for average-risk women. It is unclear if screening is appropriate for patients in their 40s. There is a small net benefit of screening from age 40 to 49 (3 deaths avoided per 10,000 women screened for 10 years, compared with 8 to 21 deaths avoided for women age 50 to 75 years).[23] The American Cancer Society (ACS) argues that women age 45 to 50 have a more similar breast cancer risk to those 50 to 54 years old (0.9% vs 1.1% 5-year risk respectively) and that 45 may be a more appropriate starting age.[24] This could be an acceptable option for women who wish to start screening in their 40s.

For patients in their 40s, the risk of early screening must be balanced against the risk of false-positive imaging. Over 10 years of screening, 61% of women in their 40s will have a false-positive mammogram.[25] Moving the screening age from 40 to 50 showed a reduction in false-positive imaging of more than 50%.[23] Patients who have experienced a false-positive mammogram are less likely to return to screening (return to screening within 36 months HR 1.36, 95% CI 1.35 to 1.37) and are at higher risk of presenting with late-stage breast cancer (0.4% vs 0.3% for false-positive vs true negative, $P = .001$).[26]

Moving the screening interval from annual to biennial is recommended by the United States Preventative Service Task Force (USPSTF) and the ACS for women in their 50s.[24,27] By moving the screening interval the 80% mortality reduction was maintained but the false-positive test rate dropped from 61.3% to 42%.[23] For average-risk patients a biennial screening model is effective at preventing breast cancer deaths but limits the risk of false-positive imaging.

The decision to stop screening should be based on age, overall life expectancy, and patient screening goals. The USPSTF recommends that screening stop at age 75.[27] The ACS recommends screening until the patient's life expectancy is less than

Table 3
Risk calculators

Calculator	Risk Calculated	Personal History Considered	Family History Considered	Comments and Access
Gail Model or NIH Breast Cancer Risk Assessment Tool (BCRAT)	• 5-y risk • Lifetime risk	• Biopsy history • Reproductive history	First-degree relatives with breast cancer	Widely available Simple Does not consider:LCIS or DCISExtensive family history Increased breast density www.mdcalc.com/gail-modelbreast-cancer-risk or https://bcrisktool.cancer.gov/calculator.html
Breast Cancer Surveillance Consortium (BCSC)	• 5-y risk • 10-y risk	• Breast density • LCIS • Biopsy history	First-degree relatives with breast cancer	Does not consider:Reproductive historyDCIS https://tools.bcsc-scc.org/BC5yearRisk/calculator.htm
International Breast Cancer Intervention Study (IBIS) or Tyrer-Cuzick model	• 5-y risk • 10-y risk • Lifetime risk	• Reproductive history • Menopause • Biopsy history • BRCA testing • Breast density	• ≥2 relatives with cancer • Ashkenazi Jewish heritage • Male breast cancer • Ovarian cancer • Second- or third-degree relatives with breast cancer	Most comprehensivehttps://ibis-risk-calculator.magview.com/ www.ems-trials.org/riskevaluator

5-y risk is used to determine whether a patient should be offered chemoprevention. Lifetime risk is used to determine whether to offer MRI in addition to annual mammography for screening.

Table 4
Screening guidelines for average-risk patients

Guideline	When to Start Screening	Screening for Over Age 45 to 50
USPSTF	• 40 to 49, individualized decision • If screening, biennial	• 50+ biennial screen • Stop at age 75
ACOG	• 40 to 49, individual decision • Annual or biennial based on SDM	• Start screening everyone by 50 • Annual or biennial based on SDM • Start to discuss stopping at age 75
ACS	• 40 to 44 discuss annual screen • 45 to 54 annual screen	• 45 to 54 annual screen • 55+ biennial screen • Stop life expectancy <10 years
ACR	• 40 annual screen	• Annual screen • No upper age cut off

Abbreviations: United States Preventative Services Task Force (USPSTF), American College of Obstetrics and Gynecology (ACOG), American Cancer Society (ACS), American College of Radiology (ACR).

10 years.[24] This is an individual decision that requires shared decision-making between the patient and provider.

Our recommendation for screening average-risk patients is to start the discussion between age 40 and 45. Inform patients of the risk of false-positive imaging in early screening and start screening if the patient is comfortable with this risk. Everyone should start screening by age 50 and a biennial approach is appropriate if it aligns with your patient's goals. Discuss stopping screening at age 75 but consider screening until a 10-year life expectancy in otherwise healthy women.

Moderate risk: screening for those with dense breast tissue
Screening guidelines should be adjusted for patients with moderate breast cancer risk. This includes women with dense breasts, a history of a non-proliferative breast lesion, one, first-degree relative with postmenopausal breast cancer, or a calculated 15% to 19% lifetime risk of breast cancer. These patients should start screening with mammography at age 40.

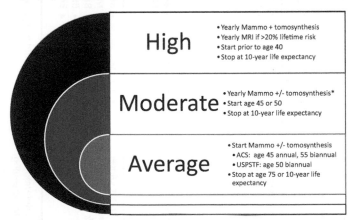

Fig. 2. Risk-based screening recommendations. Based on the patient's risk group an individualized screening strategy should be discussed with the patient. This figure can be used to guide that discussion. [a]Although current guidelines do not recommend supplemental imaging for dense breast tissue, women with extremely dense breasts may benefit from the additions of breast MRI or ultrasound given the limitations of tomosynthesis in this population. A risk calculation can be used to guide this decision.

Breast density is the proportion of glandular tissue to fat on a mammogram. Dense breasts confer a higher risk of breast cancer compared with those with normal density (RR 1.29 extremely, 1.23 heterogeneously dense).[23] Dense breasts may also decrease the sensitivity of mammography. Although no major screening guidelines support supplemental screening for dense breast tissue, there is legislation in most states that women must be notified of their breast density status.

Three main supplemental screening options have been proposed for women with dense breast tissue: tomosynthesis, ultrasound, and breast MRI. Tomosynthesis is a mammogram with additional pictures to provide a three-dimensional image of the breast. This option reduces recall rates but it is unclear if this is a useful option for women with extremely dense breasts. Whole breast ultrasound is not a suitable option due to high rates of false positives and unnecessary biopsies. Breast MRI is reserved for those with an more than 20% lifetime risk of breast cancer. All patients with dense breasts should have a risk calculation performed to see if they qualify for breast MRI. The USPSTF 2016 review concluded there is insufficient evidence for supplemental screening in patients with dense breasts.[27]

High risk
Those with a more than 20% lifetime risk of breast cancer are considered high-risk. This includes women with a history of childhood chest radiation, known high-risk genetic mutation, and prior high-risk breast lesions. Patients in this group should have a yearly mammogram. They should also be offered an annual breast MRI in addition to mammography.[22] Ideally, the mammogram and MRI are spaced 6 months apart to effectively screen twice a year. These patients may need to initiate screening before age 40. Mammography can be offered as early as age 30 and MRI at age 25. The recommended age to start screening high-risk individuals depends on each person's criteria for being high-risk and should be managed in conjunction with a breast cancer specialist.

Primary prevention
Counseling on breast cancer prevention and breast awareness should be offered to women in all risk categories. Below is a detailed outline of methods to reduce breast cancer risk.

General Counseling for all Patients

Breast awareness
It is important to counsel women on breast awareness to learn what normal breast tissue feels like. Although routine self-examinations are no longer recommended, women should be encouraged to seek care if they notice lumps, discharge, localized pain, or any other concerning change.

Personalized screening and prevention plan
All patients and providers should develop an individualized screening and prevention plan based on the patient's level of risk. This should include age to initiate screening, frequency of screening, and need for advanced imaging. If appropriate, a risk calculation should be included to guide this discussion. This is should be repeated yearly and updated with changes in personal or family history. All patients should be counseled on modifiable risk factors (see Risk Factor Review and Counseling section).

Additional Options for High-Risk Patients

Risk-reducing medications
The ACS and NCCN recommend the use of risk-reducing medications for women over the age of 35 with a greater than 1.66% 5-year risk of breast cancer and at least a 10-

year life expectancy.[20,21] Alternatively, the USPSTF advises using a 3% 5-year risk cutoff as it identifies the patients most likely to benefit from these agents.[6]

There are two selective estrogen receptor modulators (SERMs) approved for breast cancer prevention: tamoxifen and raloxifene (**Table 5**). Tamoxifen has an estrogen antagonist effect in the breast and an estrogen agonist effect on the bones and uterus. Thus, it improves bone density but is also associated with an increased risk of endometrial cancer and should not be used in postmenopausal women with a uterus. Raloxifene blocks the effects of estrogen in the breast and uterus and has a pro-estrogen effect on the bone. The STAR trial directly compared the efficacy of the two SERMs and found that although tamoxifen is superior to raloxifene in breast cancer prevention (RR 1.24, 95% CI 1.05 to 1.47), raloxifene is associated with fewer side effects.[28] SERMs are contraindicated in women with a history of pulmonary embolism or venous thromboembolism, stroke, hypercoagulable state (ie, clotting disorder, recent surgery, immobilization, pregnancy), or breastfeeding.

Although not US Food and Drug Administration (FDA)-approved, the aromatase inhibitors (AIs) anastrozole and exemestane have been studied for breast cancer risk reduction and are recommended for use by NCCN for postmenopausal women (see **Table 5**).[20] Through inhibition of aromatase, AIs block the conversion of androgens to estrogen, which is the main method of estrogen production in post-menopause women. The MAP.3 and IBIS-II trials showed the efficacy of exemestane (HR 0.47, 95% CI 0.27 to 0.79) and anastrozole (HR 0.47, 95% CI 0.32 to 0.68), respectively. No trials are comparing the risk/benefits of AIs to SERMs.[29,30] Common side effects of AIs include osteoporosis, worsening of vasomotor symptoms, and joint pain (see **Table 5**).[31] All postmenopausal women should undergo a baseline bone density assessment before starting medication.[8] The decisions of which agent to start should be based on if the patient has a uterus, menopause status, and bone density.[31]

The recommended duration of medication for breast cancer prevention is a total of 5 years (see **Table 5** for dosing).[8,28–30] Overall, studies show that providers greatly under-utilize medications for chemoprophylaxis despite a clear benefit in high-risk patients.[32,33] Barriers to care include provider knowledge limitations and time constraints as well as patient concerns about adverse effects.[34] Primary care providers, in particular, should be aware of who is eligible for risk-reducing medications and engage in shared decision-making conversations with eligible patients to potentially prevent future disease. Premenopausal women may elect to defer treatment until completion of child-bearing or after menopause.

Table 5
Risk-reducing medications

Class	SERMs		Aromatase Inhibitors
Medications	Tamoxifen	Raloxifene	Exemestane, Anastrozole
Population	Premenopausal or No uterus	Postmenopausal	Postmenopausal
Dose	20 mg daily	60 mg	Exemestane 25 mg daily Anastrazole 1 mg daily
Duration	5 y	5 y	5 y
Side effects	Menopausal symptoms DVT/PE, TIA/CVA		Arthralgias, menopausal symptoms
Other considerations	Improved bone density Endometrial cancer Cataracts	Less effective prevention than tamoxifen	Decreased bone density, baseline DEXA recommended prior to treatment

Prophylactic surgery

Risk-reducing surgery includes prophylactic mastectomy and, for some women, bilateral oophorectomy. Surgery is offered to patients with a lifetime breast cancer risk of more than 50%.[20] This is generally limited to women with a known genetic mutation, strong family history, or prior chest radiation under the age of 30. Most often surgery is performed once childbearing is complete. NCCN recommends multi-disciplinary consultations when considering surgery to discuss the risks and benefits, treatment alternatives, and available reconstruction options.[20]

SUMMARY

Breast cancer is a preventable disease for many people through lifestyle changes, risk-reducing medications, and surgery. Screening and early detection remain important tools in the treatment of breast cancer. All women, regardless of cancer risk, should undergo a breast cancer risk assessment. Women should also be counseled on ways that they can reduce their own cancer risk, including weight loss, exercise, and reduced alcohol intake. Screening decisions should be made using an individual, risk-based approach with all women receiving mammograms by age 50. A risk calculation should be performed on those with a family history of breast cancer, dense breasts, or prior breast biopsy. This calculation should be used to identify patients that qualify for advanced screening imaging, risk-reducing medications, or surgery.

CLINICS CARE POINTS

- A breast cancer risk assessment should be performed for all women starting at age 18. This should include a review of personal and family medical history, as well as a review of modifiable risk factors.

- A breast cancer risk calculation should be performed for patients with a family history of cancers, prior breast biopsies, or dense breasts.

- All women should receive mammography screening by age 50. Higher-risk women may need to begin screening as early as age 25.

- Risk-reduction medications should be offered to all women with a history of ductal carcinoma in situ, lobular carcinoma in situ, or a more than 3% 5-year risk of breast cancer.

- Breast MRI should be offered with mammography to women with a more than 20% lifetime risk of breast cancer.

DISCLOSURE

The authors have nothing to disclose.

REFERENCES

1. Center for Disease Control. Breast Cancer Statistics. Available at: https://www.cdc.gov/cancer/breast/statistics/index.htm. Accessed May 30, 2022.
2. American Cancer Society. Key Statistics for Breast Cancer. Available at: https://www.cancer.org/cancer/breast-cancer/about/how-common-is-breast-cancer.html. Accessed May 30, 2022.
3. DeSantis C, Ma J, Bryan L, et al. Breast cancer statistics, 2013. CA Cancer J Clin 2014;64(1):52–62. https://doi.org/10.3322/caac.21203. Accessed May 30, 2022.

4. Siegel R, Ward E, Brawley O, et al. Cancer statistics, 2011: the impact of eliminating socioeconomic and racial disparities on premature cancer deaths. CA Cancer J Clin 2011;61(4):212–36.

5. Colditz GA, Bohlke K. Priorities for the primary prevention of breast cancer. CA Cancer J Clin 2014;64(3):186–94. https://doi.org/10.3322/caac.21225.

6. Nelson HD, Smith MB, Griffin JC, et al. Use of medications to reduce the risk for primary breast cancer: a systematic review for the US Preventive Services Task Force. Ann Intern Med 2013;158(8):604–14.

7. Owens DK, Davidson KW, Krist AH, et al. Risk assessment, genetic counseling, and genetic testing for BRCA-related cancer: US Preventive Services Task Force recommendation statement. Jama 2019;322(7):652–65.

8. National Comprehensive Cancer Network. NCCN clinical practice guidelines in oncology: genetic/familial high-risk assessment: breast and ovarian, version 1. 2018. Available at: https://www.nccn.org/professionals/physician_gls/pdf/genetics_screening.pdf. Published online October 3, 2017. Accessed March 11, 2018.

9. Nattinger AB, Mitchell JL. Breast cancer screening and prevention. Ann Intern Med 2016;164(11):ITC81.

10. Sprague B, et al. Proportion of invasive breast cancer attributable to risk factors modifiable after menopause. Am J Epidemiol. 168(4. Available at: https://www.ncbi.nlm.nih.gov/pmc/articles/PMC2727276/. Accessed May 30, 2022.

11. Moskowitz CS, Chou JF, Wolden SL, et al. Breast cancer after chest radiation therapy for childhood cancer. J Clin Oncol Off J Am Soc Clin Oncol 2014;32(21):2217–23.

12. Schnitt SJ. Benign breast disease and breast cancer risk: morphology and beyond. Am J Surg Pathol 2003;27(6):836–41.

13. Bernstein, L et al. Lifetime recreational exercise activity and breast cancer risk among black women and white women. J Natl Cancer Inst. 97(22).

14. Marmot M, Atinmo T, Byers T, et al. Food, nutrition, physical activity, and the prevention of cancer: a global perspective. Published online 2007.

15. Chen WY, Rosner B, Hankinson SE, et al. Moderate alcohol consumption during adult life, drinking patterns, and breast cancer risk. Jama 2011;306(17):1884–90.

16. Chlebowski RT, Anderson GL, Gass M, et al. Estrogen plus progestin and breast cancer incidence and mortality in postmenopausal women. Jama 2010;304(15):1684–92.

17. Chen WY, Manson JE, Hankinson SE, et al. Unopposed estrogen therapy and the risk of invasive breast cancer. Arch Intern Med 2006;166(9):1027–32.

18. Barańska A, Błaszczuk A, Kanadys W, et al. Oral contraceptive use and breast cancer risk assessment: a systematic review and meta-analysis of case-control studies, 2009–2020. Cancers 2021;13(22):5654.

19. Owens DK, Davidson KW, Krist AH, et al. Medication use to reduce risk of breast cancer: US Preventive Services Task Force recommendation statement. Jama 2019;322(9):857–67.

20. National Comprehensive Cancer Network. NCCN clinical practice guideline in oncology: breast cancer risk reduction. 2018;Version 2. 2018. Available at: https://www.nccn.org/professionals/physician_gls/PDF/breast_risk.pdf. Accessed August 13, 2018.

21. Visvanathan K, Hurley P, Bantug E, et al. Use of pharmacologic interventions for breast cancer risk reduction: American Society of Clinical Oncology clinical practice guideline. J Clin Oncol 2013;31(23):2942–62.

22. Saslow D, Boetes C, Burke W, et al. American Cancer Society guidelines for breast screening with MRI as an adjunct to mammography. CA Cancer J Clin 2007;57(2):75–89.
23. Mandelblatt JS, Stout NK, Schechter CB, et al. Collaborative modeling of the benefits and harms associated with different US breast cancer screening strategies. Ann Intern Med 2016;164(4):215–25.
24. Oeffinger KC, Fontham ET, Etzioni R, et al. Breast cancer screening for women at average risk: 2015 guideline update from the American Cancer Society. Jama 2015;314(15):1599–614.
25. Nelson HD, Pappas M, Cantor A, et al. Harms of breast cancer screening: systematic review to update the 2009 US Preventive Services Task Force recommendation. Ann Intern Med 2016;164(4):256–67.
26. Dabbous FM, Dolecek TA, Berbaum ML, et al. Impact of a false-positive screening mammogram on subsequent screening behavior and stage at breast cancer diagnosis. Cancer Epidemiol Prev Biomark 2017;26(3):397–403.
27. Siu AL, US Preventive Services Task Force. Screening for breast cancer: US Preventive Services Task Force recommendation statement. Ann Intern Med 2016; 164(4):279–96.
28. Vogel VG, Costantino JP, Wickerham DL, et al. Update of the national surgical adjuvant breast and bowel project study of tamoxifen and raloxifene (STAR) P-2 trial: preventing breast cancer. Cancer Prev Res (Phila Pa 2010;3(6):696–706.
29. Goss PE, Ingle JN, Alés-Martínez JE, et al. Exemestane for breast-cancer prevention in postmenopausal women. N Engl J Med 2011;364(25):2381–91.
30. Cuzick J, Sestak I, Forbes JF, et al. Anastrozole for prevention of breast cancer in high-risk postmenopausal women (IBIS-II): an international, double-blind, randomised placebo-controlled trial. The Lancet 2014;383(9922):1041–8.
31. Farkas A, Vanderberg R, Merriam S, et al. Breast cancer chemoprevention: a practical guide for the primary care provider. J Womens Health 2020;29(1): 46–56.
32. Waters E, et al. Use of tamoxifen and raloxifene for breast cancer chemoprevention in 2010. Breast Cancer Res Treat. 134(2). Available at: https://www.ncbi.nlm.nih.gov/pmc/articles/PMC3771085/. Accessed May 30, 2022.
33. Crew K. Addressing barriers to uptake of breast cancer chemoprevention for patients and providers. In: American society of clinical oncology educational book. Vol 35. Available at: https://ascopubs.org/doi/10.14694/EdBook_AM.2015.35. e50. Accessed May 30, 2022.
34. Ropka ME, et al. Patient decisions about breast cancer chemoprevention: a systematic review and meta-analysis. J Clin Oncol. 28(18). Available at: https://www.ncbi.nlm.nih.gov/pmc/articles/PMC2903338/#B31. Accessed May 30, 2022.

Breast Cancer Risk Assessment and Management of the High-Risk Patient

Victoria L. Green, MD, JD, MBA[a,b,c,*]

KEYWORDS

- High-risk breast disease • Breast cancer • Breast cancer risk assessment
- Risk assessment models • Genetic testing • Breastfeeding
- Risk reduction strategies • Pharmacologic prevention

KEY POINTS

- Identifying women at the highest risk of disease can facilitate provision of targeted prevention strategies and direct individualized clinical management to those likely to benefit most.
- Through a framework of shared decision-making, health providers can assist women in balancing their personal values, goals, and objectives through information gathering and generation of a breast cancer risk profile. This information aids providers and patients in articulating and implementing evidence-based risk reduction strategies, including enhanced screening, lifestyle interventions, genetic evaluation with cascade testing of family members, use of preventive medication, and risk-reducing surgery.
- Models are designed to either estimate a women's risk of *developing* breast cancer or an estimation of the likelihood of harboring a heritable genetic mutation such as the BRCA gene. However, although there is convincing evidence that available models can predict the number of cases of breast cancer expected to develop in a population, the tools perform modestly in discriminating between individual women who will or will not develop breast cancer over time.
- Known or likely pathogenic gene mutations conferring high risk for breast cancer include BRCA1/2, P53, PTEN, PALB2, and CDH1 among others. Markedly increased risk is also noted with ATM, BARD 1, BRIP1, CHEK2, and others. Moderate penetrance genes have been elucidated; however, management recommendations require further data analysis.
- Clinical decisions regarding preventive therapies involve more considerations than medical evidence alone because of concerns of cost, reproductive and hormonal considerations, quality of life issues, baseline comorbidities and medication contraindications, and toxicity profiles.

This article previously appeared in Obstetrics & Gynecology Clinics volume 49 issue 1 March 2022.
[a] Department of Gynecology and Obstetrics, Emory University, Glenn Building 4th Floor, Atlanta, GA 30303, USA; [b] Gynecology Comprehensive Breast Center, Winship Cancer Institute at Grady Memorial Hospital; [c] Avon Breast Center
* Corresponding author: Department of Gynecology and Obstetrics, Glenn Building, 4th Floor, Atlanta, GA 30303.
E-mail address: vgree01@emory.edu

Breast cancer is the most commonly diagnosed nonskin cancer in women, with an estimated 281,550 new cases diagnosed in 2021, resulting in 43,600 deaths. Male breast cancer will account for 2650 cases and 530 deaths in 2021.[1] There are currently more than 3.8 million breast cancer survivors in the United States and it is estimated that this will increase to more than 4.9 million survivors by the year 2030, indicating the significant importance of breast and breast health.[2] Unfortunately, despite tremendous progress in early screening, diagnosis, and advancements in chemotherapeutics, racial disparities exist. In the United States, 2020 resulted in the largest single-year decline in cancer deaths overall,[3] with improved 90% 5-year relative survival, yet African American women have mortality rates that are 41% higher than white women and nearly $2\times$ that of other minority populations.

To decrease the breast cancer burden, conserve resources, and decrease unnecessary treatments, guidelines suggest interventions be reserved for those women at greatest risk for disease. Women at high risk are likely to gain the most benefit from risk-reducing interventions. Discovering new strategies to identify women at the highest risk, facilitating provision of targeted prevention strategies and directing individualized clinical management, is of critical importance in this effort. Through a framework of shared decision-making, health providers can assist women in balancing their personal values, goals, and objectives through information gathering and generation of a breast cancer risk profile. This information aids providers and patients in articulating and implementing evidence-based risk reduction strategies, including enhanced screening, lifestyle interventions, genetic evaluation with cascade testing of family members, use of preventive medication, and risk-reducing surgery.

BREAST CANCER RISK ASSESSMENT
Breast Cancer Risk Factors

Risk assessment can determine if a woman is at average or increased risk for breast cancer. Risk stratification facilitates appropriate breast cancer surveillance, discussion of risk reduction methods, and provision of applicable genetic testing (**Box 1**). Assessment begins with gathering patient genetic, familial, personal, reproductive, and lifestyle information into an individualized risk estimate (**Box 2**).

For women *without* a personal history of breast cancer, assessment begins with evaluation of the family lineage. The family history should be assessed for first-degree, second-degree, and third-degree relatives on both the maternal and paternal sides of the family with a focus on ethnicity (specifically Ashkenazi Jewish ancestry), types of cancer, laterality, age of diagnosis, and subtypes with pathology report confirmation when available. Efforts should be centered on cases of breast, ovarian, colon, fallopian tube or primary peritoneal cancer, prostate, pancreatic, and other types of germline mutation-associated cancers, documenting age of diagnosis. The magnitude of risk increases with the number of affected relatives.

A history of affected first-degree relatives and disease onset in the premenopausal period is suggestive of genetic predisposition and genetic testing should be considered as discussed in Cecelia A. Bellcross' and article, "Hereditary Breast and Ovarian Cancer: An Updated Primer for OB/GYNs," in this issue. Known or likely pathogenic gene mutations conferring high risk for breast cancer include BRCA1/2, P53, PTEN, PALB2, and CDH1 among others. Markedly increased risk is also noted with ATM, BARD 1, BRIP1, CHEK2, and others. Moderate penetrance genes have been elucidated; however, management recommendations require further data analysis. Women of Ashkenazi Jewish descent are more likely to harbor BRCA 1/2 mutations with a rate of 1:40.

Box 1
Breast cancer risk assessment

- Gather information
  - Risk factors
  - Family history
- Shared decision-making framework
- Develop risk profile and counseling
  - Risk assessment models
- Implement risk reduction strategies
  - Healthy lifestyle
  - Genetic testing
  - Enhanced surveillance
    - Imaging
      - MRI
    - Clinical examinations
  - Risk-reducing agents
    - Tamoxifen
    - Raloxifene
    - AI
  - Risk-reducing surgeries
    - Prophylactic mastectomy
    - Prophylactic oophorectomy
    - Bilateral salpingectomy

In women *without* a pedigree suggestive of genetic predisposition, other reproductive and demographic factors should be reviewed, including , age, nulliparity, hormone replacement therapy,[4] recent use of oral contraceptives, proliferative breast disease (atypical ductal hyperplasia [ADH] and atypical lobular hyperplasia [ALH]), lobular carcinoma in situ (LCIS),[5] postmenopausal obesity,[6] mammographic breast density,[7] alcohol intake,[8] smoking,[9] physical inactivity,[10] exposure to ionizing radiation (particularly between 10 and 30 years of age),[11,12] and women with higher socioeconomic status. Reproductive risk factors include prolonged exposure to endogenous estrogens, such as early menarche (before age 12 years), late menopause (after age 53 years), and delayed childbearing (childbirth before age 18 years portends one-third the risk of breast cancer of a woman delivering at age 35 years). Flat epithelial atypia is added per the National Comprehensive Cancer Network (NCCN) guidelines; however, data are not strong with respect to the degree of risk or the benefits of risk-reducing therapy in this population.[13] In some studies, breastfeeding[14,15] and exercise[16] have been shown to reduce breast cancer risk.

Although multiple risk factors have been elucidated, 80% of women with breast cancer have no risk factors other than age and female gender. The median age of breast cancer diagnosis in white women is 62 years although 36% of female breast cancer survivors are younger than 65 years.[17] By contrast, the median age is 59 years for black women and the risk of premenopausal breast cancer is greater than in white women.[18]

As mentioned, racial disparities exist as African American women have a greater risk of dying from breast cancer than Caucasian women. The reasons for the disparity are complex including African American women are more likely to present at stage IV, have lower frequency of screening,[18] have longer time between screenings, have limited follow-up after abnormal screening results[19] (despite financial or insurance coverage or resources[20]), and have comorbidities resulting in worsening survival.[21] In addition, African American women have a greater likelihood of more aggressive

---

Box 2
Breast cancer risk factors

- Increasing age
- Female gender
- Personal history of breast cancer
- Known deleterious gene mutation
- Family history of breast, ovarian, colon, prostate, pancreatic, and other types of germline mutation-associated cancers
- Nulliparity
- Hormone replacement therapy
- Recent use of oral contraceptives
- Proliferative breast disease (atypical ductal hyperplasia, atypical lobular hyperplasia)
- Lobular carcinoma in situ
- Postmenopausal obesity
- Mammographic breast density
- Alcohol intake
- Smoking
- Physical inactivity
- Exposure to ionizing radiation (particularly in women aged 10–30 years)
- Higher socioeconomic status
- Early menarche (before age 12 years)
- Late menopause (after age 53 years)
- Delayed childbearing
- Breastfeeding (protective in certain literature)
- Race—increased mortality in African American women
- Ethnicity—increased risk of BRCA ½ in Ashkenazi Jewish women
- Flat epithelial atypia (FEA) (NCCN)

---

breast cancer subtypes such as inflammatory, basal cell, luminal B, and triple-negative disease.[22] Many studies have found that equitable access to timely quality care eliminates racial disparities in cancer outcomes[23]; however, others note persistence of disparities[24] possibly implicating systemic racism and implicit bias.

Research suggests that individuals who identify as gay, lesbian, bisexual, queer, or same-gender-loving may have a higher risk of breast cancer compared with heterosexual women because of higher rates of nulliparity, alcohol consumption, smoking, and obesity.[25] In addition, these individuals have a lower lifetime prevalence of mammogram usage than heterosexual women and less timely screening because of lower perceived severity and perceptions of heterosexism and homophobia among providers.[26] Detailed information regarding past surgeries and hormonal intake is critical.

Risk Assessment Models

Risk assessment models are integral to risk stratification (**Box 3**; **Table 1**). A simple inventory of risk factors fails to identify a majority of women at high risk as 80% of

> **Box 3**
> **Common breast cancer risk assessment models**
>
> - Gail model/BCRAT (NCI Breast Cancer Risk Assessment Tool)
> - Claus
> - BRCAPRO
> - BOADICEA
> - Tyrer-Cuzick

women with breast cancer have no identifiable risk factors other than age and gender.[27,28] Models use traditional risk factors to elucidate an individualized risk estimate, which is then used in a shared decision-making framework to counsel regarding risk reduction strategies. Models are designed to either estimate a women's risk of *developing* breast cancer or an estimation of the likelihood of harboring a heritable genetic mutation such as the BRCA gene. However, although there is convincing evidence that available models can predict the number of cases of breast cancer expected to develop in a population, the tools perform modestly in discriminating between individual women who will or will not develop breast cancer over time.[29] Addition of other risk factors including breast density and polygenic risk scores have the potential to increase the discriminatory accuracy.

Important differences exist between the models, including risk factors used in the analysis; United States versus European rates of breast cancer used as baseline calibrations; consideration of invasive breast cancer and ductal carcinoma in situ (DCIS) versus invasive cancers only in prediction estimation; incorporation or exclusion of LCIS, incorporation of competing mortality rates from nonbreast cancer causes versus breast cancer mortality solely; and validation in the general population versus in the high-risk population alone. Each difference modifies the predicted absolute risk of breast cancer, particularly over long prediction intervals. These distinctions can be critical in deciding which model to use in specific family scenarios and in interpreting the studies that assess the validity of the model.[30] In addition to their differences, the models have important limitations. Most models are based on different combinations of traditional risk factors, although studies have shown that a majority of women with breast cancer do not have a known risk factor(other than age and female gender).[31] In addition, the specific risk factor may portend divergent risks for different ethnic groups.[32] Importantly, many well-established risk factors are not typically included in models. For instance, mammographic breast density is only incorporated in the Tyrer-Cuzick and Tice models. As each model incorporates substantially different risk factors, these models may result in substantially different estimates of risk for breast cancer. Additional translational research is needed to expand our knowledge of molecular and genetic markers of risk, which may modify and improve risk assessment and risk assessment models.

MANAGEMENT OF THE HIGH-RISK PATIENT

Women at high risk for breast cancer have many concerns including risk prevention and the impact on their families. Of particular focus for women's health practitioners is consideration of the impact of these conditions on reproductive and hormonal health. Thus, providers must supplement risk stratification and cancer prevention strategies with the wealth of emerging opportunities for family building, genetic testing,

Table 1
Differences between breast cancer risk assessment models

Name	Prediction/Estimation	Factors	Benefits	Target Group	Limitations
Gail/BCRAT[a]	5 y and lifetime risk for development of breast cancer Five-year risk assessment >1.67 denotes eligibility for chemoprevention	Patients' age Patients' race (modified Gail model) Age at menarche Age at first live birth First-degree relatives with breast cancer Breast biopsies History of ADH	Validated in white women >35 years in both the general population and those at high risk	Women >35 y	Does not address risk • below age 35 y • on paternal family side • second degree or more distantly related family members • family history of nonbreast cancer (ie, ovarian, prostate, colon) known to be associated with genetic mutations • LCIS, ALH • Age of diagnosis • Ashkenazi Jewish ancestry • History suggestive of germline mutation • Personal history of breast cancer • Male breast cancer • Flat epithelial atypia Accurate in population studies; however, poorly discriminates between individual risk As the model does not focus on family history, it is *not* recommended for determining eligibility for MRI assessment in high-risk women.

Claus	Risk of invasive and noninvasive breast cancer	Age of diagnosis Number of first- and second-degree relatives with breast cancer	Focused on family history Addresses maternal and paternal lineage	Underestimates risk in known or suspected carriers of breast cancer susceptibility genes Does not include hormonal and reproductive factors
Tyrer-Cuzick (IBIS[b]) Graham-Colditz	Risk of breast cancer and the likelihood of harboring a genetic mutation	Gail model variables plus alcohol intake, age at menopause, genetic mutation status, use of hormones, extended family history of breast or ovarian cancer, age of onset, laterality of breast cancer, BMI	Incorporates endocrine, familial, and personal risk factors and allows for the presence of multiple genes of differing penetrance.	As model considers age of onset of cancer and second-degree relatives, it is more appropriate to use when these features are present in families.[57]
BRCAPRO	Likelihood of possessing a BRCA ½ mutation	Personal history of breast cancer Premenopausal or postmenopausal age of affected relatives History of breast and ovarian cancer		
BOADICEA[c]	Likelihood of harboring a genetic mutation			
Pedigree Assessment Tool[d]	Identifies patients appropriate for genetic referral. Not everyone who is identified for referral will be a candidate for genetic testing			

[a] NCI breast cancer risk assessment tool.
[b] International Breast Cancer Intervention Studies (IBIS).
[c] Breast and Ovarian Analysis of Disease Incidence and Carrier Estimation Algorithm (BOADICEA).
[d] Other less commonly used mutation probability models include Manchester, Penn II, Myriad II, and FHAT. Penn II is studied with greater than 2 cases of cancer in the family and thus may not be appropriate for women with fewer than 2 cases of cancer in the family.

and management of surgical menopause. Patients may be considered high risk based on history, model risk estimate, dysplastic lesions on biopsy, early exposure to irradiation, and/or pedigree suggestive of hereditary cancer (**Box 4**).

Women with a personal history of invasive breast cancer or DCIS should follow the cancer surveillance recommendations of their oncologist.

Women at all levels of risk should always have a discussion regarding options for participation in clinical research for screening, risk assessment, or other risk-reducing interventions.

Genetic Testing

Genetic counseling should be offered to women at high risk secondary to a strong family history of very early onset of breast and/or ovarian cancer and triple negative breast cancer. Genetic testing should be offered where it is likely to impact the risk management and/or treatment of the tested individuals and/or their at-risk family members. Women with hereditary cancers often have an early age of onset of the disease and exhibit an autosomal dominant pattern of inheritance. Known pathogenic or likely pathogenic gene mutations confer a 65% to 74% lifetime risk for breast cancer (and a 39%–46% [BRCA1] or a 12% to 20% [BRCA2] risk of ovarian cancer[33]). There are also known moderate penetrance genes such as ATM or CHEK2 that confer intermediate risks of cancer with a lifetime risk of 30% compared with 12% in the general population.[34] Women without known patterns of inheritance may show familial clustering of cancer where cancer appears in families more frequently than expected based on statistics but generally not exhibiting inheritance patterns or onset age suggestive of hereditary cancer. Familial cancers share some but not all features of hereditary cancer. Familial clustering is multifactorial although it may occur by chance clustering, genetic variations in lower penetrance genes, due to shared environmental factors, and/or small family size. Management of women with hereditary cancers is reviewed in chapter 6.

Risk Reduction Strategies

Although there has been significant evolution and advancements in the field of breast cancer diagnosis and prevention, the state of the science is far from exact in predicting who will develop or die from breast cancer. Risk reduction strategies have both benefits and harms that should be discussed with women during consideration. Clinicians must weigh medication side effects, procedure risks and harms, patient-specific comorbidities, and lifestyle preferences to understand the true risk for each individual. Although each has been shown to reduce the incidence and/or risk of death from breast cancer, various study biases warrant caution in broadly applying results.

Box 4
Increased breast cancer risk

Prior history of breast cancer

Age ≥ 35 y with 5-year Gail Model risk ≥ 1.7%

Lifetime risk greater than 20% based on history of LCIS or ADH/ALH

Lifetime risk greater than 20% based on *models largely dependent on family history*

Age 10 to 30 y with prior mantle irradiation

Pedigree suggestive of or known genetic predisposition

Even among BRCA mutation carriers, who likely have the most to gain from any risk reduction strategy, options need to be presented along with other risk-management strategies including healthy dietary habits, risk-reducing salpingoophorectomy (RRSO), risk-reducing mastectomy (RRM), pharmacologic prevention, and enhanced surveillance.

Although multiple risk reduction strategies are available, patient uptake is often limited. In patients eligible for genetic counseling, only 11% choose RRM and 21% chose RRSO. Women with a prior history of cancer and/or younger than 50 years were more likely to choose risk reduction surgery.[35] In addition, although health professionals express confidence in the effectiveness of risk-reducing medications, providers felt initiation of pharmacologic prevention was the role of cancer specialists rather than a primary care preventive activity.[36] Thus, it is critical that women's health care practitioners become familiar with advancments in the field.

Lifestyle modification/healthy lifestyle

Although the literature is replete with evidence of personal characteristics, which are associated with an elevated risk of breast cancer, the association between modification of that factor and a correlative change in breast cancer risk is not as clear. Yet, in observational studies, healthy behaviors have been associated with at least a 20%–30% reduction in breast cancer incidence irrespective of the risk level.[37,38] Discussion of healthy lifestyle options is a critical approach not only for the promotion of overall health but also for the encouragement of healthy choices in *all* women, *regardless* of their breast cancer risk. Thus, all women should be counseled regarding healthy lifestyle recommendations (**Box 5**).

Studies have demonstrated that an amount of alcohol equal to 1 to 2 drinks per day is associated with an increased risk of breast cancer. However, even smaller amounts modestly increase risk.[39] Yet, the effect of a reduction in alcohol consumption on the incidence of breast cancer has not been well established.[40] According to the NCCN Breast Cancer Risk Reduction Panel, alcohol consumption should be limited to ≤ 1 drink per day defined as 1 ounce of liquor, 6 ounces of wine, or 8 ounces of beer.[41]

There is considerable evidence that moderate physical activity reduces breast cancer risk. The greatest benefit has been noted with a longer duration of activity. These benefits have been demonstrated with physical activity both as an adult,[42] during childhood[43] and in adolescence.[44] One prospective study showed the greatest risk reduction in women reporting walking or hiking for ≥ 10 h/wk[45]

Anthropometric factors including height, weight, and adiposity modify breast cancer risk. Studies have shown a high risk of postmenopausal breast cancer in women who are overweight or obese, women who gain weight in the postmenopausal period, as well as an increased risk of dying from the disease.[46] A plausible mechanism is the increased circulating endogenous estrogen levels in adipose tissue. Analogously, the association between weight and risk is stronger for hormone receptor-positive

---

Box 5
Risk Reduction/Healthy Lifestyle Counseling for overall health promotion

1. Limit alcohol consumption to ≤ 1 drink per day

2. Encourage women to stay active and exercise

3. Maintain a healthy body weight and BMI and avoid weight gain

4. Breastfeeding reduces the risk of breast cancer

cancers. Other theories favor hyperinsulinemia and insulin resistance[47] or increased insulin-like growth factor I (IGF-I)[48] associated with obesity and physical inactivity as important determinants. Furthermore, unlike other epidemiologic factors that have not been shown to reduce risk, if modified, reduction in weight of greater than 10.0 kg in postmenopausal women who were naïve to postmenopausal hormone therapy was associated with a significantly lower risk of breast cancer compared with women who maintained their weight.[49] Interestingly, evidence shows a lower risk of premenopausal breast cancer in women who are overweight compared with women who are not overweight.[39]

A wide variety of dietary factors have been examined, including intake of red meat, processed meat, animal fat, calcium, soy, and antioxidants such as beta-carotene, vitamins D, C, and E, and decreased consumption of fruits and vegetables. Epidemiologic studies of specific dietary components have provided inconsistent or inconclusive results. Some prospective studies note no association between total fruit and vegetable intake and overall risk of breast cancer; however, there is some evidence of decreased risk with a diet high in fruits and vegetables.[50] In addition, naturally occurring vitamin D (from dietary sources and the sun) may be protective in decreasing the risk of breast cancer.[51] Beneficial effects of soy have been touted; however, the protective effects have only been observed among Asian populations.[52] Importantly, overall dietary effects on breast cancer risk may be much greater during adolescence and early adulthood. Further studies are in progress to evaluate the specific role of dietary factors.

Breastfeeding is a critical modifiable preventive behavior that is inversely associated with breast cancer risk. Dose-response has been demonstrated with a longer duration associated with a greater reduction in risk.[53] As African American women have significantly lower rates of breastfeeding, authors have theorized that this may be a reason for the increased risk of receptor-negative tumors.[54] Unfortunately, the association with slavery and forced wet-nursing of white children, continues to plague the cultural acceptance of this feeding method.[55]

Pharmacologic prevention

As the understanding of genetic and epigenetic alterations involved in breast cancer initiation has deepened, evidence-based pharmacology, which alters the chain of molecular events in the pathogenesis of cancer, has evolved. Pharmacologic agents provide opportunities to address individuals at higher risk for breast cancer with effective, molecular-targeted interventions to reverse, suppress, or prevent premalignant and invasive carcinoma. This follows the example of other medical disciplines, such as cardiology, whereby it is standard practice to treat individuals at higher risk for cardiovascular disorders *before* established clinical evidence of disease, which has contributed to decreased mortality in this patient population. Although practicing healthy behaviors such as reducing obesity, breastfeeding, moderating alcohol intake, and increasing physical activity should be encouraged regardless of risk level, pharmacologic interventions are reserved for those at significantly increased risk, particularly those with elevated risk model estimates and with LCIS, ADH, ALH for whom the benefits of risk reduction generally outweigh risks and harms.

National medical organizations, including the National Comprehensive Cancer Network (NCCN),[56] the American Society of Clinical Oncology (ASCO),[57] and the United States Preventive Services Task Force (USPSTF),[29] recommend that clinicians offer risk-reducing medications to decrease the risk of estrogen receptor-positive breast cancer to asymptomatic women aged 35 years and older who are at increased risk for breast cancer and low risk for adverse medication effects. There is no single risk threshold for which pharmacologic prevention for breast cancer risk reduction should be considered. The USPSTF recommends a 5-year risk of at least 3% (based on the National Cancer Institute Breast Cancer Risk Assessment Tool [BCRAT]) and the European National Institute for Health and Care Excellence (NICE) recommends an age-dependent 10-year risk of ≥5% (based on the IBIS/Tyrer-Cuzick Risk Calculator). Initial prevention studies used a Gail/BCRAT model risk score ≥ 1.7 as an eligibility criterion; however, the mean 5-year breast cancer risk in the STAR (the Study of Tamoxifen And Raloxifene) trial was 4.03%. Currently, the BCRAT (https://bcrisktool.cancer.gov.) and Tyrer-Cuzick (http://www.ems-trials.org/riskevaluator/) models are the most frequently used models to calculate breast cancer risk in phase III prevention trials and in clinical practice.

Clinical decisions regarding preventive therapies involve more considerations than medical evidence alone because of concerns of cost, reproductive and hormonal considerations, quality of life issues, baseline comorbidities and medication contraindications, and toxicity profiles. For instance, women with AH (atypical hyperplasia) and LCIS have a 3% to 5% BCRAT risk score thus ASCO recommends these women older than 35 years, who have completed childbearing, and who have no medical contraindications should be offered pharmacologic prevention. According to ASCO, this also applies to women of African descent, whose risk for breast cancer is increased to an equal degree by atypical lesions; however, whose BCRAT estimate may be lower than discussed thresholds.[57] Women's health practitioners should individualize counseling along with principles of shared decision-making while incorporating policy and insurance coverage information when appropriate. Importantly, health care practitioners should consider patients' overall health; age; menopause status; desires for pregnancy; risk factors for venous thromboembolic events (VTEs), including smoking, cancer history, mobility, recent surgery, obesity, family history of VTE, and age more than 60 years; hysterectomy status; bone density; prior history of VTE, stroke, or transient ischemic attack; medical comorbidities; and current use of hormones or antidepressants. It is postulated that lower dosages for a shorter duration may reduce breast cancer risk with fewer adverse outcomes in postmenopausal women; however, these findings need to be validated in future trials.[58] Models are available, which assist in making decisions regarding pharmacologic intervention.[59]

Treatment of early-stage breast cancer with tamoxifen revolutionized the field of cancer care citing 40% higher disease-free survival, reduced risk of recurrence, reduced incidence of new primaries, and reduced mortality in tamoxifen-treated patients. Assessment of tamoxifen and other selective estrogen receptor modulators (SERMs) in the prevention arena became an obvious ensuing succession. The initial tamoxifen randomized prevention trial, by the National Surgical Adjuvant Breast and Bowel Project (NSABP P1) or Breast Cancer Prevention Trial (BCPT) noted a highly statistically significant 49% reduction in ER + invasive breast cancer in 13,388 healthy unaffected women enrolled between ages 35 and 60 years with Gail model risk greater than 1.66 or history of lobular carcinoma in situ (LCIS). No difference was observed in overall rates of mortality with a follow-up period of up to 7 years. An increased risk of vascular events was noted. The study also showed a reduction in hip fractures.[60] These results were supported by the International Breast Cancer Intervention Study (IBIS-1) showing a 32% reduction in all breast cancer events, 34% lower risk of ER-positive cancer in 7152 high-risk women after long-term follow-up.[61–63]

The Royal Marsden Tamoxifen Prevention Trial demonstrated a significant reduction in ER-positive breast cancer risk with tamoxifen use, however, predominantly during the post-treatment follow-up in 2471 women selected based solely on a family history of breast cancer (Gail model risk assessment was not used).[64,65] Conversely, the

Italian National Trial demonstrated no significant difference in breast cancer occurrence in the overall study population after 109 months follow-up in healthy hysterectomized women aged 35 to 70 years.[66,67] Women were allowed to receive hormonal replacement therapy. Family history of breast cancer nor Gail model risk score was used in the selection criteria. Possible reasons for the lack of benefit in the later trial include concurrent use of hormone therapy and different study populations including lower risk population due to required hysterectomy for inclusion in the study and oophorectomy may have occurred during the procedure, and possibly lower-risk women as Gail model assessment was not required. Subset analysis of women classified as increased risk based on reproductive and hormonal characteristics was noted to have a significantly reduced risk of breast cancer in the tamoxifen group; however, only 13% of patients were classified as high risk.[67,68]

Although not an initial aim of the study, a second-generation SERM, raloxifene, was associated with a 62% reduction in breast cancer risk in 7705 postmenopausal women (breast cancer risk was not considered in accrual) studied in the Multiple Outcomes of Raloxifene Evaluation (MORE) for prevention of osteoporosis.[69] Reduction in vertebral fraction risk and increase in bone mineral density was also noted. These results prompted additional studies in the Continuing Outcomes Relevant to Evista (CORE)[70] and Raloxifene Use for the Heart (RUTH)[71] trials. Both latter trials demonstrated a reduction in invasive breast cancer incidence in the raloxifene arm at 66% and 44% respectively (although there was no reduction in cardiovascular events).

The benefits in these studies prompted a head-to-head comparison of tamoxifen and raloxifene in the study of tamoxifen and raloxifene (STAR) NSABP P2 trial.[72] A total of 19,000 high-risk women were randomized to either 20 mg of tamoxifen or 60 mg of raloxifene daily. Both drugs were shown to reduce the risk of developing *invasive* breast cancer by about 50%; however, Raloxifene was shown to have 36% fewer uterine cancers and 29% fewer blood clots than the women assigned to tamoxifen. In the initial study, tamoxifen and raloxifene are equally efficacious in reducing the risk of *invasive* breast cancer; however, raloxifene was less effective in *noninvasive* breast cancer prevention than tamoxifen although the observed difference was not statistically significant. Updated STAR trial results show diminished benefits of raloxifene compared with tamoxifen after cessation of therapy.[72] Thus, absent concerns for toxicity, tamoxifen may be the superior choice for most postmenopausal women desiring nonsurgical risk reduction. The mechanism of action is not well understood. The toxicity profile is more favorable with raloxifene. Although both drugs increase a women's risk of deep vein thrombosis (DVT), stroke, ischemic heart disease, and PE, only tamoxifen is associated with an increased risk of uterine cancer and cataract formation.[73] The tamoxifen side effects are greatest in women older than 50 years (particularly the risk of uterine cancer), thus risk-benefit analysis is greatest for tamoxifen in premenopausal women, particularly those high-risk women with precancerous risk factors such as ADH, ALH, or LCIS. Often, for women at increased risk for breast cancer, the reduction in the number of breast cancer events exceeds that of the increase in the number of uterine cancer events. Raloxifene may be most efficacious in the postmenopausal women with osteoporosis for the reduction of invasive breast cancer. Unlike tamoxifen, raloxifene is FDA approved for osteoporosis prevention, and thus can be used for this reason for longer than the 5 years recommended for breast cancer prevention.

Tamoxifen, at a lower dose (5 mg daily), has demonstrated efficacy in breast cancer risk reduction in a randomized trial in women with AH, LCIS, or DCIS treated for 3 years (median follow-up 5 years); however, there are no data on the equivalency of the 2 dosages (5 mg vs 20 mg). Compared with placebo, lower dose tamoxifen was not associated with an increase in the number of serious adverse effect, including DVT and endometrial cancer. As concern for adverse effects is a major reason for limited acceptance of pharmacologic therapy, low dose tamoxifen may be an alternative for breast cancer risk reduction specifically for women with AH, LCIS, or DCIS.[74]

Generally with SERMs, there are conflicting studies regarding breast cancer risk reduction, and overall no survival benefit has been shown. In addition to uterine cancer, tamoxifen is also associated with thromboembolic events, cataract formation, increased vaginal discharge/bleeding, hot flashes, leg cramps, and bladder control problems primarily stress urinary incontinence.[75] Information regarding the influence of tamoxifen on cognition comes from reports of NSABP B14 and B20, where although negative effects are suggested, they were not able to adequately control for potential confounding factors. Thus, the reported effects of tamoxifen on cognition are inconclusive at this stage. Conversely, raloxifene is more likely to be associated with increased musculoskeletal problems (joint pain, muscle stiffness), dyspareunia (vaginal dryness), and weight gain. Although tamoxifen has been used for 5 years in the oncology field for women with breast cancer, we do not know if 5 years is the optimal therapy duration for *preventive* therapy in the unaffected high-risk individual, although this is the current standard pattern of preventive use. Moreover, studies have not determined the proper age to start therapy nor the risk level suggested for initiation of therapy. Many authors have suggested a 10-year risk of 4% to 8% for developing breast cancer to initiate preventive therapy; however, this is theoretic.[76]

A similar reduction of breast cancer *in tamoxifen-treated BRCA mutation* carriers has also been shown. Preliminary data in BRCA mutation carriers *affected* with breast cancer showed tamoxifen protected against contralateral breast cancer for carriers of BRCA 1 mutations (62%) and for those with BRCA 2 mutations (37% reduction). Overall, in women who used tamoxifen for 2 to 4 years, the risk of contralateral breast cancer was reduced by 75%. Therefore, in this study, tamoxifen use reduced the risk of contralateral breast cancer in women with pathogenic mutations in either the BRCA 1 or BRCA 2 gene.[77] Other studies have shown benefit in only BRCA 2 carriers. The lack of benefit in BRCA 1 mutation carriers is thought to be secondary to a higher likelihood of ER-negative tumors in BRCA 1 carriers. There are currently no data regarding the efficacy of raloxifene risk reduction in BRCA 1/2 mutation carriers and women who have received prior thoracic radiation. In addition, the utility of raloxifene or tamoxifen as a breast cancer risk reduction agent in women younger than 35 years is not known.

Aromatase inhibitors (AIs) reduce the biosynthesis of estrogen and have shown superior efficacy to tamoxifen in decreasing contralateral breast cancer events in patients with early-stage breast cancer. Generally, AIs have overtaken tamoxifen as the treatment of choice in the postmenopausal patient with hormone-responsive breast cancer secondary to improved efficacy over tamoxifen in reduction of breast cancer recurrence and contralateral tumors. However, there are no data comparing the benefits and risks of AIs to those of tamoxifen or raloxifene in the prevention arena.[78–82] The Mammary Prevention trial 3 (MAP 3) found a 65% relative reduction in the annual occurrence of invasive breast cancer compared with placebo and a 53% reduction in invasive plus noninvasive breast cancer in a randomized double-blind placebo-controlled multicenter, multinational trial in 4560 high-risk postmenopausal women using exemestane at 25 mg daily for a median of 3 years.[83] Although exemestane is not currently FDA approved for breast cancer risk reduction, it is included as one of the choices for breast cancer risk reduction agents by NCCN and ASCO.[13,57]

Another AI, anastrozole, was studied at 1 mg daily for 5 years in the IBIS II trial in 3864 postmenopausal women at high risk for breast cancer based on family history or prior diagnosis of DCIS, LCIS, or ADH. This study again demonstrated safety and efficacy to reduce the incidence of breast cancer in postmenopausal women.[84] There are no data on the use of anastrozole for breast cancer risk reduction in women with a germ line mutation; however, similar to tamoxifen, AIs in the adjuvant setting have also been shown in retrospective analysis to reduce the risk of contralateral breast cancer in BRCA 1/2 patients with ER-positive disease.[85] At present, studies with tamoxifen, raloxifene, exemestane, nor anastrozole show survival benefits. It is unclear whether we will ever have the ability to detect survival advantage because of low numbers of breast cancer events, limited statistical power, and use of preventive agents by women in the placebo group after the trial conclusion. However, a reduction in breast cancer incidence, in itself, is an important end point.

AIs are associated with an increased risk of musculoskeletal side effects as compared with tamoxifen. The specific effects of exemestane on bone were demonstrating a 3-fold age-related bone loss comparing baseline bone mineral density scores to 2 years post-treatment. During the study, women had adequate calcium and vitamin D intake. There was no increased fracture rate compared with placebo; thus, the clinical significance of the finding is not clear; however, authors suggest women considering exemestane for breast cancer prevention have their bone health monitored during treatment and maintain adequate calcium and vitamin D intake.[86] NCCN also supports baseline BMD (bone mineral density) evaluation in postmenopausal women choosing an AI for risk reduction.[13] Other adverse effects from exemestane are generally mild, with the most common being diarrhea, joint pain, and menopausal-related symptoms. Importantly, exemestane did not increase the risks of endometrial cancers, thromboembolism, cardiovascular events, or cataracts. However, joint stiffness and arthralgia were more common when compared with tamoxifen or raloxifene.[87] Thus, pharmacologic preventive therapy may be associated with side effects that must be assessed to determine if the benefits are greater than the risks.

As with raloxifene, the use of AIs is restricted to postmenopausal women at present, since in premenopausal women, high levels of androstenedione compete with the AI at the enzyme complex such that estrogen synthesis is not completely blocked. In addition, the initial decrease in estrogen levels causes a reflex increase in gonadotropin levels, provoking ovarian hyperstimulation, thereby increasing aromatase in the ovary and consequently overcoming the initial aromatase blockade.

Considering current information regarding pharmacologic risk reduction (despite conflicting results and known side effects), the ASCO recommends discussion of pharmacologic intervention with tamoxifen, raloxifene, or exemestane for breast cancer risk reduction in high-risk women (Gail model >1.66% or diagnosis of LCIS) at risk for ER-positive breast cancer, as part of a shared decision-making process with careful consideration of individually calculated risks and benefits.[88] Anastrozole should be considered an alternative in postmenopausal women with a diagnosis of ADH/ALH or LICS, an estimated 5-year risk (according to the National Cancer Institute Breast Cancer Risk Assessment Tool [BCRAT]) of at least 3%, a 10-year risk (IBIS/Tyrer-Cuzick Risk Calculator) of at least 5%, or a relative risk of at least 4 times the population risk for their age group if they are aged 40 to 44 years or 2 times the population risk for their age group If they are aged 45 to 69 years.[57] Eligibility criteria have changed with anastrozole based on those used for inclusion in the pivotal study.

Overall, the women in the raloxifene trials were older (median age 67–67.5 years) than women in the other trials as the target population was postmenopausal women *not* at increased risk of breast cancer (the primary aim was for prevention of osteoporosis and decreased fracture risk, ie, an aim other than breast cancer risk reduction).

By contrast, women in the tamoxifen trials were slightly younger, as these trials also included premenopausal women (median age range, 47–53 years).[89] Tamoxifen has been evaluated in premenopausal *and* postmenopausal women at increased risk for breast cancer. The AIs (exemestane and anastrozole) have been evaluated solely in postmenopausal women at increased risk for breast cancer. Raloxifene (a SERM) was evaluated in postmenopausal women *not* at increased risk for breast cancer. Thus, only tamoxifen is indicated for risk reduction in premenopausal women but is also efficacious in postmenopausal women.

Follow-up of women treated with risk reduction medications should focus on the early detection of breast cancer and the management of adverse symptoms or complications. NCCN and ASCO recommend a gynecologic examination before initiation of tamoxifen or raloxifene and to continue annually thereafter. Prompt evaluation of abnormal vaginal bleeding is critical although routine endometrial assessment with ultrasound or endometrial biopsy is not required in the asymptomatic patient. The NCCN also recommends an ophthalmology examination if cataracts or vision problems exist or develop while on tamoxifen.

Before initiation of an AI, clinicians should evaluate baseline fracture risk and measure bone mineral density. As AIs cause an increased rate of bone loss, practitioners should use anastrozole with caution in postmenopausal women with moderate bone mineral density loss. Bone protective agents such as bisphosphonates and RANKL inhibitors may be considered if moderate bone loss is noted. Patients should be encouraged to exercise regularly and take adequate calcium and vitamin D supplements. A history of osteoporosis and/or severe bone loss is a relative contraindication to anastrozole and these women were excluded in the trial. Patients should make physicians aware of joint stiffness, arthralgias, vasomotor symptoms, hypertension, dry eyes, and vaginal dryness. AIs are a better alternative than tamoxifen and raloxifene in women with a history of DVT, PE, TIA, or stroke.

It is important to note that certain selective serotonin reuptake inhibitors (SSRIs) interfere with the enzymatic conversion of tamoxifen to its more active metabolite, endoxifen, through the cytochrome P450 2D6 (CYP2D6) pathway. Thus, alternatives such as SNRIs should be substituted in these women whose quality of life diminishes because of hot flashes, when possible.[90] In addition, certain CYP2D6 genotypes are markers of poor tamoxifen metabolism, and by analogy, efficacy, nevertheless this biomarker should not be used in patient selection until further validation.[91] As estrogens and/or progestins have the potential to interact with SERMs, they are not recommended for treatment of hot flashes for women on risk reduction agents.

In summary, multiple multicenter trials across the United States, United Kingdom, and Europe have shown a benefit for tamoxifen, raloxifene, and AIs in reducing invasive and ER-positive cancer but not ER-negative breast cancer when studied in predominantly white women (84%–97% white in studies that reported this information).[92] Specifically, tamoxifen reduced the incidence of invasive breast cancer by 7 events per 1000 women over 5 years of use and raloxifene reduced the incidence by 9 events per 1000 women over 5 years. In the tamoxifen trials, benefits for risk reduction of both invasive and ER-positive cancer persisted for up to 8 years after discontinuation of the medication associated with a 43% risk reduction overall and 86% reduction in women with ADH.[63,65,93] Conversely, AIs reduced the incidence by 16 events per 10,000 women over 5 years. The absolute benefits are likely even higher for those with 3% or greater predicted risk for breast cancer (including those with a history of atypical hyperplasia or LCIS). Exemestane specifically reduced the risk of invasive breast cancer by 65% and anastrozole by 53% after 3 and 5 years of use, respectively. In addition, tamoxifen and raloxifene reduced the risk of nonvertebral and vertebral fractures, respectively. However, these SERMS are associated with an increased risk for venous thromboembolism and vasomotor symptoms. Moreover, tamoxifen increased the risk for endometrial cancer and cataracts. These risks are principally noted in older women although women who have had a hysterectomy are not at risk for endometrial cancer. The toxicity profile of AIs includes vasomotor symptoms, gastrointestinal symptoms, and musculoskeletal pain. Although long-term studies are limited, some AI trials have shown a trend toward increased cardiovascular events (such as transient ischemic attack and cerebrovascular accident); however, this risk is lowered in younger women.[94,95] No reduction in risk of fracture was seen with AIs and bone density monitoring is recommended for women on AI therapy.

Comparisons of effectiveness cannot be made between tamoxifen, raloxifene, and AIs as the placebo-controlled trials had differing participant characteristics including risk criteria, benign breast pathology, or predicted breast cancer risk as gauged by a risk assessment tool. However, the STAR trial directly compared tamoxifen with raloxifene for breast cancer risk reduction and found that tamoxifen provided a greater risk reduction for invasive breast cancer on long-term follow-up by 5 fewer cases per 10,000 women over 5 years.

Enhanced surveillance

The goal of enhanced surveillance is to decrease morbidity and mortality from breast cancer by detecting early cancers requiring less invasive therapies. Because 80% of patients with breast cancer have no risk factors other than gender and age, early identification of those at highest risk for developing the disease is difficult. Thus, one of the most important aspects in combating this disease is prevention and diagnosis at an early stage when the prognosis for cure is greatest. The 3-pronged approach of breast imaging, clinical breast examination (CBE), and breast awareness has become the hallmark of early breast cancer detection in high-risk women. According to the NCCN guidelines, enhanced surveillance begins with a clinical encounter to include a complete medical history, breast cancer risk assessment, discussion of breast awareness, and a CBE to detect the disease as early as possible and to reduce associated morbidity and mortality in high-risk women.[96] The frequency of the clinical encounter depends on the patient's age, medical and family history. Although there are multiple categories for high-risk breast cancer status, this review only focuses on those at high risk based on risk assessment models (Gail $\geq$ 1.7 or family history models >20%), mantle irradiation, or with precancerous lesions.[97] Those with pedigrees suggestive of or known genetic predispositions or those with a personal history of breast cancer are covered in other chapters within this text.

Breast awareness is a component of early breast cancer detection where women should be familiar with their breasts and immediately report any changes to their health care practitioner. Ideology regarding patient breast examination has transformed from systematic and consistent self-breast examination (BSE) on a regular basis in the average risk asymptomatic women, toward the concept of patient breast self-awareness of the normal appearance, composition (ie, topography, structure, design), and feel of the breast tissue, which may heighten awareness of changes that may be detected during their personal evaluation of their breast tissue. The value of heightened awareness, however it may be achieved, is commonly acknowledged based on the value of earlier treatment of both nonpalpable and palpable breast cancers, with a 98% 5-year survival for localized breast disease.[98] Studies show that breast cancers detected while practicing BSE (and by analogy possibly breast awareness) are diagnosed at an earlier stage and tend to be smaller than those diagnosed in the absence of any screening. In addition, women are more likely to find their tumor themselves when practicing BSE regularly.[99] Specifically, nearly half of all cancer lesions in women aged 50 years and older and more than 70% of cases of cancer in women younger than 50 years are self-detected.[100,101] However, data documenting the efficacy of BSE in reducing breast cancer mortality are lacking.[100] It may, however, represent the only viable alternative for women who do not meet mammographic screening eligibility guidelines or for whom mammography services are simply unavailable based on geography or cost prohibition. Furthermore, Shen and Zelen analyzed data from selected mammography screening trials and found the sensitivity of BSE to be appreciable (39%-59%).[102] However, most studies do not reveal such robust results. A Cochrane review concluded that screening by BSE cannot be recommended and that women who desire to be taught to perform such examinations should be informed of the lack of supporting evidence to make an informed choice. Yet, authors recommend that women should be aware of breast changes.[103] Of note, neither self-awareness patient education strategy nor its effect has been studied to determine the impact on breast cancer morbidity or mortality.

CBE seeks to detect breast abnormalities at an earlier stage of disease, when treatment options are more numerous, including less invasive alternatives, and are generally more effective than treatment options for cancers detected at later stages. Moreover, CBE may detect early-stage palpable cancer, especially those that are mammographically occult including lobular carcinomas. However, of the commonly used methods of breast cancer screening, CBE has received the least attention in the medical literature although sensitivity and specificity have been found to be 54% and 94%, respectively.[104] Yet, randomized trials comparing CBE to no screening have not been done. According to the American College of Obstetrics and Gynecology (ACOG), CBE may be offered every 1 to 3 years for average-risk women aged 25 to 39 years and annually for women aged 40 years and older, within the principles of shared decision-making and knowledge of the uncertainty of benefits and harms beyond screening mammography.[105] Although CBE in the asymptomatic average-risk women remains controversial, CBE continues to be recommended for diagnostic evaluation of high-risk women and those with signs and symptoms of breast disease and appropriate imaging as necessary. Moreover, for low-income and middle-income countries, CBE remains a core component of early detection strategies, particularly where it is combined with education on awareness and early signs and symptoms of breast disease. Studies of CBE in developing countries have been undertaken; however, they have been inconclusive and problematic.[106] In these areas, mammography screening is very costly and a complex undertaking, thus mammographic screening is generally only recommended for those countries with suitable infrastructure making long-term programs realizable.

Although CBE recommendation is variable, breast cancer risk assessment is recommended by most professional organizations including the ACOG,[107] the USPSTF, The American College of Physicians, and the American Academy of Family Physicians.

Breast cancer mortality has been declining nearly 2% each year over the last decade. This decline has been attributed to mammographic screening and treatment advances.[108] Morality rates have continued to decline in women aged 40 to 79 years, yet recent retrospective analysis shows breast cancer mortality rates have stopped declining in US women younger than 40 years.[109] Specifically, after 2010, breast cancer mortality rates demonstrated nonsignificant increases in women aged 20 to 29 and 30 to 39 years. These results are primarily attributable to change in mortality rates in White women as African American, Asian, Native American, and Hispanic women in this age group continued to decline significantly between 1990 and 2017. In addition, this transition is, at least in part, explained by rapidly rising distant-stage disease after

2000 in women aged 20 to 39 years.[110] Thus, likely contributing to ending the decline in mortality rates in women younger than 40 years. A similar increased rate of distant disease was noted in women aged 70 to 79 years. Authors surmise a possible contributor to noted trends is largely absent mammography use in women younger than 40 years and guideline changes that have discouraged screening in older women, suggesting continued screening in these age cohorts may be beneficial.[111] It is well known that women in this younger age group are more likely to experience aggressive forms of breast cancer including triple-negative or HER2-positive breast cancer; however, as treatments do not differ based solely on younger age, differences in treatment do not explain noted trends, and thus underlying causality cannot be assigned. Importantly, younger women are more likely to detect breast cancers themselves at a more advanced stage at presentation than women with screen-detected cancers.[112]

Despite the intense controversy surrounding the efficacy of mammographic screening, it remains the only imaging study that has been extensively evaluated in randomized controlled trials and has been shown, in many cases, to reduce breast cancer mortality. No reduction in mortality has been proven for any screening method other than mammography.[113] The magnitude of benefit has varied in the literature because of the diversity of study designs and screening frequency. However, data may not reflect the benefits of current mammographic technology, interpretation, and oncologic care.

Although guidelines from professional societies vary, the ACOG recommends women at average risk for breast cancer have an opportunity to initiate screening every 1 to 2 years at age 40 years or no later than age 50 years. Screening should continue until age 75 years or as long as there is a life expectancy of at least 10 years.[105] The NCCN recommends annual screening beginning at age 40 years "as it results in the greatest mortality reduction, most lives saved, and most life years gained."[96] Screening should continue as long as interventions would be recommended based on the screening findings and comorbidities.

For women at *high risk* for breast cancer based on Gail model risk greater than 1.7, mantle irradiation exposure, lifetime risk greater than 20% based on history of ADH/ALH/LCIS or risk assessment model largely dependent on family history, recommendations generally include breast awareness, a clinical encounter q 6 to 12 months, and annual imaging beginning 10 years before the affected relative, or 8 to 10 years after radiation exposure or at age identified as high risk or age of diagnosis of high-risk lesion (however not before age 30 years) (**Table 2**). MRI may also be recommended annually with similar eligibility criteria; however, not before age 25 years.[114] American Cancer Society guidelines expand the eligible categories suggesting annual MRI (in addition to mammography surveillance) for BRCA mutation carriers, as yet untested first-degree family members of BRCA mutation carriers, women with a lifetime risk of breast cancer ≥ 20%, women with a history of chest wall irradiation between age 10 and 30 years, and patients (or first-degree relatives of patients) with other genetic syndromes including Li-Fraumeni syndrome, Cowden syndrome, or Bannayan-Riley-Ruvalcaba syndrome.[115] It is important to note that women obtaining more than 4 MRIs have been shown to have retention of gadolinium-based contrast agents in the brain[116] and bone[117]; however, FDA guidelines have not identified any harmful effects to date. The clinical significance and practice implications are unclear; thus, MRI remains an option in select populations of high-risk women after shared decision-making.[118]

At present, there is insufficient evidence to recommend for or again MRI screening in women with a lifetime risk between 15% and 20%, women with atypical hyperplasia,[97] or women with heterogeneously or extremely dense breast until larger studies

Table 2
Breast cancer screening recommendations for high-risk patients

Risk Category[a]	Breast Awareness	Clinical Encounter (Not Before Age 21 y)	Mammographic Imaging[b]	MRI
Age >35 y with 5 y Gail Model risk ≥ 1.7%[d]	Yes	Q 6–12 mo	Begin at age identified as increased risk; Annually	
Lifetime risk >20% based on history of LCIS or ADH/ALH	Yes	Q 6–12 mo	Begin at age of diagnosis but not <30 y of age; Annually	Consider annually beginning at age of diagnosis but not before age 25 y
Lifetime risk >20% based on models largely dependent on family history[c]	Yes	Q 6–12 mo	Begin at age identified as increased risk; Annually beginning 10 y before the youngest affected family member but not <25 y of age	Annually beginning 10 y before the youngest affected family member but not <25 y of age
Age >25 y with prior mantle irradiation between age 10 and 30 y	Yes	Q 6–12 mo	Begin 8–10 y after radiation exposure; Annually beginning 10 y after radiation exposure but not before age 30 y	Annually beginning 10 y after radiation exposure but not before age 25 y
Age <25 y with prior mantle irradiation between age 10 and 30 y	Yes	Q 12 mo beginning 10 y after radiation therapy		
Pedigree suggestive of or known genetic predisposition	See chapter 6			

[a] Women in this group should be counseled for consideration of risk reduction strategies.
[b] The NCCN recommends mammographic imaging with consideration of tomosynthesis.
[c] Models largely dependent on family history include Claus, Tyrer-Cuzick.
[d] Gail model for use in women aged 35 years and older.

Data from National Comprehensive Cancer Network. NCCN Clinical Practice Guidelines in Oncology: Breast Cancer Screening and Diagnosis. Version 1.2020. https://www.nccn.org/professionals/physician_gls/pdf/breast_screening.pdf; with permission.

are performed. MRI has been reported to have increased sensitivity as compared with mammography specifically in high-risk women; however, less specificity frequently resulted in false-positive diagnoses and unnecessary biopsies, nearly 3 times increased in one study.[119,120] In addition, MRI has decreased ability to detect micro-calcifications, which may be an early sign of breast cancer development.[121] This limits its positive predictive value; however, this depends on pathology. Specifically, the likelihood of a false-positive diagnosis, including high-risk atypical and complex pro-liferative changes, was twice as high in women undergoing biopsy for MRI findings as for those with digital mammography (DM) with tomosynthesis.[122] Similar to screening ultrasound, the impact of MRI on survival has not been addressed in randomized clin-ical trials. Ultimately, careful patient selection is needed based on the false-negative and false-positive rates as well as cost-effectiveness of routine screening in the average risk population needs to be addressed before consideration of generalized use of MRI.

Digital breast tomosynthesis (DBT) allows multiple electronically created digital im-ages to be combined into a three-dimensional view as compared to the two-dimensional view of conventional screen film and DM. DBT has been shown to in-crease the conspicuity of many lesions while reducing false-positive findings through reduction of obscuration by overlying structures.[123] US data show that integrated 2D/3D mammography significantly increased cancer detection in population cancer screening.[124] Detailed discussion of DBT in high-risk women Is reviewed in Cimmie L. Shahan, MD and Ginger P. Layne' and article, "Advances in Breast Imaging with Current Screening Recommendations and Controversies," in this issue.

Emerging evidence suggests screening molecular imaging (breast specific gamma imaging, sestamibi scan, or positron emission mammography) may improve breast cancer detection particularly in high-risk women; however, effective radiation dosage to the whole body with these modalities remains substantially higher than mammog-raphy. In addition, there have been no studies in large screening populations with MBI.[125] Current evidence does not support thermography or ductal lavage as screening procedures in breast cancer evaluation. In addition, further studies are required to support contrast-enhanced spectral mammography for routine screening in the high-risk population although it has been shown to reduce benign biopsies in BI-RADS 4a/4b lesions[126] as well as suggested per NCCN guidelines in women who are eligible but cannot undergo MRI. Moreover, background parenchymal enhancement at CESM was associated with breast density and increased odds for breast cancer, independent of other risk factors.[127]

For diagnostic management of pregnant patients, ultrasound and age-appropriate mammogram with shielding are recommended for palpable abnormalities. MRI with gadolinium and its potential risk to the fetus are discussed in a separate chapter.

Risk-reducing mastectomy

Bilateral RRM has been shown in case series and retrospective cohort studies, to be effective in reducing both incidence and death from breast cancer.[128] Studies have shown reduction of cancer incidence in high-risk women greater than 90%, which holds true whether the nipple-areolar complex is preserved or reconstructed.[129] How-ever, studies estimate that most high-risk women (determined by strong family history but not necessarily BRCA1/2 mutation carriers) who had RRM would *not* have died from breast cancer even without the surgery (overtreatment).[128] Thus, as RRM is a radical surgical procedure with conceivable overtreatment, surgical risks, and poten-tial psychosocial effects. RRM should generally be reserved only for women at signif-icantly high risk, as with a genetic mutation conferring a high risk for breast cancer.

The paradox is that many women with breast cancer have breast-*conserving* surgery, whereas RRM *removes* the breasts of those who (at present) are unaffected with breast cancer. In northern Europe, RRM is also performed in specialist breast units for women with a lifetime risk of 25% or greater (without genetic predisposition).[130] Proactive surgery based on risk and predisposition may reduce psychological distress and anxiety. Consultations with surgeons familiar with the risks and benefits of surgery, nipple-sparing procedures, and surgical reconstruction are recommended. In addition, psychological consultations may also be considered.

Risk-reducing salpingoophorectomy

RRSO has also been shown to reduce breast cancer risk in BRCA 1/2 mutation carriers by 50%; however, there are now conflicting reports that challenge that observation where a European study that maximally eliminated bias found no evidence for a protective effect indicating previously studies may have been overestimated because of bias.[131] Although RRSO lowers the risk of ovarian cancer, it may increase the risk of cardiovascular disease, cancer other than ovarian cancer, osteoporosis, cognitive impairment, and all-cause mortality. Thus, providing detailed information is critical.

Opportunistic salpingectomy (OS) is a strategy available to all women already undergoing pelvic surgery for benign disease in an effort to decrease the risk of ovarian cancer (not breast cancer). Although the procedure offers the opportunity to significantly lower the risk of ovarian cancer, it does not completely eliminate the risk. Salpingectomy performed at the time of scheduled benign procedures or as a means of tubal sterilization, appears to safely reduce risk without concomitant increase in the risk of complications such as blood transfusions, readmissions, postoperative complications, infection, or fever compared specifically with hysterectomy alone or tubal ligation. In addition, ovarian function does not appear to be affected based on surrogate serum markers or response to in vitro fertilization. OS can be offered whether the planned hysterectomy is scheduled as minimally invasive, vaginal, or abdominal. The benefits and risks of OS should be discussed with eligible patients planning a pelvic procedure or tubal ligation.[132,133]

SUMMARY

Noted trends in increasing mortality among certain subsets of patients with breast cancer are prompting experts to call for greater awareness among practitioners. Risk assessment is of paramount importance in identifying women who have the greatest benefit from risk reduction strategies. Principles of shared decision-making should guide practitioners to incorporate patients' values, goals, and objectives. Patients will then be able to make informed choices regarding pharmacologic prevention of breast cancer, enhanced surveillance, and other risk reduction strategies. Through this process, women and clinicians share information, including potential benefits and risks and expressed preferences, and then agree on a plan. In efforts to advance personalized medicine and limit harms, strategies among women of high-risk status need to be elucidated, discussed, and offered. Allowing women to capitalize on these added benefits and education.

CLINICS CARE POINTS

- Discussion of healthy lifestyle options is a critical approach not only for the promotion of overall health but also for the encouragement of healthy choices in *all* women, *regardless* of their breast cancer risk.

- Genetic testing should be offered where it is likely to impact the risk management and/or treatment of the tested individuals and/or their at-risk family members.

- Breastfeeding is a critical modifiable preventive behavior that is inversely associated with breast cancer risk. Dose-response has been demonstrated with longer duration associated with a greater reduction in risk.

- Research suggests that individuals who identify as gay, lesbian, bisexual, queer, or same-gender-loving may have a higher risk of breast cancer compared with heterosexual women because of higher rates of nulliparity, alcohol consumption, smoking, and obesity.

- The reasons for racial disparities are complex, including African American women are more likely to present at stage IV, have lower frequency of screening, longer time between screenings, limited follow-up after abnormal screening results (despite financial or insurance coverage or resources), and comorbidities resulting in worsening survival. In addition, African American women have a greater likelihood of more aggressive breast cancer subtypes such as inflammatory, basal cell, luminal B, and triple-negative disease.

- Many studies have found that equitable access to timely quality care eliminates racial disparities in cancer outcomes; however, others note persistence of disparities possibly implicating systemic racism and implicit bias.

- Risk reduction strategies have both benefits and harms that should be discussed with women before consideration. Clinicians must weigh medication side effects, procedure risks and harms, patient-specific comorbidities, and lifestyle preferences to understand the true risk for each individual.

DISCLOSURE

The author has nothing to disclose.

REFERENCES

1. American Cancer Society. Cancer facts & figures 2021. Atlanta (GA): American Cancer Society; 2021. Available at: https://www.cancer.org/research/cancer-facts-statistics/all-cancer-facts-figures/cancer-facts-figures-2021.html. Accessed February 8, 2021.
2. American Cancer Society. Cancer treatment & survivorship facts & figures 2019-2021. Atlanta (GA): American Cancer Society; 2019.
3. Siegel RL, Miller KD, Jemal A. Cancer Statistics, 2020. CA Cancer J Clin 2020; 70(1):7–30.
4. Chlebowski RT, Rohan TE, Manson JE, et al. Breast cancer after use o of estrogen plus progestin and estrogen alone: analyses of data from two women's health initiative randomized clinical trials. JAMA Oncol 2015;1:296–305 (Level I).
5. Rungruang B, Kelley JL. Benign breast diseases: epidemiology, evaluation, and management. Clin Obstet Gynecol 2011;54:110–24 (Level III).
6. Lauby-Secretan B, Scoccianti C, Loomis D, et al. Body fatness and cancer. Viewpoint of the IARC working group. N Engl J Med 2016;375:794–8.
7. Green VL. Mammographic breast density and breast cancer risk: Implications of density legislation for practice. Clin Obstet Gynecol 2016;59(2):419–38.
8. Bagnardi V, Rota M, Botteri E, et al. Light alcohol drinking and cancer: a meta-analysis. Ann Oncol 2013;24(2):301–8.
9. Gaudet MM, Gapstur SM, Sun J, et al. Active smoking and breast cancer risk: original cohort data and meta-analysis. J Natl Cancer Inst 2013;105:515–25.

10. Pizot C, Boniol M, Mullie P, et al. Physical activity, hormone replacement therapy and breast cancer risk: A meta-analysis of prospective studies. Eur J Cancer 2016;52:138–54.

11. Henderson TO, Amsterdam A, Bhatia S, et al. Systematic review: surveillance for breast cancer in women treated with chest radiation for childhood, adolescent, or young adult cancer. Ann Intern Med 2010;152:444–55. W144-455. (Systematic Review).

12. Bhatia S, Yasui Y, Robison LL, et al. High risk of subsequent neoplasms continues with extended follow up of childhood Hodgkin's disease: report from the Late Effects Study Group. J Clin Oncol 2003;21:4386–94.

13. National Comprehensive Cancer Network. NCCN Clinical Practice Guidelines in Oncology: Breast Cancer Risk Reduction. Version 1.2020. Available at: https://www.nccn.org/professionals/physician_gls/pdf/breast_risk.pdf. Accessed February 15, 2021.

14. Collaborative group on hormonal factors in breast cancer and breastfeeding: collaborative reanalysis of individual data from 47 epidemiological studies in 30 countries, including 50302 women with breast cancer and 96973 women without disease. Lancet 2002;360:187–95.

15. Chowdhury R, Sinha B, Sankar MJ, et al. Breastfeeding and maternal health outcomes: a systematic review and meta-analysis. Acta Paediatr 2015;104:96–113.

16. Goncalves AK, Dantas Florencio GL, Maisonnette de Atayde Silva MJ, et al. Effects of physical activity on breast cancer prevention: a systematic review. J Phys Act Health 2014;11:445–54.

17. Noone AM, Howlander N, Krapcho M, et al. SEER cancer statistics review, 1975-2015. Bethesda (MD): National Cancer Institute; 2018. Available at: http://seer.cancer.gov.csr/1975_2015/. based on November 2017 SEER data submission.

18. American Cancer Society. Cancer facts & figures for African Americans 2019-2021. Atlanta (GA): American Cancer Society; 2019. p. 12.

19. McCarthy AM, Kim JJ, Beaber EF, et al. Follow –up of abnormal breast and colorectal cancer screening by race/ethnicity. Am J Prev Med 2016;51:507–12.

20. Selove R, Kilbourne B, Fadden MK, et al. Time from screening mammography to biopsy and from biopsy to breast cancer treatment among black and white women Medicare beneficiaries not participating in a health maintenance organization. Womens Health Issues 2016;26:642–7.

21. Jemal A, Robbins AS, Lin CC, et al. Factors that contributed to black-white disparities in survival among nonelderly women with breast cancer between 2004 and 2013. J Clin Oncol 2018;36:14–24.

22. Danforth DN JR. Disparities in breast cancer outcomes between Caucasian and African American women: a model for describing the relationship of biological and nonbiological factors. Breast Cancer Res 2013;15:208.

23. Ellis L, Canchola AJ, Spiegel D, et al. Racial and ethnic disparities in cancer survival: the contribution of tumor, sociodemographic, institutional and neighborhood characteristics. J Clin Oncol 2018;36(1):25–33.

24. Singh GK, Jemal A. Socioeconomic and racial/ethnic disparities in cancer mortality, incidence, and survival in the United States, 1950-2014: over six decades of changing patterns and widening inequalities. J Environ Public Health 2017;2017:2819372.

25. Committee on lesbian, gay, bisexual and transgender health issues and research gaps and opportunities, board of the health of select populations, Institute of Medicine. The health of lesbian, gay, bisexual and transgender people:

building a foundation for better understanding. Washington, DC: National Academies Press; 2011.

26. Malone J, Snguon S, Dean LT, et al. Breast cancer screening and care among black sexual minority women: a scoping review of the literature from 1990 to2017. J Womens Health 2019;28(12):1650–60.

27. Collaborative group on hormonal factors in breast cancer. Familial breast cancer: collaborative reanalysis of individual data from 52 epidemiological studies including 58.209 women with breast cancer and 101,986 women without the disease. Lancet 2001;358(9291):1389–99.

28. Green VL. Breast Diseases: Benign and Malignant. In: Rock JA, Jones HW III, editors. TeLinde's Operative Gynecology. 10th edition. Philadelphia: Lippincott Williams & Wilkins; 2008.

29. Nelson HD, Fu R, Zakher B, et al. Medication use to reduce risk of breast cancer US Preventive Services task force recommendation statement. JAMA 2019;322: 857–67.

30. Gail MH, Mai PL. Comparing breast cancer risk assessment models. J Natl Cancer Inst 2010;102(10):665–8.

31. Madigan MR, Ziegler RG, Benichou J, et al. Proportion of breast cancer cases in the United States explained by well-established risk factors. J Natl Cancer Inst 1995;87(22):1681–1685/.

32. McCullough ML, Feigelson HS, Diver WR, et al. Risk factors for fatal breast cancer in African American women and white women in a large US prospective cohort. Am J Epidemiol 2005;162(8):734–42.

33. Antoniou A, Pharoah PD, Narod S, et al. Average risks of breast and ovarian cancer associated with BRCA1or BRCA2 mutations detected in case series unselected for family history: a combined analysis of 22 studies. Am J Hum Genet 2003;72:1117–30.

34. Tung N, Domchek SM, Stadler Z, et al. Counselling framework for moderate penetrance cancer susceptibility mutations. Nat Rev Clin Oncol 2016;13:581–8.

35. Ray JA, Loescher LJ, Brewer M. Risk-reduction surgery decisions in high-risk women seen for genetic counseling. J Gen Couns 2005;14(6):473–84.

36. Sutherland S, Meiser B, Kaur R, et al. Assessing the medical workforces perceived barriers to the prescription of risk-reducing medication for women at high-risk of breast cancer. Breast J 2019;25:34–40.

37. Maas P, Barrdahl M, Joshi AD, et al. Breast cancer risk from modifiable and non-modifiable risk factors among white women in the United States. JAMA Oncol 2016;2:1295–302.

38. Song M, Giovannucci E. Preventable incidence and mortality of carcinoma associated with lifestyle factors among white adults in the United States. JAMA Oncol 2016;2:1154–61.

39. Mahoney MC, Bevers T, Linos E, et al. Opportunities and strategies for breast cancer prevention through risk reduction. CA Cancer J Clin 2008;58:347–71.

40. Chen WY, Rosner B, Hankingon SE, et al. Moderate alcohol consumption during adult life, drinking patterns, and breast cancer risk. JAMA 2011;306:1884–90.

41. National Comprehensive Cancer Network. NCCN Clinical Practice Guidelines in Oncology: Breast Cancer Risk Reduction. Version 1.2020. Available at: https://www.nccn.org/professionals/physician_gls/pdf/breast_risk.pdf. Accessed November 23, 2020.

42. Bernstein L, Patel V, Ursin G, et al. Lifetime recreational exercise activity and breast cancer risk among black women and white women. J Natl Cancer Inst 2005;97(22):1671–9.

43. Neihoff NM, White AJ, Sandler DP. Childhood and teenage physical activity and breast cancer risk. Breast Cancer Res Treat 2017;164:697–705.

44. Boeke CE, Eliassen AH, Oh H, et al. Adolescent physical activity in relation to breast cancer risk. Breast Cancer Res Treat 2014;145:715–24.

45. Howard RA, Leitzmann MF, Linet MS, et al. Physical activity and breast cancer risk among pre- and postmenopausal women in the U.S. Radiologic Technologists cohort. Cancer Causes Control 2009;20:323–33.

46. Calle EE, Rodriguez C, Walker-Thurmond K, et al. Overweight, obesity, and mortality from cancer in a prospectively studies cohort of US adults. J Engl J Med 2002;348:1625–38.

47. Bruning PF, Bonfrer JM, van Noord PA, et al. Insulin resistance and breast cancer risk. Int J Cancer 1992;52:511–6.

48. Talamini R, Franceschi S, Favero A, et al. Selected medical conditions and risk of breast cancer. Br J Cancer 1997;75:1699–703.

49. Eliassen AH, Colditz GA, Rosner B, et al. Adult weight change and risk of postmenopausal breast cancer. JAMA 2006;296:193–201.

50. Farvid MS, Chen WY, Michels KB, et al. Fruit and vegetable consumption in adolescence and early adulthood and risk of breast cancer: population based cohort study. BMJ 2016;353:i2343.

51. Linos E, Willett WC. Diet and breast cancer risk reduction. J Natl Compr Canc Netw 2007;5:711–8.

52. Dong JY, Qin LQ. Soy isoflavones consumption and risk of breast cancer incidence or recurrence: a meta-analysis of prospective studies. Breast Cancer Res Treat 2011;125:315–23.

53. Zhou Y, Chen J, Li Q, et al. Association between breastfeeding and breast cancer risk: evidence from a meta-analysis. Breastfeed Med 2015;10(3):175–82.

54. Palmer JR, Boggs DA, Wise LA, et al. Parity and lactation in relation to estrogen reception negative breast cancer in African American women. Cancer Epidemiol Biomarkers Prev 2011;20:1883–91.

55. Green VL, Killings NL, Clare CA. The historical, psychosocial, and cultural context of breastfeeding in the African American community. Breastfeed Med 2021;16(2):1–5.

56. National Comprehensive Cancer Network. NCCN Clinical Practice Guidelines in Oncology: Breast Cancer risk reduction. Version 1.2020. Available at: https://www.nccn.org/professionals/physician_gls/pdf/breast.pdf. Accessed February 1, 2021.

57. Visvanathan K, Fabian CJ, Bantug E, et al. Use of endocrine therapy for breast cancer risk reduction: ASCO clinical practice guideline. J Clin Oncol 2019; 37(33):3152–65.

58. DeCensi A, Gandini S, Serrano D, et al. Randomized dose ranging trial of tamoxifen in low doses in hormone replacement therapy users. J Clin Oncol 2007;25:4201–9.

59. Freedman AN, Yu B, Gail MH, et al. Benefit/risk assessment for breast cancer chemoprevention with raloxifene or tamoxifen for women age 50 years or older. J Clin Oncol 2011;29:2327–33.

60. Fisher B, Costantino JP, Wickerham DL, et al. Tamoxifen for prevention of breast cancer: report of the National Surgical Adjuvant Breast and Bowel Project P-1 Study. J Natl Cancer Inst 1998;90(18):1371–88.

61. Cuzick J, Forbes J, Edwards R, et al. First results from the International Breast Cancer Intervention Study (IBIS-1) a randomized prevention trial. Lancet 2002; 360(9336):817–24.

62. Cuzick, Forbes JF, Sestak I, et al. Long-term results of tamoxifen prophylaxis for breast cancer – 96 month follow up of the randomized IBIS-1 trial. J Natl Cancer Inst 2007;99(4):272–82.
63. Cuzick J, Sestak I, Cawthorn S, et al. IBIS-I Investigators. Tamoxifen for prevention of breast cancer: extended long –term follow-up of the IBIS-I breast cancer prevention trial. Lancet Oncol 2015;16(1):67–75.
64. Powles TJ, Eeles R, Ashley S. Interim analysis of the incidence of breast cancer in the Royal Marsden Hospital tamoxifen randomized chemoprevention trial. Lancet 1998;352:98–101.
65. Powles TJ, Ashley S, Tidy A, et al. Twenty-year follow up of the Royal Marsden randomized, double –blinded tamoxifen breast cancer prevention trial. J Natl Cancer Inst 2007;99(4):283–90.
66. Veronesi U, Maisonneuve P, Costa A, et al. Prevention of breast cancer with tamoxifen: preliminary findings from the Italian randomized trial among hysterectomised women. Italian tamoxifen prevention study. Lancet 1998;352:93–7.
67. Veronesi U, Maisonneuve P, Rotmensz N, et al. Tamoxifen for the prevention of breast cancer: late results of the Italian randomized tamoxifen prevention trial among women with hysterectomy. J Natl Cancer Inst 2007;99:727–37.
68. Veronesi U, Maisonneuve P, Rotmensz N, et al. Italian randomized trial among women with hysterectomy: Tamoxifen and hormone-dependent breast cancer in high risk women. J Natl Cancer Inst 2003;95:160–5.
69. Cummings SR, Eckert S, Krueger KA, et al. The effect of raloxifene on risk of breast cancer in postmenopausal women: results from the MORE randomized trial. Multiple outcomes of raloxifene evaluation. JAMA 1999;281:2189–97.
70. Martino S, Cauley JA, Barrett-Connor E, et al. Continuing outcomes relevant to evista: breast cancer incidence in postmenopausal osteoporotic women in a randomized trial of raloxifene. J Natl Cancer Inst 2004;96:1751–61.
71. Grady D, Cauley JA, Geiger MF, et al. Reduced incidence of invasive breast cancer with raloxifene among women at increased coronary risk. J Natl Cancer Inst 2008;100:854–61.
72. Vogel VG, Costantino JP, Wickerham DL, et al. Update of the national Surgical Adjuvant Breast and Bowel Project Study of Tamoxifen and Raloxifene (STAR) P2 trial: Preventing breast cancer. Cancer Prev Res 2010;3:696–706.
73. Wickerham DL, fisher B, Wolmark N, et al. Association of tamoxifen and uterine sarcoma. J Clin Oncol 2002;20:4403.
74. DeCensi A, Putoni M, Guerrieri-Gonzaga A, et al. Randomized placebo controlled trial of low dose tamoxifen to prevent local and contralateral recurrence in breast intraepithelial neoplasia. J Clin Oncol 2019;37:1629–37.
75. Land SR, Wickerham DL, Costantino JRP, et al. Patient-reported symptoms and quality of life during treatment of tamoxifen and Raloxifene for breast cancer prevention: the NSABP Study of Tamoxifen and Raloxifene (STAR) P-2 trial. JAMA 2006;295(23):2742–51.
76. Cuzick J, DeCensi a, Banu A, et al. preventive therapy for breast cancer: a consensus statement. Lancet 2011;12:496–503.
77. Narod SA, Brunet JS, Ghadirian P, et al. Tamoxifen and risk of contralateral breast cancer in BRCA1 and BRCA2 mutation carriers: a case control study. Hereditary Breast Cancer Clinical Study Group. Lancet 2000;356:1876–81.
78. Baum M, Budzar AU, Cuzick J, et al. Anastrozole alone or in combination with tamoxifen versus tamoxifen alone for adjuvant treatment of postmenopausal women with early breast cancer: first results of the ATAC randomized trial. Lancet 2002;359:2131–9.

79. Baum M, Budzar AU, Cuzick J, et al. Anastrozole alone or in combination with tamoxifen versus tamoxifen alone for adjuvant treatment of postmenopausal women with early breast cancer: results of the ATAC Arimidex, Tamoxifen Alone or in Combination: trial efficacy and safety update analyses. Cancer 2003;98: 1802–10.

80. Coombes RC, Hall E, Gibson LJ, et al. A randomized trial of exemestane after two to three years of tamoxifen therapy in postmenopausal women with primary breast cancer. N Engl J Med 2004;350:1081–92.

81. Goss PE, Ingle JN, Martino S, et al. A randomized trial of letrozole in postmenopausal women after five years of tamoxifen therapy for early-stage breast cancer. N Engl J Med 2003;349:1793–802.

82. Thurlimann B, Keshaviah A, Coates AS, et al. A comparison of letrozole and tamoxifen in postmenopausal women with early breast cancer. N Engl J Med 2005;353:2747–57.

83. Goss PE, Ingle JN, Ales-Martinez JE, et al. Exemestane for breast cancer prevention in postmenopausal. N Engl J Med 2011;364:2381–91.

84. Cuzick J, Sestak I, Forbes JF, et al. Anastrozole for prevention of breast cancer in high risk postmenopausal women (IBISII): an international, double blind, randomized placebo controlled trial. Lancet 2014;383:1041–8.

85. Nemati Shafaee M, Gutierrez-Barrera AM, Lin HY, et al. Aromatase inhibitors and the risk of contralateral breast cancer in BRCA mutation carriers. J Clin Oncol 2015;33:3–13.

86. Cheung AM, Tile L, Cardew S, et al. Bone density and structure in healthy postmenopausal women treated with Exemestane for the primary prevention of breast cancer: a nested substudy of the MAP 3 randomised controlled trial. Lancet Oncol 2012;13(3):275–84.

87. Yang Z, Simondsen K, Kolesar J. Exemestane for primary prevention of breast cancer in postmenopausal women. Am J Health Syst Pharm 2012;69(16): 1384–8.

88. Visvanathan K, Lippman SM, Hurley P, et al. American Society of Clinical Oncology clinical practice guideline update on the use of pharmacologic interventions including Tamoxifen, raloxifene, and aromatase inhibition for breast cancer risk reduction. Gynecol Oncol 2009;115(1):132–4.

89. Nelson HD, Fu R, Zakher B, et al. Medication use for the risk reduction of primary breast cancer in women: a systematic review for the U.S. preventive services task force. Rockville (MD): Agency for Healthcare Research and Quality; 2019.

90. Sideras K, Ingle JN, Amer MM, et al. Coprescription of tamoxifen and medications that inhibit CYP2D6. J Clin Oncol 2010;28:2768–76.

91. Lash TL, Rosenberg CL. Evidence and practice regarding the role for CYP2D6 inhibition in decisions about tamoxifen therapy. J Clin Oncol 2010;28:1273–5.

92. Nelson HD, Fu R, Zakher B, et al. Medication use for the risk reduction of primary breast cancer women: updated evidence report and systematic review for the US Preventive Services task force. JAMA 2019;322:868–86.

93. Pruthi S, Heisey RE, Bevers TB. Chemoprevention for breast cancer. Ann Surg Oncol 2015;22:3230–5.

94. Forbes JF, Sestak I, Howell A, et al. IBIS-II investigators. Anastrozole versus tamoxifen for the prevention of locoregional and contralateral breast cancer in postmenopausal women with locally excised ductal carcinoma in situ (IBIS-II DCIS): a double-blind, randomized controlled trial. Lancet 2016;387(10021): 866–73.

95. Goldvaser H, Barnes TA, Seruga B, et al. Toxicity of extended adjuvant therapy with aromatase inhibitors in early breast cancer: a systematic review and meta-analysis. J Natl Cancer Inst 2018;110(1). https://doi.org/10.1093/jnci/djx141.

96. National Comprehensive Cancer Network. NCCN Clinical Practice Guidelines in Oncology: Breast Cancer Screening and Diagnosis. Version 1.2020. Available at: https://www.nccn.org/professionals/physician_gls/pdf/breast_ screening. pdf. Accessed February 1, 2021.

97. Port ER, Park A, Borgen PI, et al. Results of MRI screening for breast cancer in high risk patients with LCIS and atypical hyperplasia. Ann Surg Oncol 2007;14: 1051–7.

98. American Cancer Society. Breast cancer facts & figures 2019-2021. Atlanta (GA): American Cancer Society, Inc; 2019.

99. Smith RA, Saslow D, Sawyer KA, et al. American Cancer Society guidelines for breast cancer screening: update 2003. CA Cancer J Clin 2003;53:141–69.

100. Coates RJ, Uhler RJ, Brogan DJ, et al. Patterns and predictors of the breast cancer detection methods in women under age 45 years of age (United States). Cancer Causes Control 2001;12(5):431–42.

101. Newcomer L, Mewcomb P, Trentham-Dietz A, et al. Detection method and breast carcinoma histology. Cancer 2002;95(3):470–7.

102. Shen Y, Zelen M. Screening sensitivity and sojourn time from breast cancer early detection clinical trials: mammograms and physical examinations. J Clin Oncol 2001;19:3490–9.

103. Kosters JP, Gotzsche PC. Regular self-examination or clinical examination early detection of breast cancer. Cochrane Database Syst Rev 2003;(2):CD003373.

104. Barton MB, Harris R, Fletcher SW. The rational clinical examination. Does this patient have breast cancer: The screening clinical breast examination: should it be done: How. JAMA 1999;282:1270–80.

105. Breast cancer risk assessment and screening in average risk women. Practice Bulletin No. 179. American College of Obstetricians and Gynecologists. Obstet Gynecol 2017;130:e1–16.

106. Pisani P, Parkin DM, Ngelangel C, et al. Outcome of screening by clinical examination of the breast in a trial in the Philippines. Int J Cancer 2006;118:149–54.

107. Hereditary cancer syndromes and risk assessment. ACOG Committee Opinion No. 793. American College of Obstetricians and Gynecologists. Obstet Gynecol 2019;134(6):e143–9.

108. Humphrey LL, Helfand M, Chan BK, et al. Breast cancer screening: a summary of the evidence for the U.S. Preventive Services Task Force. Ann Intern Med 2002;137:347–60.

109. Hendrick RE, Helvie MA, Monticciolo DL. Breast cancer mortality rates have stopped declining in U.S. women younger than 40 years. Radiology 2021; 00:1–7.

110. Johnson RH, Anders CK, Litton JK, et al. Breast cancer in adolescents and young adults. Pediatr Blood Cancer 2018;65(12):e27397.

111. Carlos RC, Fendrick AM, Kolenic G, et al. Breast screening utilization and cost sharing among employed insured women after the Affordable Care Act. J Am Coll Radiol 2019;16(6):788–96.

112. Ruddy KJ, Gelber S, Tamimi RM, et al. Breast cancer presentation and diagnostic delays in young women. Cancer 2014;120(1):20–5.

113. Berg WA. Tailored supplemental screening for breast cancer: what now and what next? AJR Am J Roentgenol 2009;192:390–9.

114. Warner E, Messersmith H, Causer P, et al. Systematic review: using magnetic resonance imaging to screen women at high risk for breast cancer. Ann Intern Med 2008;148:671–9.
115. Saslow D, Boetes C, Burke W, et al. American Cancer Society guidelines for breast screening with MRI as an adjunct to mammography. CA Cancer J Clin 2007;57:75–89.
116. McDonald RJ, McDonald JS, Kallmes DF, et al. Gadolinium deposition in human brain tissues after contrast enhanced MR imaging in adult patients without intracranial abnormalities. Radiology 2017;285:546–54.
117. Darrah TH, Prutsman-Pfeiffer JJ, Poreda RJ, et al. Incorporation of excess gadolinium into human bone from medical contrast agents. Metallomics 2009;1: 479–88.
118. FDA Drug Safety Communication: FDA identifies no harmful effects to date with brain retention of gadolinium-based contrast agents for MRIs; review to continue issued on May 22, 2017. https://www.fda.gov/drugs/drug-safety-and-availability/fda-drug-safety-communication-fda-warns-gadolinium-based-contrast-agents-gbcas-are-retained-body. Accessed 1/6/22.
119. Lord SJ, Lei W, Craft P, et al. A systematic review of the effectiveness of magnetic resonance imaging (MRI) as an addition to mammography and ultrasound in screening young women at high risk of breast cancer. Eur J Cancer 2007;43: 1905–17.
120. Leach MO, Boggis CR, Kixon AK, et al. Screening with magnetic resonance imaging and mammography of a UK population at high familial risk of breast can: a prospective multicenter cohort study (MARIBS). Lancet 2005;365:1769–78.
121. Mann RM, Kuhl CK, Kindel K, et al. Breast MRI: guidelines from the European Society of Breast Imaging. Eur Radiol 2008;18:1307–18.
122. Kuhl CK, Keulers A, Strobel K, et al. Not all false positive diagnoses are equal: On the prognostic implications of false-positive diagnoses made in breast MRI versus in mammography/digital tomosynthesis screening. Breast Cancer Res 2018;20:13–21.
123. Niklason LT, Christia BT, Niklason LE, et al. Digital tomosynthesis in breast imaging. Radiology 1997;205(2):399–406.
124. Caumo F, Bernardi D, Ciatto S, et al. Incremental effect from integrating 3D mammography (tomosynthesis) with 2D mammography: increased breast cancer detection evident for screening centres in population based trial. Breast 2014;23(1):76–80.
125. Mainiero MB, Moy L, Baron P, et al. ACR appropriateness criteria breast cancer screening. ACR 2017;14(11S):s383–92.
126. Zuley ML, Bandos AI, Abrams GS, et al. contrast enhanced digital mammography (CEDM) health to safely reduce benign breast biopsies for low to moderately suspicious soft tissue lesions. Acad Radiol 2020;27:969–76.
127. Sorin V, Yagil Y, Shalmon A, et al. Background parenchymal enhancement at contrast enhanced spectral mammography (CESM) as a breast cancer risk factor. Acad Radiol 2020;27:1234–40.
128. Carbine NE, Lostumbo L, Wallace J, et al. Risk-reducing mastectomy for the prevention of primary breast cancer (review). Cochrane Database Syst Rev 2018;4.
129. Baildam AD. Current knowledge of risk reducing mastectomy: Indications, techniques, results, benefits, harms. Breast 2019;46:48–51.
130. Evans DG, Baildam AD, Anderson E, et al. Risk reducing mastectomy outcomes in 10 European Centres. J Med Genet 2009;46(4):354–8.

131. Heemskerk-Gerritsen BAM, Seynaeve C, van Asperen CJ, et al. Breast cancer risk after salpingo-oophorectomy in healthy BRCA 1/2 mutation carriers: revisiting the evidence for risk reduction. J Natl Cancer Inst 2015;107(5).
132. Chapman JS, Powell CB. Surveillance of survivors: follow up after risk reducing salpingo-oophorectomy in BRCA 1/2 mutation carriers. Gynecol Oncol 2011; 122(2):339–43.
133. Opportunistic salpingectomy as a strategy for epithelial ovarian cancer prevention. ACOG Committee Opinion No. 774. American College of Obstetricians and Gynecologists. Obstet Gynecol 2019;133:e279–84.

Advances in Breast Imaging with Current Screening Recommendations and Controversies

Cimmie L. Shahan, MD[a,b,*], Ginger P. Layne, MD[a,c]

KEYWORDS

- Breast imaging • Mammography • Ultrasound • Breast MRI • Breast biopsy
- Stereotactic • Tomosynthesis

KEY POINTS

- Mammography, the gold standard for breast cancer screening, is heavily regulated and involves the use of small amounts of radiation to obtain x-ray images of the breast.
- Supplemental screening modalities, such as tomosynthesis, whole breast ultrasound, and breast MRI, serve as important adjuncts to mammography, particularly in certain populations of women, including those with dense breasts and those with a high risk for breast cancer.
- Diagnostic breast imaging, used to evaluate clinical signs and symptoms or to evaluate a finding on a screening mammogram or other imaging study, commonly includes mammography, including tomosynthesis, and ultrasound. Breast MRI is a useful modality in appropriate diagnostic settings.
- Breast imagers perform several procedures, including biopsies that lead to a diagnosis of benign and malignant lesions, as well as localization procedures to guide the surgeon to an area of interest during surgery.

INTRODUCTION

Mammography is arguably one of the most important innovations in the history of women's health care. After its widespread implementation, the rate of breast cancer

This article previously appeared in Obstetrics & Gynecology Clinics volume 49, issue 1 March 2022.
Disclosure: The authors have nothing to disclose.
[a] WVU Department of Radiology, West Virginia University School of Medicine, PO Box 9235, Morgantown, WV 26506, USA; [b] Medical Director of the Betty Puskar Breast Care Center; Section Chief of Breast Imaging WVU Department of Radiology; Assistant Professor of Radiology, West Virginia University School of Medicine; [c] Breast Imaging Fellowship Director, WVU Department of Radiology; Associate Professor of Radiology, West Virginia University School of Medicine
* Corresponding author.
E-mail addresses: cshahan@hsc.wvu.edu (C.L.S.); glayne@hsc.wvu.edu (G.P.L.)

https://doi.org/10.1016/j.ccol.2024.02.007
2352-7986/24/

deaths dropped for the first time in decades.[1] In this article, we will discuss the importance not only of mammography, which is the gold standard of breast imaging,[2] but also of other modalities that are used to complement mammography in the diagnosis of breast cancer. We have divided the article into 3 parts in order to mirror the way radiologists look at imaging: screening, diagnostic, and procedures.

BREAST CANCER SCREENING
Mammography

Background and physics
When mammography first began, it was performed as a screen-film study, like traditional x-rays.[3] The film had to be processed in a dark room, like photos. This process was time-consuming with little room for error.

With the invention of digital mammography (DM) came better contrast resolution,[4] faster access to the studies,[5] and much more latitude with technique. This increased the number of studies that could be performed and interpreted. Increased contrast resolution improved the sensitivity of mammography in dense breasts.[6] In addition, the technologists had more freedom with technique, as the images could be digitally improved after they were acquired.[7]

Why is contrast resolution so important in mammography? When you look at a mammogram, you will see various shades of gray. Fatty tissue appears darker, and fibroglandular tissue appears lighter. As cancer is also radiopaque, we need good contrast resolution to be able to discern the subtle differences between normal fibroglandular tissue and cancer. Compression also helps with finding abnormalities. It not only spreads out the tissue so that we can see more clearly, but it also decreases the number of photons needed to penetrate the breast tissue, thereby decreasing the radiation dose.[8]

Radiation dose is very low in mammography. A person will get about the same amount of radiation from one screening full-field digital mammogram (FFDM) as flying for ~13,000 miles,[9] or as simply living for approximately 7 weeks[10] (background radiation). The radiation dose from FFDM is about 27% lower than that of screen-film (30%–40% lower for dense breasts).[11] Combining both FFDM and three-dimensional (3D; tomosynthesis) images increases the dose to about 2.5 mGy for a standard phantom,[12] which is well below the ACR cut-off of 3 mGy per film.[13] New technology is allowing many imaging centers to perform only 3D images, from which the two-dimensional (2D) images are reconstructed. This drops the dose by an estimated 43%.[14] No matter whether your facility performs DM ± tomosynthesis ± reconstructed 2D views, rest assured that mammography is a very low dose procedure.

Regulation of mammography
Radiation dose and image quality in mammography are heavily regulated. The MQSA (Mammography Quality and Standards Act) Program is run by the Food and Drug Administration (FDA) and requires all facilities and personnel involved to meet certain standards for certification in order to be able to perform and interpret mammography. Also, the ACR (American College of Radiology) evaluates both phantom and patient images from each machine that performs mammography to ensure that minimum quality standards are being met. If your facility is an ACR Breast Imaging Center of Excellence, it means it has received full accreditation by the ACR in all breast imaging modalities.[15]

How a mammogram is performed and interpreted
When a mammogram is performed, the patient's breast is placed in compression, and photons travel through the breast and onto a detector. The information from the

detector is sent to a computer for processing and then to the radiologist for interpretation. Screening mammograms are performed on the asymptomatic breast.[16] Most screening mammograms involve 2 images, the craniocaudal (CC) view and the mediolateral oblique (MLO) view, of each breast (**Figs. 1** and **2**). Each view obtains its name from the direction the x-rays travel through the breast. For the CC view, the x-ray beam travels head-to-foot through a breast that is compressed horizontally; with the MLO view, the breast is compressed at an angle so as to image as much of the pectoralis muscle as possible, and the x-rays travel in the MLO direction.[17] When looking at a mammogram on a monitor, the MLO is intuitive (superior is superior, inferior is inferior), and for the CC view, the lateral breast is placed superior on the screen, and the medial breast is inferior. In general, radiologists report the location of abnormal findings either as a clock position or by quadrant, as well as mentioning the distance from the nipple.

When interpreting a mammogram, a radiologist uses the BI-RADS (Breast Imaging-Reporting and Data System) lexicon.[39] Each mammogram is given a final BI-RADS assessment category (0–6) to allow for unambiguous understanding between clinicians and radiologists of what, if anything, needs to be done next (**Table 1**). Screening mammograms with potential abnormalities are typically given a BI-RADS category 0 assessment and are routinely further evaluated with a diagnostic mammogram and/or ultrasound (US) as specified by the radiologist.[19]

Screening recommendations and controversy

There is much debate as to how frequently and at what age a patient should begin getting mammograms. This was brought to light nationally when the United States Preventive Services Task Force (USPSTF) released their updated mammography guidelines in 2016, recommending biennial screening beginning at age 50 years.[20] This recommendation conflicted with those of the most prominent organizations at

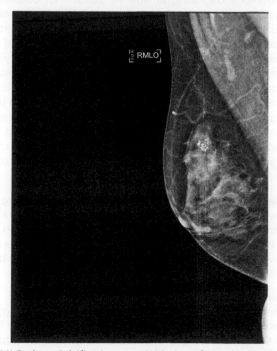

Fig. 1. Screening MLO view. Calcifications at 10:00, 4 cm from the nipple.

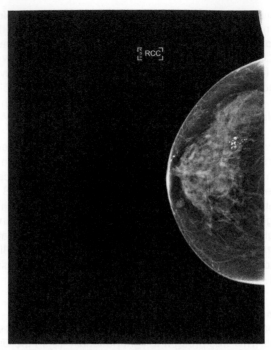

Fig. 2. Screening CC view. Calcifications at 10:00, 4 cm from the nipple.

the time. However, the data are clear: the greatest mortality benefit is seen from annual screening mammography beginning at age 40 years.[18] Of course, more frequent screening studies mean a greater likelihood of false positives, which would mean additional imaging and maybe even a biopsy.[21] This would, in turn, lead to patient anxiety and higher medical costs. Therefore, a conversation should be had with the patient about her priorities for screening: would she rather risk the possibility of additional imaging and/or biopsies for the return of decreased mortality and detecting cancer at a lower stage, or would she rather forego the anxiety and medical costs associated with potential additional testing with the possibility of finding cancer at a later stage? Only the patient can truly decide what is best for her. However, as the greatest number of lives are saved with annual screening mammography beginning at age 40 years,[18] these are the guidelines recommended by the American College of Radiology and many breast imaging centers. Mammography screening guidelines of various organizations are summarized in **Table 2**.

Frequency of screening mammograms recalled for abnormal findings

For every 1000 women screened with mammography, approximately 100 will be recalled for additional images, about 81 will either be called benign and returned to annual screening mammography or asked to return in 6 months for a short-term interval follow-up, 19 will be recommended for minimally invasive needle biopsy, and 5 will have breast cancer.[24]

When should screening mammography stop?

As a mortality benefit is seen 5 to 7 years after the onset of screening,[25] a patient may benefit from screening as long as she is expected to live another 5 to 10 years and is in good health. She should be willing and able to undergo treatment for breast cancer, including possible surgery. If the patient's life expectancy is below 10 years and she

Table 1
BI-RADS assessment categories

Category	Description	Management
0	Incomplete	Mammography: Incomplete, needs additional imaging or old films for comparison Ultrasound or MRI: Incomplete, needs additional imaging
1	Negative	Annual screening mammography
2	Benign	Annual screening Mammography
3	Probably benign, <2% chance of malignancy	Short-term interval follow-up (usually in 6 mo)
4	Suspicious 4a: Low suspicion 4b: Moderate suspicion 4c: High suspicion	Biopsy
5	Highly suggestive of malignancy (>95% chance)	Biopsy
6	Known, biopsy-proven malignancy	Follow-up as recommended by the surgeon and/or medical oncologist. BI-RADS 6 assessment usually only given when following disease during neoadjuvant chemotherapy.

Table 2
Mammography screening guidelines for average-risk patients

Organization	Age to Start	Frequency	Age to Stop
American College of Radiology and Society of Breast Imaging[22]	Age 40 y	Annually	Tailor to patient based on health and life expectancy
American College of Obstetrics and Gynecology[23]	Offer to patient beginning at age 40 y. Recommend no later than age 50 y[a]	Annually or biennially[a]	Continue until age 75 y. At age 75 y, the decision to continue should be based on a discussion between physician and patient regarding health status and longevity
United States Preventive Services Task Force[20]	Age 50 y	Biennially	Age 74 y
American Cancer Society[18]	Recommend by age 45 y, but the patient should have the option to choose at age 40 y	Annually, with the option to transition to biennially beginning at age 55 y	Continue as long as the patient is in good health and has a life expectancy of 10+ y

[a] Decision should be made by the patient after appropriate counseling.

would not be willing or able to undergo treatment, the discussion should be had about the benefits and risks of stopping screening.

Screening in the high-risk population

Another population that might have different screening recommendations is the high-risk population. If the patient has a first-degree relative with a history of breast cancer, she should be offered annual screening mammography beginning 10 years before the age at which the relative was diagnosed, or at age 40 years, whichever comes first. The American College of Radiology recommends that all patients, especially black women and those of Ashkenazi Jewish descent, be evaluated for breast cancer risk no later than age 30 years. There are multiple versions of risk-calculation software that can be used to calculate a patient's lifetime risk of breast cancer. Some breast clinics use these to screen their patients and to assess the need for supplemental or earlier screening. Patients with a 20% or greater lifetime risk of breast cancer and patients with a genetics-based risk (as well as their untested first-degree relatives) should be offered adjunctive screening with annual screening breast MRI beginning at age 25 to 30 years, as well as screening mammography beginning at age 30 years. High-risk screening recommendations are summarized in **Table 3**. Any patient who should be screened with MRI but is unable to do so could alternatively be screened with US.[22]

Digital Breast Tomosynthesis for Supplemental Screening

Conventional DM produces a 2D image of the breast, and the resulting superimposition of normal tissue may obscure features of malignancy.[26] Overlapping tissue may also mimic malignancy, leading to false-positive recalls for additional imaging.[27]

Digital breast tomosynthesis (DBT), FDA-approved in February 2011, allows the breast to be viewed in a 3D format and addresses limitations of 2D mammography.[28] During DBT imaging, the breast is compressed and imaged as it is with 2D DM. Low-dose x-ray projection images are acquired in an arc and are used to reconstruct a 3D image set with thin sections.[29,30] The images are displayed on a dedicated workstation where the radiologist can scroll through the images individually.

In the screening setting, DBT combined with DM is associated with reduced false-positive recall rates and increased breast cancer detection rates as compared with DM alone. Importantly, invasive cancers are better detected with DBT.[29–34]

Frequently, suspicious findings seen at DM are due to the superimposition of complex normal areas of breast tissue. By scrolling through the sections of the 3D image set, the reader is often able to determine that the appearance is due to summation of superimposed normal breast tissue [35](**Fig. 3**).

The conspicuity and characterization of lesions is improved with DBT.[35–37] DBT is particularly superior to 2D mammography in detecting architectural distortion, which is a common imaging manifestation of invasive breast cancer (**Fig. 4**).

Although some investigators have concluded that DBT may result in earlier detection of smaller breast cancers, it remains to be determined whether detection of DBT-only cancers will confer overall survival benefit.[38]

Breast Density and Whole-Breast Ultrasound for Supplemental Screening

Breast density is a mammographic assessment referring to the amount of fibroglandular tissue (white) relative to fat (gray) in the breast. The BI-RADS atlas[39] classifies breast composition into 4 categories (**Table 4**). It is required by the MQSA that the radiologist reports the breast density for every mammogram.

Table 3
Screening recommendations for high-risk patients

High-Risk Feature	Screening Mammography Digital Mammography ± Digital Breast Tomosynthesis	Screening MRI
Genetics-based risk and first-degree untested relatives	Annually, starting at age 30 y	Annually, beginning age 25–30 y
Calculated lifetime risk >20%	Annually, starting at age 30 y	Annually, beginning age 25–30 y
History of chest radiation therapy before age 30 y, with a cumulative dose of >10 Gy	Annually, beginning at age 25 or 8 y after radiation, whichever is later	Annually, beginning age 25–30 y
Personal history of breast cancer with dense breast tissue	Annually, starting at age 40 y or at age of diagnosis, whichever is earlier	Annually, beginning at age of diagnosis
Personal history of breast cancer diagnosed before age 50 y	Annually, starting at age 40 or at age of diagnosis, whichever is earlier	Annually, beginning at age of diagnosis
Personal history of breast cancer, atypical ductal hyperplasia, or lobular neoplasia before age 40 y	Annually, starting at age of diagnosis	Annually, beginning at age of diagnosis, should be considered, especially if other risk factors

"Dense" breasts are those that generally have more fibroglandular tissue relative to fat and fall into the categories of heterogeneously dense or extremely dense. Nearly half of women age 40 years and older who get mammograms have dense breasts.[40,41]

Greater breast density is associated with up to 3 to 6 times increased chance of breast cancer. Density is being incorporated into some risk assessment models.[41,42]

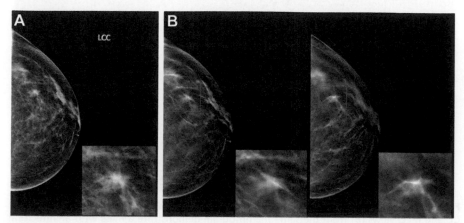

Fig. 3. Screening left CC view (*A*) demonstrates an asymmetry in the outer location (zoomed-lower right). Contiguous left CC tomosynthesis images (*B*) demonstrate the asymmetry to represent overlapping fibroglandular tissue (zoomed-lower right).

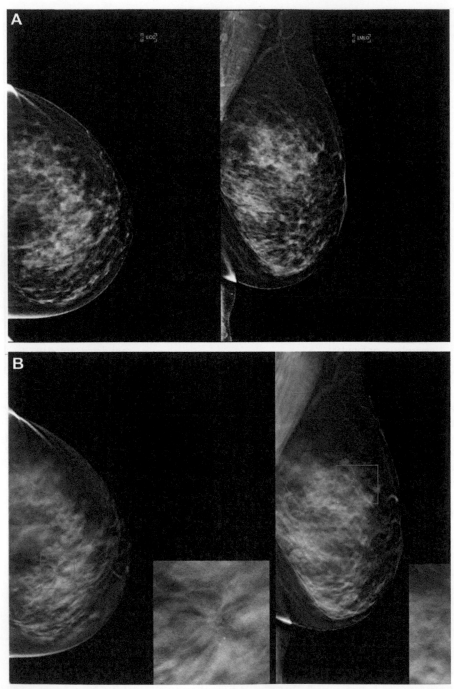

Fig. 4. Screening left CC and MLO views (*A*) demonstrate no abnormality. Tomosynthesis left CC and MLO views (*B*) from the same mammogram demonstrate a mass with architectural distortion at 11:00. Subsequent ultrasound-guided biopsy revealed this to represent invasive ductal carcinoma.

Table 4
BI-RADS fifth edition breast composition categories

a	Almost entirely fatty
b	Scattered areas of fibroglandular density
c	Heterogeneously dense, which may obscure small masses
d	Extremely dense, which lowers the sensitivity of mammography

Another implication of breast density is the masking effect, the reduced sensitivity of mammography in women with dense breasts (**Fig. 5**). The sensitivity of mammography in the detection of breast cancer is up to 90% for fatty breasts versus 60% or lower for women with extremely dense breasts.[43,44] Owing to the masking effect, the number of interval cancers, those that manifest within 1 year of a normal mammogram, is increased in women with dense breasts. Also, cancers detected on screening mammography in women with dense breasts tend to be larger and higher stage.[41] Both DM (compared to screen-film mammography) and DBT help to improve the detection of breast cancer in women with dense breasts.[6,45]

Breast density legislation was first passed in Connecticut in 2009. Since then, numerous additional states have followed, requiring patients to be notified about their breast density and what it means if they have dense breasts.[43] In 2019, the FDA announced proposed amendment to the MQSA, including mandatory reporting of breast density for patient letters and health care provider reports. This will require all mammography facilities in all states to have breast density notification to patients.[44]

Whole-breast ultrasound (WBUS) in addition to screening mammography has been shown to increase breast cancer detection compared with mammography alone in women with dense breasts. Studies have shown that WBUS in women with dense breasts will yield an additional 2.3 to 4.6 mammographically occult cancers per 1000 women. Mammographically occult cancers detected on WBUS are generally small invasive cancers.[46,47] However, WBUS is also shown to have high recall rates and low positive predictive values.[41,42,46]

Handheld WBUS is operator-dependent and potentially time-consuming. Automated whole-breast ultrasound (ABUS) is a more recently developed alternative in which standardized image sets may be obtained by a technologist (**Fig. 6**). ABUS uses a computer-driven 15 cm transducer to scan the entire breast. The radiologist uses specialized software to view the acquired images in multiple planes. Studies on ABUS show similar rates of cancer detection and recalls to those with handheld WBUS.[48,49]

Major organizations do not currently recommend for or against screening breast US as a supplement to mammography with women with dense breasts. Supplemental screening breast MRI is preferred for women at high risk for breast cancer regardless of breast density, but screening WBUS should be considered in these women who cannot tolerate breast MRI.[46] For women who are not deemed at high risk, ACR and SBI report that supplemental WBUS may be useful, but the balance between increased detection and increased risk of false positives should be discussed with the patient.[50]

DIAGNOSTIC BREAST IMAGING

Screening mammography and supplemental screening modalities are used in asymptomatic patients. Diagnostic breast imaging is used to evaluate clinical signs and symptoms or to evaluate a finding on a screening mammogram or other imaging

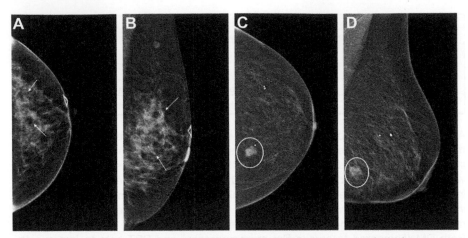

Fig. 5. Diagnostic left CC (*A*) and lateromedial (*B*) views demonstrate the dense breast tissue obscuring the palpable biopsy-proven breast cancer. Screening left CC (*C*) and MLO (*D*) views demonstrate that it is much easier to detect a smaller cancer (circle) in a fatty breast.

study. Mammography, including tomosynthesis, and US are routinely used in the diagnostic setting. Breast MRI can be a useful modality in the diagnostic setting, but the benefits of breast MRI should be weighed against its drawbacks. Other less frequently used breast imaging modalities in the diagnostic setting include contrast-enhanced mammography (CEM) and molecular breast imaging.

Mammography

Diagnostic mammography is used to evaluate findings detected at screening mammography or another imaging study, investigate the etiology of signs or symptoms of breast disease, and provide short-term follow-up of patients with probably benign (BI-RADS 3) findings.[13]

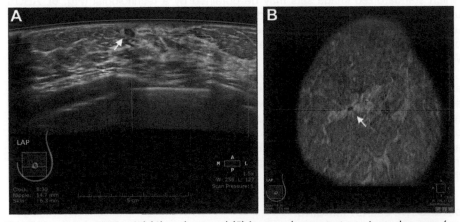

Fig. 6. Screening ABUS axial (*A*) and coronal (*B*) images demonstrate an irregular mass (*arrow*) in the lower inner left breast. This mass was occult on mammography in this patient with dense breasts. Subsequent ultrasound-guided core biopsy of the mass demonstrated invasive ductal carcinoma.

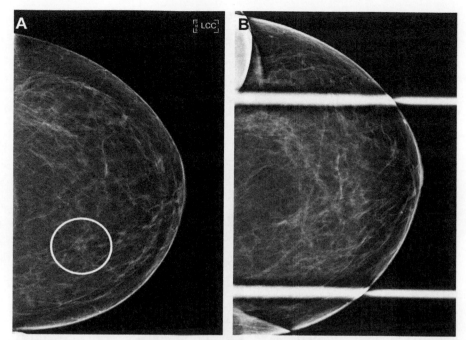

Fig. 7. Screening left CC view (*A*) demonstrates an asymmetry (circle) in the inner region. The asymmetry is not visible on the subsequent diagnostic spot compression view (*B*), indicating the asymmetry represented overlapping tissue.

Spot compression mammography is commonly performed to evaluate masses, asymmetries, and architectural distortions.[39] Spot compression applies focused pressure to determine if the finding is a true lesion or the summation of overlapping breast tissue (**Fig. 7**). Spot compression may help depict the shape, density, margins, and size of a mass.[51]

Microcalcifications are best evaluated with magnification mammography. With magnification, the distribution and morphology of calcifications are depicted more clearly than on a conventional mammogram view[52] (**Fig. 8**).

Additional supplemental views may be included in a diagnostic mammogram to evaluate and localize findings that are one-view mammogram findings and/or are not included or are at the periphery of conventional CC and MLO views.[52]

Common clinical abnormalities for which diagnostic mammography is performed include palpable lumps, concerning skin or nipple changes, and pathologic nipple discharge. Focal noncyclical breast pain may also be an indication for a diagnostic mammogram.[13] If a clinical abnormality is present, the referring clinician must describe the location and clinical specifics in detail to optimize imaging protocol and interpretation. Special imaging techniques, such as a skin marker for a palpable lump, can be used for clinical abnormalities as well.

Tomosynthesis

DBT is increasingly recognized as beneficial in the diagnostic environment. The performance of DBT has been found to be equivalent or superior to diagnostic DM in the evaluation of noncalcified lesions.[35,38]

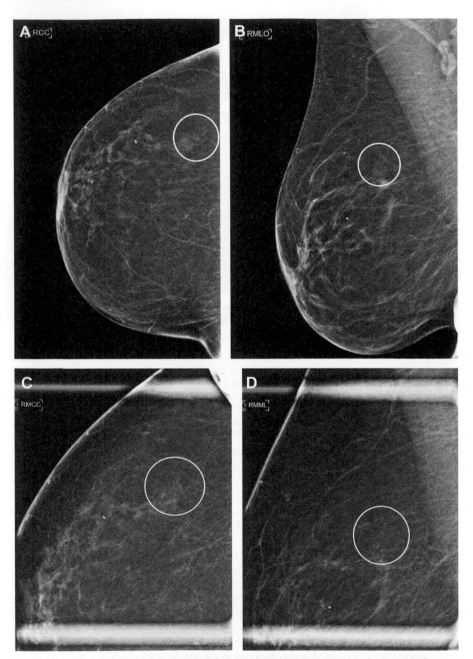

Fig. 8. Screening right CC (*A*) and MLO (*B*) views demonstrate a group of microcalcifications (circle) at 10:00. Magnification CC (*C*) and mediolateral (*D*) views better depict their suspicious features (circle)—fine pleomorphic and fine linear branching morphology with a segmental distribution.

DBT assists in differentiating benign from malignant imaging features and increases reader confidence in assigning a BI-RADS assessment. Mass features of shape, margin, and density are often better depicted at DBT, and the reader can develop a more accurate degree of suspicion before performing US.[53,54] Improved assessment of lesion size is a reported advantage of DBT.[35]

DBT + DM compared with diagnostic DM can abbreviate the diagnostic work-up. With improved lesion visibility on routine DBT + DM, additional 2D spot compression or supplemental views are less often necessary. Many masses, focal asymmetries, or architectural distortions, identified on DBT + DM, can proceed directly to diagnostic assessment with US.[38,55] If a finding is seen on only one view or is located in the skin, DBT aids in localization.[56]

If necessary, spot compression can be performed with tomosynthesis. Magnification views can only be performed with 2D technique.[38]

Ultrasound

Breast US is an integral imaging tool in the diagnostic setting. The most common indications for diagnostic breast US include evaluation of potential abnormalities detected on mammography, breast MRI, or other imaging modalities; evaluation of palpable masses and other breast-related clinical findings; and evaluation of extent of disease, including identification of abnormal axillary lymph nodes, in patients with suspected or newly diagnosed breast cancer.[19,57]

Diagnostic breast US is performed with a high-resolution transducer operating at a minimum frequency of 12 MHz. Other transducers may be used in special circumstances.[57] Proper transducer pressure and optimal patient positioning are essential. Medial lesions should generally be scanned in the supine position, and lateral lesions, including the axilla, are usually scanned with the patient in the contralateral oblique position with the arm flexed behind the head to aid in compression of the breast tissue. Images in the radial and antiradial views should be captured and laterality, clock face position, and distance from nipple annotated.[46]

Breast US is operator-dependent. Although breast US scanning may be performed by a technologist, the radiologist also benefits greatly from hands-on scanning. Real-time permits detailed lesion evaluation and analysis compared with analyzing static images on a workstation.[46,57] When searching for a lesion identified at mammography, breast MRI, or another imaging modality, careful correlation with lesion depth and surrounding anatomic structures is imperative. Lesion location may be affected by the patient's position, which differs during mammography, US, and MRI examinations. Similarly, careful attention to the region of clinical concern is necessary when scanning a palpable lump or other clinical abnormality to ensure that the correct area is scanned.[46]

Breast US is complementary to mammography because of its ability to identify or exclude the presence of an underlying mass and/or differentiate and characterize cystic and solid lesions[19,46] (**Figs. 9** and **10**).

ACR Appropriateness Criteria[58] are evidence-based guidelines to assist providers in making the most appropriate imaging or treatment decisions. There are ACR Appropriateness Criteria for a variety of breast topics, including clinical abnormalities. These criteria are an important reference for referring clinicians when ordering breast imaging examinations and also serve as valuable tools for breast imaging radiologists.[58] In women younger than 30 years, with a palpable lump, focal breast pain, or other concerning breast sign and/or symptom, US is the primary imaging test, with a high sensitivity and negative predictive value. Symptomatic women older than 30 years often require evaluation with both US and mammography.[46,58] (**Fig. 11**). US focused in

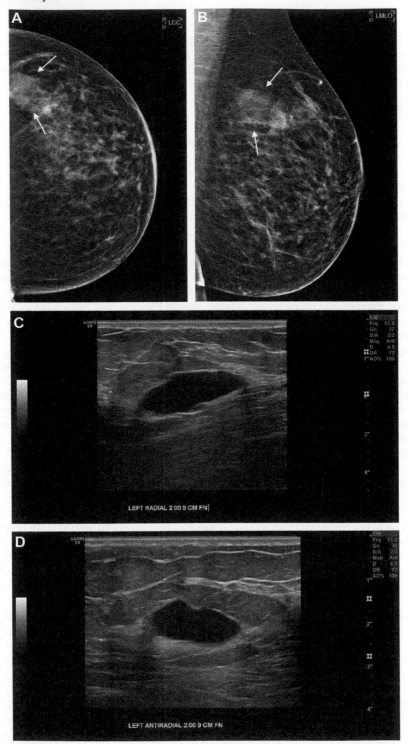

Fig. 9. Screening left CC (*A*) and MLO (*B*) views demonstrate a partially obscured oval mass (circle) at 2:00. Targeted ultrasound radial (*C*) and antiradial (*D*) images demonstrate a benign simple cyst at 2:00, which corresponds to the mammographic finding.

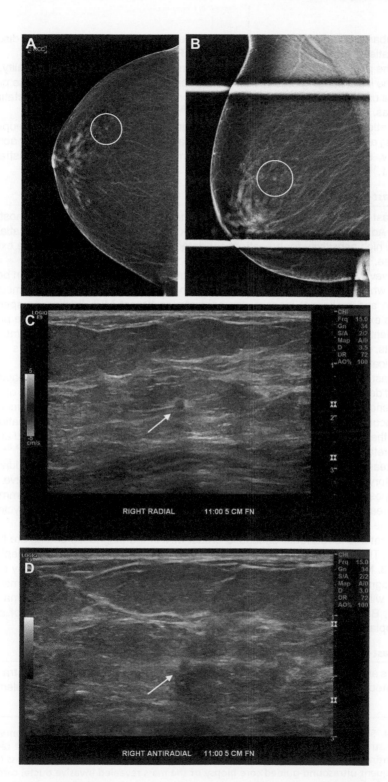

RIGHT RADIAL   11:00 5 CM FN

RIGHT ANTIRADIAL   11:00 5 CM FN

the subareolar region is routinely used in the evaluation of pathologic nipple discharge in a patient with a negative mammogram[46] (**Fig. 12**).

In the pregnant or lactating patient who presents with a clinical abnormality, US is also the initial imaging modality of choice. Targeted US examination in these patients can be used to identify masses, including fibroadenomas, galactoceles, lactating adenomas, abscesses, and invasive cancers.[59,]

In patients with known or suspected malignancy, US can be useful in preoperative staging and assessment of the extent of disease. US can be used to identify abnormal axillary, supraclavicular, and internal mammary lymph nodes as demonstrated in **Fig. 11**.[19,46]

Contrast-Enhanced Breast MRI

Contrast-enhanced breast MRI is a useful imaging tool in appropriate diagnostic settings. Advantages of breast MRI include lack of ionizing radiation, good spatial resolution, high sensitivity for breast cancer detection, and ability to assess the extent of disease.[60,61]

However, breast MRI also has disadvantages which require that discretion be exercised when determining when and for whom breast MRI should be performed. Both benign and malignant masses can enhance on breast MRI, limiting its specificity. MRI is expensive, requires the use of intravenous contrast, and may not be possible in patients who cannot lie prone, have large girth measurements, have extremely large breasts, or are claustrophobic. Tissue expanders and some metallic implants are contraindications to breast MRI.[60,61]

Breast MRI is performed with a woman in the prone position with the breasts positioned dependently in a breast coil. After precontrast imaging sequences are obtained, intravenous gadolinium contrast is administered. Postcontrast imaging sequences are then acquired at specified intervals, which allow for analysis of kinetic information, aiding in the assessment of lesions. Computer-aided detection software is used at image interpretation to manage large data sets and highlight kinetic information.[61,62]

Increased parenchymal enhancement has been observed normally during the secretory phase of the menstrual cycle. This normal enhancement may give rise to false-positive and false-negative MRI examinations. It is therefore recommended that breast MRI be performed during the second week of the menstrual cycle when possible.

Indications for contrast-enhanced breast MRI in the diagnostic setting are listed in **Box 1**. The utility of breast MRI in the setting of a known breast cancer is depicted in **Fig. 13**. MRI should not precede or replace problem-solving mammography or US in the diagnostic setting (**Fig. 14**). Because MRI will miss some cancers that mammography will detect, it also should not be used as a substitute for screening mammography. Breast MRI may be performed without contrast for assessment of silicone gel implant integrity.[61]

Contrast-Enhanced Mammography

CEM is an emerging modality that combines DM with the administration of intravenous iodinated contrast material.[63] The FDA approved CEM in 2011 as a supplement to

Fig. 10. Screening right CC view (*A*) and diagnostic right MLO spot compression view (*B*) demonstrate an oval mass in the upper outer right breast (circle). Right breast radial (*C*) and antiradial (*D*) ultrasound images demonstrate a corresponding irregular mass (*arrow*). Subsequent ultrasound-guided core biopsy of the mass revealed invasive ductal carcinoma.

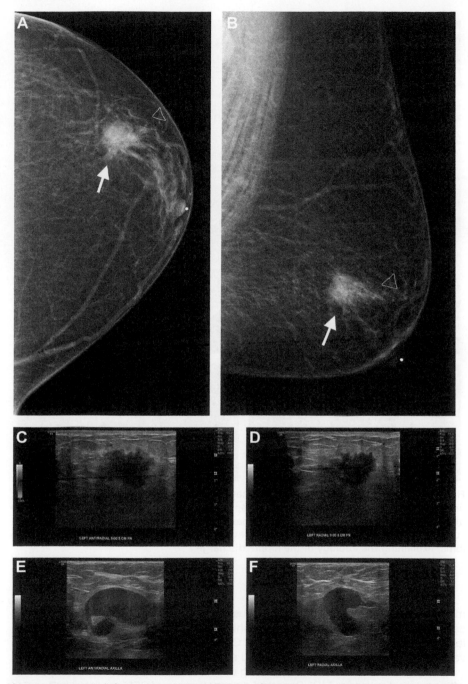

Fig. 11. Diagnostic left CC (*A*) and MLO (*B*) views demonstrate a spiculated mass in the left breast at 3:00, corresponding to the palpable lump indicated by a triangle skin marker. Radial (*C*) and antiradial (*D*) ultrasound images demonstrate a corresponding spiculated mass, representing invasive ductal carcinoma by ultrasound-guided biopsy. Ultrasound imaging of the left axilla before the biopsy demonstrated a morphologically abnormal left axillary lymph node with eccentric cortical thickening (*E, F*). Ultrasound-guided biopsy of this lymph node confirmed the pathology of metastatic breast cancer.

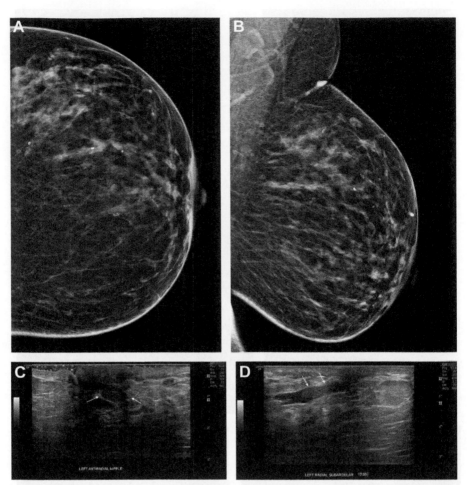

Fig. 12. Diagnostic left CC (*A*) and MLO (*B*) images in a patient with spontaneous bloody left nipple discharge demonstrate no mammographic abnormality. Antiradial (*C*) and radial (*D*) ultrasound images of the subareolar left breast demonstrate an intraductal mass (*arrows*). Subsequent ultrasound-guided core biopsy revealed this mass to represent a benign papilloma, explaining the etiology of the nipple discharge.

mammography and US to help identify suspected breast cancers.[64] Breast cancers can be identified at CEM by mammographic characteristics as well as by neovascularity.[63,] Studies report the performance of CEM is similar to breast MRI. Additional advantages of CEM include lower costs and shorter imaging time than breast MRI.[64]

Currently, CEM is most commonly being used to evaluate disease extent in patients with contraindications to MRI. Reported diagnostic uses of CEM are listed in **Box 2**.[67]

CEM is not yet widely used, and practice parameters and recommendations for CEM have not yet been created. This may be attributed to the challenges of CEM, which include risk of allergic reactions and extravasation associated with contrast administration, unavailability of CEM-directed biopsy, and higher radiation dose than conventional mammography.[63,64]

Box 1
Indications for contrast-enhanced breast MRI

Assessment of the extent of disease in a patient with known breast malignancy

Assessment of response to neoadjuvant chemotherapy

Concern for cancer recurrence with inconclusive clinical, mammographic, and/or US findings inconclusive

Identification of mammographically occult primary tumor in patients presenting with metastatic disease

Lesion characterization in select cases

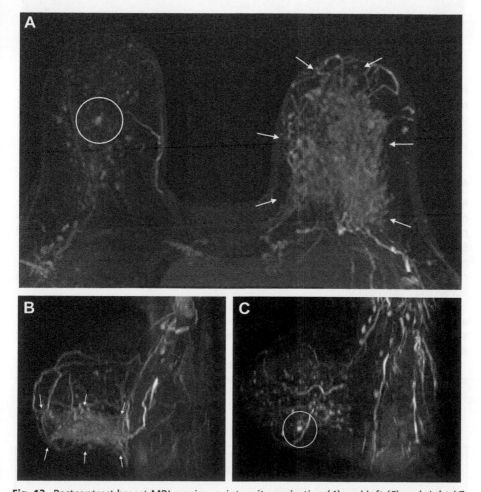

Fig. 13. Postcontrast breast MRI maximum intensity projection (*A*) and left (*B*) and right (*C*) sagittal images demonstrate extensive segmental nonmass enhancement throughout the lower left breast (*arrows*) and a 6 mm enhancing oval mass in the right breast at 6:00 (*circle*) in this patient with 2 cm of microcalcifications in the lower-left breast on mammography. Pathology on the left was high-grade ductal carcinoma in situ and on the right was invasive ductal carcinoma.

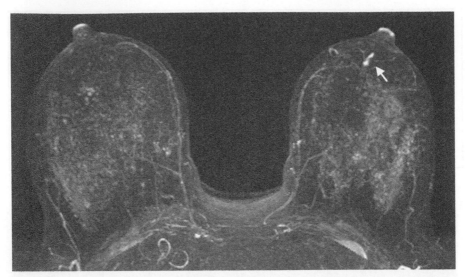

Fig. 14. Postcontrast breast MRI maximum intensity projection demonstrates 12 mm linear nonmass enhancement in the retroareolar left breast in a patient with spontaneous left bloody nipple discharge. No abnormality was seen on previous diagnostic mammogram or targeted ultrasound. MRI-guided biopsy demonstrated the finding to represent a benign papilloma, explaining the etiology of the nipple discharge.

Molecular Breast Imaging

Molecular breast imaging (MBI) has emerged because of recent advances in nuclear medicine. Breast-specific gamma imaging (BSGI) and positron emission mammography (PEM) are functional breast imaging techniques that image cellular activity.[68] BSGI uses gamma cameras to visualize the uptake of Technetium-99m (^{99m}Tc) sestamibi, an FDA-approved radiopharmaceutical that accumulates selectively in breast tumors. A BSGI examination consists of 4 views that are identical in positioning to a screening mammogram.[65]

PEM uses the radiopharmaceutical 18F-fluorodeoxyglucose (18F-FDG) that measures metabolic activity, which is typically greater in breast tumors than in normal tissue. Planar detectors are placed on either side of the breast with the patient positioned analogous to mammography.[68]

Potential uses of breast MBI are listed in **Box 3**.[69] Sensitivity and specificity of MBI are reportedly high for lesions ≥1 cm. An advantage of MBI is that its sensitivity is not affected by dense breast tissue.[66]

Box 2
Diagnostic uses of contrast-enhanced mammography

Workup of abnormal screening mammogram

Symptomatic patients

Surgical planning and extent of disease

Response to neoadjuvant systemic therapy

Box 3
Potential indications for breast MBI

Extent of disease/preoperative staging in newly diagnosed breast cancer

Evaluation of response to neoadjuvant chemotherapy

Detection of local breast cancer recurrence

Evaluation for primary breast cancer in women with unknown primary

Adjunct to conventional breast imaging for problem solving in indeterminate cases

Breast cancer screening for high-risk women who cannot undergo MRI

The radiation exposure associated with radiotracer injection, which is over 10 times greater than that from 2-view mammography, is a drawback of MBI. Efforts to reduce radiation dose are being explored and are critical to MBI's further evolution.[68]

BREAST IMAGING PROCEDURES

Image-guided procedures (aspirations, biopsies, localization procedures for surgery) can be performed using any of the imaging modalities that are used to evaluate the breasts. Common image-guided biopsies include US-, mammography-, and MRI-guided biopsies. There are benefits and drawbacks to each of these modalities.

If an US-guided biopsy is feasible for a particular lesion, it is the first choice of the radiologist. Ultrasound-guided biopsies require no radiation, are more comfortable for the patient, and take the least time. In addition, since US allows for real-time imaging of the lesion during biopsy, and the most suspicious portion of the lesion can be targeted, this leads to less upstaging of malignancies during surgery.[70] This has the potential to decrease the number of surgeries for the patient, as upstaging during surgery often means the patient has to return for another surgery (sentinel node biopsy). Ultrasound also allows us to assess the axillary nodes at the time of biopsy.

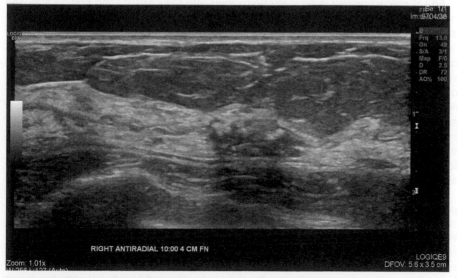

Fig. 15. Calcifications from **Figs. 1** and **2**, as seen with ultrasound.

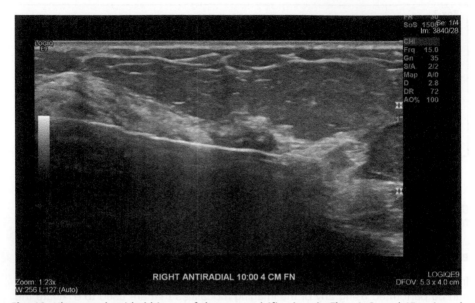

Fig. 16. Ultrasound-guided biopsy of the same calcifications in **Figs. 1, 2,** and **15**, using ultrasound guidance. The vacuum-assisted biopsy device is inserted with the bowl open just under the area of calcifications.

Calcifications can sometimes be biopsied using US, such as when they are associated with a mass or when there are enough calcifications to be appreciated with US (**Figs. 15** and **16**). In this case, the biopsy specimen is typically imaged with mammography during the procedure to confirm that calcifications are within the specimen (**Fig. 17**). Finally, US can also be used to aspirate fluid-filled lesions for diagnosis or symptomatic relief. Such lesions include painful cysts, complicated cysts (to confirm cystic nature), galactoceles, abscesses, hematomas, and seromas.

An US-guided biopsy is typically performed with the patient lying supine and with her arm raised above her head. The area of interest is visualized with US, and the skin is marked. The skin is prepped and draped, and a local anesthetic is used to numb the skin and deeper soft tissues. A small incision is made in the skin, and a biopsy device is used to obtain several samples. Of note, the smallest gauge biopsy device (usually 13G or 14G) is used in US, as real-time imaging allows confidence in obtaining the samples. However, biopsy devices as large as 9G can be used, if needed, to obtain adequate samples of calcifications or to remove most of a small suspected papilloma or fibroadenoma. After specimens are collected, a biopsy marker is placed at the biopsy site for future reference. After pressure is held and the incision is closed with either adhesive or Steri-Strips, a mammogram is obtained to confirm clip placement and to confirm the correlation between the mammographic and US findings.

Mammography-guided procedures can be performed using either stereotactic guidance or tomosynthesis guidance.[17] This modality is typically used to sample calcifications, masses, or other lesions that cannot be visualized with US. First, a scout image (**Fig. 18**) is used to confirm that the lesion is in the field of view. Once the lesion is visualized, 2 images are obtained, each at opposite 15° angles from the scout image. The lesion is targeted on each of these images, and the computer uses this to triangulate and to give coordinates for the lesion. If using tomosynthesis, the lesion

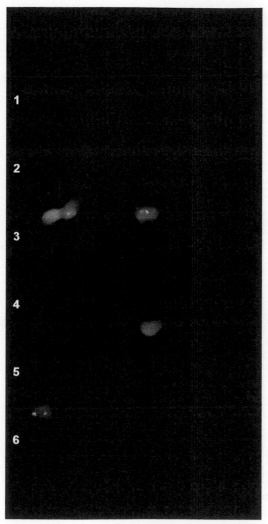

Fig. 17. Radiograph of biopsy specimens from US-guided biopsy shown in **Figs. 15** and **16**, showing calcifications within the specimen.

is targeted on the image on which it is seen best, and the computer again calculates the coordinates. During either procedure, the skin is cleaned, and a local anesthetic is administered. The biopsy device is placed proximal to the lesion with images to confirm. The biopsy device is quickly advanced or "fired" into the target lesion. Again, more images are obtained to confirm placement (**Figs. 19** and **20**), and the biopsy is performed. The specimens are imaged to confirm the presence of the target in the specimens. A biopsy marker is then placed (**Fig. 21**), and a mammogram is performed to confirm appropriate marker placement. Of note, the biopsy device used in stereotactic/tomosynthesis biopsy (8G to 12G) is usually larger than that used in US.

MRI biopsy generally involves a very similar biopsy device to that used in stereotactic/tomosynthesis biopsy, and the device is typically the largest of all of the devices (8G or 9G). However, MRI-guided biopsy is reserved for lesions only seen by MRI

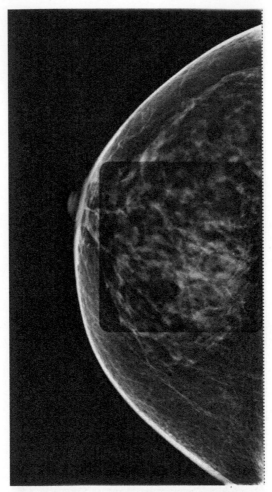

Fig. 18. Scout image of calcifications during a stereotactic biopsy.

and not seen with any other modality, as they are the most uncomfortable for the patient, take the longest time, and are the most costly of all breast biopsies.[71]

During biopsy, the patient is placed in the MRI scanner in a similar position as when she received the original MRI. The breast that is being biopsied is held in compression to keep it from moving during imaging and biopsy. Images are obtained both before and after administration of contrast and are compared to the prior MRI. Most institutions use a form of computer-aided detection software when performing MRI-guided biopsies. A fiducial is present on the compression device on the breast to provide a reference point for calculating the coordinates for the biopsy. When the abnormality is found on the biopsy scan (**Fig. 22**), the radiologist indicates to the software the location of both the fiducial and the abnormality so that the software can give the coordinates for biopsy. The skin is cleansed, and the breast is locally anesthetized. A plastic placeholder is placed at the target, and additional MRI images are obtained to confirm that the biopsy will occur in the correct location (**Fig. 23**). Adjustments can be made, if necessary, then the biopsy device is used to obtain samples, a biopsy marker is

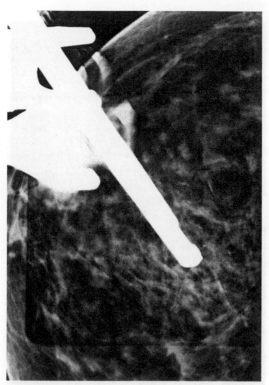

Fig. 19. Stereotactic image taken 15° from the position seen in the scout image, after firing, with calcifications adjacent to the biopsy device bowl.

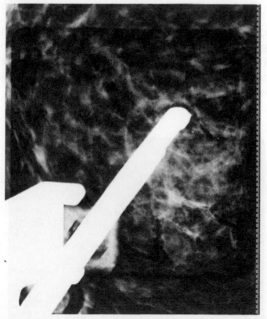

Fig. 20. Stereotactic image taken 15° from the position seen in the scout image, in the opposite direction from that seen in Figure 20, after firing, with calcifications adjacent to the biopsy device bowl.

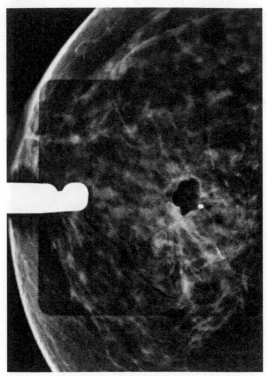

Fig. 21. Removal of biopsy device from breast, after placement of a biopsy clip during stereotactic biopsy.

placed, and additional images are obtained to confirm clip placement. After appropriate care is taken to hold pressure and to close the incision, the patient should have a mammogram to confirm clip placement. Six-month follow-up MRIs are frequently recommended after benign MRI-guided biopsy,[72] as this is the only modality on which the lesion was seen.

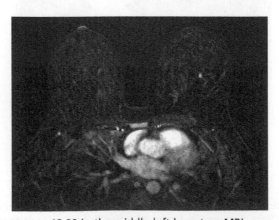

Fig. 22. Enhancing mass at 12:00 in the middle left breast on MRI.

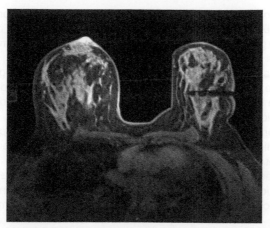

Fig. 23. MRI-guided biopsy of the mass seen in **Fig. 22**. Of note, the biopsy device is inserted into the breast either from lateral (as in this case) or from medial.

Localization wires or radioactive seeds can also be placed in the breast using any of these modalities before surgery. Both wires and radioactive seeds can be used to guide the surgeon to the area of interest in the breast or in the axilla during excisional biopsy or lumpectomy.

Postbiopsy recommendations vary from institution to institution, but common recommendations include icing the biopsied area the day of biopsy to minimize bruising and hematoma formation, no lifting of anything heavier than 5 pounds with the ipsilateral arm for 3 days, and wearing a sports bra continuously for 3 days after the procedure. Although there is no scientific data to show that blood thinners must be stopped

Table 5		
Pathology types and their management		
Type of Pathology	**Possible Pathology Results**	**Management**

Benign	Cysts
	Fibrocystic changes
	Usual ductal hyperplasia
	Fibroadenoma
	Pseudoangiomatous stromal hyperplasia
	Fat necrosis
	Benign lymph nodes
		Return to screening or 6-mo
		  follow-up imaging, based
		  on radiologist recommendation

High Risk	Fibroepithelial lesions
	Papillomas
	Radial scars
	Phyllodes tumors
	Atypical ductal hyperplasia
	Lobular neoplasia ()(lobular carcinoma
	  in situ, atypical lobular hyperplasia)
	Flat epithelial atypia
		Referral to surgeon for
		  possible excisional biopsy

Malignant	Ductal carcinoma in situ Invasive ductal carcinoma Invasive lobular carcinoma	Referral to surgeon and medical oncologist

before percutaneous breast biopsy to prevent hematoma formation,[73] most institutions recommended holding anticoagulants before the procedure, if possible. However, if the risk is too great for the patient to stop anticoagulants, or if time does not allow, the biopsy can be performed while the patient is anticoagulated.

Any time a breast biopsy is performed, using any modality, radiology-pathology correlation should be assessed by the radiologist.[74] If there is no radiology-pathology concordance, the biopsy should be repeated, or the patient should be referred to a surgeon for excisional biopsy.

Several common pathology results may be seen after a breast biopsy. These can be stratified into benign lesions, high-risk lesions, and cancer. These pathologies and their management will be briefly described in **Table 5**.

In summary, breast imaging is a vast field that involves several different imaging modalities. In this article, we have set the stage to allow the referring physician to understand why and how common studies and procedures are performed in the breast imaging clinic.

CLINICS CARE POINTS

- Screening mammography performed annually beginning at the age of 40 years saves the most lives.
- Supplemental screening modalities, such as whole breast ultrasound in women with dense breasts and breast MRI in the high-risk setting, may be used in addition to but should not replace mammography.
- When indicating the location of a palpable breast lump, it is best to document the clock position and the distance from the nipple.
- Ultrasound is the first step in a diagnostic work-up for patients younger than 30 years with a concerning breast sign and/or symptom.
- Mammography is the first step in a diagnostic work-up for patients aged 40 years and older with a concerning breast sign and/or symptom.
- Although an ultrasound may be performed first in the diagnostic work-up of patients aged 30 to 39 years, a mammogram will also often be performed.
- Contrast-enhanced breast MRI may be used in select diagnostic settings but should not precede or replace appropriate work-up with mammography and ultrasound.
- Breast MRI may also be used to evaluate silicone implant integrity. Saline implant rupture can be detected on clinical examination.
- Unilateral, clear or bloody, spontaneous nipple discharge may be caused by malignancy and should be worked up with imaging. Bilateral, manual, milky, or green discharge is not typically associated with malignancy but may be associated with serum hormone abnormalities (prolactin, thyroid-stimulating hormone).

REFERENCES

1. Hendrick RE, Baker JA, Helvie MA. Breast cancer deaths averted over 3 decades. Cancer 2019;125(9):1482–8.
2. Miller MG. Breast cancer screening: can we talk? J Gen Intern Med 2001;16(3):206–7.
3. IARC Working Group on the Evaluation of Cancer-Preventive Interventions. Breast cancer screening. Lyon (France): IARC; 2016. p. 2. Screening Techniques.

4. Digital compared with screen-film mammography: performance measures in concurrent cohorts within an organized breast screening program. Radiology 2013; 268:684–93.
5. Haygood T, Wang J, Atkinson N, et al. Timed efficiency of interpretation of digital and film-screening mammograms. AJR Am J Roentgenol 2009;192(1):216–20.
6. Pisano ED, Gatsonis C, Hendrick E, et al, for DMISTInvestigatorsGroup. Diagnostic performance of digital versus film mammography. N Engl J Med 2005; 353:1773–83.
7. Obenauer S, Luftner-Nagel S, von Heyden D, et al. Screen film vs full-field digital mammography: image quality, detectability and characterization of lesions. Eur Radiol 2002;12(7):1697–702.
8. Brnić Z, Hebrang A. Breast compression and radiation dose in two different mammographic oblique projections: 45 and 60 degrees. Eur J Radiol 2001; 40(1):10–5.
9. Calculate Your Radiation Dose. EPA. Available at: https://www.epa.gov/radiation/calculate-your-radiation-dose.
10. Radiation Dose to Adults from Common Imaging Examinations. ACR. Available at: https://www.acr.org/-/media/ACR/Files/Radiology-Safety/Radiation-Safety/Dose-Reference-Card.pdf.
11. Gennaro G, di Maggio C. Dose comparison between screen/film and full-field digital mammography. Eur Radiol 2006;16(11):2559–66.
12. Feng SS, Sechopoulos I. Clinical digital breast tomosynthesis system: dosimetric characterization. Radiology 2012;263(1):35–42.
13. ACR practice guidelines for the performance of screening and diagnostic mammography. Available at: https://www.acr.org/-/media/ACR/Files/Practice-Parameters/screen-diag-mammo.pdf.
14. Garayoa J, Hernandez-Giron I, Castillo M, Valverde J, Chevalier M. Digital Breast Tomosynthesis: Image Quality and Dose Saving of the Synthesized Image. In: Fujita H, Hara T, Muramatsu C, editors. Breast Imaging. IWDM 2014. Lecture Notes in Computer Science, vol 8539. Springer, Cham; 2014. https://doi.org/10.1007/978-3-319-07887-8_22.
15. Breast Imaging Center of Excellence. ACR. Available at: https://www.acraccreditation.org/breast-imaging-center-of-excellence.
16. BCSC Standard Definitions. NCI;2009.[Dec 10, 2015]. Available at: https://www.bcsc-research.org/application/files/4516/0096/5722/BCSC_Data_Definitions_v3__2020.09.23.pdf.
17. Brant WE, Helms CA, Klein JS, et al. Fundamentals of diagnostic radiology. 3th ed. Philadelphia: LWW; 2019.
18. Oeffinger KC, Fontham ET, Etzioni R, et al. Breast cancer screening for women at average risk: 2015 guideline update from the ACS. JAMA 2015;314(15): 1599–614.
19. Stavros. Introduction to breast ultrasound. breast ultrasound. Philadelphia: LWW; 2004. p. 1–15.
20. Siu, on behalf of the USPSTF. Screening for Breast Cancer: USPSTF Recommendation Statement. Ann Intern Med 2016;164:279–96.
21. Tosteson ANA, Fryback DG, Hammond CS, et al. Consequences of false-positive screening mammograms. JAMA Intern Med 2014;174(6):954–61.
22. Monticciolo DL, Newell MS, Moy L, et al. Breast cancer screening in women at higher-than-average risk: recommendations from the ACR. J Am Coll Radiol 2018;15:408–14.

23. Breast Cancer Risk Assessment and Screening in Average Risk Women. ACOG Practice Bulletin. Number179.July2017.
24. Mammography Screening: Facts and Figures. SBI. Available at: https://www.sbi-online.org/endtheconfusion/FactsFigures.aspx.
25. Kopans. An open letter to panels that are deciding guidelines for breast cancer screening. 2015. Available at: https://www.sbi-online.org/Portals/0/KOPANS%20ON%20BREAST%20CANCER%20SCREENING%20GUIDELINES.pdf.
26. Carney PA, Miglioretti DL, Yankaskas BC, et al. Individual and combined effects of age, breast density, and hormone replacement therapy use on the accuracy of screening mammography. Ann Intern Med 2003;138:168–75.
27. Brewer NT, Salz T, Lillie SE. Systematic review: the long-term effects of false-positive mammograms. Ann Intern Med 2007;146(7):502–10.
28. Facility Certification and Inspection (MQSA): Digital Accreditation. USFDA Website. Available at: http://www.fda.gov/Radiation-EmittingProducts/MammographyQualityStandardsActandProgram/FacilityCertificationandInspection/ucm114148.htm.
29. Rafferty EA, Park JM, LE Philpotts, et al. Assessing radiologist performance using combined digital mammography and breast tomosynthesis compared with digital mammography alone: results of a multicenter, multireader trial. Radiology 2013; 266(1):104–13.
30. Skaane P, Bandos AI, Gullien R, et al. Comparison of digital mammography alone and digital mammography plus tomosynthesis in a population-based screening program. Radiology 2013;267(1):47–56.
31. Ciatto S, Houssami N, Bernardi D, et al. Integration of 3D digital mammography with tomosynthesis for population breast-cancer screening (STORM): a prospective comparison study. Lancet Oncol 2013;14(7):583–9.
32. Durand MA, Haas BM, Yao X, et al. Early clinical experience with digital breast tomosynthesis for screening mammography. Radiology 2015;274(1):85–92.
33. Haas BM, Kalra V, Geisel J, et al. Comparison of tomosynthesis plus digital mammography and digital mammography alone for breast cancer screening. Radiology 2013;269(3):694–700.
34. Friedewald SM, Rafferty EA, Rose SL, et al. Breast cancer screening using tomosynthesis in combination with digital mammography. JAMA 2014;311(24): 2499–507.
35. Peppard HR, Nicholson BE, Rochman CM, et al. Digital breast tomosynthesis in the diagnostic setting: indications and clinical applications. Radiographics 2015; 35(4):975–90.
36. Poplack SP, Tosteson TD, Kogel CA, et al. Digital breast tomosynthesis: initial experience in 98 women with abnormal digital screening mammography. AJR Am J Roentgenol 2007;189(3):616–23.
37. Tagliafico A, Astengo D, Cavagnetto F, et al. One-to-one comparison between digital spot compression view and digital breast tomosynthesis. Eur Radiol 2012;22(3):539–44.
38. Butler R, Conant E, Philpotts L. Digital Breast Tomosynthesis, what we have learned. JBI 2019;1(1):9–22.
39. D'Orsi CJ, Sickles EA, Mendelson EB, et al. ACR BI-RADS® atlas, breast imaging reporting and data System. Reston (VA): ACR; 2013.
40. Persson I, Thurfjell E, Holmberg L. Effect of estrogen and estrogen-progestin replacement regimens on mammographic breast parenchymal density. J Clin Oncol 1997;15:3201–7.
41. Freer PE. Mammographic breast density: Impact on breast cancer risk and implications for screening. Radiographics 2015;35(2):302–15.

42. Boyd NF, Guo H, Martin LJ, et al. Mammographic density and the risk and detection of breast cancer. N Engl J Med 2007;356(3):227–36.
43. DenseBreast-Info. Legislation and regulation. 2015. Available at: https://densebreast-info.org/legislation.aspx.
44. DenseBreast-Info. Is there a national reporting standard? 2019March 28. Available at: https://densebreast-Info.org/is-there-a-federal-law.aspx.
45. Rose SL, Shisler JL. Tomosynthesis impact on breast cancer screening in patients younger than 50 years old. AJR Am J Roentgenol 2018;210(6):1401–4.
46. Hooley RJ, Scoutt LM, Philpotts LE. Breast ultrasonography: state of the art. Radiology 2013;268(3):642–59.
47. Berg WA, Blume JD, Cormack JB, et al. Combined screening with ultrasound and mammography vs mammography alone in women at elevated risk of breast cancer. JAMA 2008;299(18):2151–63.
48. Brem RF, Tabár L, Duffy SW, et al. Assessing improvement in detection of breast cancer with three-dimensional automated breast US in women with dense breast tissue:the SomoInsight Study. Radiology 2015;274(3):663–73.
49. van Zelst JCM, Mann RM. Automated three-dimensional breast US for screening: technique, artifacts, and lesion characterization. Radiographics 2018;38(3): 663–83.
50. Mainiero,et al. ACR Appropriateness Criteria® Breast Cancer Screening. Available at: https://acsearch.acr.org/docs/70910/Narrative/.
51. Chesebro AL, Winkler NS, Birdwell RL, et al. Developing asymmetries at mammography: A multimodality approach to assessment and management. Radiographics 2016;36(2):322–44.
52. Kopans. Chapter 10: mammographic positioning. Breast imaging. 3rd edition. Philadephia: LWW; 2007. p. 281–322.
53. Lei J, Yang P, Zhang L, et al. Diagnostic accuracy of digital breast tomosynthesis versus digital mammography for benign and malignant lesions in breasts: a meta-analysis. Eur Radiol 2014;24(3):595–602.
54. Andersson I, Ikeda DM, Zackrisson S, et al. Breast tomosynthesis and digital mammography: a comparison of breast cancer visibility and BIRADS classification in a population of cancers with subtle mammographic findings. Eur Radiol 2008;18(12):2817–25.
55. Lourenco AP, Barry-Brooks M, Baird GL, et al. Changes in recall type and patient treatment following implementation of screening digital breast tomosynthesis. Radiology 2015;274:337–42.
56. Conant EF. Clinical implementation of digital breast tomosynthesis. Radiol Clin North Am 2014;52(3):499–518.
57. ACR practice guideline for the performance of a breast ultrasound examination. Available at: https://www.acr.org/-/media/ACR/Files/Practice-Parameters/US-Breast.pdf.
58. ACR Appropriateness Criteria®. Available at: https://acsearch.acr.org/list.
59. diFlorio-Alexander,et al. ACR Appropriateness Criteria® Breast imaging of pregnancy and lactating women. Available at: https://acsearch.acr.org/docs/3102382/Narrative/.
60. Molleran M. Setting up and optimizing a breast MRI practice. Breast MRI. Philadelphia: Elsevier; 2014. p. 1–9.
61. ACR Practice Parameter for the performance of contrast-enhanced MRI of the breast. Available at: https://www.acr.org/-/media/ACR/Files/Practice-Parameters/MR-Contrast-Breast.pdf.

62. Mann RM, Cho N, Moy L. Breast MRI: state of the art. Radiology 2019;292: 520–36.
63. Ghaderi KF, Phillips J, Perry H, et al. Contrast-enhanced mammography: current applications and future directions. Radiographics 2019;39:1907–20.
64. Phillips J, Fein-Zachary VJ, Slanetz PJ. Pearls and pitfalls of contrast-enhanced mammography. JBI 2019;1(1):64–72.
65. Rechtman LR, Lenihan MJ, Lieberman JH, et al. Breast-specific gamma imaging for the detection of breast cancer in dense versus nondense breasts. AJR Am J Roentgenol 2014;202(2):293–8.
66. Berg WA, Madsen KS, Schilling K, et al. Breast cancer: comparative effectiveness of positron emission mammography and MR imaging in presurgical planning for the ipsilateral breast. Radiology 2011;258(1):59–72.
67. Lewin JM, Patel BK, Tanna A. Contrast-enhanced mammography: a scientific review. JBI 2020;2(1):7–15.
68. Narayanan D, Berg WA. Dedicated breast gamma camera imaging and breast positron emission tomography: current status and future directions. PET Clin 2018;13(3):363–81.
69. ACR Practice Parameter for the performance of MBI using a dedicated gamma camera. Available at: https://www.acr.org/~/media/ACR/Documents/PGTS/guidelines/MBI.pdf.
70. Dillon MF, Hill ADK, Quinn CM, et al. The accuracy of ultrasound, stereotactic, and clinical core biopsies in the diagnosis of breast cancer, with an analysis of false-negative cases. Ann Surg 2005;242(5):701–7.
71. Chesebro AL, Chikarmane SA, Ritner JA, et al. Troubleshooting to overcome technical challenges in image-guided breast biopsy. Radiographics 2017; 37(3):705–18.
72. Sung JS, Lee CH, Morris EA, et al. American patient follow-up after concordant histologically benign imaging-guided biopsy of MRI-detected lesions. AJR Am J Roentgenol 2012;198(6):1464–9.
73. Somerville P, Seifert PJ, Destounis SV, et al. Anticoagulation and Bleeding Risk After Core Needle Biopsy. AJR Am J Roentgenol 2008;191(4):1194–7.
74. Oluwaseyi Olayinka, Gagandeep Kaur MD, Ana Rebelo. Rad-path correlate: concordance and discordance rates in danbury hospital patient population. Am J Clin Pathol 2019;152(1):S48.

Molecular Breast Imaging and Positron Emission Mammography

Miral M. Patel, MD[a],*, Beatriz Elena Adrada, MD, FSBI[a],
Amy M. Fowler, MD, PhD, FSBI[b,c],
Gaiane M. Rauch, MD, PhD, FSBI, FSABI[d,e]

KEYWORDS

- Molecular breast imaging • Breast Specific gamma imaging • Dedicated breast PET
- Positron emission mammography • FDG • ^{99m}Tc-sestamibi

KEY POINTS

- Molecular breast imaging (MBI) is a promising adjunct breast imaging modality for breast cancer screening, staging, treatment response evaluation and problem solving, with performance similar to breast MRI.
- Current effective dose for MBI performed with 240 to 300 MBq of ^{99m}Tc-sestamibi is 2 to 2.5 mSv and can be decreased to 1.2 mSv with administration of half-dose ^{99m}Tc-sestamibi (150 MBq) and use of image-processing software, making it comparable to an effective dose of 1.2 mSv for digital mammography combined with tomosynthesis.
- Breast-specific positron imaging systems provide higher sensitivity than whole-body positron emission tomography for breast cancer detection.

INTRODUCTION

Molecular imaging methods for evaluation of breast cancer have been investigated since the 1970s, when the first report was published about accumulation of the bone imaging radiopharmaceutical technetium 99m-methyl diphosphonate (Tc99m-MDP) in the primary breast cancer of patients imaged for metastatic disease.[1] Additional reports about avid uptake of the cardiac perfusion agent ^{99m}Tc-sestamibi in breast tumors followed in the 1980s and early 1990s,[2] and led to the development

This article previously appeared in *PET Clinics* volume 18 issue 4 October 2023.

[a] Department of Breast Imaging, The University of Texas MD Anderson Cancer Center, 1515 Holcombe, CPB5.3208, Houston, TX 77030, USA; [b] Department of Radiology, Section of Breast Imaging and Intervention, University of Wisconsin – Madison, 600 Highland Avenue, Madison, WI 53792-3252, USA; [c] Department of Medical Physics, University of Wisconsin Carbone Cancer Center, University of Wisconsin-Madison, 600 Highland Avenue, Madison, WI 53792-3252, USA; [d] Department of Abdominal Imaging, The University of Texas MD Anderson Cancer Center, 1515 Holcombe, Unit 1473, Houston, TX 77030, USA; [e] Department of Breast Imaging, The University of Texas MD Anderson Cancer Center, 1515 Holcombe, Unit 1473, Houston, TX 77030, USA

* Corresponding author.

E-mail address: MPatel6@mdanderson.org

of scintimammography, a nuclear medicine method for breast cancer imaging. However, scintimammography utilized large field-of-view gamma cameras used for general nuclear medicine imaging resulting in poor spatial resolution with low sensitivity for nonpalpable lesions (30%–60%).[3]

New types of dedicated single- or dual-headed nuclear medicine breast imaging systems for single photon emitting radiotracers, jointly referred to as molecular breast imaging (MBI) systems, have been developed in recent years. Additionally, there has been emergence of dedicated breast-specific imaging systems for positron emitting radiopharmaceuticals: positron emission mammography (PEM) with detectors in mammographic configuration, and dedicated breast PET (dbPET) with detectors in ring configuration. These improvements in technology led to increased utilization of both single photon and coincidence detection dedicated breast imaging systems. They have been shown to be useful for multiple indications, such as detection of mammographically occult breast cancer, breast cancer local staging, monitoring of the response to neoadjuvant systemic therapy, and evaluating indeterminate imaging findings visualized on conventional breast imaging.[4–8] The purpose of this article is to review the available dedicated breast-specific nuclear medicine imaging modalities and discuss their role in the diagnosis and management of breast cancer.

MOLECULAR BREAST IMAGING
Equipment and Procedure

There are 2 types of MBI-dedicated gamma camera systems currently available for breast imaging. The first-generation system on the market was a single-headed gamma camera with a sodium iodide or cesium iodide detector (Eve Clear Scan e680, SmartBreast, previously known as Dilon 6800, Dilon Technologies) commonly known as breast-specific gamma imaging (BSGI). Advances in technology led to introduction of dual-headed gamma cameras with cadmium zinc telluride semiconductor detectors, usually referred as MBI, that improved spatial resolution, lesion detection, and count sensitivity: LumaGem 3200s (CMR Naviscan, Carlsbad, CA, USA); and Eve Clear Scan e750 (SmartBreast, Pittsburgh, PA, USA).[9]

Recently published Society of Nuclear Medicine and Molecular Imaging (SNMMI)/ European Association of Nuclear Medicine (EANM) Procedure Standard/Practice Guidelines and American College of Radiology (ACR) Practice Parameters describe MBI technique in detail.[10,11] Therefore, we provide a brief description of the procedure in this section. Fasting for at least 3 hours and having a warm blanket around their torso is advised to patients before proceeding with the intravenous injection of the radiotracer ^{99m}Tc-sestamibi. The goal is to decrease blood flow to the liver, and increase delivery of the radiotracer to the breast.[12] The dose of ^{99m}Tc-sestamibi initially used for MBI was 740 to 1100 MBq (20–30 mCi). However, equipment optimization allowed reduction of the administered dose to 240 to 300 MBq (6.5–8 mCi).[13] The image acquisition usually starts 5 to 10 minutes after radiotracer injection. During the imaging process, the patient sits comfortably with the breast gently immobilized between 2 gamma cameras for the MBI system, or a gamma camera and a paddle for the BSGI system. The images are obtained in standard mammographic views (craniocaudal and mediolateral oblique), with an acquisition time of 10 min/view, and a total imaging time for both breasts of 40 minutes.[10]

MBI interpretation is usually performed by a fellowship-trained breast radiologist with additional training in the evaluation of MBI. MBI images are reviewed together with available standard-of-care breast imaging, such as mammogram and ultrasound. Published MBI lexicon is used for interpretation and reporting of MBI.[14,15]

Biopsy

A suspicious MBI finding should be correlated with mammography and a second look ultrasound. If conventional breast imaging does not show a correlate for the MBI finding, MBI-guided biopsy is recommended. Before the development of the MBI biopsy device, the lack of MBI biopsy capability was a barrier to the integration of MBI into the breast imaging workflow.

Direct biopsy is available for Eve Clear Scan e680 (previously Dilon 6800, Dilon), has been approved by the US Food and Drug Adminstration for Eve Clear Scan e750 (formerly Discovery NM 750b, by GE) in 2016, and is in development for the Luma-Gem.[16] The MBI biopsy device uses the stereotactic principle for lesion localization. The ^{99m}Tc-sestamibi dose for MBI biopsy is recommended to be increased to 600 to 800 MBq to improve lesion conspicuity. No special precautions are needed for the personnel performing the MBI biopsy procedure or when the specimen is transported and subsequently analyzed. The ability to obtain a specimen to confirm lesion retrieval during the MBI-guided biopsy is one of the main advantages over breast MRI-guided biopsy. The second advantage is the lower cost of an MBI-guided biopsy ($1500) versus MRI-guided biopsy ($3500).[17] Additional advantages of MBI-guided biopsy are the lack of contraindications to MBI, a claustrophobic-free device with good patient tolerance. Limitations of MBI-guided biopsy are comparable to the stereotactic-guided biopsy related to lesion localization in the posterior and retroareolar regions.

Clinical Indications

Screening

Mammography is the accepted gold standard for breast cancer screening. However, it has limited sensitivity in patients with dense breast tissue. Approximately three-quarters of women younger than age 50 and over one-third of women age 50 and older have dense breast tissue.[18] The presence of dense breast tissue itself also confers a 1.2 to 2 times increased risk of developing breast cancer.[19] The overall sensitivity of digital mammography has been shown to be 84%[20]; however, clinical trials in women with dense breast tissue or increased risk of breast cancer demonstrate the sensitivity of mammography to be reduced to as low as 25% to 50%.[21] Therefore, supplemental screening modalities are recommended in these patient populations which may consist of whole breast ultrasound, MRI, or MBI, with MRI historically considered the most sensitive examination available. Unlike mammography, MBI detection of breast cancer is not affected by tissue density[22] (**Fig. 1**).

Since 2011, there have been 3 studies evaluating MBI as a supplemental screening modality in women with dense breast tissue[4,23,24] and one study evaluating BSGI detecting mammographically occult breast cancer in women at increased lifetime risk of breast cancer[25] (**Table 1**). In the initial 2011 study by Rhodes and colleagues[4] evaluating the role of supplemental screening MBI in women with dense breast tissue, MBI demonstrated an incremental cancer detection rate of 7.5 cases per 1000 women screened compared to a cancer detection rate of 3.2 cases per 1000 for patient screening with mammography alone. The addition of MBI resulted in a sensitivity increase from 27% (mammography alone) to 91% (mammography and MBI). Specificity for combined mammography and MBI was 85%. A subsequent study was performed to evaluate supplemental screening with MBI in women with dense breast tissue utilizing a lower radiation dose and demonstrated similar results with an incremental CDR of 8.8 per 1000 and increase in sensitivity from 23.8% (mammography alone) to 90.5% (mammography and MBI).[23] The recall rate was noted to increase from 11%

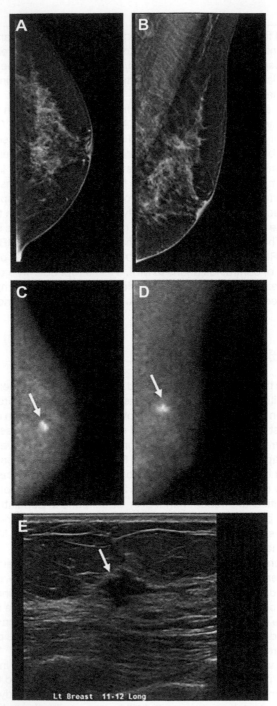

Fig. 1. A 48-year-old woman presents for routine screening. (*A, B*) CC and MLO views from screening mammogram examination demonstrate heterogeneously dense breast tissue, and the examination was read as negative. (*C, D*) CC and MLO views from subsequent MBI

(mammography alone) to 17.6% (mammography and MBI).[23] The 2016 study by Shermis and colleagues[24] also demonstrated a similar incremental cancer detection rate of 7.7 per 1000. The first multicenter prospective ongoing trial, Density MATTERS (Molecular Breast Imaging and Tomosynthesis to Eliminate the Reservoir of Cancers, NCT03220893), compares breast cancer detection between screening with digital breast tomosynthesis (DBT) and DBT combined with MBI. Preliminary results from this trial demonstrate a similar increase in CDR with initial MBI screening showing incremental CDR of 9.3 per 1000.[26] With recent increased emphasis on detection of *clinically significant* breast cancer, it is important to note that in the 2015 study performed by Rhodes and colleagues,[23] 80% of cancers detected by MBI alone were invasive and 82% were node negative.

To date, one retrospective review of 849 patients evaluating the incremental increase in breast cancer detection amongst high-risk women undergoing BSGI has been performed.[25] BSGI demonstrated an incremental cancer detection rate of 16.5 cancers per 1000 women screened. The most recent study published in 2022 evaluated 716 patients who underwent supplemental MBI examination for *either* dense breast tissue or increased lifetime risk and outcomes of abnormal MBI findings combining the 2 common indications for supplemental screening MBI. They reported high overall cancer detection rate of 15.4 per 1000, and 11.2 per 1000 for invasive cancers.[27]

Potential advantages for MBI compared to MRI as a supplemental screening modality include similar imaging projection to mammography (craniocaudal and mediolateral oblique views) facilitating comparison, faster interpretation time, claustrophobia-free modality, and safe in patients with renal disease, pacemakers, metallic implants, and gadolinium-based contrast agent allergies. Disadvantages include limited evaluation of lesions along the chest wall, potential difficulty with insurance coverage, and increased recall rates. An additional potential cited concern is radiation exposure which will be discussed further in subsequent sections.

Breast cancer staging

Staging of breast cancer routinely includes diagnostic mammography, ultrasound, and possibly breast MRI in certain clinical settings. The goal of complete local staging is detecting additional sites of malignancy within the ipsilateral breast or contralateral breast for accurate baseline evaluation of disease extent and surgical planning (**Fig. 2**). Although MRI demonstrates high sensitivity, it has moderate specificity and higher costs which may limit its use and lead to additional imaging evaluation and biopsies.

A meta-analysis of the use of breast MRI in staging of patients with breast cancer demonstrated that mammographically occult ipsilateral lesions were detected by MRI in 16% to 20% of women along with contralateral malignancies in 3% to 9% of women.[28] However, a high number of false positives associated with MRI require verification of MRI findings with tissue sampling which may result in treatment delays. In addition, certain patient populations including patients with claustrophobia, large body habitus, renal insufficiency, or implanted devices may not be able to undergo MRI. MBI can be especially useful for these patient populations.[29]

---

demonstrate 1.1 cm homogeneous mass uptake at 12:00 position 4.4 cm from the nipple (*arrow*). (*E*) US demonstrates a corresponding irregular, hypoechoic mass in the 11 to 12 o'clock position. US-guided biopsy was performed yielding invasive ductal carcinoma, low nuclear grade, ER+, PR−, HER2+.

Table 1
Molecular breast imaging and breast-specific gamma imaging performance in supplemental breast cancer screening

Study	Design	Total Enrolled	Incremental Cancer Detection Rate	Recall Rate	Sensitivity MBI	MBI + Mammo	Specificity MBI	MBI + Mammo	PPV1	PPV3
Rhodes et al,[4] 2011	Prospective, single academic institution	936 (dense breast)	7.5 per 1000 (7/936)	8%	82%	91%	93%	85%	12%	28%
Rhodes et al,[23] 2015	Prospective, single academic institution	1585 (dense breast)	8.8 per 1000 (14/1485)	7.5%	80%	91%	93%	83%	14.3%	33.3%
Brem et al,[25] 2016	Retrospective	849 (increased risk)	16.5 per 1000 (14/849)	25%	-	-	-	-	6.7%	14.4%
Shermis et al,[24] 2016	Retrospective, single community-based	1696 (dense breast)	7.7 per 1000 (13/1696)	8.4%	-	-	-	-	9.1%	19.4%
Maimone et al,[27] 2022	Retrospective, single institution	716 (dense breast + increased risk)	9.8 per 1000 (7/716)	13%	-	-	-	-	11.8%	27.5%

Data Source.[4,23–25]

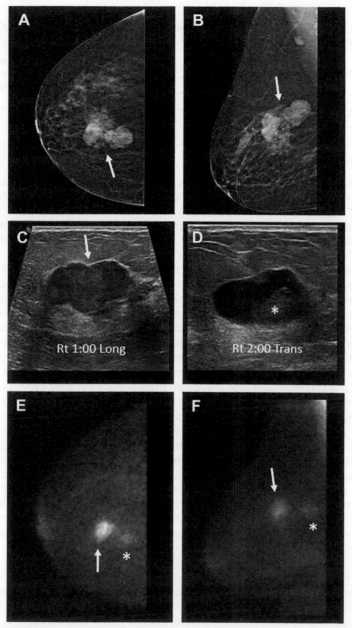

Fig. 2. A 60-year-old woman presenting with abnormal mammogram. (*A*, *B*) CC and MLO mammogram images demonstrate 2 adjacent masses in the upper inner quadrant of the right breast (*arrows*). (*C*) Longitudinal grayscale sonographic image demonstrates an irregular, hypoechoic mass in the right breast 1 o'clock position, 9 cm from nipple (*arrow*). Core biopsy demonstrated invasive ductal carcinoma with apocrine features, grade 2. (*D*) Transverse grayscale sonographic image demonstrates a circumscribed complex cystic and solid mass in the right breast 2 o'clock position, 12 cm from nipple. Associated increased color Doppler flow was noted in the hypoechoic component (*). Fine needle aspiration targeting the hypoechoic component demonstrated fibrocystic change versus intraductal papilloma.

Table 2 Molecular breast imaging/breast-specific gamma imaging versus MRI: evaluation of treatment response after neoadjuvant chemotherapy		MBI		MRI	
Study	Patient Number	Sensitivity	Specificity	Sensitivity	Specificity
Lee et al,[38] 2014	122	74%	72.2%	81.7%	72.2%
Kim et al,[37] 2019	114	70.2%	90%	83.3%	60%
Hunt et al,[7] 2019	102	58.9%	82.4%	82.8%	69.4%

Data Source.[7,37,38]

A 2019 prospective study compared staging of newly diagnosed breast cancer with 3 imaging modalities, MRI, contrast-enhanced mammography (CEM), and MBI. They found that all 3 modalities were effective in the local staging of breast cancer by demonstrating similar visualization of index cancers; however, MRI demonstrated a lower positive predictive value (PPV) for lesions undergoing biopsy compared to MBI and CEM (PPV MRI 28%, MBI 44%, CEM 52%).[30]

In a 2018 retrospective study published by Collarino and colleagues[6] of 287 women with biopsy-proven breast malignancy who underwent MBI for local staging, MBI detected larger tumor extent and/or additional sites of malignancy in 14% (40/287 patients). Previous studies have also demonstrated that MBI may be useful in detecting ipsilateral or contralateral malignancy with one series of 159 women with clinically suspicious breast lesions noted to have 6% additional ipsilateral foci and 5% contralateral foci detected by MBI.[31] Another study demonstrated that MBI detected larger extent of disease or additional ipsilateral of contralateral foci in 10.9% of subjects.[32]

Certain breast cancer subtypes are known to be better evaluated by MRI compared to routine staging examinations. For example, invasive lobular carcinoma (ILC) is more challenging to diagnose by mammography and ultrasound due to the infiltrative pattern of growth. For this reason, MRI is frequently used to evaluate extent of disease in patients with ILC due to its high sensitivity ranging from 77% to 100%.[33] In earlier studies, MBI has been reported to have a sensitivity of 89% to 93% and a specificity of 79% in diagnosis of ILC with Brem and colleagues[34] reporting the sensitivity of MBI to be higher than that of MRI (93% vs. 83%).[35] However, more recent studies have demonstrated limitations of MBI in detecting invasive lobular carcinoma with sensitivities for ILC noted to be 69% to 85%.[30,36] An additional limitation of MBI in staging of breast cancer is the limited ability to evaluate chest wall disease and evaluate axillary lymph nodes.

Response to neoadjuvant chemotherapy

Neoadjuvant chemotherapy (NAC; **Table 2**) is widely used in locally advanced breast cancer to reduce disease burden and potentially make a patient a candidate for breast conservation surgery as opposed to mastectomy. Imaging plays a key role by determining the baseline extent of disease, monitoring response to chemotherapy, and

---

(*E*, *F*) CC and MLO MBI images demonstrate marked mass uptake in the mass at the 1 o'clock position, 9 cm from nipple (*arrow*) and moderate mass uptake in the mass at the 2 o'clock position, 12 cm from nipple (*). Given the uptake, US-guided core biopsy of the 2 o'clock position mass was recommended. Final pathology was invasive ductal carcinoma with apocrine features, grade 2.

evaluation of residual disease after completion of therapy prior to surgery. Currently breast MRI is the primary imaging modality utilized with sensitivities for residual disease noted to be 86% to 92%, specificity 60% to 89%, and accuracy 76% to 90%.[7] MBI is a promising imaging modality for evaluation of residual disease after neoadjuvant treatment (**Fig. 3**).

A 2019 study by Hunt and colleagues[7] prospectively evaluated the accuracy of MBI and MRI to evaluate for residual disease relative to final pathologic analysis. Although both imaging modalities in the study showed comparable measurements on baseline pre-treatment imaging, variability in prediction of residual disease post-treatment was noted with MRI demonstrating sensitivity 82.8%, specificity 69.4%, MBI sensitivity 58.9%, and specificity 82.4% and neither demonstrated high enough accuracy to replace the need to evaluate residual tumor burden on final surgical pathology specimen.

Another study by Kim and colleagues[37] in 2019 retrospectively evaluated BSGI and MRI to compare assessment of treatment response and noted similar sensitivities for both modalities (BSGI 70.2% and MRI 83.3%) with increased specificity for BSGI (BSGI 90% and MRI 60%).

A 2014 study by Lee and colleagues[38] retrospectively evaluated the performance of BSGI with MRI in the assessment of residual tumor after NAC. In the 122 patients evaluated, both modalities demonstrate similar sensitivity and specificity in residual tumor detection (MBI sensitivity and specificity 74%, 72.2% and MRI sensitivity and specificity 81.7%, 72.2%). However, there was variability in estimation of residual tumor size based on the molecular subtype of breast cancer. Although relatively accurate measurements were noted for triple negative breast cancer, residual tumor size was underestimated by BSGI in luminal subtypes and by MRI in both luminal and HER2 subtypes.[38] Overall, no available breast imaging modality is capable of accurate evaluation of residual disease after NAC.

MBI may be utilized during NAC to predict nonresponsiveness to chemotherapy. In a meta-analysis by Collarino and colleagues,[39] 3 studies investigated the ability of MBI to predict lack of response to chemotherapy before or early during NAC and demonstrated a sensitivity of 74% and a specificity of 92%. However, it was noted that there was heterogeneity amongst the study design and further investigation of MBI utilization for prediction of response was needed.[39]

Problem solving

Conventional imaging with mammogram and ultrasound is often adequate to render a final Breast Imaging Reporting and Data System (BI-RADS) category for work-up of clinical, mammographic, and ultrasound findings. In rare instances, advanced functional imaging is needed as a problem-solving imaging modality.[10,11] The role of MBI in this scenario is similar to breast MRI but at a lower cost.[40] MBI has been shown to be valuable in the resolution of complex clinical and imaging cases by mammography and ultrasound (**Fig. 4**). Siegal and colleagues[41] evaluated 416 patients in whom MBI was performed for problem solving of various findings including 56% for asymmetries, 14% for calcifications, 6% for mass, and 7% for evaluation of a palpable finding with negative mammography and ultrasound. A benign or negative BI-RADS was assigned in 70% of those patients helping with the resolution of the case. Sixty-eight cases (14%) resulted in biopsy. Of those, malignant pathology was present in 43%, high risk lesion in 15% and 42% were benign.[41] Only 2 cases out of 289 (0.07%) were false negatives in this study.

Weigert and colleagues[42] evaluated 1042 patients who underwent MBI for different indications. MBI was recommended in 38% of patients due to a mammographic abnormality such as asymmetry, subtle calcifications, discordant results between

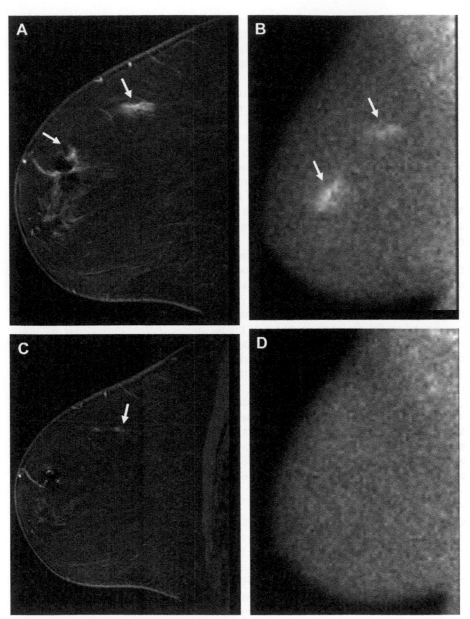

Fig. 3. A 60-year-old woman with multifocal invasive ductal breast cancer, low nuclear grade, ER-, PR-, and HER2- undergoing neoadjuvant chemotherapy. (*A*) Baseline post-contrast sagittal MR image demonstrates 2 irregular enhancing masses with associated susceptibility artifact from biopsy clips consistent with sites of biopsy-proven multifocal breast cancer. (*B*) Correlating multifocal uptake is noted on the MLO MBI image. (*C*) Post-neoadjuvant chemotherapy sagittal post-contrast MR image demonstrates residual linear non-mass enhancement (*arrow*) associated with the posterior site of biopsy-proven malignancy. (*D*) Post-neoadjuvant chemotherapy MLO MBI image demonstrates no residual uptake. Final surgical pathology demonstrated fibrosis with no invasive cancer.

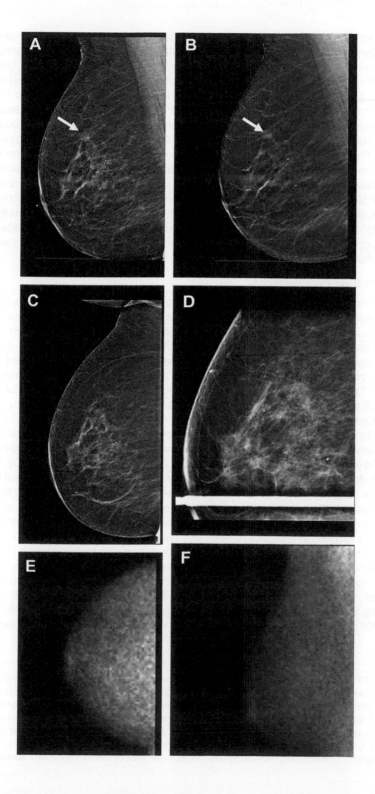

multiple studies, and in 11% of patients for a palpable mass with negative mammography. Comparison of the ultrasound versus MBI for workup of mammographic findings showed that MBI had higher sensitivity (80% vs. 70%), specificity (76% vs. 47%), PPV (53% vs. 32%), and negative predictive value (NPV; 92% vs. 81%) than ultrasound (US). For patients with negative or indeterminate mammographic findings, BSGI overall significantly increased detection of malignant and high-risk lesions. A retrospective study of 381 MBI results in patients with low suspicion mammographic or ultrasound findings showed the NPV of MBI to be 99.7% and false-negative rate (FNR) 2.7%, which resulted in 67.5% reduction in number of biopsies. The clinical application of the high NPV of MBI for problem solving requires further evaluation in larger patient populations.[8] Other scenarios where MBI is useful as a problem-solving imaging modality are patients with direct silicone injections, MRI incompatible implants, or with other contraindications for MRI. Approximately 15% of patients are unable to undergo breast MRI due to implantable devices, body habitus, renal insufficiency, contrast medium reaction, and claustrophobia.[40,43] MBI could be a viable option for these patients.

Radiation Dose Considerations

The misconception about the high radiation dose of MBI has been an impediment to the widespread acceptance of MBI as a breast imaging modality. The radiation dose varies among breast imaging modalities, and although the radiation during mammography is delivered directly to the breast, the ^{99m}Tc-sestamibi used for MBI is distributed systemically in the body with the highest radiation doses absorbed by the kidneys, colon, small intestine, and bladder and a smallest radiation dose to the breast.[44] The effective dose equivalent, a metric reported in milliSieverts (mSv), is better suited to assess radiation to the organs and compare different imaging modalities.[45] Early gamma cameras used relatively high ^{99m}Tc-sestamibi doses of 740 to 1100 MBq (20–30 mCi), with effective doses of 5.9 to 9.4 mSv, which are above the background radiation level (3.1 mSv/y). However, with recent equipment optimization, the ^{99m}Tc-sestamibi doses have decreased to 240 from 300 MBq (6.5–8 mCi), with an effective dose of MBI of 2 to 2.5 mSv, far lower than the background radiation level.[45] There are ongoing attempts to reduce the effective dose of MBI close to digital mammography. Tao and colleagues[46] developed an image processing algorithm which provided acceptable quality MBI images with half-dose ^{99m}Tc-sestamibi (150 MBq). This resulted in an effective dose of 1.0 mSv, which is comparable to an effective dose from 2-view digital mammography combined with tomosynthesis (1.2 mSv).

The benefit-to-radiation risk ratio, defined as the ratio of estimated cancer death averted to the estimated radiation-caused cancer death per 100,000 women screened, has been shown to be lower for supplemental screening MBI than for screening mammography.[47] Brown and Covington[48] found that the benefit-to-risk ratio for MBI might overlap with mammography if variations in mammographic technique

Fig. 4. A 75-year-old woman with history of left breast cancer. (A, B) MLO mammography 2D and 3D images demonstrate an asymmetry (arrow) in the superior region of the right breast. (C, D) Right LM and LM spot compression views demonstrate the asymmetry is not seen. Ultrasound was negative. Given her history of breast cancer, MBI was recommended for further evaluation. (E, F) CC and MLO MBI views show no suspicious uptake. The examination was given a BI-RADS 1: Negative for malignancy and the patient resumed annual mammogram. Subsequent mammogram follow-up (not shown) has been negative for 4 years.

are accounted for (tomosynthesis-synthetic views, 2D full-field digital mammography), compression thickness, and age. They reported a further increase in the benefit-to-radiation risk ratio for MBI with ultra-low dose (150 MBq) of ^{99m}Tc-sestamibi as proposed by Tao and colleagues.[49]

POSITRON EMISSION MAMMOGRAPHY
Equipment and Procedure

The positron emitting radiopharmaceutical, 2-deoxy-2-[^{18}F]fluoro-D-glucose (FDG), is the most commonly used molecular imaging agent for breast cancer. Whole-body positron emission tomography/computed tomography (PET/CT) with FDG can be used clinically for initial systemic staging, restaging, and therapy response assessment for patients with breast cancer.[50] However, whole-body PET/CT is not recommended for primary breast cancer detection or for distinguishing benign from malignant breast lesions due to limited spatial resolution for subcentimeter lesions.[51,52] This technical limitation of whole-body scanners led to the development of dedicated breast imaging devices which bring the detectors closer to the breast for improved spatial resolution.[53]

There are 2 main designs for breast specific positron imaging systems.[3,54,55] The planar design consists of 2 opposing parallel planar detectors and has been termed positron emission mammography (PEM). For PEM, the patient is seated with the breast in mild compression with images acquired in the same views as conventional X-ray mammography. The other design uses a ring-shaped detector configuration in which the patient lies in the prone position. This design is typically referred to as dedicated breast PET (dbPET) and provides full tomographic images. The in plane spatial resolution of breast specific positron imaging systems is typically 1 to 2 mm compared to 4 to 6 mm with whole-body PET scanners which enables smaller lesion detection.

Clinical practice guidelines for the performance of high-resolution breast PET have been published by the Japanese Society of Nuclear Medicine.[56] As with whole-body FDG PET/CT, patients are instructed to fast for at least 4 to 6 hours. The intravenously injected activity of FDG is typically 10 mCi (370 MBq) for PEM and 3 to 5 mCi (111–185 MBq) for dbPET. Image acquisition typically begins 60 minutes after FDG injection or 90 minutes post-injection if dbPET is performed after whole-body PET. For PEM, craniocaudal and mediolateral oblique views of each breast are acquired for 10 minutes per view (40-minute total scan time). For dbPET, images are acquired for 5 to 7 minutes per ring position with the total scan time depending on breast length.

Standardized terminology has been developed to describe and interpret findings on breast-specific positron imaging.[57,58] The lexicon follows a similar organization as the American College of Radiology Breast Imaging Reporting and Data System for breast MRI.[59] Breast-specific positron imaging exams should be interpreted with other conventional breast imaging available, together with information about previous biopsy and treatment history. Experienced breast imaging radiologists who completed a 2-hour training module in PEM interpretation for a multi-institutional clinical trial in the Unites States achieved high diagnostic accuracy and interobserver agreement.[60]

An important feature of breast-specific positron imaging systems is the capability to biopsy lesions that may be only seen with PET. A PEM-guided biopsy system is commercially available that uses a stereotactic method for lesion targeting.[61–63] Biopsy systems for dbPET remain in technical development.[64]

Clinical Indications

The diagnostic performance of breast-specific positron imaging systems has been evaluated in several studies. A meta-analysis of 8 studies including 873 women with known or suspected breast cancer imaged with PEM found an overall pooled sensitivity of 85% and pooled specificity of 79% with an area under the curve (AUC) of 0.88.[65] In 2020, a subsequent meta-analysis of 5 studies including 722 women with breast cancer demonstrated better sensitivity, NPV, and accuracy of PEM compared to whole-body PET for primary breast cancer detection.[66] Specificity and PPV were similar between the 2 imaging modalities. For dbPET, recent large studies involving up to 938 women also found increased sensitivity for breast cancer detection compared to whole-body PET/CT, particularly for T1 stage tumors (<2 cm), subcentimeter tumors, lower grade tumors, and ductal carcinoma in situ.[67,68]

Potential clinical applications for breast-specific positron imaging include local staging of newly diagnosed breast cancer for surgical planning, evaluating neoadjuvant therapy response, and detecting local disease recurrence within the breast. For preoperative local staging, there have been 2 prospective studies comparing PEM with breast MRI.[5,69] Both studies showed that the sensitivity of PEM was comparable to breast MRI for detecting additional unsuspected cancers in the ipsilateral breast.[5,69] The specificity of PEM was comparable[69] or better[5] than breast MRI. For detection of residual disease after completion of neoadjuvant chemotherapy, PEM and dbPET have been shown to be more sensitive and more accurate than whole-body PET/CT.[70–72] As an early biomarker of therapy response, a decrease in FDG uptake on PEM after the first cycle of neoadjuvant chemotherapy has been shown to correlate with final pathologic response.[73] Thus, breast-specific positron imaging has similar clinical indications as breast MRI and may be a feasible alternative for patients who have contraindications for breast MRI.

In contrast to MBI, there is very limited literature regarding the use of breast-specific positron imaging as a supplemental screening modality for women with mammographically dense breasts or those with elevated lifetime risk of breast cancer. One study reported a 2.3% cancer detection rate using PEM in 265 women (165 without breast symptoms) participating in an FDG PET cancer screening program in Japan.[74]

Additional Considerations and Challenges

A barrier to the use of breast-specific positron imaging for supplemental breast cancer screening is the current radiation exposure associated with the examination (3.5 mSv effective dose equivalent from 185 MBq FDG).[56] Although this amount is comparable to natural background radiation and considered negligible risk, it is more than other breast imaging modalities, including MBI (2–2.5 mSv from 300 MBq ^{99m}Tc-sestamibi). Research efforts to reduce the radiation dose have shown clinically acceptable image quality using 25% injected FDG activity, which corresponds to a radiation dose of 0.9 mSv.[75,76]

There are additional technical and practical challenges with breast-specific positron imaging. These devices have inherently limited evaluation of the axilla and difficulty visualizing far posterior lesions near the chest wall, particularly with the prone design.[5,77,78] However, modifications to the imaging table have been shown to increase the amount of breast tissue in the field of view.[79,80] Furthermore, some indolent tumors may not have sufficient levels of glucose metabolism to be detected using FDG.[81]

SUMMARY

Recent advances in nuclear breast imaging technology with development of the dual-headed direct conversion gamma imaging systems and biopsy capability led to increased interest in this emerging nuclear medicine modality in the breast imaging community. There is a growing body of literature demonstrating similar performance of MBI in comparison with MRI for breast cancer screening, staging, treatment response assessment, and problem solving. Recently published ACR Practice Parameters and SNMMI/EANM Practice Guidelines, as well as ongoing efforts to reduce radiation dose, further support increased incorporation of MBI in the breast imaging practice. Breast-specific positron imaging systems are not widely used in clinical practice in the United States; however, there is growing clinical data published by international sites including Japan, Spain, and the Netherlands supporting its use for multiple indications. Further research is needed focused on the appropriate clinical applications for breast-specific positron imaging to provide impactful information to guide treatment decisions for patients with breast cancer. The use of radiopharmaceuticals beyond FDG may also expand the potential applications of this technology.[82,83]

CLINICS CARE POINTS

- MBI demonstrates increased incremental cancer detection rates when utilized as a supplemental screening modality in women with dense breast tissue or increased lifetime risk of breast cancer.

- MBI is a useful alternative in local staging for breast cancer demonstrating similar sensitivity to MRI and CEM and may play a role in predicting response to neoadjuvant chemotherapy.

- MBI may be used for problem-solving evaluation of mammographic asymmetries, subtle or multiple groups of calcifications, palpable findings with negative conventional imaging, discordant results between multiple studies and in patients with implants or direct silicone injections.

- Potential applications of breast-specific positron imaging are local staging, neoadjuvant treatment response evaluation, and detection of local disease recurrence in the breast.

DISCLOSURE

A.M. Fowler receives book chapter royalty from Elsevier, Inc and has served on an advisory board for GE Healthcare. The Department of Radiology at the University of Wisconsin School of Medicine and Public Health receives research support from GE Healthcare. G.M. Rauch received research grant support from GE Healthcare.

ACKNOWLEDGMENTS

The authors acknowledge the University of Wisconsin Carbone Cancer Center Support Grant P30 CA014520 and the Department of Radiology, University of Wisconsin School of Medicine and Public Health for support. The authors acknowledge the National Institutes of Health/National Cancer Institute Cancer Center Support Grant P30 CA016672 and the Department of Breast Imaging, The University of Texas MD Anderson Cancer Center. The authors also acknowledge the work of many others that could not be discussed due to space limitations.

REFERENCES

1. Berg GR, Kalisher L, Osmond JD, et al. 99mTc-diphosphonate concentration in primary breast carcinoma. Radiology 1973;109(2):393–4.

2. Aktolun C, Bayhan H, Kir M. Clinical experience with Tc-99m MIBI imaging in patients with malignant tumors. Preliminary results and comparison with Tl-201. Clin Nucl Med 1992;17(3):171–6.

3. Hruska CB, O'Connor MK. Nuclear imaging of the breast: translating achievements in instrumentation into clinical use. Med Phys 2013;40(5):050901.

4. Rhodes DJ, Hruska CB, Phillips SW, et al. Dedicated dual-head gamma imaging for breast cancer screening in women with mammographically dense breasts. Radiology 2011;258(1):106–18.

5. Berg WA, Madsen KS, Schilling K, et al. Breast cancer: comparative effectiveness of positron emission mammography and MR imaging in presurgical planning for the ipsilateral breast. Radiology 2011;258(1):59–72.

6. Collarino A, Valdes Olmos RA, van Berkel L, et al. The clinical impact of molecular breast imaging in women with proven invasive breast cancer scheduled for breast-conserving surgery. Breast Cancer Res Treat 2018;169(3):513–22.

7. Hunt KN, Conners AL, Goetz MP, et al. Comparison of (99m)Tc-sestamibi molecular breast imaging and breast MRI in patients with invasive breast cancer receiving neoadjuvant chemotherapy. AJR Am J Roentgenol 2019;213(4): 932–43.

8. Jain R, Katz DR, Kapoor AD. The clinical utility of a negative result at molecular breast imaging: initial proof of concept. Radiol Imaging Cancer 2020;2(5): e190096.

9. Hunt KN. Molecular breast imaging: a scientific review. Journal of Breast Imaging 2021;3(4):416–26.

10. Hruska CB, Corion C, de Geus-Oei L-F, et al. SNMMI procedure standard/EANM practice guideline for molecular breast imaging with dedicated γ-Cameras. J Nucl Med Technol 2022;50(2):103–10.

11. American College of Radiology. ACR practice parameter for the performance of molecular breast imaging (MBI) using a dedicated gamma camera. Available at: https://www.acr.org/-/media/ACR/Files/Practice-Parameters/MBI.pdf. Accessed January 24, 2023.

12. Swanson T, Tran TD, Ellingson L, et al. Best practices in molecular breast imaging: a guide for technologists. J Nucl Med Technol 2018. https://doi.org/10.2967/jnmt.117.204263.

13. Hruska CB, Weinmann AL, Tello Skjerseth CM, et al. Proof of concept for low-dose molecular breast imaging with a dual-head CZT gamma camera. Part II. Evaluation in patients. Med Phys 2012;39(6):3476–83.

14. Conners AL, Maxwell RW, Tortorelli CL, et al. Gamma camera breast imaging lexicon. AJR Am J Roentgenol 2012;199(6):W767–74.

15. Conners AL, Hruska CB, Tortorelli CL, et al. Lexicon for standardized interpretation of gamma camera molecular breast imaging: observer agreement and diagnostic accuracy. Eur J Nucl Med Mol Imaging 2012;39(6):971–82.

16. Hruska CB. Updates in molecular breast imaging. Semin Roentgenol 2022;57(2): 134–8.

17. Adrada BE, Moseley T, Kappadath SC, et al. Molecular breast imaging-guided percutaneous biopsy of breast lesions: a new frontier on breast intervention. J Breast Imaging 2020;2(5):484–91.

18. Checka CM, Chun JE, Schnabel FR, et al. The relationship of mammographic density and age: implications for breast cancer screening. AJR Am J Roentgenol 2012;198(3):W292–5.

19. Sickles EA. The use of breast imaging to screen women at high risk for cancer. Radiol Clin North Am 2010;48(5):859–78.

20. Kerlikowske K, Hubbard RA, Miglioretti DL, et al. Comparative effectiveness of digital versus film-screen mammography in community practice in the United States: a cohort study. Ann Intern Med 2011;155(8):493–502.
21. Hruska CB. Molecular breast imaging for screening in dense breasts: state of the art and future directions. AJR Am J Roentgenol 2017;208(2):275–83.
22. Rechtman LR, Lenihan MJ, Lieberman JH, et al. Breast-specific gamma imaging for the detection of breast cancer in dense versus nondense breasts. AJR Am J Roentgenol 2014;202(2):293–8.
23. Rhodes DJ, Hruska CB, Conners AL, et al. Journal club: molecular breast imaging at reduced radiation dose for supplemental screening in mammographically dense breasts. AJR Am J Roentgenol 2015;204(2):241–51.
24. Shermis RB, Wilson KD, Doyle MT, et al. Supplemental breast cancer screening with molecular breast imaging for women with dense breast tissue. AJR Am J Roentgenol 2016;207(2):450–7.
25. Brem RF, Ruda RC, Yang JL, et al. Breast-specific gamma-imaging for the detection of mammographically occult breast cancer in women at increased risk. J Nucl Med 2016;57(5):678–84.
26. Rhodes D, Hunt K, Conners A, et al. Abstract PD4-05: molecular breast imaging and tomosynthesis to eliminate the reservoir of undetected cancer in dense breasts: the Density MATTERS trial. Cancer Res 2019;79(4_Supplement). PD4-05-PD04-05.
27. Maimone S, Hatcher KM, Tavana A, et al. Downstream imaging following abnormal molecular breast imaging, lessons learned and suggestions for success. Clin Imaging 2022;92:44–51.
28. Plana MN, Carreira C, Muriel A, et al. Magnetic resonance imaging in the preoperative assessment of patients with primary breast cancer: systematic review of diagnostic accuracy and meta-analysis. Eur Radiol 2012;22(1):26–38.
29. Rauch GM, Adrada BE. Comparison of breast MR imaging with molecular breast imaging in breast cancer screening, diagnosis, staging, and treatment response evaluation. Magn Reson Imaging Clin N Am 2018;26(2):273–80.
30. Sumkin JH, Berg WA, Carter GJ, et al. Diagnostic performance of MRI, molecular breast imaging, and contrast-enhanced mammography in women with newly diagnosed breast cancer. Radiology 2019;293(3):531–40.
31. Brem RF, Shahan C, Rapleyea JA, et al. Detection of occult foci of breast cancer using breast-specific gamma imaging in women with one mammographic or clinically suspicious breast lesion. Acad Radiol 2010;17(6):735–43.
32. Zhou M, Johnson N, Gruner S, et al. Clinical utility of breast-specific gamma imaging for evaluating disease extent in the newly diagnosed breast cancer patient. Am J Surg 2009;197(2):159–63.
33. Mann RM. The effectiveness of MR imaging in the assessment of invasive lobular carcinoma of the breast. Magn Reson Imaging Clin N Am 2010;18(2):259–76, ix.
34. Brem RF, Ioffe M, Rapelyea JA, et al. Invasive lobular carcinoma: detection with mammography, sonography, MRI, and breast-specific gamma imaging. AJR Am J Roentgenol 2009;192(2):379–83.
35. Kelley KA, Crawford JD, Thomas K, et al. A comparison of breast-specific gamma imaging of invasive lobular carcinomas and ductal carcinomas. JAMA Surg 2015;150(8):816–8.
36. Conners AL, Jones KN, Hruska CB, et al. Direct-conversion molecular breast imaging of invasive breast cancer: imaging features, extent of invasive disease, and comparison between invasive ductal and lobular histology. AJR Am J Roentgenol 2015;205(3):W374–81.

37. Kim S, Plemmons J, Hoang K, et al. Breast-specific gamma imaging versus MRI: comparing the diagnostic performance in assessing treatment response after neoadjuvant chemotherapy in patients with breast cancer. AJR Am J Roentgenol 2019;212(3):696–705.

38. Lee HS, Ko BS, Ahn SH, et al. Diagnostic performance of breast-specific gamma imaging in the assessment of residual tumor after neoadjuvant chemotherapy in breast cancer patients. Breast Cancer Res Treat 2014;145(1):91–100.

39. Collarino A, de Koster EJ, Valdes Olmos RA, et al. Is technetium-99m sestamibi imaging able to predict pathologic nonresponse to neoadjuvant chemotherapy in breast cancer? A meta-analysis evaluating current use and shortcomings. Clin Breast Cancer 2018;18(1):9–18.

40. Dibble EH, Hunt KN, Ehman EC, et al. Molecular breast imaging in clinical practice. AJR Am J Roentgenol 2020;215(2):277–84.

41. Siegal E, Angelakis E, Morris P, et al. Breast molecular imaging: a retrospective review of one institutions experience with this modality and analysis of its potential role in breast imaging decision making. Breast J 2012;18(2):111–7.

42. Weigert JM, Bertrand ML, Lanzkowsky L, et al. Results of a multicenter patient registry to determine the clinical impact of breast-specific gamma imaging, a molecular breast imaging technique. AJR Am J Roentgenol 2012;198(1):W69–75.

43. Huppe AI, Mehta AK, Brem RF. Molecular breast imaging: a comprehensive review. Semin Ultrasound CT MR 2018;39(1):60–9.

44. O'Connor MK, Li H, Rhodes DJ, et al. Comparison of radiation exposure and associated radiation-induced cancer risks from mammography and molecular imaging of the breast. Med Phys 2010;37(12):6187–98.

45. Hruska CB. Let's get real about molecular breast imaging and radiation risk. Radiol Imaging Cancer 2019;1(1):e190070.

46. Tao AT, Hruska CB, Conners AL, et al. Dose reduction in molecular breast imaging with a new image-processing algorithm. AJR Am J Roentgenol 2020;214(1):185–93.

47. Hendrick RE, Tredennick T. Benefit to radiation risk of breast-specific gamma imaging compared with mammography in screening asymptomatic women with dense breasts. Radiology 2016;281(2):583–8.

48. Brown M, Covington MF. Comparative benefit-to-radiation risk ratio of molecular breast imaging, two-dimensional full-field digital mammography with and without tomosynthesis, and synthetic mammography with tomosynthesis. Radiol Imaging Cancer 2019;1(1):e190005.

49. Covington MF, Brown M. Molecular breast imaging at ultra-low radiation dose. AJR Am J Roentgenol 2020;215(2):W30.

50. Fowler AM, Cho SY. PET imaging for breast cancer. Radiol Clin North Am 2021;59(5):725–35.

51. Kumar R, Chauhan A, Zhuang H, et al. Clinicopathologic factors associated with false negative FDG-PET in primary breast cancer. Breast Cancer Res Treat 2006;98(3):267–74.

52. Avril N, Rose CA, Schelling M, et al. Breast imaging with positron emission tomography and fluorine-18 fluorodeoxyglucose: use and limitations. J Clin Oncol 2000;18(20):3495–502.

53. Thompson CJ, Murthy K, Weinberg IN, et al. Feasibility study for positron emission mammography. Med Phys 1994;21(4):529–38.

54. Surti S. Radionuclide methods and instrumentation for breast cancer detection and diagnosis. Semin Nucl Med 2013;43(4):271–80.

55. Hsu DF, Freese DL, Levin CS. Breast-dedicated radionuclide imaging systems. J Nucl Med 2016;57(Suppl 1):40S–5S.
56. Satoh Y, Kawamoto M, Kubota K, et al. Clinical practice guidelines for high-resolution breast PET, 2019 edition. Ann Nucl Med 2021;35(3):406–14.
57. Narayanan D, Madsen KS, Kalinyak JE, et al. Interpretation of positron emission mammography: feature analysis and rates of malignancy. AJR Am J Roentgenol 2011;196(4):956–70.
58. Miyake KK, Kataoka M, Ishimori T, et al. A proposed dedicated breast PET lexicon: standardization of description and reporting of radiotracer uptake in the breast. Diagnostics 2021;11(7):1267.
59. Morris EA, Comstock C, Lee C, et al. ACR BI-RADS magnetic resonance imaging. In: ACR BI-RADS atlas, breast imaging reporting and data system. Reston (VA): American College of Radiology; 2013.
60. Narayanan D, Madsen KS, Kalinyak JE, et al. Interpretation of positron emission mammography and MRI by experienced breast imaging radiologists: performance and observer reproducibility. AJR Am J Roentgenol 2011;196(4):971–81.
61. Raylman RR, Majewski S, Weisenberger AG, et al. Positron emission mammography-guided breast biopsy. J Nucl Med 2001;42(6):960–6.
62. Kalinyak JE, Schilling K, Berg WA, et al. PET-guided breast biopsy. Breast J 2011; 17(2):143–51.
63. Argus A, Mahoney MC. Positron emission mammography: diagnostic imaging and biopsy on the same day. AJR Am J Roentgenol 2014;202(1):216–22.
64. Hellingman D, Teixeira SC, Donswijk ML, et al. A novel semi-robotized device for high-precision (18)F-FDG-guided breast cancer biopsy. Rev Esp Med Nucl Imagen Mol 2017;36(3):158–65.
65. Caldarella C, Treglia G, Giordano A. Diagnostic performance of dedicated positron emission mammography using fluorine-18-fluorodeoxyglucose in women with suspicious breast lesions: a meta-analysis. Clin Breast Cancer 2014;14(4): 241–8.
66. Keshavarz K, Jafari M, Lotfi F, et al. Positron Emission Mammography (PEM) in the diagnosis of breast cancer: a systematic review and economic evaluation. Med J Islam Repub Iran 2020;34:100.
67. Sueoka S, Sasada S, Masumoto N, et al. Performance of dedicated breast positron emission tomography in the detection of small and low-grade breast cancer. Breast Cancer Res Treat 2021;187(1):125–33.
68. Sasada S, Kimura Y, Masumoto N, et al. Breast cancer detection by dedicated breast positron emission tomography according to the World Health Organization classification of breast tumors. Eur J Surg Oncol 2021;47(7):1588–92.
69. Schilling K, Narayanan D, Kalinyak JE, et al. Positron emission mammography in breast cancer presurgical planning: comparisons with magnetic resonance imaging. Eur J Nucl Med Mol Imaging 2011;38(1):23–36.
70. Noritake M, Narui K, Kaneta T, et al. Evaluation of the response to breast cancer neoadjuvant chemotherapy using 18F-FDG positron emission mammography compared with whole-body 18F-FDG PET: a prospective observational study. Clin Nucl Med 2017;42(3):169–75.
71. Koyasu H, Goshima S, Noda Y, et al. The feasibility of dedicated breast PET for the assessment of residual tumor after neoadjuvant chemotherapy. Jpn J Radiol 2019;37(1):81–7.
72. Sasada S, Masumoto N, Goda N, et al. Dedicated breast PET for detecting residual disease after neoadjuvant chemotherapy in operable breast cancer: a prospective cohort study. Eur J Surg Oncol 2018;44(4):444–8.

73. Soldevilla-Gallardo I, Medina-Ornelas SS, Villarreal-Garza C, et al. Usefulness of positron emission mammography in the evaluation of response to neoadjuvant chemotherapy in patients with breast cancer. Am J Nucl Med Mol Imaging 2018;8(5):341–50.

74. Yamamoto Y, Tasaki Y, Kuwada Y, et al. A preliminary report of breast cancer screening by positron emission mammography. Ann Nucl Med 2016;30(2):130–7.

75. Satoh Y, Sekine T, Omiya Y, et al. Reduction of the fluorine-18-labeled fluorodeoxyglucose dose for clinically dedicated breast positron emission tomography. EJNMMI Phys 2019;6(1):21.

76. MacDonald LR, Hippe DS, Bender LC, et al. Positron emission mammography image interpretation for reduced image count levels. J Nucl Med 2016;57(3): 348–54.

77. Teixeira SC, Rebolleda JF, Koolen BB, et al. Evaluation of a hanging-breast PET system for primary tumor visualization in patients with stage I-III breast cancer: comparison with standard PET/CT. AJR Am J Roentgenol 2016;206(6):1307–14.

78. Iima M, Nakamoto Y, Kanao S, et al. Clinical performance of 2 dedicated PET scanners for breast imaging: initial evaluation. J Nucl Med 2012;53(10):1534–42.

79. O'Connor MK, Tran TD, Swanson TN, et al. Improved visualization of breast tissue on a dedicated breast PET system through ergonomic redesign of the imaging table. EJNMMI Res 2017;7(1):100.

80. Hashimoto R, Akashi-Tanaka S, Watanabe C, et al. Diagnostic performance of dedicated breast positron emission tomography. Breast Cancer 2022;29(6): 1013–21.

81. Grana-Lopez L, Herranz M, Dominguez-Prado I, et al. Dedicated breast PET value to evaluate BI-RADS 4 breast lesions. Eur J Radiol 2018;108:201–7.

82. Jones EF, Ray KM, Li W, et al. Initial experience of dedicated breast PET imaging of ER+ breast cancers using [F-18]fluoroestradiol. NPJ Breast Cancer 2019;5:12.

83. Thakur ML, Zhang K, Berger A, et al. VPAC1 receptors for imaging breast cancer: a feasibility study. J Nucl Med 2013;54(7):1019–25.

Treatment

Incorporating Value-Based Decisions in Breast Cancer Treatment Algorithms

Ton Wang, MD, MS[a], Lesly A. Dossett, MD, MPH[b,c],*

KEYWORDS

- Breast cancer • De-implementation • Overtreatment • Value in health care
- Cancer care continuum

KEY POINTS

- Patients with early-stage breast cancer have an excellent prognosis and are at risk of overtreatment.
- There are many evidence-based opportunities to improve value across the breast cancer care continuum, requiring thoughtful approaches to breast cancer screening, diagnostics, surgical oncology, medical oncology, and radiation oncology.
- Value-based decisions in breast cancer care offer the opportunity to improve patient outcomes while minimizing the risks associated with low-value services.

INTRODUCTION: DEFINING "VALUE" IN BREAST CANCER CARE

Value in health care is measured by improvements in patient health outcomes relative to the cost of achieving that result.[1] This definition is centered around the patient, with the expectation that health-care services rendered provide a measurable benefit. While the goal of achieving high-value care is often mistaken for pure cost-saving efforts, the emphasis is on the delivery of appropriate but not excessive or potentially harmful care.

The United States spends $760 to 935 billion annually on health-care waste.[2] A significant and avoidable sector of waste is low-value care, defined as unnecessary tests, procedures, medications, or other services resulting in increased health-care expenditures without a clinically meaningful benefit. This issue is particularly important in cancer care which was estimated in 2019 to cost Americans over $21 billion annually

This article previously appeared in Surgical Oncology Clinics volume 32 issue 4 October 2023.
ᵃ Department of Surgery, Cedars-Sinai Medical Center, Los Angeles, CA, USA; ᵇ Department of Surgery, University of Michigan, Ann Arbor, MI, USA; ᶜ Institute for Healthcare Policy and Innovation, University of Michigan, 1500 East Medical Center Drive, Ann Arbor, MI 48109, USA
* Corresponding author.
E-mail address: ldossett@umich.edu

Clinics Collections 14 (2024) 241–261
https://doi.org/10.1016/j.ccol.2024.02.019
2352-7986/24/© 2024 Elsevier Inc. All rights reserved.

in out-of-pocket costs and lost wages.[3] Of all cancer types, the costs associated with breast cancer diagnosis and survivorship is the greatest, with risks of financial toxicity present long after the initial diagnosis.[4,5]

There are numerous opportunities to improve value in breast cancer care. The delivery of high-value care requires balancing patient preferences with evidence-based practice to develop a high-value approach. This review summarizes the current literature and recommends strategies to avoid overtreatment throughout the breast cancer care continuum with the goal of improving patient outcomes while minimizing the risks associated with low-value services.

IMPROVING VALUE-BASED DECISIONS IN SCREENING AND DIAGNOSTICS
Genetic Testing

Although most breast cancers are sporadic, approximately 5% to 10% are associated with a heritable syndrome.[6] The implications of diagnosing a pathogenic mutation have evolved with the introduction of new breast cancer therapies. Consequently, identifying high-penetrance mutations (BRCA1, BRCA2, CDH1, PALB2, PTEN, and TP53) has the potential to affect screening, surgical, and medical decision-making for patients and their family members. However, the potential benefits of genetic testing must be balanced against the overall low prevalence of high-penetrance pathogenic or likely variants (PGVs) and the potential consequences associated with identifying nonactionable mutations or variants of unknown significance (VUS).

Proponents of multigene panel testing for all breast cancer patients argue clear utility in identifying high-penetrance PGVs. In a prospective study of newly diagnosed breast cancer patients, results from genetic testing changed clinical management in more than 75% of patients.[7] While the majority of these changes were risk-reducing strategies such as high-risk screening, chemoprevention, or specialist referrals, patients with PGVs were also found to have alterations in surgical and chemotherapy strategies for their primary breast cancer. Notably, this study found similar numbers of PGVs and subsequent changes in clinical management in patients who both did and did not meet National Comprehensive Cancer Network (NCCN) screening guidelines. This is consistent with studies showing that traditional screening strategies relying on family history, patient age, or other risk factors miss up to 50% of all potentially actionable genetic mutations.[8,9]

While it was previously difficult to directly link genetic testing to improved patient survival, the OlympiA trial demonstrated improved progression-free survival with the Poly ADP-ribose polymerase (PARP) inhibitor Olaparib for germline BRCA1/2 patients with early-stage breast cancer.[10] This trial was particularly groundbreaking for utilizing targeted therapy in the adjuvant setting rather than in metastatic disease, underscoring a need to identify patients with actionable mutations earlier in their clinical course. In addition, the potential impact of diagnosing a PGV is not limited to a patient's initial breast cancer treatment. Patients with high-penetrance mutations for breast cancer are known to be at risk of other cancer types and should be counseled on the need for risk-reducing surgeries (eg, bilateral salpingo-oophorectomy for patients with BRCA1/2 mutations or total gastrectomy for patients with CDH1 mutations) and modified screening protocols for other cancer types.[11] Finally, the identification of a PGV in a breast cancer patient can trigger cascade genetic testing, in which relatives of an index patient are offered genetic testing. Although cascade testing is infrequently implemented, it is a cost-effective cancer-prevention strategy with the potential to exponentially impact surveillance and management strategies of at-risk individuals.[12]

Despite the potential advantages, there are several risks of universal multigene panel testing. Pretest and posttest genetic counseling provides patients with detailed risk assessments and has been shown to improve accuracy of risk perception and decrease cancer-related worry, anxiety, and depression.[13] As a result, candidates for genetic testing should be referred for appropriate counseling. The expanding indications for genetic testing have led to a national shortage of trained genetic counselors; estimates suggest there is only 1 genetic counselor per 300,000 people in the United States.[14] A fully implemented universal multigene panel testing strategy would exacerbate this issue and result in many patients who do not receive appropriate counseling about the implications of their testing results. Some strategies to expand the reach of genetic counseling include telemedicine visits, web-based patient education platforms, and specialized training of selected medical providers to serve as genetic counselor extenders.[15]

The costs of genetic testing have decreased significantly, and contemporary analyses suggest that a universal testing strategy can be cost-effective.[16] However, the costs of genetic testing are not limited to the test itself, and the indirect costs associated with identifying PGVs in low- to moderate-penetrance genes or VUS must be considered. In studies of multigene panel testing, up to 50% of patients can be found to have a VUS.[8] The identification of mutations for which guidelines do not support a change in breast cancer management has been shown to result in overtreatment, unindicated high-risk surveillance, and patient anxiety, all of which are costly and potentially harmful.[17] In one study of patients with BRCA1/2 VUS, nearly 40% of patients without a diagnosis of breast cancer received prophylactic bilateral mastectomies. In follow-up, 22% of patients underwent reclassification of their VUS, with 95% of reclassifications as benign.[18] Similarly, while current guidelines support bilateral mastectomy in patients with high-penetrance mutations, best practice for management of moderate-penetrance genes such as *ATM* and *CHEK2* (2- to 4-fold increased risk of breast cancer) are less clear. Despite a lack of evidence to support prophylactic surgery in these patients, studies suggest nearly a third of patients without breast cancer and half of patients with breast cancer who have mutations in moderate-penetrance genes receive bilateral mastectomies, equivalent to that of patients with high-penetrance mutations.[19,20]

Breast Magnetic Resonance Imaging for Screening in Women at Average Risk

Breast magnetic resonance imaging (MRI) has emerged as an important imaging adjunct for patients because of its high sensitivity for cancer detection (95% vs 55% for mammogram).[21] Meta-analyses demonstrate that MRI can increase identification of additional malignancies, with the finding of a synchronous ipsilateral or contralateral cancer in up to 16% and 4% of patients, respectively.[22,23] While the role of MRI for breast cancer screening in high-risk patients (defined as >20% lifetime breast cancer risk) is well-established and cost-effective, population-based studies suggest more than 80% of patients undergoing screening breast MRI are patients at average risk.[24,25]

A potential reason why breast MRI utilization has increased dramatically in the last two decades is conflicting evidence as to whether breast MRI is a better screening tool in patients with dense breasts. Legislation in the United States requires patients to be notified if they have heterogeneously or extremely dense breasts; however, this includes nearly 50% of women in the age range of 40 to 74 years.[26] The DENSE trial in the Netherlands was the first randomized, controlled trial to specifically evaluate the role of breast MRI as an adjunct in patients with extremely dense breasts and normal screening mammograms.[27] Although this study demonstrated breast MRI results in increased detection of breast cancer over mammography alone, the variable sensitivity of breast MRI resulted in a false-positive rate of 8%.

Breast MRI is a costly study with an average payment of $1200, compared to $350 for diagnostic mammography, $130 for tomosynthesis, and $130 for ultrasound.[28] Abbreviated breast MRI has been proposed as a solution to decrease the time of image acquisition, study reading time, and subsequent cost of breast MRI to increase its value as a screening tool.[29] Abbreviated breast MRI, which relies on rapid protocols capturing the very early postcontrast phase, has equal sensitivity and specificity to traditional breast MRI in detecting breast cancer at a fraction of the time and cost. However, breast MRI is associated with significant care cascades that must be considered before widespread implementation of screening MRI. Studies have consistently demonstrated that receipt of breast MRI is an independent risk factor for surgical overtreatment with unilateral and contralateral mastectomy.[30,31] In addition, breast MRI recipients have significantly greater mammary and extramammary cascade events including additional imaging, procedures, clinic visits, hospitalizations, and new diagnoses with higher total and out-of-pocket spending.[32]

Screening in Asymptomatic Patients with a Limited Life Expectancy

None of the randomized controlled trials that established the efficacy of screening mammography included patients older than 74 years, and thus the value of breast cancer screening in elderly patients is unknown.[33] For breast cancer screening, meta-analyses demonstrate a lag-time of approximately 10 years to prevent 1 death per 1000 people screened, suggesting minimal utility of breast cancer screening in patients with a limited life expectancy.[34] Consequently, national guidelines recommend cessation of routine screening mammography in patients with a less than a 5- to 10-year life expectancy. Despite these recommendations, studies show that up to 53% of women with a high 9-year mortality risk receive screening mammography.[35]

The harms associated with breast cancer screening in women with limited life expectancy result from care cascades associated with a false-positive result and overdiagnosis of in-situ or low-risk carcinomas. Estimates suggest that over a 10-year screening period, 20% of women aged ≥ 75 years will experience a false-positive mammogram, which can result in additional imaging, unnecessary biopsies, and significant anxiety and distress.[36] In addition, women with a limited life expectancy are at high risk of overdiagnosis for low-risk breast cancers that may have never become symptomatic or otherwise impacted their quality of life.

The reasons for persistent breast cancer screening despite limited life-expectancy are multifactorial. Obtaining an annual mammogram as part of routine health care is an entrenched habit developed over several decades, and physician recommendation for screening cessation is insufficient to influence patient behavior.[37,38] This is supported by studies showing that among individuals who recall having had a discussion about screening cessation with their physician, 40% plan to continue cancer screening.[39] At least some patient hesitancy to trust recommendations for screening cessation is related to poor accuracy of clinician and patient survival predictions, with studies showing both groups overestimate life expectancy.[40,41] This bias is compounded by a tendency to overestimate the benefits and underestimate the risks of receiving a particular medical intervention.[42,43] Some strategies to deimplement breast cancer screening in older women with limited life expectancies include the incorporation of validated life-expectancy calculators, decision-aids, and reframing screening cessation from "taking something away" from patients to "redistributing health-care priorities".[44,45]

IMPROVING VALUE-BASED DECISIONS IN BREAST SURGICAL ONCOLOGY
Utilization of Outpatient Mastectomy and Enhanced Recovery After Surgery Protocols

The safety of outpatient mastectomy in patients undergoing bilateral mastectomies, modified radical mastectomy, and immediate implant-based breast reconstruction is well established, with systematic reviews showing no difference in major or minor complications, including rates of hematoma, seroma, reoperations, or readmissions for patients undergoing same-day unilateral or bilateral mastectomy with or without implant-based immediate reconstruction.[46] Outpatient surgery offers many benefits to health-care systems including significant cost savings and the opportunity to increase inpatient capacity for other admissions, an advantage that was notable during the COVID-19 pandemic.[47] In addition to financial benefits, outpatient surgery is associated with improved patient satisfaction, decreased opioid usage, decreased anxiety, and improved time to independence.[47,48]

Although same-day mastectomy has been shown to be feasible for over 20 years, only approximately 20% of mastectomies nationally are performed as outpatient procedures.[49] Unlike many other cancer operations such as pancreatectomies that are largely centralized in major medical centers, breast cancer operations are decentralized and therefore subject to significant variations in performance patterns. A recent study of facilities across the state of Michigan demonstrated that only 16% of mastectomies without reconstruction were performed as an outpatient procedure, and 23% of patients were admitted for 2 days or more.[50] These variations in practice patterns accounted for a nearly 2-fold difference in 30- and 90-day episode cost.

A commonly cited barrier to same-day mastectomy is the concern about inadequate pain control in the outpatient setting. This concern has largely been addressed through protocols for multimodal pain management based on Enhanced Recovery After Surgery principles.[51,52] There are several instances in which institutional implementation of outpatient protocols for same-day mastectomy with or without reconstruction have been highly successful. A notable example is the Kaiser Permanente Northern California group which instituted a pilot project across 21 medical centers to Implement same-day unilateral or bilateral mastectomy with or without immediate breast reconstruction over a 6-month time period.[53] The protocol included preoperative patient education, multimodal analgesia, and a defined postoperative care plan and was highly successful, increasing same-day mastectomy rates from 16% to 75%.

De-escalation of Axillary Surgery in Breast Cancer Patients

Lymphedema occurs in 20% of patients after axillary lymph node dissection (ALND), with the risk doubling when combined with adjuvant chemotherapy or radiotherapy.[54,55] While the risks associated with ALND are well-accepted, long-term studies demonstrate that up to 5% of patients undergoing sentinel lymph node biopsy (SLNB) also develop lymphedema.[54] Long-term consequences of lymphedema include infectious complications, frequent utilization of outpatient medical services, significantly restricted mobility, reduced quality of life, and decreased psychosocial well-being.[56,57] In addition, lymphedema is a leading cause of financial toxicity in breast cancer survivors, accounting for decreased ability to return to work and up to 112% higher out-of-pocket costs up to 10 years after breast cancer diagnosis.[5,58] As a result, de-escalation of axillary surgery in appropriate circumstances has the potential to significantly improve long-term outcomes for breast cancer survivors.

Current evidence supports the de-escalation of axillary surgery in three circumstances. The first is avoiding ALND in patients with limited nodal disease who are undergoing breast-conserving surgery (BCS) with adjuvant radiotherapy. This recommendation is based on results from the ACOSOG Z0011 trial which demonstrated no improvement in disease-free or overall survival with completion ALND for patients with 1 to 2 positive sentinel lymph nodes.[59] The second is avoiding upfront ALND without attempting SLNB in patients with previously positive axillary lymph nodes who become clinically node negative (cN0) following neoadjuvant chemotherapy. This is based on the SENTINA and ACOSOG Z1071 trials which demonstrated the feasibility and accuracy of SLNB for axillary staging in these patients.[60,61] The final is avoiding routine SLNB in cN0 women ≥70 years old with estrogen-receptor-positive (ER+), HER2-negative (HER2−) early-stage breast cancer. This is based on the CALGB 9343 trial which demonstrated no improvement in breast-cancer-specific or overall survival with nodal staging.[62]

Current national trends suggest appropriate omission of completion ALND for patients undergoing BCS is excellent, with recent studies showing only 14% of patients who are potential candidates for omission of ALND receiving this procedure.[63] Similarly, national rates of SLNB in clinically node-positive patients who become cN0 following neoadjuvant chemotherapy have increased significantly from 30% in 2012 to 50% in 2015 following dissemination of clinical trial results, and the current rate of SLNB is likely much higher.[64] However, SLNB in older women with low-risk, cN0 breast cancer continues to be performed at high rates, with estimates suggesting that up to 87% of patients who are eligible of SLNB omission continue to receive this procedure.[63] In addition to the risk for lymphedema and other surgical complications associated with SLNB in women ≥70 years old, axillary staging at the time of breast cancer resection is associated with a 65% increase in 90-day episode cost and increased likelihood of care cascades, including a nearly 2-fold increase in postoperative radiotherapy for women who may have been candidates for omission of both axillary staging and radiotherapy.[65]

Potential patient-level barriers to the deimplementation of SLNB in older patients include a desire to know their pathological axillary status for "peace of mind," the perception they are healthier than average patient and more likely to benefit from additional therapies, and concern that age-based guidelines are discriminatory.[66] Some strategies to reduce low-value SLNB at the patient level include emphasizing the excellent prognosis associated with early-stage, ER+ breast cancer; educating patients on the risks of overtreatment; and improved decision-making tools such as decision aids.[66–68] Potential provider-level barriers to the deimplementation of SLNB in older patients with early-stage breast cancer include the belief that it is a low-risk procedure that adds minimal time to an operation and the misperception that the result of the biopsy will change adjuvant chemotherapy or radiotherapy recommendations.[69] However, the results of RxPONDER and supporting retrospective studies have increasingly emphasized that nodal status does not predict tumor biology and that recurrence scores based on genomic tests such as Oncotype Dx and Mammaprint more accurately predict benefit from adjuvant therapies.[70,71]

Contralateral Prophylactic Mastectomy in Average-Risk Patients with Unilateral Breast Cancer

The utilization of contralateral prophylactic mastectomy (CPM) has increased over the last two decades, with a greater proportion of patients electing for bilateral mastectomy after a diagnosis of breast cancer without a clear indication. Recent estimates suggesting that bilateral mastectomies comprise 10% to 13% of all breast cancer procedures and 28% to 30% of all mastectomy cases.[72] Notably, this trend includes patients with early stage or in situ breast cancers who would otherwise be excellent candidates for breast conservation therapy.[73]

The single greatest factor contributing to widespread utilization of CPM is the increasing availability of breast reconstruction.[73,74] In one analysis of women with unilateral breast cancer, 46% of patients who received CPM underwent breast reconstruction compared with 17% of patients who received unilateral mastectomy.[74] Compared with unilateral mastectomy, bilateral mastectomy with breast reconstruction is known to be an independent risk factor for major and minor postoperative complications including wound complications, need for reoperation, flap loss for patients undergoing autologous reconstruction, and longer length of stay.[75,76] In addition, despite more extensive oncologic surgery and potential history of radiation to the therapeutic side, the risk associated with a postoperative complication after bilateral mastectomy has been shown to be equivalent between the therapeutic and prophylactic side, with nearly 20% of patients experiencing a complication on the prophylactic breast.[77]

Unsurprisingly, CPM is associated with significantly higher costs than unilateral mastectomy during the index oncologic procedure and additional reconstructive procedures, particularly given the average patient requires 2 to 3 operations to complete breast reconstruction.[78–80] Cost-effectiveness studies have attempted to justify CPM given the potential savings associated with cessation of life-long screening surveillance.[81] However, the literature suggests many patients continue to receive non-evidence-based imaging surveillance following bilateral mastectomy.[82] Importantly, the financial burden of CPM is not limited to costs to the health-care system; compared with BCS, patients undergoing bilateral mastectomy report higher incurred debt, altered employment, and financial toxicity.[83]

The reasons for the increased popularity and high utilization of CPM are complex. Multiple studies have shown the decision for bilateral mastectomy to be preference sensitiveness and that patient-level factors driving an increase in CPM rates include a desire for "peace of mind," the misperception that a more intensive surgery will improve survival, and potential for improved symmetry.[84,85] No single strategy for the deimplementation of CPM exists. However, current evidence suggests definite gaps in patient preoperative education; studies suggest patients have poor understanding of the risks of bilateral mastectomy including increased postoperative complications, loss of skin and nipple sensation, and financial toxicity while simultaneously overestimating the oncologic benefit.[86,87]

IMPROVING VALUE-BASED DECISIONS IN MEDICAL ONCOLOGY
Routine Staging of Asymptomatic Patients at Low Risk of Metastatic Breast Cancer

National organizations advise against routine staging with CT, positron emission tomography (PET), or bone scans for asymptomatic patients with early-stage breast cancer based on evidence that only 0.2% and 1.2% of patients with stage I or II breast cancer, respectively, are found to have distant metastases on preoperative staging.[88] However, the risk of false-positive results or incidental findings associated with unnecessary diagnostic testing is costly and can result in harmful care cascades. Despite these recommendations, routine staging scans remain prevalent. In one study evaluating the utilization of staging chest CTs in patients with clinical stage I or II breast, 11% of stage I breast cancer patients and 36% of stage II breast cancer patients underwent a staging chest CT.[89] Although 23% of stage I patients were found to have pulmonary nodules, only 1% of all patients had pulmonary metastases. However, the finding of a pulmonary nodule resulted in an average of 2.3 follow-up CTs, with some patients followed up for several years with up to 16 additional CT scans.

Efforts from Choosing Wisely and American Society of Clinical Oncology to reduce unnecessary staging for patients diagnosed with early-stage breast cancer have had a modest impact, with time-series analyses of national data showing a 16% decline in imaging overutilization following the release of guidelines to avoid routine staging scans.[90] Similarly, state-wide registries have shown a significant decrease over time in utilization of staging scans for patients with stage 0-IIA breast cancer, but not stage IIB.[91] Greater deimplementation of routine staging for asymptomatic, early-stage breast cancer patients will require more than published guidelines; although studies suggest over 80% of physicians treating breast cancer are aware of guidelines recommending against routine staging, they are not influenced to order less imaging.[92] While this finding has been attributed to patient preferences, studies evaluating physician-level variation associated with overutilization found the odds of a patient receiving staging scans were 3-fold higher if the ordering physician's prior patient also received scans, suggesting provider-driven overutilization.[93]

Personalized Decision-Making for Adjuvant Chemotherapy

While the development of novel chemotherapeutic agents has resulted in improved survival for breast cancer patients, an equally ground-breaking advance has been the ability to leverage genomic testing to identify patients who can safely omit adjuvant chemotherapy. The TAILORx and RxPONDER trials demonstrated the utility of the 21-gene Oncotype Dx recurrence score in predicting the absolute benefit of adjuvant chemotherapy in patients with ER+/HER2− disease, shifting this decision from one that was largely based on anatomical staging to one based on tumor biology.[70,94] As a result, there has been a decrease in national rates of chemotherapy utilization, with one study showing a decline from 27% in 2013 to 14% in 2015 among patients with stage I-II ER+/HER2− disease and a decline from 81% to 64% among patients with node-positive disease.[95] This decrease in adjuvant chemotherapy administration has occurred concurrently with increased utilization of recurrence score tests.[96]

The routine incorporation of genomic tests into practice offers a key opportunity for improving value in breast cancer care. The benefit of this personalized approach is greatest in older patients who are the most vulnerable to the toxicities of chemotherapy. Simulations suggest older patients with hormone receptor (HR) positive breast cancer may experience negative quality-adjusted life-years if they receive chemotherapy compared with endocrine therapy alone.[97] Before RxPONDER, postmenopausal patients with node-positive disease would likely have been considered to be at high risk and recommended adjuvant chemotherapy. However, incorporating recurrence risk scores into the decision-making algorithm has significantly improved the likelihood that an individual patient will benefit from adjuvant chemotherapy.

IMPROVING VALUE-BASED DECISIONS IN RADIATION ONCOLOGY
Radiotherapy Omission in Older Patients with Low-Risk Breast Cancer

Although all breast cancer patients have traditionally been treated with the same combination of therapies, modern evidence suggests older women are more likely to be diagnosed with ER+ breast cancers with favorable tumor biology.[98] These tumors are associated with an excellent long-term prognosis, and the probability of a woman aged ≥70 years dying from breast cancer is less than 1%.[99] As a result, substantial evidence exists to support the de-escalation of certain adjuvant therapies, including radiotherapy, in this low-risk population.

There are two key trials supporting radiotherapy omission for older women with small, ER+ breast cancers. The CALGB 9343 trial randomized cN0 breast cancer patients aged ≥70 years with ER+ tumors ≤2 cm to endocrine therapy alone or whole-breast radiotherapy and endocrine therapy.[62] This was followed by the PRIME II trial, which randomized pathologically node-negative breast cancer patients aged ≥65 years with ER+ tumors ≤3 cm to endocrine therapy alone or whole-breast radiotherapy and endocrine therapy.[100] The findings from both trials confirmed an expected higher rate of locoregional recurrence for the cohorts treated without radiotherapy, but no difference in rates of salvage mastectomy, distant metastases, or breast-cancer-specific and overall survival. In fact, the 10-year breast-cancer-specific survival in the CALGB 9343 trial was >97%, regardless of radiotherapy receipt. These findings have led to additional efforts to expand the indications for adjuvant radiotherapy omission; the preliminary results of the LUMINA trial suggest patients aged ≥55 years with stage I, low- to intermediate-grade luminal A tumors receiving endocrine therapy can safely omit adjuvant radiotherapy after BCS with a 5-year local recurrence rate of only 2.3%.[101]

While the improvement in locoregional recurrence is often cited to justify adjuvant radiotherapy in this low-risk population, it is notable that the locoregional recurrence rate at 10 years in both CALGB 9343 and PRIME II, was 10%, which is within the accepted range for locoregional recurrence following breast cancer treatment.[62,100] In addition, the modern rate of locoregional recurrence is likely lower than reported in these trials, given these trials used tamoxifen for endocrine therapy rather than the more efficacious aromatase inhibitors typically used today.[102]

Importantly, women aged ≥70 years with cN0, stage I ER+ breast cancer should not be required to undergo SLNB to be considered for omission of adjuvant radiotherapy. CALGB 9343 did not require pathological confirmation of negative nodal status as an inclusion criterion.[62] This trial predated widespread utilization of SLNB, and two-thirds of patients did not undergo any axillary staging given the morbidity of ALND for staging purposes. This is further supported by retrospective studies suggesting adjuvant radiotherapy does not improve survival even in patients with pathologically node-positive lymph nodes if they receive endocrine therapy.[103]

Despite the strong data supporting the safety of radiotherapy omission in cN0 breast cancer patients aged ≥70 years with stage I ER+ tumors, up to 65% of patients eligible for omission continue to receive adjuvant radiotherapy after BCS, a trend that has remained stable since 2005 when the NCCN guidelines were updated to allow for radiotherapy omission in this low-risk population.[104] The overutilization of radiotherapy is costly; the estimated cost of radiotherapy ranges from $5300 per patient for accelerated partial-beam irradiation (APBI) to $13,000 for whole-breast radiation.[65,105] In addition to the financial consequences, older patients are at higher risk of experiencing significant decreases in quality of life with adjuvant radiotherapy, which is supported by studies showing that older women heavily consider the frequency of appointments required for radiotherapy and its impact on their caregivers.[66,106] While there are likely some patient-level factors contributing to the persistent utilization of radiotherapy in older women with low-risk breast cancer, studies have shown that if given the choice, most patients would decline radiotherapy.[66,107] Rather, the decision is heavily influenced by provider recommendations and a tendency for both patients and providers to overestimate the potential benefit of radiotherapy in improving locoregional recurrence rates.[106,108]

Shorter Radiation Therapy Schedules in Appropriate Patients

The original studies supporting adjuvant whole-breast irradiation following BCS used a conventional fractionation schedule delivering 1.8 to 2 Gy per fraction over 5 to 7 weeks. Since that time, multiple trials have demonstrated the efficacy of hypofractionation of whole-breast irradiation, which delivers a higher dose per fraction over 3 to 4 weeks, at providing equivalent locoregional control, cosmesis, and potentially reduced acute toxicities. In addition to improved patient convenience, hypofractionation is significantly cheaper.[109] Although the initial American Society for Radiation Oncology (ASTRO) guidelines in 2011 endorsed hypofractionation only for patients aged ≥50 years with pT1-2N0 tumors, updated guidelines in 2018 expanded the indications to recommend hypofractionated whole-breast irradiation delivered in 15 to 16 fractions as the preferred regimen for all breast cancer patients, regardless of age or tumor characteristics.

Despite the significant advantages of hypofractionated regimens, adoption in the United States has been slow, with studies showing conventional fractionation remains the most common method of delivery, with under 40% of patients receiving hypofractionation.[110] This contrasts significantly with the relatively quick adoption of hypofractionation schedules internationally, with shorter radiotherapy schedules the current standard of care in Canada and the United Kingdom.[110] Although there are relatively little data on national practice patterns over the last few years, there is some evidence that the resource-limited environment of the COVID-19 pandemic may have encouraged more widespread adoption of hypofractionation in the United States.[111]

Similarly, APBI offers another opportunity to personalize adjuvant radiotherapy for a subset of patients with low-risk tumor features. While randomized trials comparing APBI techniques via brachytherapy, external beam, or intraoperative radiation have demonstrated noninferiority when compared with whole-breast radiotherapy, APBI has been associated with poorer long-term cosmetic outcomes and worse long-term locoregional control for patients with higher-risk tumor features.[112,113] However, APBI is associated with significant cost savings compared with whole-breast irradiation, the shorter treatment schedule is more convenient for patients, and patients who are reluctant to accept adjuvant radiotherapy due to the concern for side effects may find APBI acceptable. As a result, ASTRO allows for APBI as an alternative to whole-breast irradiation following BCS in patients aged ≥50 years with Tis-T1 breast cancer and negative margins.[114]

IMPROVING VALUE-BASED DECISIONS IN POSTCANCER SURVEILLANCE
Breast Cancer Surveillance Recommendations for Detecting Locoregional Recurrence

Current national guidelines recommend annual mammography for locoregional surveillance for patients undergoing BCS. The recommendation for when to obtain the first mammogram after surgery differs, with some organizations suggesting that the first mammogram be obtained 6 months after surgery to establish a baseline and confirm removal of the imaging abnormality.[115] Although some institutions routinely perform semi-annual mammography for the first 2 to 5 years after BCS because of the higher risk of locoregional recurrence in the early postoperative years, there are no data to suggest this improves detection of locoregional recurrence compared with annual mammography.[116]

For patients undergoing mastectomy with or without reconstruction, there is some controversy about the appropriateness of imaging surveillance, with most national guidelines recommending against any routine imaging. An exception is the American College of Radiology, which states that surveillance mammography with or without digital breast tomosynthesis may be appropriate for patients undergoing mastectomy with tissue-based reconstruction.[117] No studies have demonstrated the cost-effectiveness of routine postmastectomy surveillance with mammography, breast ultrasound, or breast MRI when compared with clinical breast exam alone. A recent systematic review and meta-analysis demonstrated low yield of imaging surveillance following mastectomy with or with reconstruction, with an overall pooled cancer detection rate ranging from 1.9 per 1000 examinations for mammography to 5.2 per 1000 examinations for MRI.[82] For all imaging modalities, the rates of imaging-detected cancers were lower than the overall cancer detection rates, suggesting most cancers were clinically detected on physical exam.

Breast Cancer Surveillance Recommendations for Detecting Distant Recurrence

To date, there is no evidence that early detection of breast cancer metastasis improves breast-cancer-specific or overall survival.[118] Consequently, national guidelines recommend against routine imaging or laboratory testing for asymptomatic patients treated with a curative intent.[119] While it is notable these recommendations are based on older studies that predate current imaging techniques, improved understanding of tumor biology, and modern systemic therapies, an updated Cochrane review in 2016 again did not support routine surveillance imaging.[120] A recent study evaluating outcomes of patients with recurrent disease detected on surveillance imaging versus symptoms showed a potential survival benefit with detection of recurrence on imaging for patients with high-risk tumor subtypes (HER2+, triple negative breast cancers), but no benefit for patients with ER+, HER2− breast cancers.[121]

Utilization of surveillance imaging such as PET-CT scans and radionuclide bone scans vary widely among providers. In addition to being costly and associated with false-positive findings, these studies are frequently no better than physical exam alone. For example, most bony metastases are diagnosed based on symptoms rather than imaging.[122] Similarly, tumor markers such as CA 1503, CA 27.29, CEA, and "liquid biopsies" have not been shown to be sensitive nor specific and can lead to either false reassurance or significant anxiety if elevated without an imaging correlate.[123] Despite the lack of utility, tumor markers continue to be used at high rates by providers, with recent surveys suggesting over 40% of oncologists routinely order tumor marker testing.[124] One study found that 42% of patients aged 65 years and older with stage I-III breast cancer received at least 1 tumor marker test within 2 years of diagnosis.[125] Tumor marker testing was associated with increased receipt of advanced imaging and subsequent biopsy. In addition, patients who underwent tumor marker testing had significantly increased overall cost of care by 35% in the first 12 months after diagnosis and by 28% in months 13 to 24 after diagnosis.

SUMMARY

In conclusion, breast cancer treatment has evolved significantly in the last few decades with an increasing emphasis on tailoring treatment recommendations based on tumor biology. With this has come a natural de-escalation of care for patients with favorable tumor characteristics, with multiple clinical trials in surgical, medical, and radiation oncology supporting the safety of omitting previously routine care in selected patients. The ability to personalize cancer therapies based on a patient's tumor biology offers a key opportunity to ensure that patients receive high-value services across the breast cancer care continuum.

CLINICS CARE POINTS

Recommendations	
Screening and diagnostics	
Genetic testing	There is significant variability in recommendations from major organizations on which patients genetic testing should be ordered.

	National Comprehensive Cancer Network (NCCN) guidelines are the most restrictive and suggest testing for high-penetrance breast cancer susceptibility genes under limited circumstances based on patient age, tumor type, family history, and probability models.
	American Society of Clinical Oncology (ASCO) guidelines recommend genetic testing be offered to individuals with a personal or family history with features suggestive of a genetic cancer susceptibility gene if the results will influence management of the patient or at-risk family members. ASCO recommends that all genetic testing be accompanied by pretest and posttest counseling.
	The American Society of Breast Surgeons (ASBrS) has advocated for genetic testing in all individuals diagnosed with breast cancer.
Breast magnetic resonance imaging (MRI) for breast cancer screening in average-risk women	NCCN, ASBrS, and American College of Surgeons (ACS) agree that breast MRI should not be used for routine breast cancer screening in average-risk women.
	Indications for screening breast MRI include: • Screening in patients at high risk for breast cancer, defined as a high-risk germline genetic mutation, a history of chest wall irradiation, or >20-25% lifetime risk of breast cancer based on a probability model. • As a diagnostic adjunct to mammography after weighing the risks vs benefits.
Breast cancer screening cessation in asymptomatic women with limited life expectancy	ASBrS and ACS recommend cessation of screening mammography in women with a less than 5–10 y life expectancy, even among women with a personal history of breast cancer.
	The United States Preventive Services Task Force (USPSTF) recommends breast cancer screening for patients up to the age of 74 years. For patients aged $\geq$75 y, USPSTF concludes that there is insufficient evidence to assess the risks vs benefits of continued screening.
Breast surgical oncology Breast surgery in the outpatient setting	Unilateral and bilateral mastectomy with or without immediate reconstruction is safe in the outpatient setting and should be performed concurrently with the implementation of an Enhanced Recovery After Surgery (ERAS) protocol.
	An appropriate ERAS protocol should include: • Preoperative education to set expectations for the patient and their family. • Multimodal analgesia in the preoperative and postoperative setting to limit opioid utilization and improve likelihood of discharge from the recovery suite. • A plan for close postoperative follow-up.
De-escalation of axillary surgery	Current evidence supports de-escalation of axillary surgery in three circumstances: 1. Avoid axillary lymph node dissection (ALND) in patients with cT1-T2, cN0 invasive breast cancer with 1–2 positive lymph nodes who are undergoing breast-conserving surgery (BCS) with adjuvant radiotherapy. 2. Avoid ALND without first performing sentinel lymph node biopsy (SLNB) in patients with previously

clinically node-positive breast cancer who become cN0 following neoadjuvant chemotherapy.

3. Avoid SLNB in cN0 women aged ≥70 years with ER+, HER2− early-stage breast cancer.

Contralateral prophylactic mastectomy

Major organizations including ASBrS recommend against bilateral mastectomy for patients with unilateral breast cancer at average risk of contralateral breast cancer. Patients who strongly desire this procedure should be fully educated on the lack of survival benefit associated with contralateral prophylactic mastectomy, increased postoperative risks of bilateral surgery, higher potential for financial toxicity, and uncertainty regarding long-term patient-reported outcomes.

Breast medical oncology

Staging for patients with early-stage breast cancer

<1% of patients with early-stage breast cancer have metastatic disease at diagnosis. ASCO and NCCN recommend against routine staging for asymptomatic patients with stage 0-II breast cancer.

Personalizing recommendations for adjuvant chemotherapy

Patients with ER+/HER2− breast cancer should be considered for genomic tests such as Oncotype Dx to evaluate recurrence risk and potential benefit associated with chemotherapy administration. Patients who are not candidates for or who would decline chemotherapy regardless of genomic test results should not undergo testing.

Breast radiation oncology

Radiotherapy in older patients with low-risk breast cancer

NCCN guidelines allow for omission of adjuvant radiotherapy in women aged ≥70 years with pT1, cN0, ER+, HER2− breast cancer who plan to receive adjuvant endocrine therapy.

Patients should be informed of the potential for radiotherapy omission prior to decision-making for BCS vs mastectomy, as this may encourage patients to undergo BCS rather than mastectomy.

The decision to omit SLNB should be independent of the decision to omit radiotherapy in eligible patients.

Shorter adjuvant radiotherapy schedules

ASTRO guidelines support hypofractionation rather than conventional fractionation as the standard of care for all breast cancer patients requiring adjuvant whole breast irradiation.

ASTRO guidelines support accelerated partial-beam irradiation (APBI) as an acceptable alternative to whole breast irradiation in patients ≥ 50 y with T1 invasive breast cancer and negative margins. APBI can also be considered in patients with low-risk ductal carcinoma in situ (DCIS), defined as screen-detected, low to intermediate nuclear grade, ≤ 2.5 cm, and resected with negative margins ≥ 3 mm.

Post-breast-cancer surveillance

Detection of locoregional recurrence

NCCN and ASCO guidelines recommend asymptomatic patients receive routine surveillance with annual mammography, with the first mammogram obtained between 6 and 12 months after breast conserving therapy for breast cancer.

Following mastectomy with or without reconstruction for breast cancer, annual clinical breast exam without any routine imaging is sufficient for surveillance of asymptomatic patients.

Detection of distant recurrence	NCCN and ASCO guidelines recommend against routine surveillance imaging and laboratory markers in asymptomatic patients following breast cancer treatment with curative intent.

DISCLOSURES

The authors have nothing to disclose.

REFERENCES

1. Porter ME. What is value in health care? N Engl J Med 2010;363(26):2477–81.
2. Shrank WH, Rogstad TL, Parekh N. Waste in the US Health Care System: Estimated Costs and Potential for Savings. JAMA 2019;322(15):1501–9.
3. Yabroff KR, Mariotto A, Tangka F, et al. Annual report to the nation on the status of cancer, Part 2: patient economic burden associated with cancer care. J Natl Cancer Inst 2021;113(12):1670–82.
4. Mariotto AB, Enewold L, Zhao J, et al. Medical Care Costs Associated with Cancer Survivorship in the United States. Cancer Epidemiol Biomarkers Prev 2020; 29(7):1304–12.
5. Dean LT, Moss SL, Ransome Y, et al. "It still affects our economic situation": long-term economic burden of breast cancer and lymphedema. Support Care Cancer 2019;27(5):1697–708.
6. Tung N, Lin NU, Kidd J, et al. Frequency of Germline Mutations in 25 Cancer Susceptibility Genes in a Sequential Series of Patients With Breast Cancer. J Clin Oncol 2016;34(13):1460–8.
7. Whitworth PW, Beitsch PD, Patel R, et al. Clinical Utility of Universal Germline Genetic Testing for Patients With Breast Cancer. JAMA Netw Open 2022;5(9): e2232787.
8. Beitsch PD, Whitworth PW, Hughes K, et al. Underdiagnosis of Hereditary Breast Cancer: Are Genetic Testing Guidelines a Tool or an Obstacle? J Clin Oncol 2019;37(6):453–60.
9. Yadav S, Hu C, Hart SN, et al. Evaluation of Germline Genetic Testing Criteria in a Hospital-Based Series of Women With Breast Cancer. J Clin Oncol 2020; 38(13):1409–18.
10. Tutt ANJ, Garber JE, Kaufman B, et al. Adjuvant Olaparib for Patients with BRCA1- or BRCA2-Mutated Breast Cancer. N Engl J Med 2021;384(25):2394–405.
11. National Comprehensive Cancer Network. Genetic/Familial High-Risk Assessment: Breast, Ovarian, and Pancreatic (Version 1.2023). Available at: https://www.nccn.org/professionals/physician_gls/pdf/genetics_bop.pdf.   Published 2022. Accessed December 29, 2022.
12. Roberts MC, Dotson WD, DeVore CS, et al. Delivery Of Cascade Screening For Hereditary Conditions: A Scoping Review Of The Literature. Health Aff 2018; 37(5):801–8.
13. Nelson HD, Pappas M, Zakher B, et al. Risk assessment, genetic counseling, and genetic testing for BRCA-related cancer in women: a systematic review to update the U.S. Preventive Services Task Force recommendation. Ann Intern Med 2014;160(4):255–66.
14. Raspa M, Moultrie R, Toth D, et al. Barriers and Facilitators to Genetic Service Delivery Models: Scoping Review. Interact J Med Res 2021;10(1):e23523.

15. Kinney AY, Steffen LE, Brumbach BH, et al. Randomized Noninferiority Trial of Telephone Delivery of BRCA1/2 Genetic Counseling Compared With In-Person Counseling: 1-Year Follow-Up. J Clin Oncol 2016;34(24):2914–24.

16. Sun L, Brentnall A, Patel S, et al. A Cost-effectiveness Analysis of Multigene Testing for All Patients With Breast Cancer. JAMA Oncol 2019;5(12):1718–30.

17. Murphy BL, YI M, Arun BK, et al. Contralateral Risk-Reducing Mastectomy in Breast Cancer Patients Who Undergo Multigene Panel Testing. Ann Surg Oncol 2020;27(12):4613–21.

18. Welsh JL, Hoskin TL, Day CN, et al. Clinical Decision-Making in Patients with Variant of Uncertain Significance in BRCA1 or BRCA2 Genes. Ann Surg Oncol 2017;24(10):3067–72.

19. Reid S, Roberson ML, Koehler K, et al. Receipt of Bilateral Mastectomy Among Women With Hereditary Breast Cancer. JAMA Oncol 2022;9(1):143–5.

20. Comeaux JG, Culver JO, Lee JE, et al. Risk-reducing mastectomy decisions among women with mutations in high- and moderate- penetrance breast cancer susceptibility genes. Mol Genet Genomic Med 2022;10(10):e2031.

21. Aristokli N, Polycarpou I, Themistocleous SC, et al. Comparison of the diagnostic performance of Magnetic Resonance Imaging (MRI), ultrasound and mammography for detection of breast cancer based on tumor type, breast density and patient's history: A review. Radiography 2022;28(3):848–56.

22. Houssami N, Ciatto S, Macaskill P, et al. Accuracy and surgical impact of magnetic resonance imaging in breast cancer staging: systematic review and meta-analysis In detection of multifocal and multicentric cancer. J Clin Oncol 2008; 26(19):3248–58.

23. Brennan ME, Houssami N, Lord S, et al. Magnetic resonance imaging screening of the contralateral breast in women with newly diagnosed breast cancer: systematic review and meta-analysis of incremental cancer detection and impact on surgical management. J Clin Oncol 2009;27(33):5640–9.

24. Taneja C, Edelsberg J, Weycker D, et al. Cost effectiveness of breast cancer screening with contrast-enhanced MRI in high-risk women. J Am Coll Radiol 2009;6(3):171–9.

25. Stout NK, Nekhlyudov L, Li L, et al. Rapid increase in breast magnetic resonance imaging use: trends from 2000 to 2011. JAMA Intern Med 2014;174(1): 114–21.

26. Kerlikowske K, Miglioretti DL, Vachon CM. Discussions of Dense Breasts, Breast Cancer Risk, and Screening Choices in 2019. JAMA 2019;322(1):69–70.

27. Bakker MF, de Lange SV, Pijnappel RM, et al. Supplemental MRI Screening for Women with Extremely Dense Breast Tissue. N Engl J Med 2019;381(22): 2091–102.

28. Vlahiotis A, Griffin B, Stavros AT, et al. Analysis of utilization patterns and associated costs of the breast imaging and diagnostic procedures after screening mammography. Clinicoecon Outcomes Res 2018;10:157–67.

29. Tollens F, Baltzer PAT, Dietzel M, et al. Economic potential of abbreviated breast MRI for screening women with dense breast tissue for breast cancer. Eur Radiol 2022;32(11):7409–19.

30. Pettit K, Swatske ME, Gao F, et al. The Impact of Breast MRI on Surgical Decision-Making: Are Patients at Risk for Mastectomy? J Surg Oncol 2009; 100(7):553–8.

31. Kuritzky AM, Lee MC. Long-term impact of staging breast magnetic resonance imaging-a risk for overtreatment? Transl Cancer Res 2017;6:S476–8.

32. Ganguli I, Keating NL, Thakore N, et al. Downstream Mammary and Extramammary Cascade Services and Spending Following Screening Breast Magnetic Resonance Imaging vs Mammography Among Commercially Insured Women. JAMA Netw Open 2022;5(4):e227234.

33. Chen TH, Yen AM, Fann JC, et al. Clarifying the debate on population-based screening for breast cancer with mammography: A systematic review of randomized controlled trials on mammography with Bayesian meta-analysis and causal model. Medicine (Baltim) 2017;96(3):e5684.

34. Lee SJ, Boscardin WJ, Stijacic-Cenzer I, et al. Time lag to benefit after screening for breast and colorectal cancer: meta-analysis of survival data from the United States, Sweden, United Kingdom, and Denmark. Bmj-Brit Med J 2013;346: e8441.

35. Royce TJ, Hendrix LH, Stokes WA, et al. Cancer screening rates in individuals with different life expectancies. JAMA Intern Med 2014;174(10):1558–65.

36. Walter LC, Schonberg MA. Screening Mammography in Older Women A Review. Jama-J Am Med Assoc 2014;311(13):1336–47.

37. Torke AM, Schwartz PH, Holtz LR, et al. Older adults and forgoing cancer screening: "I think it would be strange". JAMA Intern Med 2013;173(7):526–31.

38. Housten AJ, Pappadis MR, Krishnan S, et al. Resistance to discontinuing breast cancer screening in older women: A qualitative study. Psycho Oncol 2018;27(6): 1635–41.

39. Kotwal AA, Walter LC, Lee SJ, et al. Are We Choosing Wisely? Older Adults' Cancer Screening Intentions and Recalled Discussions with Physicians About Stopping. J Gen Intern Med 2019;34(8):1538–45.

40. White N, Reid F, Harris A, et al. A Systematic Review of Predictions of Survival in Palliative Care: How Accurate Are Clinicians and Who Are the Experts? PLoS One 2016;11(8):e0161407.

41. Allen LA, Yager JE, Funk MJ, et al. Discordance between patient-predicted and model-predicted life expectancy among ambulatory patients with heart failure. JAMA 2008;299(21):2533–42.

42. Hoffmann TC, Del Mar C. Patients' expectations of the benefits and harms of treatments, screening, and tests: a systematic review. JAMA Intern Med 2015; 175(2):274–86.

43. Hoffmann TC, Del Mar C. Clinicians' Expectations of the Benefits and Harms of Treatments, Screening, and Tests: A Systematic Review. JAMA Intern Med 2017; 177(3):407–19.

44. Schoenborn NL, Boyd CM, Lee SJ, et al. Communicating About Stopping Cancer Screening: Comparing Clinicians' and Older Adults' Perspectives. Gerontol 2019;59(Suppl 1):S67–76.

45. Schoenborn NL, Bowman TL 2nd, Cayea D, et al. Primary Care Practitioners' Views on Incorporating Long-term Prognosis in the Care of Older Adults. JAMA Intern Med 2016;176(5):671–8.

46. Marxen T, Shauly O, Losken A. The Safety of Same-day Discharge after Immediate Alloplastic Breast Reconstruction: A Systematic Review. Plast Reconstr Surg Glob Open 2022;10(7):e4448.

47. Specht MC, Kelly BN, Tomczyk E, et al. One-Year Experience of Same-Day Mastectomy and Breast Reconstruction Protocol. Ann Surg Oncol 2022;29(9): 5711–9.

48. Marla S, Stallard S. Systematic review of day surgery for breast cancer. Int J Surg 2009;7(4):318–23.

49. Sibia US, Klune JR, Turcotte JJ, et al. Hospital-Based Same-Day Compared to Overnight-Stay Mastectomy: An American College of Surgeons National Surgical Quality Improvement Program Analysis. Ochsner J 2022;22(2):139–45.

50. Hughes TM, Ellsworth B, Berlin NL, et al. Statewide Episode Spending Variation of Mastectomy for Breast Cancer. J Am Coll Surg 2022;234(1):14–23.

51. Jogerst K, Thomas O, Koslorek HE, et al. Same-Day Discharge After Mastectomy: Breast Cancer Surgery in the Era of ERAS((R)). Ann Surg Oncol 2020; 27(9):3436–45.

52. Offodile AC 2nd, Gu C, Boukovalas S, et al. Enhanced recovery after surgery (ERAS) pathways in breast reconstruction: systematic review and meta-analysis of the literature. Breast Cancer Res Treat 2019;173(1):65–77.

53. Vuong B, Graff-Baker AN, Yanagisawa M, et al. Implementation of a Post-mastectomy Home Recovery Program in a Large, Integrated Health Care Delivery System. Ann Surg Oncol 2019;26(10):3178–84.

54. DiSipio T, Rye S, Newman B, et al. Incidence of unilateral arm lymphoedema after breast cancer: a systematic review and meta-analysis. Lancet Oncol 2013; 14(6):500–15.

55. Kwan JYY, Famiyeh P, Su J, et al. Development and Validation of a Risk Model for Breast Cancer-Related Lymphedema. JAMA Netw Open 2020;3(11):e2024373.

56. Shih YC, Xu Y, Cormier JN, et al. Incidence, treatment costs, and complications of lymphedema after breast cancer among women of working age: a 2-year follow-up study. J Clin Oncol 2009;27(12):2007–14.

57. Jorgensen MG, Toyserkani NM, Hansen FG, et al. The impact of lymphedema on health-related quality of life up to 10 years after breast cancer treatment. NPJ Breast Cancer 2021;7(1):70.

58. Boyages J, Kalfa S, Xu Y, et al. Worse and worse off: the impact of lymphedema on work and career after breast cancer. SpringerPlus 2016;5:657.

59. Giuliano AE, Ballman KV, McCall L, et al. Effect of Axillary Dissection vs No Axillary Dissection on 10-Year Overall Survival Among Women With Invasive Breast Cancer and Sentinel Node Metastasis: The ACOSOG Z0011 (Alliance) Randomized Clinical Trial. JAMA 2017;318(10):918–26.

60. Kuehn T, Bauerfeind I, Fehm T, et al. Sentinel-lymph-node biopsy in patients with breast cancer before and after neoadjuvant chemotherapy (SENTINA): a prospective, multicentre cohort study. Lancet Oncol 2013;14(7):609–18.

61. Boughey JC, Suman VJ, Mittendorf EA, et al. Sentinel lymph node surgery after neoadjuvant chemotherapy in patients with node-positive breast cancer: the ACOSOG Z1071 (Alliance) clinical trial. JAMA 2013;310(14):1455–61.

62. Hughes KS, Schnaper LA, Bellon JR, et al. Lumpectomy plus tamoxifen with or without irradiation in women age 70 years or older with early breast cancer: long-term follow-up of CALGB 9343. J Clin Oncol 2013;31(19):2382–7.

63. Wang T, Bredbeck BC, Sinco B, et al. Variations in Persistent Use of Low-Value Breast Cancer Surgery. JAMA Surg 2021;156(4):353–62.

64. Wong SM, Weiss A, Mittendorf EA, et al. Surgical Management of the Axilla in Clinically Node-Positive Patients Receiving Neoadjuvant Chemotherapy: A National Cancer Database Analysis. Ann Surg Oncol 2019;26(11):3517–25.

65. Bredbeck BC, Baskin AS, Wang T, et al. Incremental Spending Associated with Low-Value Treatments in Older Women with Breast Cancer. Ann Surg Oncol 2022;29(2):1051–9.

66. Wang T, Mott N, Miller J, et al. Patient Perspectives on De-Escalation of Breast Cancer Treatment Options in Older Women with Hormone-Receptor Positive

Breast Cancer: A Qualitative Study. JAMA Netw Open 2020;3(9):e2017129. Under Review.

67. Baskin A, Wang T, Hawley ST, et al. Gaps in Breast Cancer Treatment Information for Older Women. Ann Surg Oncol 2020;28(2):950–7. Manuscript in progress.

68. Schonberg MA, Freedman RA, Recht AR, et al. Developing a patient decision aid for women aged 70 and older with early stage, estrogen receptor positive, HER2 negative, breast cancer. J Geriatr Oncol 2019;10(6):980–6.

69. Smith ME, Vitous CA, Hughes TM, et al. Barriers and Facilitators to De-Implementation of the Choosing Wisely((R)) Guidelines for Low-Value Breast Cancer Surgery. Ann Surg Oncol 2020;27(8):2653–63.

70. Kalinsky K, Barlow WE, Gralow JR, et al. 21-Gene Assay to Inform Chemotherapy Benefit in Node-Positive Breast Cancer. N Engl J Med 2021;385(25):2336–47.

71. Bello DM, Russell C, McCullough D, et al. Lymph Node Status in Breast Cancer Does Not Predict Tumor Biology. Ann Surg Oncol 2018;25(10):2884–9.

72. Wang T, Baskin AS, Dossett LA. Deimplementation of the Choosing Wisely Recommendations for Low-Value Breast Cancer Surgery: A Systematic Review. JAMA Surg 2020;155(8):759–70.

73. Baskin AS, Wang T, Bredbeck BC, et al. Trends in Contralateral Prophylactic Mastectomy Utilization for Small Unilateral Breast Cancer. J Surg Res 2021;262:71–84.

74. Agarwal S, Kidwell KM, Kraft CT, et al. Defining the relationship between patient decisions to undergo breast reconstruction and contralateral prophylactic mastectomy. Plast Reconstr Surg 2015;135(3):661–70.

75. Osman F, Saleh F, Jackson TD, et al. Increased postoperative complications in bilateral mastectomy patients compared to unilateral mastectomy: an analysis of the NSQIP database. Ann Surg Oncol 2013;20(10):3212–7.

76. Momoh AO, Cohen WA, Kidwell KM, et al. Tradeoffs Associated With Contralateral Prophylactic Mastectomy in Women Choosing Breast Reconstruction: Results of a Prospective Multicenter Cohort. Ann Surg 2017;266(1):158–64.

77. Sergesketter AR, Marks C, Broadwater G, et al. A Comparison of Complications in Therapeutic versus Contralateral Prophylactic Mastectomy Reconstruction: A Paired Analysis. Plast Reconstr Surg 2022;149(5):1037–47.

78. Boughey JC, Schilz SR, Van Houten HK, et al. Contralateral Prophylactic Mastectomy with Immediate Breast Reconstruction Increases Healthcare Utilization and Cost. Ann Surg Oncol 2017;24(10):2957–64.

79. Billig JI, Duncan A, Zhong L, et al. The Cost of Contralateral Prophylactic Mastectomy in Women with Unilateral Breast Cancer. Plast Reconstr Surg 2018;141(5):1094–102.

80. Eom JS, Kobayashi MR, Paydar K, et al. The number of operations required for completing breast reconstruction. Plast Reconstr Surg Glob Open 2014;2(10):e242.

81. Zendejas B, Moriarty JP, O'Byrne J, et al. Cost-effectiveness of contralateral prophylactic mastectomy versus routine surveillance in patients with unilateral breast cancer. J Clin Oncol 2011;29(22):2993–3000.

82. Smith D, Sepehr S, Karakatsanis A, et al. Yield of Surveillance Imaging After Mastectomy With or Without Reconstruction for Patients With Prior Breast Cancer: A Systematic Review and Meta-analysis. JAMA Netw Open 2022;5(12):e2244212.

83. Greenup RA, Rushing C, Fish L, et al. Financial Costs and Burden Related to Decisions for Breast Cancer Surgery. J Oncol Pract 2019;15(8):e666–76.

84. Buchanan PJ, Abdulghani M, Waljee JF, et al. An Analysis of the Decisions Made for Contralateral Prophylactic Mastectomy and Breast Reconstruction. Plast Reconstr Surg 2016;138(1):29–40.

85. Sando IC, Billlg JI, Ambani SW, et al. An Evaluation of the Choice for Contralateral Prophylactic Mastectomy and Patient Concerns About Recurrence in a Reconstructed Cohort. Ann Plast Surg 2018;80(4):333–8.

86. Offodile AC 2nd, Hwang ES, Greenup RA. Contralateral Prophylactic Mastectomy in the Era of Financial Toxicity: An Additional Point for Concern? Ann Surg 2020;271(5):817–8.

87. Rosenberg SM, Tracy MS, Meyer ME, et al. Perceptions, knowledge, and satisfaction with contralateral prophylactic mastectomy among young women with breast cancer: a cross-sectional survey. Ann Intern Med 2013;159(6):373–81.

88. Brennan ME, Houssami N. Evaluation of the evidence on staging imaging for detection of asymptomatic distant metastases in newly diagnosed breast cancer. Breast 2012;21(2):112–23.

89. Dull B, Linkugel A, Margenthaler JA, et al. Overuse of Chest CT in Patients With Stage I and II Breast Cancer: An Opportunity to Increase Guidelines Compliance at an NCCN Member Institution. J Natl Compr Canc Netw 2017;15(6):783–9.

90. Baltz AP, Siegel ER, Kamal AH, et al. Clinical Impact of ASCO Choosing Wisely Guidelines on Staging Imaging for Early-Stage Breast Cancers: A Time Series Analysis Using SEER-Medicare Data. JCO Oncol Pract 2022;19(2):e274–85.

91. Henry NL, Braun TM, Breslin TM, et al. Variation in the use of advanced imaging at the time of breast cancer diagnosis in a statewide registry. Cancer 2017;123(15):2975–83.

92. Simos D, Hutton B, Graham ID, et al. Imaging for metastatic disease in patients with newly diagnosed breast cancer: are doctor's perceptions in keeping with the guidelines? J Eval Clin Pract 2015;21(1):67–73.

93. Lipitz-Snyderman A, Sima CS, Atoria CL, et al. Physician-Driven Variation in Nonrecommended Services Among Older Adults Diagnosed With Cancer. JAMA Intern Med 2016;176(10):1541–8.

94. Sparano JA, Gray RJ, Makower DF, et al. Adjuvant Chemotherapy Guided by a 21-Gene Expression Assay in Breast Cancer. N Engl J Med 2018;379(2):111–21.

95. Kurian AW, Bondarenko I, Jagsi R, et al. Recent Trends in Chemotherapy Use and Oncologists' Treatment Recommendations for Early-Stage Breast Cancer. J Natl Cancer Inst 2018;110(5):493–500.

96. Schaafsma E, Zhang B, Schaafsma M, et al. Impact of Oncotype DX testing on ER+ breast cancer treatment and survival in the first decade of use. Breast Cancer Res 2021;23(1):74.

97. Chandler Y, Jayasekera JC, Schechter CB, et al. Simulation of Chemotherapy Effects in Older Breast Cancer Patients With High Recurrence Scores. J Natl Cancer Inst 2020;112(6):574–81.

98. Van Herck Y, Feyaerts A, Alibhai S, et al. Is cancer biology different in older patients? Lancet Healthy Longev 2021;2(10):e663–77.

99. Giaquinto AN, Sung H, Miller KD, et al. Breast Cancer Statistics, 2022. CA Cancer J Clin 2022;72(6):524–41.

100. Kunkler IH, Williams LJ, Jack WJL, et al. Breast-Conserving Surgery with or without Irradiation in Early Breast Cancer. N Engl J Med 2023;388(7):585–94.

101. Whelan T, Smith S, Nielsen T, et al. LUMINA: A prospective trial omitting radiotherapy (RT) following breast conserving surgery (BCS) in T1N0 luminal A breast cancer (BC). J Clin Oncol 2022;40(17).

102. Early Breast Cancer Trialists' Collaborative G. Aromatase inhibitors versus tamoxifen in early breast cancer: patient-level meta-analysis of the randomised trials. Lancet 2015;386(10001):1341–52.

103. McKevitt E, Cheifetz R, DeVries K, et al. Sentinel Node Biopsy Should Not be Routine in Older Patients with ER-Positive HER2-Negative Breast Cancer Who Are Willing and Able to Take Hormone Therapy. Ann Surg Oncol 2021;28(11): 5950–7.

104. Taylor LJ, Steiman JS, Anderson B, et al. Does persistent use of radiation in women > 70 years of age with early-stage breast cancer reflect tailored patient-centered care? Breast Cancer Res Treat 2020;180(3):801–7.

105. Greenup RA, Camp MS, Taghian AG, et al. Cost comparison of radiation treatment options after lumpectomy for breast cancer. Ann Surg Oncol 2012;19(10): 3275–81.

106. Shumway DA, Griffith KA, Hawley ST, et al. Patient views and correlates of radiotherapy omission in a population-based sample of older women with favorable-prognosis breast cancer. Cancer 2018;124(13):2714–23.

107. Dossett LA, Mott NM, Bredbeck BC, et al. Using Tailored Messages to Target Overuse of Low-Value Breast Cancer Care in Older Women. J Surg Res 2022; 270:503–12.

108. Shumway DA, Griffith KA, Sabel MS, et al. Surgeon and Radiation Oncologist Views on Omission of Adjuvant Radiotherapy for Older Women with Early-Stage Breast Cancer. Ann Surg Oncol 2017;24(12):3518–26.

109. Bekelman JE, Sylwestrzak G, Barron J, et al. Uptake and costs of hypofractionated vs conventional whole breast irradiation after breast conserving surgery in the United States, 2008-2013. JAMA 2014;312(23):2542–50.

110. Kang MM, Hasan Y, Waller J, et al. Has Hypofractionated Whole-Breast Radiation Therapy Become the Standard of Care in the United States? An Updated Report from National Cancer Database. Clin Breast Cancer 2022;22(1):e8–20.

111. Knowlton CA. Breast Cancer Management During the COVID-19 Pandemic: the Radiation Oncology Perspective. Curr Breast Cancer Rep 2022;14(1):8–16.

112. Vicini FA, Cecchini RS, White JR, et al. Long-term primary results of accelerated partial breast irradiation after breast-conserving surgery for early-stage breast cancer: a randomised, phase 3, equivalence trial. Lancet 2019;394(10215): 2155–64.

113. Whelan TJ, Julian JA, Berrang TS, et al. External beam accelerated partial breast irradiation versus whole breast irradiation after breast conserving surgery in women with ductal carcinoma in situ and node-negative breast cancer (RAPID): a randomised controlled trial. Lancet 2019;394(10215):2165–72.

114. Correa C, Harris EE, Leonardi MC, et al. Accelerated Partial Breast Irradiation: Executive summary for the update of an ASTRO Evidence-Based Consensus Statement. Pract Radiat Oncol 2017;7(2):73–9.

115. Lam DL, Houssami N, Lee JM. Imaging Surveillance After Primary Breast Cancer Treatment. AJR Am J Roentgenol 2017;208(3):676–86.

116. McNaul D, Darke M, Garg M, et al. An evaluation of post-lumpectomy recurrence rates: is follow-up every 6 months for 2 years needed? J Surg Oncol 2013;107(6):597–601.

117. Expert Panel on Breast I, Heller SL, Lourenco AP, et al. ACR Appropriateness Criteria(R) Imaging After Mastectomy and Breast Reconstruction. J Am Coll Radiol 2020;17(11S):S403–14.
118. Cheun JH, Jung J, Lee ES, et al. Intensity of metastasis screening and survival outcomes in patients with breast cancer. Sci Rep 2021;11(1):2851.
119. NCCN Clinical Practice Guidelines in Oncology: Breast Cancer Version 4.2023. Available at: https://www.nccn.org/professionals/physician_gls/pdf/breast_blocks.pdf. Published 2023. Accessed March 23, 2023.
120. Moschetti I, Cinquini M, Lambertini M, et al. Follow-up strategies for women treated for early breast cancer. Cochrane Database Syst Rev 2016;2016(5):CD001768.
121. Schumacher JR, Neuman HB, Yu M, et al. Surveillance Imaging vs Symptomatic Recurrence Detection and Survival in Stage II-III Breast Cancer (AFT-01). J Natl Cancer Inst 2022;114(10):1371–9.
122. Wickerham L, Fisher B, Cronin W. The efficacy of bone scanning in the follow-up of patients with operable breast cancer. Breast Cancer Res Treat 1984;4(4):303–7.
123. Harris L, Fritsche H, Mennel R, et al. American Society of Clinical Oncology 2007 update of recommendations for the use of tumor markers in breast cancer. J Clin Oncol 2007;25(33):5287–312.
124. Hahn EE, Munoz-Plaza C, Wang J, et al. Anxiety, Culture, and Expectations: Oncologist-Perceived Factors Associated With Use of Nonrecommended Serum Tumor Marker Tests for Surveillance of Early-Stage Breast Cancer. J Oncol Pract 2017;13(1):e77–90.
125. Ramsey SD, Henry NL, Gralow JR, et al. Tumor marker usage and medical care costs among older early-stage breast cancer survivors. J Clin Oncol 2015;33(2):149–55.

Multidisciplinary Management of Breast Cancer and Role of the Patient Navigator

Andrew Fenton, MD[a],*, Nicki Downes, DO[a],
Amanda Mendiola, MD[a], Amy Cordova, MSN, APRN-CNP, OCN[a],
Kathy Lukity, RN, BSN, CBCN[a], Julie Imani, MSN, APRN-CNS, OCN[a]

KEYWORDS

- Multidisciplinary • Breast center • Navigators • Survivorship • Fertility

KEY POINTS

- Modern breast cancer care is best provided in comprehensive breast centers.
- Optimal outcomes in the care of breast cancer patients occur with multidisciplinary care.
- Navigators imrprove outcomes and patient satisfaction.

MODERN BREAST CANCER CARE: AN INTRODUCTION

Breast cancer remains one of the most common cancers diagnosed in the United States. It stands to be the most funded and publicly highlighted cancer across the globe. With the much-needed exposure and research, changes to treatment pathways are continually evolving. The medical community has combated breast cancer with the most up-to-date recommendations by creating a multidisciplinary management model. Since the creation of the first free-standing multidisciplinary breast center in Van Nuys, California in the 1970s, this approach to breast cancer treatment has become the standard of care.[1]

What defines the term "multidisciplinary" has grown over the years to include far more than surgeons, pathologists, and oncologists. One such invaluable addition to this comprehensive team is the role of the patient navigator. Coordinated care for patients with breast cancer can be exceedingly complex, with many possible missed opportunities to improve patients' outcomes and quality of life. Patient navigators are germane to streamlining the process of diagnosis, treatments, and survivorship. Research has shown that, with the proper use of nurse navigators, patient quality of life, satisfaction with care, and length of stay in the hospital were all

This article previously appeared in Obstetrics & Gynecology Clinics volume 49, issue 1 March 2022.
[a] Cleveland Clinic Akron General, 1 Akron General Avenue, Akron, OH, USA
* Corresponding author.
E-mail address: FentonA@ccf.org

improved.[2] This article serves as a comprehensive review of the multifaceted care of breast cancer.

COMPREHENSIVE BREAST CENTER

The National Consortium of Breast Centers defines several center models, focusing on individual aspects of breast cancer care and culminating in the comprehensive breast cancer center model.[3] Combining all aspects of breast cancer management in one setting has streamlined the patient experience from diagnosis to survivorship. Gabel and colleagues[4] showed a decrease from time of diagnosis to treatment and a substantial increase in patient satisfaction after establishing a multidisciplinary breast cancer center. In this era of the new medical market, patient satisfaction and quality are metrics that are now dictating compensation and type of care. The National Accreditation Program for Breast Centers (NAPBC) through the American College of Surgeons has strived to outline evidence-based and consensus-based criteria for evaluating and managing breast disease. Multidisciplinary breast centers endeavor to provide the most up-to-date academic- and patient-centered care of breast disease with the help of several organizations such as the NABPC, The American Society of Breast Surgeons, and the American College of Radiology, to name a few.

MULTIDISCIPLINARY TEAM

Central to the modern treatment of the patient with breast cancer are surgeons, radiologists, pathologists, and medical and radiation oncologists. Gone are the days when patients go to the operating room to diagnose breast cancer. The vast majority of cases are diagnosed in the radiology suite using a stereotactic or ultrasound-guided core biopsy. These biopsies provide histologic samples for pathologic diagnosis and molecular marker assays, all critical to therapeutic planning.

The various subspecialties work hand-in-hand to provide seamless recommendations and care. Breast centers are arranged to have the patient seen by each discipline either in same-day appointments in a defined clinic or space, or seen sequentially in private offices or clinics. Each discipline requires various pretreatment evaluations, tests, and imaging. As discussed elsewhere in this article, guiding and monitoring the patient through this maze of visits and tests is a crucial task of the patient navigator.

Multidisciplinary teams that work together frequently develop specific patterns and efficiencies that can streamline care. For example, if the surgeon knows what typical workup the medical oncologist requires, testing can usually be initiated before the medical oncology visit. Professional and collegial relationships between the various disciplines ensure cutting-edge care, from the initial evaluation, radiographic workup, and biopsy to definitive treatment.

Current advances in breast cancer survival have occurred because of a shift to multidisciplinary care.[5] The modern treatment of breast cancer is the model for multimodality therapy. For example, surgery is always thought to be the first-line therapy for breast cancer, but in some instances, as discussed elsewhere in this article, it is not optimal to operate first.

BREAST RADIOLOGY

Mammographic screening recommendations have long been a topic of debate with differing opinions on when to begin, how frequently to repeat, and when to stop screening. However, early detection and thus treatment has been proven time and again to significantly alter patients' outcomes.[6] Radiologists are essentially the first multidisciplinary team members to identify an abnormality that needs further diagnostic workup. Radiologists can specialize in breast imaging by additional fellowship training. Comprehensive breast centers can achieve a special designation of "Imaging Center of Excellence" through the American College of Radiology by meeting specific standards.

Radiologists are trained in the early detection of mammographic abnormalities including masses, asymmetry, microcalcifications, and nipple discharge. Their testing modalities include screening and diagnostic mammograms, usually digital and increasingly coupled with tomosynthesis (ie, 3-dimensional mammograms), ultrasound examination, and breast MRI. Specially trained radiologists can accurately diagnose lesions with stereotactic and ultrasound-guided biopsies. Specialized centers can perform MRI-guided biopsies as well. Radiopaque markers are placed into the breast to help identify the biopsied area for future follow-up or surgical excision, depending on the pathologic findings.

After the identification of cancer or high-risk lesions, radiologists are needed to localize lesions for surgical planning. There are several tools in their armamentarium to localize lesions for operative excision. The first and most widely used is wire localization, which is placed via ultrasound, stereotactic, or MRI guidance. Newer options that are quickly being used include radioactive seeds and radiofrequency transmitters.

MEDICAL ONCOLOGY

The decision for and timing of chemotherapy is the field in breast cancer that is perhaps evolving the fastest. With every new tumor molecular marker identified, new prospective clinical trials emerge, helping to quantify its effect on patient outcomes. From the discovery of human epidermal growth factor receptor 2 (HER2) in 1987 and the more recent programmed death ligand-1 in 2018, targets of cancer destruction have become more complex. Medical oncologists are the gatekeepers of such medications. Their tools effectively alter the outcomes of breast cancer by allowing personalized care.

Although most systemic therapies are given in the postoperative setting, there are scenarios in which the timing of treatment differs. The medical oncologist treats locally advanced[7] or inflammatory breast cancers first with neoadjuvant chemotherapy, then reassesses for surgical options. Tumors greater than 2 cm, those with biopsy-proven nodal disease, or specific molecular markers determined on core biopsy are candidates for neoadjuvant therapy. For example, triple-negative (estrogen, progesterone, and HER2 negative) breast cancers are uniquely aggressive tumors that often benefit from this approach, as do HER2-enriched tumors. Patients who present with larger tumors but still prefer breast conservation therapy (partial mastectomy) are candidates for neoadjuvant chemotherapy, especially for patients with larger tumors and smaller breast size. Downstaging of the tumor can occur with chemotherapy, allowing for breast conservation therapy.

The combination of molecular markers, tumor size, nodal status, and a patient's medical and genetic history create numerous treatment options best approached by a multidisciplinary care team to ensure the best clinical outcome.

RADIATION ONCOLOGY

Radiation oncologists also provide valuable input for the management of patients with breast cancer. They are trained to identify which patient situations would benefit the most from radiation delivered in several modalities. All patients under the age of 70 treated with breast-conserving therapy require whole breast or partial breast irradiation to achieve local control equal to a simple mastectomy.[8] Also, postmastectomy radiation is indicated in patients who have tumors greater than 5 cm, or 4 or more axillary lymph nodes involved with metastatic breast cancer.[9]

Whole breast radiation can now be given over shorter time frames than traditional treatment protocols, thus decreasing unwanted side effects and increasing the therapeutic dosage. The decision to proceed with partial breast versus whole breast radiation or short versus traditional course whole breast radiation depends on many factors. The standard treatment protocol in breast conservation is approximately 5 or 6 weeks. Patients receive 1.8- to 2.0-Gy fractions of radiation at each treatment session for a total dose of approximately 50 Gy in conventional fractionated, whole breast radiation.[10] Recent data show treatment efficacy with hypofractionated radiation schedules, including a shorter course and a higher daily dosage delivered.[11]

New studies are beginning to investigate the use of radiation therapy in patients undergoing breast-conserving therapy who have received radiation therapy once and now have developed a remote in-breast ipsilateral recurrence.[12] As one can see, early collaboration with these team members allows for further specialization and tailoring of care for the patient with breast cancer.

PATHOLOGY

Pathology input can be critical to accurate diagnosis, staging, and determination of molecular subtypes (luminal, HER2-enriched, or triple-negative cancer). Pathologists play a crucial role in connecting the link between diagnosis and treatment. Pathologists have been at the forefront of altering the way we approach and treat breast cancer. Breast cancer is a biologically heterogeneous process. A pathologist's role has evolved from simple identification to providing prognostic prediction and clinicopathologic correlation.[13]

The burgeoning fields of genomics and molecular characterization provide personalized care by testing the genetic makeup of each patient's tumor cells. Several commercial tests are available that use genomic microarray analysis to prognosticate the likelihood of cancer recurrence, thus dictating when chemotherapy is potentially beneficial and therefore recommended. These tests are primarily used in ER-positive, node-negative patients, but its usefulness has been extrapolated to other more complex scenarios. Breast pathologists continually assist in clinical management decisions through their valuable input in tumor boards and case reviews.

SURGERY

Over the last 20 years, the role of the surgeon has changed immensely. Surgeons are more often than not the first person to fully evaluate the patient. This appointment involves a thorough physical examination, reviewing a patient's imaging and pathology, and discussing its implications and the pathways of treatment. General surgeons were once the only options for surgical management of breast cancer until subspecialization led to the creation of the Surgical Breast Oncology Fellowship.

The Society of Surgical Oncology has recognized the need for specialty training. Kingsmore and colleagues revealed a significant discrepancy in outcomes for women treated by breast surgeons versus nonspecialists.[14] Patients treated by nonspecialists had a 20% increase in the risk of death and a 2 times higher risk of breast and axillary recurrence.[14]

Surgical techniques have evolved with the development of breast-conserving therapy. Axillary nodal involvement remains the most important prognostic feature in breast cancer. How the axilla is evaluated has changed significantly over the last

30 years. Traditionally the axilla was most thoroughly evaluated by way of complete axillary lymph node dissection. Through Krag and colleagues'[15] pioneering work came the standardization of sentinel lymph node biopsy in breast cancer management, which is now the mainstay for evaluating clinical node-negative disease.

There has also been a more recent expansion in oncoplastic surgical techniques, bridging plastic surgical techniques (ie, mastopexy and mammoplasty) with oncologic procedures to improve aesthetic outcomes without an oncologic deficit. Nipple-sparing mastectomy, usually paired with immediate reconstruction, has been a recent addition to the surgical armamentarium for selected patients.

Outside the scope of oncoplasty lies the critical role of the plastic surgeon in breast reconstruction. In 1998, the Women's Health and Cancer Rights Act was enacted to provide insurance coverage to women who elect reconstruction in connection with their mastectomies, whether they desire prostheses or ipsilateral or contralateral tissue reconstruction.[16] A well-functioning breast center provides its patients access to reconstructive surgeons preoperatively. Most patients would prefer immediate reconstruction, but treatment requirements (ie, chemotherapy or radiation) may require delayed reconstruction. The most common options offered for reconstruction are tissue expanders, implants, autologous tissue flaps, or any combination of these. These decisions require clear communication between all treating physicians to achieve optimal oncologic and cosmetic outcomes.

ONCOLOGY PATIENT NAVIGATORS

Oncology patient navigators are facilitators of timely access to appropriate health care and resources for patients and their families. The concept of patient navigation was introduced in 1990 by Harold P. Freeman, MD. His work highlighted the benefit of navigation in following African American women with late stage breast cancer at Harlem Hospital. His work was the impetus behind a national movement to involve nurse navigators in the cancer continuum.[17] In 2002, the National Cancer Institute established funding for additional patient navigator programs in cancer care. After this, the NAPBC established patient navigation as a standard for breast center accreditation.

Patient navigation provides personalized assistance to patients, families, and caregivers. It is designed to overcome barriers and facilitate timely access to high-quality care throughout the treatment process. This role allows for the assessment of needs and coordination of care. According to the NAPBC manual, the goal is to enhance outcomes, increase satisfaction, and decrease the cost of care.[18] Research has shown decreased time to diagnostic evaluation and treatment after abnormal screening using the patient navigation process.[19]

For a navigation program to be successful, a needs assessment should be done to identify the population in need of these services. The American College of Surgeons Commission of Cancer recommends cancer programs assess their population every 3 years.[20] The needs assessment can include several measures, such as time to initiating care, time to completion of workup, or receipt of guideline-appropriate care. Once the in-need group has been identified, the navigation process can start targeting them. This can be done with patient intake forms and algorithms that will highlight these at-risk patients.

After the needs assessment, the skillset of the navigator needs to be determined. For some centers, this could be logistical needs (ie, transportation, interpreters) or clinical duties (ie, postoperative instructions, patient education). However, most programs will likely have overlapping needs and require a hybridized role that can address both by using navigators with nursing or social work backgrounds.[21]

Personal characteristics also need to be considered when choosing a navigator. Individuals with problem-solving skills with experience in diversity are very suited for this type of role. This may include those with expertise in health care, cancer survivors, or language skills specific to the target population.[22] For a navigator to be useful, they require support as they integrate into the care team. This includes information systems. These systems should help the navigator to identify patients efficiently within their working population. Patient navigators need the means to document their work and share this with clinicians.

In sum, patient navigators provide patients with education and knowledge about their illness. Patient navigation aims to overcome health system barriers and provide health education and psychosocial support across the continuum of care.[23] A wide range of navigation program models has proven to decrease the burden of cost, reduce readmission and emergency room visits, and improve the quality of life for the patients with cancer.[24] In the cancer setting, navigators work with the multidisciplinary care team as a patient advocate, care provider, educator, counselor, and facilitator. Navigators are able to fill any gaps between patients, their family members, and care providers.

SURVIVORSHIP

An increasing population of 3.8 million breast cancer survivors[25] presents many challenges as well as many opportunities for improvement in cancer care. Cancer may affect every aspect of an individual's life, including overall well-being.[26]

Transitioning to the post-treatment phase of care often causes significant anxiety or distress for patients. Breast centers must include a survivorship component to provide comprehensive services for breast cancer survivors. Benefits of a survivorship clinic include assessing long-term toxicities, expert toxicity management, and coordination of care with a multidisciplinary team.[27] A comprehensive breast cancer survivorship care plan includes details related to the cancer diagnosis, treatment received, surveillance recommendations, key symptoms to report, treatment side effects, healthy behavior recommendations, and supportive care resources (**Fig. 1**).

GENETIC COUNSELORS

Genetic counselors have become vital members of the breast cancer team owing to their vast knowledge of genetic disorders based on patients' current diagnosis and family history. They can select various gene panels and, most important, discuss the results and their implications for the patient. The results provide essential up-to-date information regarding the genetic findings, surveillance needs, and the importance of following up with their physician.

Occasionally, genetic testing results can alter the patient's treatment plan, especially BRCA 1 and 2 mutations. These patients may opt for more aggressive surgical intervention, including prophylactic or bilateral mastectomy and prophylactic oophorectomy. Some genetic findings can uncover the need to monitor other potential tumor sites and family members.

TUMOR BOARD, CANCER RESEARCH, AND TUMOR REGISTRY

Multidisciplinary care of the patient with breast cancer culminates in modern tumor boards. Multidisciplinary tumor boards are essential to review cases prospectively.[4] These meetings typically occur weekly and involve all the medical specialties discussed elsewhere in this article. The treating physician presents the cases. Then the

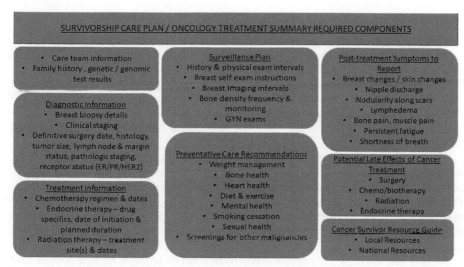

Fig. 1. Required components that encompass a survivorship care plan for use in multidisciplinary breast center.

images and pathology are reviewed, the clinical or pathologic stage is determined, and finally the treatment plans are discussed based on nationally accepted guidelines. The research personnel also present available research protocols and clinical trials. Eligibility for participation is determined. Patient accrual to clinical trials is necessary for continued accreditation by the NAPBC and American College of Surgeons Commission on Cancer.

A well-functioning tumor registry, staffed by certified tumor registrars, is critical for data abstraction of patients with cancer and participation in tumor board. Data are submitted to the National Cancer Data Base for programs accredited by the Commission on Cancer, which currently accounts for more than 70% of newly diagnosed cancer cases. This database allows programs to monitor their adherence to multiple important quality metrics (**Fig. 2**).

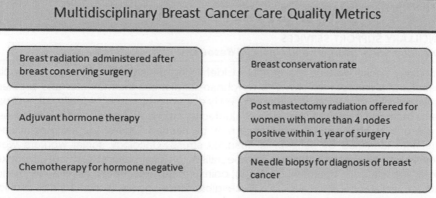

Fig. 2. Quality metrics endorsed by breast specific professional societies and accrediting programs.

FERTILITY

Breast cancer affects approximately 11,000 women under the age of 40 each year, making it the most common malignancy in women of childbearing age.[28] With 5-year survival rates approaching 90%, many of these women may desire to have children in the future, creating an essential role for fertility preservation. Several national medical organizations recommend that individuals receive information about the risks of treatment-associated infertility, a review of available options and, when interested, a referral to reproductive medicine specialists before beginning anticancer treatment.[29–31]

Although the provider cannot predict the absolute risk of post-treatment infertility, information and guidelines are available to assist patients in pursuing fertility preservation.[29–34] The type of systemic therapy is also somewhat predictive of overall infertility risk. Gonadotoxic agents include alkylating agents, anthracyclines, and taxanes.[35–38] In women with hormone receptor-positive disease, the use of tamoxifen may cause amenorrhea, but it does not increase the risk of permanent ovarian failure or infertility.[39]

Multiple options for fertility preservation exist such as embryo, mature oocyte, and ovarian tissue cryopreservation. With early referrals to reproductive medicine specialists, this process should not delay the start of anticancer treatment for most women. When other fertility preservation techniques are not feasible, ovarian suppression with gonadotropin-releasing hormone analogs can be considered.[29–31,34]

SEXUAL HEALTH

Issues regarding infertility and body image can negatively affect the overall sexual health of the patient with breast cancer. Sexual health is an integral component of a patient's quality of life. Cancer survivors whose sexual health is impacted by treatment are at increased risk of distress and diminished quality of life. Sexual function may be affected by the physical symptoms of cancer itself as well as its treatment, and has been observed in up to 60% of patients with breast cancer.[40] Dysfunction may result in changes in overall health status, body image, and view of one's sexuality.[41]

It is recommended that there be a discussion with each patient, initiated by a member of the health care team, regarding sexual health and potential dysfunction.[42] Overcoming barriers to communication about this important topic and making specialized referrals is essential to providing patients with comprehensive survivorship care.

ANCILLARY SUPPORT SERVICES
Oncology Social Workers and Financial Resources

Oncology social workers are critical in identifying patients at risk of psychosocial distress and financial toxicity. The psychosocial distress thermometer and problem list is used for screening patients with newly diagnosed cancer.[43] Ideally, all new patients receiving treatment should be evaluated by an oncology social worker to assess areas of concern or where assistance may be needed. One of the most significant stressors identified by patients is financial stress. Oncology social workers work closely with financial reimbursement specialists to assist patients with out-of-pocket expenses related to treatment costs (eg, coinsurance, prescription assistance, manufacturer assistance) when available and eligible. Oncology social workers also provide local foundations' resources when patients need assistance with rent/mortgage, utilities, and groceries while undergoing treatment for cancer.

Table 1	
Symptoms alleviated by complementary therapies	
Symptoms	**Complementary Therapy**
Anxiety	Massage, meditation, art therapy
Fatigue	Yoga, massage, art therapy
Nausea and vomiting	Acupuncture, aromatherapy, music therapy
Pain (including neuropathy)	Acupuncture, music therapy, herbal supplements, healing touch and massage
Sleep problems	Yoga, relaxation techniques

Common symptoms exhibited by patients with breast cancer and complementary therapies that can alleviate them.

COMPLEMENTARY THERAPIES

The management of breast cancer goes far beyond just surgery and medicine. There are several supplementary therapies included in a multidisciplinary team that address the patient as a whole. Providing an outlet apart from cancer treatment and correcting the side effects of treatment encompass a vast group of specialties (**Table 1**). Emotional, psychosocial, financial, wellness, and functional support complete holistic treatment paradigms.

Art therapy creates a therapeutic outlet for emotional growth and well-being. Such therapy has been shown to improve anxiety, depression, fatigue, and treatment outcomes in women diagnosed with breast cancer.[44] Pain management is a multifactorial concern and thus is best treated with multimodal and integrative approaches. Twenty percent to 80% of patients experience pain during breast cancer management. This pain significantly alters a person's quality of life.[45] The National Institute of Health outlines an evidence-based guideline to pain management by identifying and using pharmacologic and nonpharmacologic tools.[45] In a systematic review looking at the efficacy of complementary medicine on relieving cancer pain, it was found that there was a minimal, but notable, benefit using acupuncture, music, herbal supplements, healing touch, and massage.[46]

Chemotherapy-induced peripheral neuropathy is a toxicity that may persist for months to years after completing neoadjuvant or adjuvant chemotherapy for breast cancer. A short course (6–8 weeks) of acupuncture has demonstrated clinically significant improvement in subjective sensory symptoms, including paresthesia and neuropathic pain.[47] The established safety profile of acupuncture may prove beneficial for patients following completion of treatment. Furthermore, acupuncture may be considered a necessary intervention, given the lack of effective therapies for chemotherapy-induced peripheral neuropathy.

Functional medicine is an exciting and quickly expanding tool to combat cancer's negative outcome after a cancer diagnosis. Incorporating principles of integrative or lifestyle medicine may be beneficial to breast cancer survivors. Focusing on lifestyle changes, such as diet, exercise, and stress management, may help patients to feel that they are regaining control of their lives. Lasting lifestyle modifications may promote future health and well-being.

SUMMARY

The modern management of the patient with breast cancer is complex and multidisciplinary. Multiple medical specialties play important roles in the treatment and monitoring of these patients from diagnosis through survivorship. As patients with breast cancer span the age continuum, consideration of fertility and sexual health issues plays an important role, as do ancillary services involving social workers and financial resource counselors. Adjunctive services, such as art therapy, acupuncture, and functional medicine, improve long-term outcomes. Patient navigators, who are uniquely positioned to guide these patients through this maze of consultations, treatments, and services, help to bridge the gap between the medical, social, and emotional aspects of modern breast cancer care.

CLINICS CARE POINTS

- The modern management of breast cancer is multidisciplinary, involving surgeons, radiologists, pathologists, and medical and radiation oncologists
- The majority of patients are diagnosed in radiology with a core biopsy, not in the operating room.
- Breast-conserving therapy is typically the first option for early stage breast cancer, but when mastectomy is required, reconstructive surgical options must be provided to patients.
- Patient navigators bridge the gap for patients and families, assisting them in all aspects of care from diagnosis through completion of treatment.
- Patient navigators help patients to overcome barriers, and provide educational and psychosocial support.
- Regularly scheduled tumor boards allow all disciplines to review cases in a prospective fashion, thereby personalizing care, discussing accurate staging, treatment options, and eligibility for clinical trial participation.
- Comprehensive breast care includes more than physicians. Geneticists, social workers, financial resource counselors, survivorship clinics, fertility and sexual health counseling, and complementary therapies coordinate complete care of the patient with cancer.

DISCLOSURE

The authors have nothing to disclose.

REFERENCES

1. Silverstein MJ. The Van Nuys Breast Center: the first free-standing multidisciplinary breast center. Surg Oncol Clin N Am 2000;9(2):159–75.
2. Lee T, Ko I, Lee I, et al. Effects of nurse navigators on health outcomes of cancer patients. Cancer Nurs 2011;34:376–84.
3. 5 Breast Center Types. National Quality Measures for Breast Center. nqmbc.org. 2020. Available at: https://www.nqmbc.org/quality-measure-program/breast-center-types.cms. September 15, 2020.
4. Gabel M, Hilton NE, Nathanson SD. Multidisciplinary breast clinics. Do they work? Cancer 1997;79:2380–4.
5. Golledge J, Wiggins JE, Callam MJ. Effect of surgical subspecialization on breast cancer outcome. Br J Surg 2000;87(10):1420–5.
6. Nelson HD, Fu R, Cantor A, et al. Effectiveness of breast cancer screening: systematic review and meta-analysis to update the 2009 U.S. Preventive Services Task Force Recommendation. Ann Intern Med 2016;164(4):244–55.

7. Derks MGM, van de Velde CJH. Neoadjuvant chemotherapy in breast cancer: more than just downsizing. Lancet Oncol 2018;19(1):2–3.

8. Clark M, Collins R, Darby S, et al. Effects of radiotherapy and of differences in the extent of surgery for early breast cancer on local recurrence and 15-year survival: an overview of randomized trials. Lancet 2005;366:2087–106.

9. Wright JL, Parekh A. Updates in postmastectomy radiation. Surg Oncol Clin N Am 2017;26(3):383–92.

10. Moran MS. Advancements and personalization of breast cancer treatment strategies in radiation therapy. Cancer Treat Res 2018;173:89–119.

11. Whelan TJ, Pignol JP, Levine MN, et al. Long-term results of hypofractionated radiation therapy for breast cancer. N Engl J Med 2010;362(6):513–20.

12. Arthur DW, Winter KA, Kuerer HM, et al. Effectiveness of breast-conserving surgery and 3-dimensional conformal partial breast reirradiation for recurrence of breast cancer in the ipsilateral breast: the NRG Oncology/RTOG 1014 Phase 2 Clinical Trial. JAMA Oncol 2019;6(1):75–82.

13. Masood S. The changing role of pathologists from morphologists to molecular pathologists in the era of precision medicine. Breast J 2020;26(1):27–34.

14. Kingsmore D, Hole D, Gillis C. Why does specialist treatment of breast cancer improve survival? The role of surgical management. Br J Cancer 2004;90(10): 1920–5.

15. Krag DN, Weaver DL, Alex JC, et al. Surgical resection and radiolocalization of the sentinel lymph node in breast cancer using a gamma probe. Surg Oncol 1993;2(6):335–9.

16. Women's Health and Cancer Rights. Act (WHCRA). Centers for Medicare and Medicaid Services. CMS.gov. Available at: https://www.cms.gov/CCIIO/Programs-and-Initiatives/Other-Insurance-Protections/whcra_factsheet. December 18, 2020.

17. Neal CD, Weaver DT, Raphel TJ, et al. Patient navigation to improve cancer screening in underserved populations: reported experiences, opportunities, and challenges. J Am Coll Radiol 2018;15(11):1565–72.

18. National Accreditation Program for Breast Centers Standards Manual 2018 Edition. Facs.org. 2018. Available at: https://accreditation.facs.org/accreditation documents/NAPBC/Portal%20Resources/2018NAPBCStandardsManual.pdf#:~: text=The%20breast%20center%20must%20be%20in%20compliance%20with, Cancer%20Conference%20%E2%80%A2%20Standard%202.1%3A%20Multi disciplinary%20Patient%20Management. January 20, 2021.

19. Kim K, Choi JS, Choi E, et al. Effects of community-based health worker interventions to improve chronic disease management and care among vulnerable populations: a systematic review. Am J Public Health 2016;106(4):e3–28.

20. Commission on Cancer. Optimal resources for cancer care. American College of Surgeons. Commission on Cancer-Cancer Program Standards: ensuring patient-centered care. Facs.org/cancer. 2020. Available at: https://www.facs.org/-/media/files/quality-programs/cancer/coc/optimal_resources_for_cancer_care_2020_standards.ashx. January 03, 2021.

21. Gunn CM, Clark JA, Battaglia TA, et al. An assessment of patient navigator activities in breast cancer patient navigation programs using a nine-principle framework. Health Serv Res 2014;49(5):1555–77.

22. Charlot M, Santana MS, Chen CA, et al. Impact of patient and navigator race and language concordance on care after cancer screening abnormalities. Cancer 2015;121(9):1477–83.

23. Baik SH, Gallo LC, Wells KJ. Patient navigation in breast cancer treatment and survivorship: a systematic review. J Clin Oncol 2016;34(30):3686–96.

24. Balaban RB, Galbraith AA, Burns ME, et al. A patient navigator intervention to reduce hospital readmissions among high-risk safety-net patients: a randomized controlled trial. J Gen Intern Med 2015;30(7):907–15.
25. Shapiro CL. Cancer survivorship. N Engl J Med 2018;379(25):2438–50.
26. McCanney J, Winckworth-Prejsnar K, Schatz AA, et al. Addressing Survivorship in Cancer Care. J Natl Compr Canc Netw 2018;16(7):801–6.
27. Ross N. APRN-Led Clinics Enable Comprehensive Survivorship Care. 2018. Available at: https://www.ons.org/. December 30, 2020.
28. U.S. Cancer Statistics Working Group. U.S. Cancer Statistics Data Visualizations Tool, based on 2019 submission data (1999–2017): U.S. Department of Health and Human Services, Centers for Disease Control and Prevention and National Cancer Institute. Available at: www.cdc.gov/cancer/dataviz. June, 2020.
29. Waks AG, Partridge AH. Fertility preservation in patients with breast cancer: necessity, methods, and safety. J Natl Compr Canc Netw 2016;14(3):355–63.
30. Oktay K, Harvey BE, Partridge AH, et al. Fertility preservation in patients with cancer: ASCO Clinical Practice Guideline Update. J Clin Oncol 2018;36(19): 1994–2001.
31. Practice Committee of the American Society for Reproductive Medicine. Fertility preservation in patients undergoing gonadotoxic therapy or gonadectomy: a committee opinion. Fertil Sterility 2019;112:1022–33.
32. Alliance for Fertility Preservation. Available at: https://www.allianceforfertility preservation.org/advocacy/state-legislation. December 14, 2020.
33. Patel P, Kohn TP, Cohen J, et al. Evaluation of reported fertility preservation counseling before chemotherapy using the quality oncology practice initiative survey. JAMA Netw Open 2020;3(7):e2010806.
34. Ter Welle-Butalid MEE, Vriens IJHI, Derhaag JGJ, et al. Counseling young women with early breast cancer on fertility preservation. J Assist Reprod Genet 2019; 36(12):2593–604.
35. Ganz PA, Land SR, Geyer CE Jr, et al. Menstrual history and quality-of-life outcomes in women with node-positive breast cancer treated with adjuvant therapy on the NSABP B-30 trial. J Clin Oncol 2011;29(9):1110–6.
36. Zhao J, Liu J, Chen K, et al. What lies behind chemotherapy-induced amenorrhea for breast cancer patients: a meta-analysis. Breast Cancer Res Treat 2014; 145(1):113–28.
37. Bines J, Oleske DM, Cobleigh MA. Ovarian function in premenopausal women treated with adjuvant chemotherapy for breast cancer. J Clin Oncol 1996;14(5): 1718–29.
38. Petrek JA, Naughton MJ, Case LD, et al. Incidence, time course, and determinants of menstrual bleeding after breast cancer treatment: a prospective study. J Clin Oncol 2006;24(7):1045–51.
39. Lambertini M, Del Mastro L, Pescio MC, et al. Cancer and fertility preservation: international recommendations from an expert meeting. BMC Med 2016;14:1.
40. Camejo N, Castillo C, Hernandez AL, et al. Assessment of the sexual health of breast cancer survivors and their interest in discussing their difficulties with their doctors during follow-up. J Clin Oncol 2020;38(15_suppl). https://doi.org/10. 1200/jco.2020.38.15_suppl.e12542.
41. Aerts L, Christiaens MR, Enzlin P, et al. Sexual functioning in women after mastectomy versus breast conserving therapy for early-stage breast cancer: a prospective controlled study. Breast 2014;23(5):629–36.
42. Barbera L, Zwaal C, Elterman D, et al. Interventions to address sexual problems in people with cancer. Curr Oncol 2017;24(3):192.

43. Robbeson C, Hugenholtz-Wamsteker W, Meeus M, et al. Screening of physical distress in breast cancer survivors: concurrent validity of the Distress Thermometer and Problem List. *Eur J Cancer Care* (Engl) 2019;28(1):e12880.
44. Tang Y, Fu F, Gao H, et al. Art therapy for anxiety, depression, and fatigue in females with breast cancer: a systematic review. J Psychosoc Oncol 2019;37(1): 79–95.
45. PDQ® supportive and Palliative care Editorial board. PDQ cancer pain. Bethesda, MD: National Cancer Institute; 2020. Available at: https://www.cancer.gov/about-cancer/treatment/side-effects/pain/pain-hp-pdq. November 3, 2020.
46. Bardia A, Barton DL, Prokop LJ, et al. Efficacy of complementary and alternative medicine therapies in relieving cancer pain: a systematic review. J Clin Oncol 2006;24(34):5457–64.
47. Lu W, Giobbie-Hurder A, Freedman RA, et al. Acupuncture for chemotherapy-induced peripheral neuropathy in breast cancer survivors: a randomized controlled pilot trial. Oncologist 2020;25(4):310–8.

Addressing Inequalities in Breast Cancer Care Delivery

Leisha C. Elmore, MD, MPHS[a,b],
Oluwadamilola M. Fayanju, MD, MA, MPHS[b,*]

KEYWORDS

• Health equity • Health disparities • Breast cancer

KEY POINTS

- The etiology of health disparities is multifactorial and driven in large part by challenges in access to care, differential receipt of guideline-concordant care, and limited enrollment of diverse patients in clinical trials that serve as the foundation for treatment development.
- Black women diagnosed with breast cancer have a mortality rate that is 40% higher than White women. Hispanic ethnicity is associated with increased likelihood of not receiving guideline-concordant breast cancer treatment.
- Aggregate reporting of Asian American, Native Hawaiians, and Other Pacific Islanders limits subgroup analysis that may reveal within-group disparities.
- Intentional dismantling of structural barriers to equitable care requires intervention at the societal, health system, institution, and provider level.

INTRODUCTION/HISTORY/DEFINITIONS/BACKGROUND
Epidemiology of Breast Cancer

Breast cancer is the most common cancer diagnosed among women in the United States and much of the world. One in eight US women will develop breast cancer in their lifetime. Although overall incidence for breast cancer has been stable for decades, these rates fail to capture the nuance within subpopulations. When we look at trends in incidence over time, there are notable differences by race and ethnicity. Historically, incidence rates were higher among White women than Black women, but these rates have now converged and are now comparable. Incidence rates are notably lower for American Indian/Alaska Natives, Hispanic, and Asian/Pacific Islander

This article previously appeared in Surgical Oncology Clinics volume 32 issue 4 October 2023.
[a] Department of Surgery, Penn Presbyterian Medical Center, University of Pennsylvania, Perelman School of Medicine, 51 North 39th Street, 266 Wright Sanders, Philadelphia, PA 19104, USA; [b] Division of Breast Surgery, Department of Surgery, Hospital of the University of Pennsylvania, 3400 Spruce Street, Silverstein 4, Philadelphia, PA 19104, USA
* Corresponding author.
E-mail address: Oluwadamilola.fayanju@pennmedicine.upenn.edu
Twitter: @DrLolaFayanju (L.C.E.)

women, but they are increasing most significantly among Asian/Pacific Islander and American Indian/Alaska Native women.[1]

Despite the relatively stable incidence of breast cancer in the general population, mortality has declined by approximately 40% since 1975 owing to improvements in early detection, a better understanding of tumor biology, the development of targeted therapies, and improved treatment algorithms. However, this improvement in mortality has not been equally realized by all patients. In fact, in 2021, breast cancer became the leading cause of cancer death in Black women, surpassing lung cancer. Furthermore, Black women have the highest breast cancer death rate of all racial/ethnic groups, and a mortality rate that has been 40% higher than their White peers in recent years.[2] Of note, despite the rising incidence of breast cancer in the Asian/Pacific Islander population, mortality in this group remains the lowest of all racial and ethnic groups.[1]

When systemic differences emerge in any health outcome, interrogation of these differences requires an examination of how much they represent variations driven by nonmodifiable factors versus targets that are amenable to change. For example, with regard to breast cancer incidence, we know that certain factors are associated with a higher incidence; female sex is a predisposing factor, and breast cancer incidence increases steadily with age, making both biological sex and age nonmodifiable risk factors. Conversely, unequal access to care or treatment serves as potentially modifiable forces in disparate health outcomes.

Understanding Health Equity

To provide a foundation for the remainder of this article, it is important to understand the definition of the terms health disparity and health equity.

The Office of Disease Prevention and Health Promotion defines a *health disparity* as a *"... health difference that is closely linked with social, economic, and/or environmental disadvantage. Health disparities adversely affect groups of people who have systematically experienced greater obstacles to health based on their racial or ethnic group; religion; socioeconomic status; gender; age; mental health; cognitive, sensory, or physical disability; sexual orientation or gender identity; geographic location; or other characteristics historically linked to discrimination or exclusion."*[3] The key component of this definition is that the health difference disproportionally affects a historically marginalized population.

The Centers for Disease Control defines *health equity* as *"the state in which everyone has a fair and just opportunity to attain their highest level of health. Achieving this requires ongoing societal efforts to (1) Address historical and contemporary injustices (2) Overcome economic, social and other obstacles to health and (3) eliminate preventable health disparities."*[4] This definition highlights that many of the driving forces behind health inequities are the result of long-standing, systemic biases that must be dismantled. Promoting health equity does not simply mean providing the *same* care to everyone, but rather may ultimately involve allotting extra resources to elevate certain individuals to an appropriate standard of care.

Limitations in Data Reporting

The striking difference in breast cancer mortality in Black women relative to their peers represents a health disparity rooted in inequitable care at both the health system and societal levels. Although most of the existing data surrounding disparities address this pervasive and long-standing racial inequity, poor outcomes among Black women are not the only opportunity for improvement in care delivery.

In many studies on breast cancer, Asian Americans, Native Hawaiians, and Other Pacific Islanders are reported in aggregate and limit the ability to appreciate nuance within subpopulations.[5,6] This phenomenon is also true in reporting for Hispanic ethnicity, where more frequent use of disaggregated data could reveal within-group disparities along racial dimensions.[7] Furthermore, most of our data on breast cancer exclude male patients, limiting our ability to understand differences in biology, treatment response, and outcomes by sex. Finally, limited collection and availability of data on self-reported sexual orientation and gender identity in health care settings hinder attempts to quantify and mitigate disparities in access and outcome known to exist in the lesbian, gay, bisexual, transgender, queer or questioning and more (LGBTQ) community.[8]

In the remainder of this article, the authors describe the landscape of health disparities in breast cancer care delivery with a focus on racial/ethnic disparities.

Biological Differences

Black women are more likely to present with triple-negative breast cancer (TNBC), a subtype known to be more aggressive with fewer targeted therapy options and poorer disease-free and overall survival as compared with other variants. TNBC represents 21% of new breast cancer diagnoses in Black women, compared with 10% in White, Asian/Pacific Islander and 12% in Hispanic and American Indian/Alaska Native.[1]

The field of oncologic anthropology, coined by Dr Lisa Newman and Dr Linda Kaljee, studies how population migration can affect breast cancer epidemiology.[9] African American women have a combination of African, European, and indigenous ancestry as a result of their ancestors' passage to the Americas via the trans-Atlantic slave trade. An analysis of breast cancer in Africa demonstrated TNBC in 53.2% of Ghanaian/West African women. The evaluation of slave trade routes demonstrates that West Africans were predominantly routed to North America, and this understanding has prompted increased interrogation of how genetic ancestry originating in West Africa might affect rates of TNBC among African American women.[10]

The African American Breast Cancer Epidemiology and Risk Consortium, which is a collaboration of four breast cancer research programs, conducted an analysis of 3629 cases in Black women with 4648 control patients. In this analysis, they identified a novel gene (3q26.21) for estrogen receptor negative breast cancer among Black women.[11]

This work supports that there are biological contributors to variation in the epidemiology of TNBC. However, the vast majority of breast cancer, even for Black women, is hormone receptor (HR) positive, and much of the racial disparity in survival observed among Black women after breast cancer diagnosis is due to worse outcomes among those with HR-positive disease.[12] Furthermore, among women with TNBC, Black–White differences in outcome are less pronounced and can, in large part, be attributed to differential, and likely inequitable, receipt of surgery and chemotherapy.[13] Thus, although higher incidence of TNBC contributes to worse mortality among Black women relative to other groups to racial disparities in breast cancer outcomes, it is not the sole driver.

In the remainder of this article, the authors explores largely modifiable factors driving disparate and unequal breast cancer outcomes and discuss ways they can work toward a collective goal of promoting equitable health care for individuals with breast cancer.

DISCUSSION
Access to Care

Access to high-quality medical care optimizes health outcomes. Concomitantly, for many patients, the lack of access serves as a significant barrier and is a contributor to disparities in health outcomes. Below, the authors explore ways in which limited access to care impacts breast cancer outcomes.

- *Insurance Coverage, Screening, and Early Detection*
- The percentage of uninsured individuals in the United States has decreased since the passage of the Affordable Care Act in 2010, but disparities in coverage still exist. The individuals of American Indian and Alaska Natives have the highest uninsured rates, followed by Hispanic, Native Hawaiian, Pacific Islander, and Black individuals. However, Asian Americans have the lowest uninsured rates,[14] again highlighting the importance of disaggregating Asians and Pacific Islanders in research.
- Insurance coverage is associated with access to primary care providers and likelihood of receiving screening mammography. Individuals who are underinsured and uninsured are less likely to receive screening mammography, are more likely to be screened at lower resource and nonaccredited facilities, and are less likely to be screened with tomosynthesis, that is, 3D mammography. Furthermore, there is evidence that underinsured and uninsured individuals experience longer delays in follow-up of abnormal results.[15] The early detection is associated with improved survival outcomes for women diagnosed with breast cancer. Thus, challenges with access to care, in part because of disparate rates of insurance coverage, are a barrier to equitable health outcomes.
- Even with insurance, a diagnosis of cancer is associated with a significant financial burden to patients. The cost of treatment and resultant financial toxicity affect treatment decisions, adherence to recommended therapy, and posttreatment surveillance.[16] Furthermore, likelihood of experiencing financial toxicity after breast cancer diagnosis is increased among women of color.[17]
- *Treatment Location*
- Many patients do not live near health care facilities that provide screening services, and likewise, access to specialty care is not universally accessible. As a result, differential proximity to high-quality treatment facilities also facilitates disparity among patients with breast cancer with regard to stage at diagnosis and time to treatment.[18] In a study from Detroit, living in areas with greater Black segregation and limited mammography access was associated with a higher risk of advanced stage breast cancer diagnoses.[19] In a study of patients in Chicago, Black and Hispanic patients were more likely to be treated at facilities that are not accredited by the National Consortium of Breast Centers or deemed a Breast Imaging Center of Excellence by the American College of Radiology.[20] This finding was also corroborated by a Surveillance, Epidemiology, and End Results (SEER) analysis of 51,878 women undergoing breast surgery, which demonstrated that Black women were more likely to be treated at lower volume and lower quality hospitals. Black, Hispanic, and Asian patients with breast cancer were also more likely to receive care at hospitals with a higher proportion of Medicaid patients.[18] Treatment facility choice is multifactorial but in part reflects referral patterns and spatial accessibility. Elevating care in areas serving minority patients should be a public health mission and could significantly mitigate geography-related disparities in breast cancer care and outcomes.

Breast Cancer Treatment

The implementation of new technology and treatment options often reach low-resource populations at a slower rate, thereby transiently or permanently exacerbating disparities in health outcomes. Even with access to guideline-concordant care, there is evidence of systematic differences in receipt of treatment based on patient factors, such as weight, race, and ethnicity. Here, the authors briefly explore disparities in care delivery.

- *Chemotherapy*
- Chemotherapy represents a critical element in the treatment of locally advanced breast cancer and is also increasingly used in earlier stage triple-negative and HER2-positive breast cancer. The role of systemic therapy is to prolong disease-free intervals and overall survival. In select patients, systemic therapy in the neoadjuvant setting can also facilitate downstaging, thereby enabling patients to receive less extensive, less morbid locoregional treatment (ie, surgery and radiation) to the breast and axilla.
- In a study evaluating chemotherapy dosing over a 12-year period, data demonstrated that Black women were more likely to receive lower relative dose intensity compared with White women.[21] In a contemporary systematic review and meta-analysis, findings of dose intensity differences were not noted, but Black women were more likely to experiences delays in initiating therapy greater than 90 days. Furthermore, Black women with early-stage disease who were eligible for chemotherapy were significantly more likely to discontinue chemotherapy.[22] Hispanic ethnicity has also been associated with delays in time to chemotherapy.[23,24] Delays in initiating adjuvant chemotherapy are associated with worse clinical outcomes, particularly when delays are greater than 90 days.[23] Taken together, this suggests that there are both patient and provider factors that impact chemotherapy utilization and represent modifiable targets driving inequities in breast cancer care delivery.
- *Surgery*
- Surgical treatment of breast cancer represents a mainstay of curative intent therapy. Black women are more likely to experience postoperative complications and have longer length of stay compared with White women.[25,26] Hispanic women have also been shown to have higher rates of postoperative complications.[25,27] Finally, Black and Hispanic women have overall higher body mass index (BMIs) and more comorbid medical conditions that place them at higher surgical risk than White peers, and these factors are also believed to contribute to their lower rates of postmastectomy reconstruction. Although preoperative optimization and comanagement with primary care and subspecialty providers are critical, there is often limited time for medical optimization due to the need to provide timely cancer care and prevent compromise to cancer outcomes. Improvement in surgical outcomes is in part dependent on addressing disparities in health outcomes that occur before an individual's breast cancer diagnosis and requires interventions aimed at the level of primary care.
- *Radiation*
- Adjuvant radiation therapy is a critical element in the treatment of many people with breast cancer and it facilitates improvements in local regional control. Although contemporary literature supports select indications for omission of radiotherapy, adjuvant radiation has been the long-standing standard of care after partial mastectomy. Radiation is also indicated after mastectomy in select patients with locally advanced disease.
- Black women are less likely than White women to receive adjuvant radiation.[28–31] In an analysis of the SEER database over 17 years, non-Hispanic Black and Hispanic patients were less likely to receive radiation than White patients, a finding most pronounced with receipt of postmastectomy radiation therapy.[30] Significant racial disparities in utilization of radiation after breast conservation have also been

reported.[31] Treatment at a facility that is less likely to administer a treatment modality will result in lower utilization of that service. In a population-based analysis, Black women were less likely than White women to receive care at high-quality hospitals, defined as being in the top quartile for rates of radiation after breast-conserving surgery.[32]

- *Endocrine Therapy*
- In HR-positive breast cancer, adjuvant endocrine therapy for patients without contraindications is recommended to reduce the risk of breast cancer recurrence. Despite this recommendation, non-initiation, nonadherence, and non-persistence in the use of endocrine therapy are seen across all racial and ethnic groups. However, Black race and Hispanic ethnicity, as well as having low income, has been associated with especially low rates of adherence to endocrine therapy. Reasons cited include concerns about side effects, cost, and perceived patient-provider communication.[33]
- *Challenges during Survivorship*
- The early detection of breast cancer recurrence can influence clinical outcomes. Although there are no established guidelines for survivorship management, surveillance mammography is critical in women with intact breast tissue after treatment. In a systematic review and meta-analysis over a 20-year period, Black, Hispanic, and Asian American women were less likely to receive timely surveillance mammography compared with White women.[34]
- Obesity has been associated with as much as a 35% to 40% increased risk of breast cancer recurrence and with worse overall survival.[35] Rates of obesity are higher in Black women and in women of Hispanic ethnicity.[36] Targeted interventions to promote healthy weight may represent an actionable intervention, though patients may find weight loss hard to prioritize in the midst of and immediately following treatment of breast cancer.[37] Data suggest, however, that there is a much bigger public health crisis. Black and Hispanic children are twice as likely to be obese by the age of 7 years as White children are, highlighting the need for large-scale public health interventions targeting obesity in communities of color.[38,39]

Research and Clinical Trials

Although the early detection is critical and has been a major contributor to improvements in breast cancer outcomes, research and clinical trials have resulted in marked improvement in treatment approaches for women diagnosed with breast cancer. Clinical trials have provided the foundation for de-escalation of surgical management, targeted therapy for HER2-positive breast cancer, and treatment algorithms for TNBC, which represent just a few of the myriad examples of ways that care has been advanced by research.

In many clinical trials, there has been a fundamental lack of racial/ethnic and gender representation. An analysis of cell lines from two major suppliers used for preclinical and clinical trials—the American Type Culture Collection (ATCC) and European Collection of Authenticated Cell Cultures (ECACC)—was conducted to analyze representation of women of African ancestry compared with women of European ancestry. Women of European ancestry represented 80% of the ATCC cell lines and 94% of the ECACC cell lines.[40] Enrollment in clinical trials, while limited across all demographics, is also reported to be lowest in Black, Hispanic, and Asian/Pacific Islander patients, a finding that is also observed among surgical trials of patients with breast cancer.[41,42]

Patients of color are less likely to be treated at institutions where there is access to clinical trials. In addition, stringent trial exclusion criteria related to Eastern cooperative oncology group (ECOG) performance scores and the absence of particular comorbidities further decrease participation of minoritized patients, given higher chronic disease burdens in these groups.[42] Even with geographic access, limited voluntary participation in clinically trials is in part rooted in mistrust within communities of color resulting from episodes of exploitation. The US Public Health Service Syphilis Study at Tuskegee is one well-known example.[43] Black men were enrolled in an observational study of syphilis but not provided informed consent about their participation or even told about their diagnosis. Furthermore, even after treatment with penicillin became available, these men were not provided care for their diagnosis. Another well-known example is displayed in the development of HeLa cells. Henrietta Lacks was a Black mother who ultimately succumbed to cervical cancer. Cells obtained from her cervix were used without her knowledge or consent and ultimately served as the foundation for therapeutic development across a range of diseases. Furthermore, beginning in 1946, the US government conducted experiments in which over 5000 Guatemalan citizens were intentionally infected with bacteria that cause sexually transmitted infections without their informed consent.[44] Many remained untreated into the 2010s. Although these historical examples have helped fuel generations of mistrust toward the health care system, ongoing systemic racism as well as microaggression and macroaggression toward patients and communities of color persist and affect both enrollment in clinical trials and collective impressions about the institution of medicine as a whole.

In a literature review assessing minority participation in clinical trials by Clark and colleagues, five key themes emerged as barriers to enrollment in clinical trials: mistrust, lack of comfort with clinical trial process, lack of information about clinical trials, time and resource constraints associated with clinical trial participation, and lack of clinical trial awareness.[45] Understanding and overcoming these barriers are critical in encouraging diverse participation in clinical trials. Of note, a major reason many patients of color cite for nonparticipation is a failure of health care providers to ask whether they were interested. The Just Ask! program developed by Nadine Barrett, PhD, and available through the Association of Community Cancer Centers and American Cancer Society is an educational program aimed at improving the ability of investigators and research teams recruit diverse clinical trial participants.[46]

Exclusion of male patients has limited our understanding of breast cancer in patients of male sex.[47] Although male breast cancer represents only 1% of all newly diagnosed breast cancer, men typically present with advanced disease and are more likely to die from breast cancer than women are. Furthermore, treatment of men diagnosed with breast cancer is often extrapolated from trials that exclude men. Given the low prevalence of breast cancer in men, accruing a sufficient number of patients to conduct an adequately powered analysis represents a challenge to the medical community that can potentially be enhanced through targeted enrollment outreach and community engagement strategies.

Institutions and research teams can build trustworthiness through inclusion of diverse individuals on their research teams and the use of clinical trial navigators for both women and men. Clinical trial navigators, who often come from minoritized communities, not only provide patients with resources to address potential logistical barriers to participation but also serve as sources of hope and confidence for patients wary of research and health care.[48]

Social Determinants of Health

Although treating a disease process is at the core of providing appropriate health care, understanding the lived experience of a patient and potential barriers to care is important contributors to promoting health equity. Social determinants of care are defined in Health People 2030, a publication of the Office of Disease Prevention and Health Promotion, as *"the conditions in the environment where people are born, live, learn, work, play, worship and age that affect a wide range of health, functioning, and quality-of-life outcomes and risks."*[49] Housing, food, and financial insecurity affect a patient's experience of their treatment and the ability to follow a prescribed treatment plan. For example, if a patient has to choose between a prescription for endocrine therapy and a utility bill or a doctor's appointment and a day of work when financially unstable and supporting a family, they are placed in an impossible situation. Often times, these patients are met with questions about compliance rather than concern for how they can be supported in their care, promoting mistrust and undermining the patient–provider relationship.

Cumulative life stressors throughout daily life can lead to compromise in an individual's ability to cope and have health consequences, measured biologically as allostatic load. Measurements of allostatic load have been inconsistent in the literature but include biomarkers that measure the body's biological response to stress and downstream health outcomes.[50] In fact, an increase in allostatic load was associated with a 9% increase in cancer-specific mortality in a contemporary systematic review and meta-analysis.[51] Although this finding is compelling, it is worth noting that the heterogeneity in defining allostatic load in the literature limits this analysis.

In addition to psychosocial stressors, systemic racism, or political, legal, economic, health care, school, and criminal justice systems that lead to institutionalized race-based discrimination must be considered when contextualizing a patient's lived experience.[52]

How Can We Move the Needle?

An understanding of the complex contributing factors is critical to begin to dismantle health disparities in breast cancer care delivery. To make progress toward equitable care, concerted and intentional efforts must be made at the provider, institutional, health system, and societal levels.

Implicit bias is the result of rapid, unconscious stereotyping, and discriminatory behavior. Implicit bias can affect shared decision-making and patient–provider relationships as well perpetuate mistrust. In a study of 2535 physicians who took the Race Attitude Implicit Association Test (IAT), there was an overall preference for White Americans over Black Americans. Of note, individual self-reported bias and actual implicit bias were not concordant, with higher levels of implicit bias seen on IAT than self-report.[53] Implicit bias can also lead to microaggressions, which are subtle insults or prejudicial behavior toward a marginalized group, and in some cases to macroaggressions, which are overt prejudicial behavior. An awareness of individual bias and how it can affect patient care decisions and patient–provider interactions is critical to overcoming imbedded mistrust and promoting equitable care. A focus on contextualizing the experience of our patients and familiarizing ourselves with support services can help strengthen the patient–provider relationship. Routine screening for unmet social needs and evaluation of the patient experience during their course of treatment is gradually becoming more common via increased use of social need screens and patient-reported outcome measure tools.[54]

At the institutional and health system level, efforts to achieve a diverse workforce will help mitigate disparities in patient care. A diverse work environment leads to a better understanding of racial and culture differences that contributes to culturally competent care for all patients. Furthermore, providers who are traditionally underrepresented in medicine are more likely to provide care to minoritized and medically underserved communities.[55] Given the often complex financial, social, and medical needs of patients, especially from minoritized communities, receiving breast cancer treatment, having a robust suite of supportive services, including social work, financial counselors, and patient navigators may help overcome barriers to high-quality care delivery, including delays in care and perioperative support.

Public health interventions to address the root cause of higher rates of obesity and comorbid conditions within Black and Hispanic communities are a high-level and complex goal that is a critical piece of promoting health equity. Dismantling systemic and structural racism that are deeply embedded in the foundation of society are a crucial step in addressing inequities in care delivery for breast cancer and mitigating disparate health outcomes across all disease sites.

SUMMARY

The anatomy of health disparities is complex, and although this article addresses many of the contributing factors, it is not exhaustive. Health disparities affect the spectrum of the breast care experience, ranging from risk assessment, screening behavior, and early detection to treatment protocols and survivorship. Drivers of disparate breast cancer outcomes begin before a patient's stepping foot into the office a breast cancer specialist.[54] Attention to implicit bias, improving diversity in the work force, and providing robust supportive care services to treat patients in the context of their lived experience rather than their disease alone represent critical steps to promoting equity in breast cancer diagnosis, treatment, outcomes, and clinical trial participation.

DISCLOSURES

Dr O.M. Fayanju is supported by the National Institutes of Health, United States (NIH) under Award Numbers 7K08CA241390-03 (PI: Fayanju) and P50CA244690 (PIs: Beidas, Bekelman). The content of this manuscript is solely the responsibility of the authors and does not necessarily represent the official views of the NIH. Dr O.M. Fayanju also reports institutional grants from Gilead Sciences, United States, and Sanofi as well as support via philanthropic funds from the Haas family. Dr L.C. Elmore has nothing to disclose.

REFERENCES

1. American Cancer Society. Breast Cancer Facts & Figures 2019-2020. Accessed December 15, 2022. https://www.cancer.org/content/dam/cancer-org/research/cancer-facts-and-statistics/breast-cancer-facts-and-figures/breast-cancer-facts-and-figures-2019-2020.pdf.
2. American Cancer Society. Cancer Facts & Figure for African American/Black People 2022-2024. Accessed December 15, 2022. https://www.cancer.org/content/dam/cancer-org/research/cancer-facts-and-statistics/cancer-facts-and-figures-for-african-americans/2022-2024-cff-aa.pdf.
3. Office of Disease Prevention and Health Promotion. Health Equity in Healthy People 2030. Accessed January 21, 2023. https://health.gov/healthypeople/priority-areas/health-equity-healthy-people-2030.
4. Center for Disease Control and Prevention Office of Minority Health & Health Equity. What is Health Equity? Accessed January 21, 2023. https://www.cdc.gov/healthequity/whatis/index.html#anchor_09858.
5. Yu AYL, Thomas SM, DiLalla GD, et al. Disease characteristics and mortality among Asian women with breast cancer. Cancer 2022;128(5):1024–37.

6. Champion CD, Thomas SM, Plichta JK, et al. Disparities at the Intersection of Race and Ethnicity: Examining Trends and Outcomes in Hispanic Women With Breast Cancer. JCO Oncol Pract 2022;18(5):e827–38.

7. Swami N, Nguyen T, Dee EC, et al. Disparities in Primary Breast Cancer Stage at Presentation Among Hispanic Subgroups. Ann Surg Oncol 2022;29(13):7977–87.

8. Quinn GP, Sanchez JA, Sutton SK, et al. Cancer and lesbian, gay, bisexual, transgender/transsexual, and queer/questioning (LGBTQ) populations. CA: a cancer journal for clinicians 2015;65(5):384–400.

9. Newman LA, Kaljee LM. Health Disparities and Triple-Negative Breast Cancer in African American Women: A Review. JAMA Surg 2017;152(5):485–93.

10. Newman LA, Jenkins B, Chen Y, et al. Hereditary susceptibility for triple negative breast cancer associated with Western Sub-Saharan African Ancestry: results from an International Surgical Breast Cancer Collaborative. Annals of surgery 2019;270(3):484–92.

11. Huo D, Feng Y, Haddad S, et al. Genome-wide association studies in women of African ancestry identified 3q26.21 as a novel susceptibility locus for oestrogen receptor negative breast cancer. Hum Mol Genet 2016;25(21):4835–46.

12. Warner ET, Tamimi RM, Hughes ME, et al. Racial and Ethnic Differences in Breast Cancer Survival: Mediating Effect of Tumor Characteristics and Sociodemographic and Treatment Factors. J Clin Oncol 2015;33(20):2254–61.

13. Cho B, Han Y, Lian M, et al. Evaluation of Racial/Ethnic Differences in Treatment and Mortality Among Women With Triple-Negative Breast Cancer. JAMA Oncol 2021;7(7):1016–23.

14. Kaiser Family Foundation. Health Coverage by Race and Ethnicity, 2010-2021. Accessed December 15, 2022. https://www.kff.org/racial-equity-and-health-policy/issue-brief/health-coverage-by-race-and-ethnicity/.

15. Schueler KM, Chu PW, Smith-Bindman R. Factors associated with mammography utilization: a systematic quantitative review of the literature. J Womens Health (Larchmt) 2008;17(9):1477–98.

16. Greenup RA. Financial Toxicity and Shared Decision Making in Oncology. Surgical Oncology Clinics 2022;31(1):1–7.

17. Politi MC, Yen RW, Elwyn G, et al. Women Who Are Young, Non-White, and with Lower Socioeconomic Status Report Higher Financial Toxicity up to 1 Year After Breast Cancer Surgery: A Mixed-Effects Regression Analysis. Oncol 2020;26(1):e142–52.

18. Keating NL, Kouri EM, He Y, et al. Location Isn't Everything: Proximity, Hospital Characteristics, Choice of Hospital, and Disparities for Breast Cancer Surgery Patients. Health Serv Res 2016;51(4):1561–83.

19. Dai D. Black residential segregation, disparities in spatial access to health care facilities, and late-stage breast cancer diagnosis in metropolitan Detroit. Health Place 2010;16(5):1038–52.

20. Molina Y, Silva A, Rauscher GH. Racial/Ethnic Disparities in Time to a Breast Cancer Diagnosis: The Mediating Effects of Health Care Facility Factors. Med Care 2015;53(10):872–8.

21. Griggs JJ, Sorbero MES, Stark AT, et al. Racial Disparity in the Dose and Dose Intensity of Breast Cancer Adjuvant Chemotherapy. Breast Cancer Res Treat 2003;81(1):21–31.

22. Green AK, Aviki EM, Matsoukas K, et al. Racial disparities in chemotherapy administration for early-stage breast cancer: a systematic review and meta-analysis. Breast Cancer Res Treat 2018;172(2):247–63.

23. Chavez-MacGregor M, Clarke CA, Lichtensztajn DY, et al. Delayed Initiation of Adjuvant Chemotherapy Among Patients With Breast Cancer. JAMA Oncol 2016;2(3):322–9.
24. Fedewa SA, Ward EM, Stewart AK, et al. Delays in adjuvant chemotherapy treatment among patients with breast cancer are more likely in African American and Hispanic populations: a national cohort study 2004-2006. J Clin Oncol 2010; 28(27):4135–41.
25. Akinyemiju TF, Vin-Raviv N, Chavez-Yenter D, et al. Race/ethnicity and socioeconomic differences in breast cancer surgery outcomes. Cancer Epidemiology 2015;39(5):745–51.
26. Sarver MM, Rames JD, Ren Y, et al. Racial and Ethnic Disparities in Surgical Outcomes after Postmastectomy Breast Reconstruction. J Am Coll Surg 2022;234(5): 760–71.
27. Mets EJ, Chouairi FK, Gabrick KS, et al. Persistent disparities in breast cancer surgical outcomes among hispanic and African American patients. European Journal of Surgical Oncology 2019;45(4):584–90.
28. Dragun AE, Huang B, Tucker TC, et al. Disparities in the application of adjuvant radiotherapy after breast-conserving surgery for early stage breast cancer. Cancer 2011;117(12):2590–8.
29. Du XL, Gor BJ. Racial Disparities and Trends in Radiation Therapy After Breast-Conserving surgery for Early-stage Breast Cancer in Women, 1992 to 2002. Ethn Dis 2007;17(1):122–8.
30. Martinez SR, Beal SH, Chen SL, et al. Disparities in the Use of Radiation Therapy in Patients With Local-Regionally Advanced Breast Cancer. Int J Radiat Oncol Biol Phys 2010;78(3):787–92.
31. Smith GL, Shih YC, Xu Y, et al. Racial disparities in the use of radiotherapy after breast-conserving surgery: a national Medicare study. Cancer 2010;116(3):734–41.
32. Keating NL, Kouri E, He Y, et al. Racial differences in definitive breast cancer therapy in older women: are they explained by the hospitals where patients undergo surgery? Med Care 2009;47(7):765–73.
33. Roberts MC, Wheeler SB, Reeder-Hayes K. Racial/Ethnic and socioeconomic disparities in endocrine therapy adherence in breast cancer: a systematic review. Am J Public Health 2015;105(Suppl 3):e4–15.
34. Advani P, Advani S, Nayak P, et al. Racial/ethnic disparities in use of surveillance mammogram among breast cancer survivors: a systematic review. J Cancer Surviv 2022;16(3):514–30.
35. Jiralerspong S, Goodwin PJ. Obesity and Breast Cancer Prognosis: Evidence, Challenges, and Opportunities. J Clin Oncol 2016;34(35):4203–16.
36. Nayak P, Paxton RJ, Holmes H, et al. Racial and Ethnic Differences in Health Behaviors Among Cancer Survivors. Am J Prev Med 2015;48(6):729–36.
37. Fayanju OM, Greenup RA, Zafar SY, et al. Modifiable Barriers and Facilitators for Breast Cancer Care: A Thematic Analysis of Patient and Provider Perspectives. J Surg Res 2023;284:269–79.
38. Taveras EM, Gillman MW, Kleinman KP, et al. Reducing racial/ethnic disparities in childhood obesity: the role of early life risk factors. JAMA Pediatr 2013;167(8): 731–8.
39. Williams DR, Mohammed SA, Shields AE. Understanding and effectively addressing breast cancer in African American women: Unpacking the social context. Cancer 2016;122(14):2138–49.
40. Clarke S, Chin SN, Dodds L, et al. Racial disparities in breast cancer preclinical and clinical models. Breast Cancer Res 2022;24(1):56.

41. Stewart JH, Bertoni AG, Staten JL, et al. Participation in Surgical Oncology Clinical Trials: Gender-, Race/Ethnicity-, and Age-based Disparities. Ann Surg Oncol 2007;14(12):3328–34.

42. Fayanju OM, Ren Y, Thomas SM, et al. A Case-Control Study Examining Disparities in Clinical Trial Participation Among Breast Surgical Oncology Patients. JNCI Cancer Spectr 2020;4(2):pkz103.

43. Reverby SM. Ethical failures and history lessons: the US Public Health Service research studies in Tuskegee and Guatemala. Publ Health Rev 2012;34:1–18.

44. Rodriguez MA, García R. First, Do No Harm: The US Sexually Transmitted Disease Experiments in Guatemala. American Journal of Public Health 2013; 103(12):2122–6.

45. Clark LT, Watkins L, Piña IL, et al. Increasing Diversity in Clinical Trials: Overcoming Critical Barriers. Curr Probl Cardiol 2019;44(5):148–72.

46. Barrett NJ, Boehmer L, Schrag J, et al. An Assessment of the Feasibility and Utility of an ACCC-ASCO Implicit Bias Training Program to Enhance Racial and Ethnic Diversity in Cancer Clinical Trials. JCO Oncol Pract 2023;Op2200378. https://doi.org/10.1200/op.22.00378.

47. Duma N, Hoversten KP, Ruddy KJ. Exclusion of male patients in breast cancer clinical trials. JNCI Cancer Spectr 2018;2(2):pky018.

48. Guerra CE, Sallee V, Hwang WT, et al. Accrual of Black participants to cancer clinical trials following a five-year prospective initiative of community outreach and engagement. J Clin Oncol 2021;39(15_suppl):100.

49. Office of Disease Prevention and Health Promotion. Healthy People 2030: Social Determinants of Health. Accessed January 15, 2023. https://health.gov/healthypeople/priority-areas/social-determinants-health.

50. Obeng-Gyasi S, Tarver W, Carlos RC, et al. Allostatic load: a framework to understand breast cancer outcomes in Black women. NPJ Breast Cancer 2021; 7(1):100.

51. Mathew A, Doorenbos AZ, Li H, et al. Allostatic Load in Cancer: A Systematic Review and Mini Meta-Analysis. Biol Res Nurs 2021;23(3):341–61.

52. Braveman P, Arkin E, Proctor D, et al. Systemic And Structural Racism: Definitions, Examples, Health Damages, And Approaches To Dismantling. Health Aff 2022;41(2):171–8.

53. Sabin J, Nosek BA, Greenwald A, et al. Physicians' implicit and explicit attitudes about race by MD race, ethnicity, and gender. J Health Care Poor Underserved 2009;20(3):896–913.

54. Fayanju OM, Ren Y, Stashko I, et al. Patient-reported causes of distress predict disparities in time to evaluation and time to treatment after breast cancer diagnosis. Cancer 2020. https://doi.org/10.1002/cncr.33310.

55. Walker KO, Moreno G, Grumbach K. The association among specialty, race, ethnicity, and practice location among California physicians in diverse specialties. J Natl Med Assoc 2012;104(1–2):46–52.

Evaluation of Treatment Response in Patients with Breast Cancer

Saima Muzahir, MD, FCPS, FRCPE[a,b,*], Gary A. Ulaner, MD, PhD[c,d], David M. Schuster, MD, FACR[b]

KEYWORDS

- Breast cancer • Treatment response • CT • MR imaging • FDG PET-CT
- Bone scan

KEY POINTS

- In breast cancer, clinicopathologic stage and tumor biology guides the selection of appropriate imaging modalities for response assessment.
- For response monitoring FDG-PET/CT compared to CE-CT alone provides earlier detection of the first progression, leading to change or revision in treatment plans.
- FDG-PET/CT for response monitoring in patients with metastatic breast cancer may improve clinical decision-making and patient survival.

INTRODUCTION

Female breast cancer (BC) is one of the most diagnosed cancers and causes of cancer-related deaths in women, second only to lung cancer in Unites States. The American Cancer Society has estimated that 290,560 Americans wlll be diagnosed with BC and 43,780 will die of disease in the United States in 2022.[1] Management of BC not only depends on accurate diagnosis and staging but also on the best possible measures of response assessment. Imaging plays a vital role in the initial diagnosis and staging as well as in the response assessment to therapy, which is widely used to guide treatment decisions, although there are no specific recommendations for imaging procedures in the international metastatic breast cancer (MBC)

This article previously appeared in PET Clinics volume 18 issue 4 October 2023.

[a] Division of Nuclear Medicine and Molecular Imaging, Department of Radiology and Imaging Sciences, 1364 Clifton Road, Atlanta GA 30322, USA; [b] Division of Nuclear Medicine and Molecular Imaging, Department of Radiology and Imaging Sciences, Emory University Hospital, Room E152, 1364 Clifton Road, Atlanta, GA 30322, USA; [c] Molecular Imaging and Therapy, Hoag Family Cancer Institute, Newport Beach, CA, USA; [d] Radiology and Translational Genomics, University of Southern California, Los Angeles, CA, USA

* Corresponding author. Emory University Hospital, Division of Nuclear Medicine and Molecular Imaging, Department of Radiology and Imaging Sciences, 1364 Clifton Road, Atlanta GA 30322, USA

E-mail address: saima.muzahir@emory.edu

Clinics Collections 14 (2024) 289–307
https://doi.org/10.1016/j.ccol.2024.02.015

guidelines.[2,3] In this review, we will analyze and compare the diagnostic accuracy and clinical utility of conventional and molecular imaging in the assessment of tumor response to therapy.

Locally Advanced Breast Cancer

In locally advanced BC, neoadjuvant chemotherapy (NAC) is now the standard of care.[4] The goal of NAC is to downstage primary tumors, to increase the rate of breast conservation, to eliminate micrometastatic disease, and to predict prognosis using tumor response as a parameter. Studies have shown that patients who attain pathological complete response (pCR) after NAC have a longer disease-free survival and better overall survival (OS) as compared with nonresponders.[5,6] Early and accurate assessment of response to therapy can help in making timely decisions regarding change in treatment to a more effective regimen, which can increase rates of breast conservation surgery.

NEOADJUVANT THERAPY RESPONSE ASSESSMENT

These can be broadly divided into anatomic imaging and functional imaging. Anatomic imaging includes ultrasound (US), digital mammography (DM), and digital breast tomosynthesis (DBT). Functional imaging modalities include dynamic contrast-enhanced MR imaging, F-18 Fluorodeoxyglucose positron emission tomography-computed tomography (F-18 FDG PET-CT), molecular breast imaging using 99mTc-sestamibi and newer hybrid PET-MR imaging. Currently there is lack of standard approach for the imaging evaluation and follow-up of patients undergoing NAC. According to the recent NCCN guidelines, a multidisciplinary approach should be used to determine the selection of different imaging methods before surgery.[7]

ANATOMIC IMAGING TECHNIQUES
Digital Mammography and Digital Breast Tomosynthesis

Mammography is the most used imaging modality to assess tumor size after NAC. However, the accuracy of mammography in assessing residual tumor size is highly influenced by the initial mammographic appearance of the tumor. The accuracy of mammography is higher for masses with well-circumscribed margins on pretreatment mammography compared with masses with ill-defined margins.[4] Decreases in tumor size and density are the most reliable indicators of treatment response, whereas changes in calcifications can be misleading and are considered one of the challenges in image interpretation.[8] Mammography is more sensitive than clinical examination (79% vs 49%) in the prediction of residual carcinoma; it is however not accurate enough to obviate surgical biopsy.[9] DBT has higher resolution compared with conventional DM particularly in small lesions and dense breasts.[10] It is more accurate than DM in assessing response and has a good correlation with histopathology for residual tumor size after NAC.[11] Yet, there still may be limitations related to overestimation of tumor size on DBT compared with DM.[8]

Ultrasound

US is a widely used modality in assessing response to NAC and is more accurate than mammography in assessing residual tumor size after NAC.[12,13] However, there is no difference between mammography and US in predicting complete pathologic response.[12] Several studies showed that the combined use of both mammography and US improved the accuracy of predicting a pCR to NAC compared with the use of either modality alone.[14,15] Automated breast US (ABUS) using three-dimensional images featuring high reproducibility and less operator dependence allows more appropriate evaluation of large breast masses and architectural distortion compared with conventional breast US.[16] However, ABUS tends to underestimate residual tumor size resulting in lowest reliability compared with DM, DBT, and MR imaging.[8] US is also considered the most accurate predictor of response in axillary lymph nodes compared with mammography and physical examination.[17]

MR Imaging

MR imaging performs well in dense breasts and is the most sensitive imaging modality for detecting multifocality and monitoring patient response to NAC.[18,19] It outperforms mammography, US, and clinical examination in evaluating residual tumor after NAC with excellent correlation between macroscopic tumor size and the tumor established by MR imaging.[8] It remains as the most accurate imaging modality for NAC response assessment,[18] accurately assessing residual tumor after NAC with high sensitivity, specificity, and accuracy.[20] The multicenter American College of Radiology Imaging Network (ACRIN) 6657 study showed that not only functional tumor volume measurements are more accurate in predicting response but may also help in predicting recurrence-free survival.[21] Multiple studies using radiomic and deep learning have looked at predicting pCR from pretreatment MR images have found that separating tumors into their subtypes improves accuracy and that different features are predictive of response to therapy in different tumor subtypes.[22] MR imaging however has limited utility and can underestimate residual disease in tumors with nonmass morphology such as invasive lobular cancer and luminal tumors.[23,24] MR tends to overestimate response with taxane-based NAC.[25]

F-18 Fluorodeoxyglucose PET-CT

F-18 FDG evaluates glucose metabolism in BC cells, independent of breast density.[26] Decreased glucose metabolism within BC tissue on F-18 FDG PET-CT is a useful indicator to assess the effectiveness of NAC[27] and can provide information on tumor metabolic activity, which can help in distinguishing active tumor from posttherapeutic changes[28](Fig. 1). It is important to have knowledge about different BC histologic types because different histologic types vary in their FDG avidity and pattern of spread and key outcomes such as pathologic response and survival may vary by BC subtypes and type of treatment.[29,30] Estrogen receptor (ER)-negative tumors have statistically significantly higher FDG avidity compared with ER-positive tumors.[28,29] High-grade (grade 3) tumors have significantly higher FDG uptake than lower grade tumors.[31] Key outcomes such as pathologic response and survival may vary by BC subtypes and type of treatment.[32] PET parameters that best correlate with pathologic response vary based on tumor phenotype. Changes in SUVmax or total lesion glycolysis (TLG) are most adequate for triple-negative BC and for ER-positive/human epidermal growth factor receptor 2 (HER2)-negative cancers and absolute SUVmax after 2 cycles of NAC for HER2-positive BCs.[33] Schelling and colleagues showed significant differences in FDG uptake between responders and nonresponders after the first course of chemotherapy, before radiological response.[34] Large prospective multicenter evaluated changes in SUVmax at baseline and after first and second cycles of chemotherapy, their results showed that a threshold of 45% decrease in standardized uptake value (SUV) correctly identified responders, and histopathologic nonresponders were identified with a negative predictive value of 90%. Similar results were found after the second cycle when using a threshold of 55% relative decrease in SUV.[35] Another meta-analysis showed a cutoff value of SUV reduction between 55% and 65%, best correlated with pathologic condition and might potentially identify

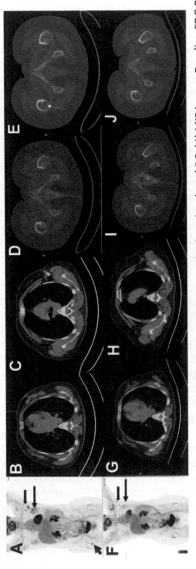

Fig. 1. A 50-year-old woman diagnosed with left breast ER-positive, HER-2-negative invasive ductal BC. (*A*) MIP image: Baseline FDG PET shows FDG avid multifocal left BC (*long black arrow*) with left axillary adenopathy (*thick black arrow*) and focal uptake in right proximal femur (*short black arrow*). (*B*) Fused transaxial FDG PET-CT image shows left primary BC, (*C*) fused transaxial image showing left axillary adenopathy, (*D*) fused transaxial image showing FDG avid right proximal femur, corresponding to a tiny lytic lesion on the CT portion of the PET examination (*E, white arrow*). (*F*) MIP image: Follow-up PET CT scan following chemotherapy shows favorable response to therapy with resolution of FDG uptake in left breast primary (*long black arrow*) and interval decrease in size, number, and metabolic activity in left axillary adenopathy (*short black arrow*), (*G*) fused transaxial image with resolution of primary lesion, (*H*) fused transaxial image showing response to therapy in left axillary adenopathy. (*I*) Fused transaxial image showing significant interval reduction in FDG uptake in right femur lytic lesion. MIP: maximal intensity projection. (*J*) CT portion of the PET CT exam, shows very minimal peripheral sclerosis in the right femur lytic lesion.

nonresponders early in the treatment course.[36] Studies have confirmed that achievement of pCR correlates with both OS and disease-free survival with the greatest benefit seen in aggressive BC subtypes.[37,38] A multicenter open label phase 2 trial in Her-2 positive early BC assessed early metabolic responses to neoadjuvant trastuzumab and pertuzumab showed that FDG PET identified patients with HER2-positive, early-stage BC who were likely to benefit from chemotherapy-free dual HER2 blockade with trastuzumab and pertuzumab.[39] PET-CT has higher sensitivity when compared with MR as FDG has the ability to offer early metabolic response prediction when compared with MR imaging. MR imaging however has a higher specificity; therefore, a combined use of these 2 imaging modalities may have better ability to improve the diagnostic performance in assessing pCR after NAC.[40,41] Cho and colleagues in a prospective study showed that FDG PET-MR imaging can help to predict non-pCR after the first cycle of NAC.[42]

Regional Axillary Node Evaluation with F-18 Fluorodeoxyglucose Positron Emission Tomography

Regional axillary node status is the most important variable to predict prognosis. There have been very few studies assessing changes in FDG uptake in axillary lymph nodes.[43,44] Rousseau and colleagues showed that FDG PET can accurately predict the pathologic status of regional axillary lymph nodes in early-stage BC (stage II and III) after one course of NAC in 52 patients who achieved a nodal pCR. One of the limitations of the study was that not all patients had biopsy confirmed lymph node metastases at baseline; this limited the calculation of true responders.[45] The early assessment of response can help in patient management and can guide clinicians to revise their treatment plans and goals of care relative to their original plans based on FDG PET-CT imaging by avoiding ineffective chemotherapy and to continue preoperative chemotherapy in responding patients.[28]

Breast-Specific Gamma Imaging

Breast-specific gamma imaging (BSGI) using Tc-99m sestamibi 99m Tc-methoxyisobutylisonitrile (MIBI) was Food and Drug Administration (FDA) approved as a second-line breast imaging agent in dense breasts or where mammography findings are equivocal.[46,47] Breast MR imaging is considered as the modality of choice in assessing response to NAC because of superior accuracy than clinical examination, mammography, and US.[48] However, BSGI using MIBI has a potential role in assessing response to NAC in patients where breast MR imaging cannot be performed or is contraindicated.[47] In a large prospective study by Hunt and colleagues compared the size of invasive BC before and after NAC using breast MR imaging and BSGI and assessed the accuracy of post-NAC BSGI and MR imaging relative to pathologic diagnosis. The results of the study showed that both modalities show similar disease extent before NAC; however, both modalities lack sufficient accuracy in predicting pathologic complete response after NAC compared with pathologic evaluation.[49] Despite its clinical utility, BSGI is, however, not widely available.

METASTATIC BREAST CANCER THERAPY RESPONSE ASSESSMENT

MBC is now considered a chronic disease with an increase in the number of women living longer with MBC due to advancements in BC treatment. The prognosis for MBC however is still low with a 5-year OS of only 25%.[50] There have been limited studies evaluating treatment response in MBC compared with studies evaluating response to NAC. This might be because histopathologic diagnosis is almost always available after NAC but is rarely present after the treatment of metastatic disease.[51]

Contrast-Enhanced CT in Metastatic Breast Cancer

Contrast-enhanced CT (CECT) using Response Evaluation Criteria in Solid Tumors (RECIST 1.1) is widely used in response evaluation in MBC.[52,53] Most current guidelines recommend RECIST 1.1 for response evaluation, treatment, and monitoring of MBC.[3] The RECIST criteria are well defined and have a high degree of repeatability. However, it suffers from major drawback because osseous metastases are considered nonmeasurable disease and in distinguishing viable from nonviable residual tumor tissue. There is also a weak correlation between degree of response and survival.[54,55] Mandrekar and colleagues published that the RECIST criteria showed poorer correlation with survival for MBC than for other cancers (colorectal and nonsmall cell lung cancer). The results remained unchanged whether patients in the stable disease group were considered as responders, or nonresponders.[56]

F-18 Fluorodeoxyglucose Positron Emission Tomography

Accurate and early response evaluation has become more important with an increase in the number of treatment options available because it can potentially affect patient survival. The randomized clinical trials evaluating response to therapy with new drugs still use new RECIST criteria.[53] The disadvantage is that several cycles of treatment are requited before cross-sectional imaging (CT or MR imaging) can detect measurable changes in tumor size and changes in tumor do not often correlate with patient outcome. A prospective study compared FDG PET-CT with CECT showed that FDG PET-CT is superior in detecting earlier disease progression with a potentially clinically relevant median delay of 6 months for CECT.[57] Kitajima and colleagues showed that FDG PET-CT accurately assessed early response and prediction of progression after one cycle of chemotherapy in recurrent or MBC.[58] There are no specific recommendations for response monitoring for patients with MBC outside clinical trials.[3] Phase I/II clinical trials applying FDG-PET/CT to evaluate response showed that early metabolic response can predict survival and can be used as a biomarker to response evaluation, especially for molecular targeted therapies.[59,60] Riedel and colleagues showed that evaluating tumor response with FDG PET/CT seems to be a superior predictor of progression-free survival (PFS) and disease-specific survival than response on CE-CT.[54] Naghavi-Behzad and colleagues showed that there is improved patient management and a survival benefit of 14 to 24 months when FDG-PET/CT was used alone or in combination with CT.[61] A semiquantitative set of response evaluation criteria for whole-body FDG-PET/CT, Positron Emission Tomography Response Criteria in Solid Tumors (PERCIST), was proposed in 2009.[62] PERCIST has many advantages. These include high degree of repeatability, less interobserver variability than in measurements with CE-CT, the ability to differentiate between metabolically viable cancer from posttherapy changes.[54] Response assessment using PERCIST criteria is not only more sensitive in detecting progressive or responding disease response but also superior in prediction of progression-free and disease-specific survival compared with RECIST 1.1.[54,63] Several studies have shown increased sensitivity of FDG PET-CT compared with CT and bone scintigraphy (BS) in staging and response evaluation.[64,65] PERCIST-based response assessment relies on standardized uptake value (SUV) normalized by lean body mass measurement either normalized to body weight or lean body mass (SUL).[62] Ulaner and colleagues in a large multicenter trial of neratinib for rare HER2-mutant malignancies (SUMMIT) showed that using PET response criteria allowed patients with nonmeasurable disease by RECIST criteria allowed recruitment of such patients that otherwise would have been denied access to the trial.[66] Tumor heterogeneity has been associated with immune infiltration, metastasis, and drug resistance. FDG PET-CT can be used for noninvasive evaluation of tumor heterogeneity and in predicting response to chemotherapy. Patients on immunotherapy can have pseudoprogression presenting as initially increased tumor lesion size and subsequently decreased tumor burden. It is recommended to get serial FDG PET-CT scan to differentiate pseudoprogression from true progression.[67,68] Recently, a study proposed a novel method to assess intratumor and intertumor heterogeneity using FDG PET-CT in patients with triple-negative BC on immunotherapy showing that baseline intertumor heterogeneity could be a predictor for first-line immunotherapy.[69] Metabolic flare (MF) characterized by transient increase in FDG avidity of lesions after endocrine therapy is usually seen within first 2 weeks after therapy and is predictive of responsiveness to endocrine therapy.[70,71] MF however does not interfere with response assessments as FDG PET scans are usually performed no earlier than 4 to 6 weeks after initiating therapy and is generally not seen with chemotherapy. Cyclin-dependent 4/6 kinase (CDK4/6) inhibitors plus endocrine therapy is standard of care in the treatment of hormone receptor-positive HER2-negative BC. Studies have shown that FDG PET-CT can help in early response assessment in patients on CDK4/6 inhibitors and can provide prognostic information.[72,73] Groheux previously summarized the data on FDG PET/CT for monitoring treatment response in patients with MBC through 2018.[30] We expand this to now include trials through 2022 (**Table 1**), which are notable for their emphasis on prospective trials.

MR Imaging

MR imaging provides information related to the differences in the cellular density and water mobility between benign and malignant tissues with the advantage of not exposing patients to ionizing radiation.[74,] Studies have demonstrated superiority of MR imaging over BS in identifying bone metastases with a pooled sensitivity of 97% versus 79% for BS and a pooled specificity of 95% versus 82%, respectively.[75] Whole body MR imaging (WBMRI) although is not routinely used in bone dominant (BD) MBC. A retrospective study assessing the utility of WBMRI in addition to CT, BS, and FDG PET-CT in influencing anticancer treatment decisions in MBC showed that WBMRI can help in earlier identification of disease progression compared with other imaging modalities.[76] MR imaging can also help in equivocal findings on BS and can guide for local therapy in sites that were negative on a BS and can also help in management decisions through identifying complications such as cord compression associated with bone metastases.

Influence of Tumor Histology on FDG PET

The 2 most common histologic subtypes are invasive ductal carcinoma (IDC) accounting for 75% to 80% of primary BC and invasive lobular cancer (ILC), this accounts for 10% to 15% of primary BC.[77] Primary ILC and metastases from ILC have low FDG uptake compared with IDC.[33,78] Osseous metastases from ILC tend to be sclerotic and are more likely to be missed by FDG PET-CT than osseous metastases from IDC because of their low FDG uptake, which is indistinguishable from background activity.[79] The pattern of metastases in ILC is unusual with a tendency to spread to the serosal surfaces such as pleura and peritoneum, retroperitoneum and gastrointestinal, genitourinary tracts and an increased rate of leptomeningeal spread than IDC.[80] These sites of metastatic spread can be challenging to identify due to the presence of overlying physiologic FDG uptake, this most likely results in lower detection rates of ILC metastases than IDC.[80,81]

Table 1
Studies evaluating F-18 fluorodeoxyglucose positron emission tomography assessing response in breast cancer 2019–2022

Reference	Type	No of Patients	Site of Metastases	Timing of PET	Main Objective	Results
Ulaner et al,[66] 2019	Prospective	81	No specific site	Baseline and follow-up every 8 wk	To determine whether FDG PET can expand eligibility in biomarker-selected clinical trials by providing a means to quantitate response in patients with nonassessable disease by RECIST	PET response criteria allowed patients with non-RECIST measurable disease access to therapy and facilitated more rapid accrual of patients to this trial of a rare biomarker
Vogsen et al,[63] 2021	Retrospective	37	No specific site	Baseline and follow-up	Assessed feasibility and potential benefit of applying PERCIST for response monitoring in metastatic breast cancer using baseline PERCIST baseline and the nadir PERCIST nadir as a reference	PERCIST nadir, can be helpful in clinical decision-making and for response monitoring in MBC
Seifert et al,[72] 2021	Retrospective	8	No specific site	Baseline and 14 d after the start of treatment	Assessed feasibility of early metabolic response assessment to predict the long-term treatment response to CDK4/6 inhibitor therapy	Elevated TLG on early FDG-PET is associated with long-term treatment failure and a poor outcome in patients undergoing CDK4/6 inhibitor therapy for MBC

		N	Site	Timepoints	Objective	Findings
Makhlin et al,[100] 2022	Prospective	23	Bone dominant metastases	Baseline, at 4 wk and 12 wk post-ET	To evaluate the role PET-CT early 4 wk PET-CT in predicting PFS	At the 4-wk time point PET responders had numerically longer PFS, OS and tSRE compared with nonresponders, suggesting the clinical utility of 4-wk ^{18}F-FDG PET/CT as an early predictor of treatment failure
Vogsen et al,[57] 2022	Prospective	87	No specific site	Every 9–12 wk	Compared CE-CT and FDG PET-CT or response monitoring in MBC using the standardized response evaluation criteria RECIST 1.1 and PERCIST	FDG PET-CT identified disease progression earlier than CE-CT in most patients with a potentially clinically relevant median 6-mo delay for CE-CT
Kitajima et al,[58] 2022	Prospective	33	No specific site	Before and after one cycle of systemic therapy	To evaluate the usefulness of early assessment of tumor response using FDG PET-CT after one cycle of systemic therapy in patients with recurrent and MBC	After one cycle of systemic therapy PET/CT was able to reflect early metabolic changes regardless of the lesion site and showed accuracy for early response evaluation and prediction of progression in patients with recurrent or MBC

Abbreviations: CECT, contrast-enhanced computed tomography; MBC, metastatic breast cancer; OS, overall survival; PERCIST, PET response criteria in solid tumor; PFS, progression-free survival; RECIST, response criteria in solid tumors; tSRE, time to skeletal-related event.

Skeletal Metastases

About 30% to 85% of patients develop bone metastases during the disease course, more commonly in ER + MBC.[82,83] Bone metastases are considered nonmeasurable by RECIST criteria[53]; therefore, clinicians usually rely on improvement in symptoms to assess response to treatment. It is challenging to evaluate changes in the size of bone metastases using conventional imaging as healed sclerotic lesions do not disappear and lytic lesions can show sclerotic changes as an indicator of treatment response.[84,85]

Bone Scintigraphy

BS performed with Tc-99m labeled diphosphonate is a low cost and widely available whole-body imaging for identifying bone metastases with good sensitivity; however, it lacks specificity and this can lead to false positives.[86] Whole body BS with single photon emission computed tomography (SPECT) including a low-dose CT scan as part of SPECT-CT examination helps in improving lesion to background ratio and low-dose CT allows for anatomic lesion localization, results in increasing the diagnostic accuracy of the examination.[87] BS however has its limitations when it is used for response assessment. Coombes and colleagues assessing response to systemic therapy in patients with bone metastases showed that only 52% of responders demonstrated scintigraphic improvement and 62% of nonresponders showed scintigraphic deterioration at 6 to 8 months.[88] Flare phenomenon is usually seen in patients receiving chemotherapy or endocrine therapy between 2 weeks to 3 months following therapy but can rarely be seen as late as 6 months after treatment.[89,90] The lag time of 3 to 6 months limits clinical utility of BS in response assessment although it has been shown that if serial bone scans confirm a flare, then it is likely to herald a favorable response to therapy.[91] Although several studies have shown the superiority of FDG PET-CT in evaluating lytic osseous metastases compared with BS; however, BS has clinical utility in assessing response if FDG exhibits minimal or no uptake.[92] Sodium fluoride PET-CT (F-18 NaF PET-CT) is similar to BS, the uptake corresponds to increased osteoblastic activity, and therefore it lacks specificity and can cause false positives; however, low-dose whole body CT acquired as part of NaF PETCT helps in improving specificity.[93] The clinical utility of F-18 NaF in monitoring response assessment is less well described in literature; however, the combined use of F-18 NaF and FDG PET-CT might be considered in selected patients with BC with suspicious sclerotic bone lesions and negative FDG PET-CT.[94]

F-18 Fluorodeoxyglucose Positron Emission Tomography

FDG PET-CT has shown superior sensitivity in the detection of bone involvement in patients with MBC than conventional imaging and is emerging as the modality of choice for treatment monitoring of bone dominant MBC[64] (**Fig. 2**). FDG uptake in viable bone metastases acts as a tumor-specific tracer rather than reflecting altered bone microenvironment.[95] Stafford and colleagues reported a correlation between changes in 18F-FDG uptake and the overall clinical assessment of a response in patients with BD MBC.[96] Multiple studies have shown that patients with MBC who showed no change in F18 FDG uptake were twice as likely to progress than patients who showed a metabolic response.[97,98] Makhlin and colleagues showed that patients with BD MBC receiving endocrine therapy, early time point FDG PET-CT imaging at 4 weeks provides prognostic information and can help in early identification of responders versus nonresponders. The data from this study have been used to support the ongoing large multicenter EA1183 trial (FEATURE) in evaluating whether FDG-PET/

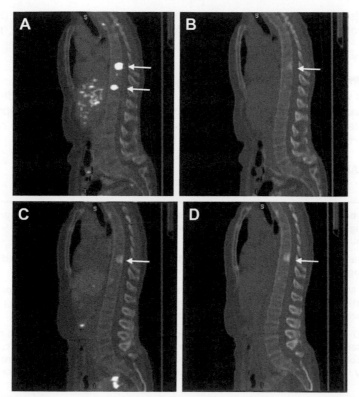

Fig. 2. A 65-year-old woman with metastatic left BC (ER positive, PR positive, HER-2 negative) with bone metastasis. (*A*) Fused sagittal image shows FDG avid lesions in the spine (*arrows*), (*B*) CT sagittal image shows sclerotic lesions on CT portion of the FDG PET/CT examination (*arrow*). (*C and D*) Follow-up scan, after CDK4/6 inhibitor and hormonal therapy. Sagittal fused FDG PET/CT image shows favorable response to therapy with interval decrease in metabolic activity in spine lesions (*arrow*). Sagittal CT image shows interval increase in sclerosis on the CT portion of the examination (*arrow*).

CT imaging can be used to serially measure and classify the response of BD MBC to systemic therapy. The study will assess if the categories of metabolic response measured by FDG-PET/CT are predictive of key clinical endpoints: PFS, time to skeletal-related events (SRE), and OS.[99,100]

OTHER FDA-APPROVED RADIONUCLIDES
F-18 Fluoroestradiol

F18 Fluoroestradiol (18F-FES) was FDA approved in 2020 to detect ER-positive lesions in patients with recurrent or MBC as an adjunct to biopsy.[101,102] FES has additional clinical utility in imaging ILC ER + metastases that show low FDG uptake.[102] Several clinical studies have evaluated the role of 18F-FES PET/CT in not only assessing in vivo ER expression but also in predicting response to therapy, evaluation of effective ER blockade and helping the clinicians in treatment strategy decisions.[103,104] There are now published Appropriate Use Criteria for FES, which do not recommend the use of FES PET for the evaluation of treatment response at this time.[105] Estrogen Receptor-targeted PET is more fully discussed in a separate article in this issue of PET

CLINICS (see Gary A Ulaner and colleagues' article, "Estrogen Receptor (ER)- and Progesterone Receptor (PR)-targeted PET for Patients with Breast Cancer,").

SUMMARY

With continued advancements in the management of BC, there will be increase in the number of women living with MBC leading to an increase in economic burden, which includes expenses related to imaging and other diagnostic testing. It is important to appropriately select different imaging modalities that can help in accurate response assessment and help with timely treatment decision-making.

CLINICS CARE POINTS

- Digital breast tomosynthesis is more accurate than conventional digital mammography in assessing response to neoadjuvant chemotherapy with good correlation with histopathology for residual tumor size.
- Combined use of both mammography and US improves the accuracy of predicting a pathologic complete response compared to use of either modality alone.
- Breast MRI is most accurate imaging modality for assessing response to neoadjuvant chemotherapy although it has to be kept in mind that MRI tends to overestimate response with taxane based neoadjuvant chemotherapy.
- FDG PET CT can accurately predict the pathologic status of regional axillary lymph nodes in early-stage BC (stage II and III) as early as after one course of chemotherapy which can guide the oncologists in patient management however the role of FDG PET in assessing response to therapy in primary breast mass largely depends upon the tumor histology and receptor status.
- FDG PET-CT has high clinical utility in assessing response to metastatic breast cancer; using PET response criteria allows patients with non-RECIST measurable access to therapy and helps in timely clinical decision making based on response assessment. FDG PET-CT also provides prognostic information and helps to early identify responders from non-responders.
- FDG PET-CT has superior sensitivity compared to conventional imaging in the detection of osseous metastases and is emerging as the modality of choice for treatment monitoring of bone dominant metastatic breast cancer.

DISCLOSURE

GAU discloses grants, consulting fees, honoraria, and/or speaker fees from Lantheus, GE Heathcare, Curium, POINT, RayzeBio, Briacell, and ImaginAb.

REFERENCES

1. Siegel RL, Miller KD, Fuchs HE, et al. Cancer statistics, 2022. CA Cancer J Clin 2022;72(1):7–33.
2. Wockel A, Festl J, Stuber T, et al. Interdisciplinary Screening, diagnosis, therapy and follow-up of breast cancer. Guideline of the DGGG and the DKG (S3-level, AWMF Registry number 032/045OL, December 2017) - Part 1 with recommendations for the Screening, diagnosis and therapy of breast cancer. Geburtshilfe Frauenheilkd 2018;78(10):927–48.

3. Cardoso F, Paluch-Shimon S, Senkus E, et al. 5th ESO-ESMO international consensus guidelines for advanced breast cancer (ABC 5). Ann Oncol 2020; 31(12):1623–49.
4. Huber S, Wagner M, Zuna I, et al. Locally advanced breast carcinoma: evaluation of mammography in the prediction of residual disease after induction chemotherapy. Antioancer Res 2000;20(1B):553–8.
5. Fisher B, Bryant J, Wolmark N, et al. Effect of preoperative chemotherapy on the outcome of women with operable breast cancer. J Clin Oncol 1998;16(8): 2672–85.
6. Fisher ER, Wang J, Bryant J, et al. Pathobiology of preoperative chemotherapy: findings from the National surgical adjuvant breast and Bowel (NSABP) protocol B-18. Cancer 2002;95(4):681–95.
7. Gradishar WJ, Moran MS, Abraham J, et al. Breast cancer, version 3.2022, NCCN clinical practice guidelines in Oncology. J Natl Compr Canc Netw 2022;20(6):691–722.
8. Park J, Chae EY, Cha JH, et al. Comparison of mammography, digital breast tomosynthesis, automated breast ultrasound, magnetic resonance imaging in evaluation of residual tumor after neoadjuvant chemotherapy. Eur J Radiol 2018;108:261–8.
9. Helvie MA, Joynt LK, Cody RL, et al. Locally advanced breast carcinoma: accuracy of mammography versus clinical examination in the prediction of residual disease after chemotherapy. Radiology 1996;198(2):327–32.
10. Mun HS, Kim HH, Shin HJ, et al. Assessment of extent of breast cancer: comparison between digital breast tomosynthesis and full-field digital mammography. Clin Radiol 2013;68(12):1254–9.
11. Murakami R, Tani H, Kumita S, et al. Diagnostic performance of digital breast tomosynthesis for predicting response to neoadjuvant systemic therapy in breast cancer patients: a comparison with magnetic resonance imaging, ultrasound, and full-field digital mammography. Acta Radiol Open 2021;10(12). 20584601211063746.
12. Keune JD, Jeffe DB, Schootman M, et al. Accuracy of ultrasonography and mammography in predicting pathologic response after neoadjuvant chemotherapy for breast cancer. Am J Surg 2010;199(4):477–84.
13. Bosch AM, Kessels AG, Beets GL, et al. Preoperative estimation of the pathological breast tumour size by physical examination, mammography and ultrasound: a prospective study on 105 invasive tumours. Eur J Radiol 2003;48(3): 285–92.
14. Peintinger F, Kuerer HM, Anderson K, et al. Accuracy of the combination of mammography and sonography in predicting tumor response in breast cancer patients after neoadjuvant chemotherapy. Ann Surg Oncol 2006;13(11):1443–9.
15. Makanjuola DI, Alkushi A, Al Anazi K. Defining radiologic complete response using a correlation of presurgical ultrasound and mammographic localization findings with pathological complete response following neoadjuvant chemotherapy in breast cancer. Eur J Radiol 2020;130:109146.
16. Shin HJ, Kim HH, Cha JH. Current status of automated breast ultrasonography. Ultrasonography 2015;34(3):165–72.
17. Herrada J, Iyer RB, Atkinson EN, et al. Relative value of physical examination, mammography, and breast sonography in evaluating the size of the primary tumor and regional lymph node metastases in women receiving neoadjuvant chemotherapy for locally advanced breast carcinoma. Clin Cancer Res 1997; 3(9):1565–9.

18. Scheel JR, Kim E, Partridge SC, et al. MRI, clinical examination, and mammography for preoperative assessment of residual disease and pathologic complete response after neoadjuvant chemotherapy for breast cancer: ACRIN 6657 trial. AJR Am J Roentgenol 2018;210(6):1376–85.

19. Londero V, Bazzocchi M, Del Frate C, et al. Locally advanced breast cancer: comparison of mammography, sonography and MR imaging in evaluation of residual disease in women receiving neoadjuvant chemotherapy. Eur Radiol 2004; 14(8):1371–9.

20. Rauch GM, Adrada BE, Kuerer HM, et al. Multimodality imaging for evaluating response to neoadjuvant chemotherapy in breast cancer. AJR Am J Roentgenol 2017;208(2):290–9.

21. Hylton NM, Blume JD, Bernreuter WK, et al. Locally advanced breast cancer: MR imaging for prediction of response to neoadjuvant chemotherapy–results from ACRIN 6657/I-SPY TRIAL. Radiology 2012;263(3):663–72.

22. Braman NM, Etesami M, Prasanna P, et al. Intratumoral and peritumoral radiomics for the pretreatment prediction of pathological complete response to neoadjuvant chemotherapy based on breast DCE-MRI. Breast Cancer Res 2017; 19(1):57.

23. Chen JH, Bahri S, Mehta RS, et al. Impact of factors affecting the residual tumor size diagnosed by MRI following neoadjuvant chemotherapy in comparison to pathology. J Surg Oncol 2014;109(2):158–67.

24. Mukhtar RA, Yau C, Rosen M, et al. Clinically meaningful tumor reduction rates vary by prechemotherapy MRI phenotype and tumor subtype in the I-SPY 1 TRIAL (CALGB 150007/150012; ACRIN 6657). Ann Surg Oncol 2013;20(12): 3823–30.

25. Schrading S, Kuhl CK. Breast cancer: Influence of taxanes on response assessment with dynamic contrast-enhanced MR imaging. Radiology 2015;277(3): 687–96.

26. Ollivier L, Balu-Maestro C, Leclere J. Imaging in evaluation of response to neoadjuvant breast cancer treatment. Cancer Imag 2005;5(1):27–31.

27. Wahl RL, Zasadny K, Helvie M, et al. Metabolic monitoring of breast cancer chemohormonotherapy using positron emission tomography: initial evaluation. J Clin Oncol 1993;11(11):2101–11.

28. Avril S, Muzic RF Jr, Plecha D, et al. (1)(8)F-FDG PET/CT for monitoring of treatment response in breast cancer. J Nucl Med 2016;57(Suppl 1):34S–9S.

29. Groheux D, Majdoub M, Sanna A, et al. Early metabolic response to neoadjuvant treatment: FDG PET/CT criteria according to breast cancer subtype. Radiology 2015;277(2):358–71.

30. Groheux D. Role of Fludeoxyglucose in breast cancer: treatment response. Pet Clin 2018;13(3):395–414.

31. Ueda S, Tsuda H, Asakawa H, et al. Clinicopathological and prognostic relevance of uptake level using 18F-fluorodeoxyglucose positron emission tomography/computed tomography fusion imaging (18F-FDG PET/CT) in primary breast cancer. Jpn J Clin Oncol 2008;38(4):250–8.

32. Schneider-Kolsky ME, Hart S, Fox J, et al. The role of chemotherapeutic drugs in the evaluation of breast tumour response to chemotherapy using serial FDG-PET. Breast Cancer Res 2010;12(3):R37.

33. Bos R, van Der Hoeven JJ, van Der Wall E, et al. Biologic correlates of (18)fluorodeoxyglucose uptake in human breast cancer measured by positron emission tomography. J Clin Oncol 2002;20(2):379–87.

34. Schelling M, Avril N, Nahrig J, et al. Positron emission tomography using [(18)F] Fluorodeoxyglucose for monitoring primary chemotherapy in breast cancer. J Clin Oncol 2000;18(8):1689–95.

35. Schwarz-Dose J, Untch M, Tiling R, et al. Monitoring primary systemic therapy of large and locally advanced breast cancer by using sequential positron emission tomography imaging with [18F]fluorodeoxyglucose. J Clin Oncol 2009;27(4): 535–41.

36. Wang Y, Zhang C, Liu J, et al. Is 18F-FDG PET accurate to predict neoadjuvant therapy response in breast cancer? A meta-analysis. Breast Cancer Res Treat 2012;131(2):357–69.

37. van der Hage JA, van de Velde CJ, Julien JP, et al. Preoperative chemotherapy in primary operable breast cancer: results from the European Organization for Research and Treatment of Cancer trial 10902. J Clin Oncol 2001;19(22): 4224–37.

38. von Minckwitz G, Untch M, Blohmer JU, et al. Definition and impact of pathologic complete response on prognosis after neoadjuvant chemotherapy in various intrinsic breast cancer subtypes. J Clin Oncol 2012;30(15):1796–804.

39. Perez-Garcia JM, Gebhart G, Ruiz Borrego M, et al. Chemotherapy de-escalation using an (18)F-FDG-PET-based pathological response-adapted strategy in patients with HER2-positive early breast cancer (PHERGain): a multicentre, randomised, open-label, non-comparative, phase 2 trial. Lancet Oncol 2021;22(6):858–71.

40. Kwong MS, Chung GG, Horvath LJ, et al. Postchemotherapy MRI overestimates residual disease compared with histopathology in responders to neoadjuvant therapy for locally advanced breast cancer. Cancer J 2006;12(3):212–21.

41. Liu Q, Wang C, Li P, et al. Corrigendum to "the role of (18)F-FDG PET/CT and MRI in assessing pathological complete response to neoadjuvant chemotherapy in patients with breast cancer: a Systematic review and meta-analysis". BioMed Res Int 2016;2016:1235429.

42. Cho N, Im SA, Cheon GJ, et al. Integrated (18)F-FDG PET/MRI in breast cancer: early prediction of response to neoadjuvant chemotherapy. Eur J Nucl Med Mol Imaging 2018;45(3):328–39.

43. Bassa P, Kim EE, Inoue T, et al. Evaluation of preoperative chemotherapy using PET with fluorine-18-fluorodeoxyglucose in breast cancer. J Nucl Med 1996; 37(6):931–8.

44. Mankoff DA, Dunnwald LK, Gralow JR, et al. Changes in blood flow and metabolism in locally advanced breast cancer treated with neoadjuvant chemotherapy. J Nucl Med 2003;44(11):1806–14.

45. Rousseau C, Devillers A, Campone M, et al. FDG PET evaluation of early axillary lymph node response to neoadjuvant chemotherapy in stage II and III breast cancer patients. Eur J Nucl Med Mol Imaging 2011;38(6):1029–36.

46. O'Connor M, Rhodes D, Hruska C. Molecular breast imaging. Expert Rev Anticancer Ther 2009;9(8):1073–80.

47. Muzahir S. Molecular breast cancer imaging in the Era of Precision Medicine. AJR Am J Roentgenol 2020;215(6):1512–9.

48. Bouzon A, Acea B, Soler R, et al. Diagnostic accuracy of MRI to evaluate tumour response and residual tumour size after neoadjuvant chemotherapy in breast cancer patients. Radiol Oncol 2016;50(1):73–9.

49. Hunt KN, Conners AL, Goetz MP, et al. Comparison of (99m)Tc-sestamibi molecular breast imaging and breast MRI in patients with invasive breast cancer

receiving neoadjuvant chemotherapy. AJR Am J Roentgenol 2019;213(4): 932–43.

50. Lim B, Hortobagyi GN. Current challenges of metastatic breast cancer. Cancer Metastasis Rev 2016;35(4):495–514.

51. Ulaner GA. PET/CT for patients with breast cancer: where is the clinical impact? AJR Am J Roentgenol 2019;213(2):254–65.

52. Bensch F, van Kruchten M, Lamberts LE, et al. Molecular imaging for monitoring treatment response in breast cancer patients. Eur J Pharmacol 2013; 717(1–3):2–11.

53. Eisenhauer EA, Therasse P, Bogaerts J, et al. New response evaluation criteria in solid tumours: revised RECIST guideline (version 1.1). Eur J Cancer 2009; 45(2):228–47.

54. Riedl CC, Pinker K, Ulaner GA, et al. Comparison of FDG-PET/CT and contrast-enhanced CT for monitoring therapy response in patients with metastatic breast cancer. Eur J Nucl Med Mol Imaging 2017;44(9):1428–37.

55. Fojo AT, Noonan A. Why RECIST works and why it should stay–counterpoint. Cancer Res 2012;72(20):5151–7 [discussion: 5158].

56. Mandrekar SJ, An MW, Meyers J, et al. Evaluation of alternate categorical tumor metrics and cut points for response categorization using the RECIST 1.1 data warehouse. J Clin Oncol 2014;32(8):841–50.

57. Vogsen M, Harbo F, Jakobsen NM, et al. Response monitoring in metastatic breast cancer - a prospective study comparing (18)F-FDG PET/CT with conventional CT. J Nucl Med 2023;64(3):355–61.

58. Kitajima K, Higuchi T, Yamakado K, et al. Early assessment of tumor response using (18)F-FDG PET/CT after one cycle of systemic therapy in patients with recurrent and metastatic breast cancer. Hell J Nucl Med 2022;25(2):155–62.

59. Lin NU, Guo H, Yap JT, et al. Phase II study of Lapatinib in combination with trastuzumab in patients with human epidermal growth factor receptor 2-positive metastatic breast cancer: clinical outcomes and predictive value of early [18F]fluorodeoxyglucose positron emission tomography imaging (TBCRC 003). J Clin Oncol 2015;33(24):2623–31.

60. Mayer IA, Abramson VG, Isakoff SJ, et al. Stand up to cancer phase Ib study of pan-phosphoinositide-3-kinase inhibitor buparlisib with letrozole in estrogen receptor-positive/human epidermal growth factor receptor 2-negative metastatic breast cancer. J Clin Oncol 2014;32(12):1202–9.

61. Naghavi-Behzad M, Vogsen M, Vester RM, et al. Response monitoring in metastatic breast cancer: a comparison of survival times between FDG-PET/CT and CE-CT. Br J Cancer 2022;126(9):1271–9.

62. Wahl RL, Jacene H, Kasamon Y, et al. From RECIST to PERCIST: Evolving Considerations for PET response criteria in solid tumors. J Nucl Med 2009;50(Suppl 1):122S–50S.

63. Vogsen M, Bulow JL, Ljungstrom L, et al. FDG-PET/CT for response monitoring in metastatic breast cancer: the Feasibility and benefits of applying PERCIST. Diagnostics 2021;11(4):723.

64. Hansen JA, Naghavi-Behzad M, Gerke O, et al. Diagnosis of bone metastases in breast cancer: lesion-based sensitivity of dual-time-point FDG-PET/CT compared to low-dose CT and bone scintigraphy. PLoS One 2021;16(11): e0260066.

65. Hildebrandt MG, Lauridsen JF, Vogsen M, et al. FDG-PET/CT for response monitoring in metastatic breast cancer: Today, Tomorrow, and beyond. Cancers 2019;11(8):1190.

66. Ulaner GA, Saura C, Piha-Paul SA, et al. Impact of FDG PET imaging for expanding patient Eligibility and measuring treatment response in a Genome-Driven Basket trial of the pan-HER kinase inhibitor, neratinib. Clin Cancer Res 2019;25(24):7381–7.

67. Ma Y, Wang Q, Dong Q, et al. How to differentiate pseudoprogression from true progression in cancer patients treated with immunotherapy. Am J Cancer Res 2019;9(8):1546–53.

68. Costa LB, Queiroz MA, Barbosa FG, et al. Reassessing patterns of response to immunotherapy with PET: from morphology to metabolism. Radiographics 2021; 41(1):120–43.

69. Xie Y, Liu C, Zhao Y, et al. Heterogeneity derived from (18) F-FDG PET/CT predicts immunotherapy outcome for metastatic triple-negative breast cancer patients. Cancer Med 2022;11(9):1948–55.

70. Dehdashti F, Mortimer JE, Trinkaus K, et al. PET-based estradiol challenge as a predictive biomarker of response to endocrine therapy in women with estrogen-receptor-positive breast cancer. Breast Cancer Res Treat 2009;113(3):509–17.

71. Mortimer JE, Dehdashti F, Siegel BA, et al. Metabolic flare: indicator of hormone responsiveness in advanced breast cancer. J Clin Oncol 2001;19(11): 2797–803.

72. Seifert R, Kuper A, Tewes M, et al. [18F]-Fluorodeoxyglucose positron emission tomography/CT to assess the early metabolic response in patients with hormone receptor-positive HER2-negative Metastasized breast cancer treated with Cyclin-dependent 4/6 kinase inhibitors. Oncol Res Treat 2021;44(7–8):400–7.

73. Taralli S, Lorusso M, Scolozzi V, et al. Response evaluation with (18)F-FDG PET/CT in metastatic breast cancer patients treated with Palbociclib: first experience in clinical practice. Ann Nucl Med 2019;33(3):193–200.

74. Miles A, Evans RE, Halligan S, et al. Predictors of patient preference for either whole body magnetic resonance imaging (WB-MRI) or CT/PET-CT for staging colorectal or lung cancer. J Med Imaging Radiat Oncol 2020;64(4):537–45.

75. Shen G, Deng H, Hu S, et al. Comparison of choline-PET/CT, MRI, SPECT, and bone scintigraphy in the diagnosis of bone metastases in patients with prostate cancer: a meta-analysis. Skeletal Radiol 2014;43(11):1503–13.

76. Bhaludin BN, Tunariu N, Koh DM, et al. A review on the added value of whole-body MRI in metastatic lobular breast cancer. Eur Radiol 2022;32(9):6514–25.

77. Li CI, Anderson BO, Daling JR, et al. Trends in incidence rates of invasive lobular and ductal breast carcinoma. JAMA 2003;289(11):1421–4.

78. Buck A, Schirrmeister H, Kuhn T, et al. FDG uptake in breast cancer: correlation with biological and clinical prognostic parameters. Eur J Nucl Med Mol Imaging 2002;29(10):1317–23.

79. Dashevsky BZ, Goldman DA, Parsons M, et al. Appearance of untreated bone metastases from breast cancer on FDG PET/CT: importance of histologic subtype. Eur J Nucl Med Mol Imaging 2015;42(11):1666–73.

80. He H, Gonzalez A, Robinson E, et al. Distant metastatic disease manifestations in infiltrating lobular carcinoma of the breast. AJR Am J Roentgenol 2014;202(5): 1140–8.

81. Hogan MP, Goldman DA, Dashevsky B, et al. Comparison of 18F-FDG PET/CT for systemic staging of newly diagnosed invasive lobular carcinoma versus invasive ductal carcinoma. J Nucl Med 2015;56(11):1674–80.

82. van Uden DJP, van Maaren MC, Strobbe LJA, et al. Metastatic behavior and overall survival according to breast cancer subtypes in stage IV inflammatory breast cancer. Breast Cancer Res 2019;21(1):113.

83. Yang H, Wang R, Zeng F, et al. Impact of molecular subtypes on metastatic behavior and overall survival in patients with metastatic breast cancer: a single-center study combined with a large cohort study based on the Surveillance, Epidemiology and End Results database. Oncol Lett 2020;20(4):87.

84. Morris PG, Lynch C, Feeney JN, et al. Integrated positron emission tomography/computed tomography may render bone scintigraphy unnecessary to investigate suspected metastatic breast cancer. J Clin Oncol 2010;28(19):3154–9.

85. Morris PG, Ulaner GA, Eaton A, et al. Standardized uptake value by positron emission tomography/computed tomography as a prognostic variable in metastatic breast cancer. Cancer 2012;118(22):5454–62.

86. Brenner AI, Koshy J, Morey J, et al. The bone scan. Semin Nucl Med 2012;42(1): 11–26.

87. Buck AK, Nekolla S, Ziegler S, et al. Spect/ct. J Nucl Med 2008;49(8):1305–19.

88. Coombes RC, Dady P, Parsons C, et al. Assessment of response of bone metastases to systemic treatment in patients with breast cancer. Cancer 1983;52(4): 610–4.

89. Schneider JA, Divgi CR, Scott AM, et al. Flare on bone scintigraphy following Taxol chemotherapy for metastatic breast cancer. J Nucl Med 1994;35(11): 1748–52.

90. Vogel CL, Schoenfelder J, Shemano I, et al. Worsening bone scan in the evaluation of antitumor response during hormonal therapy of breast cancer. J Clin Oncol 1995;13(5):1123–8.

91. Coleman RE, Mashiter G, Whitaker KB, et al. Bone scan flare predicts successful systemic therapy for bone metastases. J Nucl Med 1988;29(8):1354–9.

92. Koolen BB, Vegt E, Rutgers EJ, et al. FDG-avid sclerotic bone metastases in breast cancer patients: a PET/CT case series. Ann Nucl Med 2012;26(1):86–91.

93. Cook GJR, Goh V. Molecular imaging of bone metastases and their response to therapy. J Nucl Med 2020;61(6):799–806.

94. Taralli S, Caldarella C, Lorusso M, et al. Comparison between 18F-FDG and 18F-NaF PET imaging for assessing bone metastases in breast cancer patients: a literature review. Clinical and Translational Imaging 2020;8(2):65–78.

95. Cook GJ, Azad GK, Goh V. Imaging bone metastases in breast cancer: staging and response assessment. J Nucl Med 2016;57(Suppl 1):27S–33S.

96. Stafford SE, Gralow JR, Schubert EK, et al. Use of serial FDG PET to measure the response of bone-dominant breast cancer to therapy. Acad Radiol 2002; 9(8):913–21.

97. Specht JM, Tam SL, Kurland BF, et al. Serial 2-[18F] fluoro-2-deoxy-D-glucose positron emission tomography (FDG-PET) to monitor treatment of bone-dominant metastatic breast cancer predicts time to progression (TTP). Breast Cancer Res Treat 2007;105(1):87–94.

98. Peterson LM, O'Sullivan J, Wu QV, et al. Prospective study of serial (18)F-FDG PET and (18)F-Fluoride PET to predict time to skeletal-related events, time to progression, and survival in patients with bone-dominant metastatic breast cancer. J Nucl Med 2018;59(12):1823–30.

99. Using FDG pet ct to assess response of bone dominant metastatic breast. cancer 2020. NCT04316117.

100. Makhlin I, Korhonen KE, Martin ML, et al. (18)F-FDG PET/CT for the evaluation of therapy response in hormone receptor-positive bone-dominant metastatic breast cancer. Radiol Imaging Cancer 2022;4(6):e220032.

101. Ulaner GA, Jhaveri K, Chandarlapaty S, et al. Head-to-Head evaluation of (18)F-FES and (18)F-FDG PET/CT in metastatic invasive lobular breast cancer. J Nucl Med 2021;62(3):326–31.
102. Chae SY, Son HJ, Lee DY, et al. Comparison of diagnostic sensitivity of [(18)F]fluoroestradiol and [(18)F]fluorodeoxyglucose positron emission tomography/computed tomography for breast cancer recurrence in patients with a history of estrogen receptor-positive primary breast cancer. EJNMMI Res 2020; 10(1):54.
103. Linden HM, Kurland BF, Peterson LM, et al. Fluoroestradiol positron emission tomography reveals differences in pharmacodynamics of aromatase inhibitors, tamoxifen, and fulvestrant in patients with metastatic breast cancer. Clin Cancer Res 2011;17(14):4799–805.
104. Liao GJ, Clark AS, Schubert EK, et al. 18F-Fluoroestradiol PET: current status and potential Future clinical applications. J Nucl Med 2016;57(8):1269–75.
105. Ulaner GA, Mankoff DA, Clark AS, et al. Appropriate use criteria for estrogen receptor–targeted PET imaging with 16α-^{18}F-Fluoro-17β-Fluoroestradiol. J Nuc Med 2023;64(3):351–4.

Chemotherapy

Adjuvant Systemic Therapy for Postmenopausal, Hormone Receptor-Positive Early Breast Cancer

Stephen R.D. Johnston, MA, FRCP, PhD

KEYWORDS

- Hormone receptor-positive breast cancer • Adjuvant endocrine therapy
- Recurrence score • Aromatase inhibitor

KEY POINTS

- Optimal selection of adjuvant therapy in HR+ early breast cancer requires accurate assessment of an individual's risk of recurrence.
- Clinical-pathologic staging and biological factors including genomic signatures combine to provide both prognostic and predictive information.
- Endocrine therapy (ET) with aromatase inhibitors for between 5 and 10 years is the mainstay of adjuvant therapy.
- De-escalation of chemotherapy use in HR+ EBC has followed integration of genomic profiling in node-negative/1 to 3 node-positive disease.
- In high-risk node-positive HR+ EBC, adjuvant abemaciclib for 2 years combined with ET further reduces recurrence risk.

INTRODUCTION

Hormone receptor-positive (HR+) breast cancer is the most common subset of the disease in postmenopausal women presenting with early-stage disease, accounting for 75% of all cases.[1] HR+ breast cancer has a risk for both early and late recurrence, with at least half of all disease recurrences occurring more than 5 years after initial diagnosis, including a significant number more than 10 years after diagnosis.[2] Following locoregional breast surgery with/without radiotherapy, adjuvant systemic therapy is given to reduce the risk of recurrence (ROR) and enhance the chances of cure, and for HR+ early breast cancer (EBC) this has centered on endocrine therapy

This article previously appeared in *Hematology/Oncology Clinics* volume 37 issue 1 February 2023.

Department of Medicine, Royal Marsden NHS Foundation Trust, Fulham Road, Chelsea, London, SW3 6JJ, UK

E-mail address: Stephen.johnston@rmh.nhs.uk

(ET) and chemotherapy. Twenty-five years ago, ET consisted of the antiestrogen tamoxifen given for up to 5 years to all patients with HR+ EBC regardless of menopausal status, and combination chemotherapy was recommended to patients based on clinical staging features such as node-positive disease, or those with node-negative disease but high tumor grade or large tumor size. Although tamoxifen alone for 5 years (compared with no ET) reduced ROR by 39% and improved survival by 30%,[3] the additional gains from chemotherapy were always much more modest. Despite that, chemotherapy was often given to all women with HR+ tumors larger than 1 cm, or to those with node-positive disease, albeit older patients (>75 years) tended not to be offered chemotherapy due to the short-term toxicity impact negating the minimal impact on recurrence risk and overall survival (OS).

Over the subsequent quarter of a century, there have been significant advances made in our understanding of HR+ breast cancer and its heterogeneous biology, together with improved ET options and longer durations of treatment, and more recently de-escalation strategies to identify those postmenopausal patients with HR+ EBC who do not need chemotherapy. The modern management of HR+ breast cancer involves a more in-depth assessment of an individual's ROR based on both clinical and biological features. The foundation of this assessment relies on the American Joint Committee for Cancer staging criteria, including tumor size and nodal involvement,[4] with a higher ROR being associated with higher anatomic stage and increased numbers of nodes.[5] The staging system has now been updated to incorporate biological factors such as tumor grade, receptor status, and also prognostic/predictive information provided by multigene assays.[4] This article reviews the criteria that are now used in clinical practice to assess ROR in HR+ EBC, the optimal ET strategies that are used for individual patients, and the role of systemic chemotherapy and the regimens used, together with the new developments including adjuvant CDK 4 and 6 inhibitors for high-risk node-positive EBC. In addition, future directions that may further individualize recurrence risk with a view to personalizing adjuvant therapies are discussed.

PROGNOSTIC FACTORS AND ASSESSING RISK OF RECURRENCE

Optimal selection of adjuvant systemic therapy in HR+ EBC requires an accurate assessment of an individual's risk for disease recurrence. After primary surgery, this can now be easily assessed by using both clinical and pathologic features that include tumor size, histologic grade, presence of vascular invasion, and extent of lymph node involvement, together with the biological information provided by estrogen receptor (ER) status, progesterone receptor (PgR) status, human epidermal growth factor receptor-2 (HER2) status, and information provided by various gene expression assays. Expression of the biomarkers ER and PgR assessed by immunohistochemistry (IHC), and HER2 assessed by IHC or in situ hybridization, combine to identify the breast cancer subtype and inform prognosis and the degree of benefit from adjuvant ET. High ER and/or PgR expression is predictive of benefit from ET, whereas lack of these markers is considered a poor prognostic marker.[5] Guidelines from the American Society of Clinical Oncology (ASCO) and College of American Pathologists recommend designating tumors as ER low positive if ER expression is 1% to 10%.[6] Expression of ER in the absence of PgR is associated with tumors that have higher grade and cell proliferation (so-called luminal B-like tumors) and have a worse prognosis, compared with tumors in which both ER and PgR are expressed at high levels, which are more likely to be grade 1 or 2 (luminal A tumors) (Table 1).[2] HER2 serves as both a prognostic marker and predictive marker for HER2-targeted therapies, and half of all HER2-positive tumors coexpress hormone receptors, albeit often at a lower quantitative level.

Table 1
Characteristics of intrinsic subtypes and the spectrum in-between for hormone receptor-positive, human epidermal growth factor receptor-2-negtive early breast cancer

Characteristic	Luminal a Subtype ⟵	⟶ Luminal B Subtype
Tumor grade	1 (Well	2 (Moderately	3 (Poorly
ER expression	differentiated)	differentiated)	differentiated)
PgR expression	+++ (Strong)	++ to +++	+ to ++ (Weak to
Ki67 index, %	++ to +++ (Strong)	0 to +++	moderate)
21-Gene recurrence	<10 (Low)	10–20	0 to ++ (Negative to
score[a]	<11 (Low)	11 to 25	weak)
Other	Lower	(Intermediate)	>20 (High)
genomic	Low (<10%	Lower to higher	>25 (High)
signatures[b]	risk over 10 years)	Lower to higher	Higher
Breast cancer			Higher (>20% risk
recurrence			over 10 years)
risk			

[a] The 21-gene recurrence score ranges from 0-100, with higher scores indicating a greater chance of recurrence and chemotherapy benefit.
[b] Other genomic signatures include the 7-gene signature (MammaPrint), PAM50 Risk of Recurrence (Prosigna), Breast Cancer Index, and EndoPredict.
Adapted from Harbeck N, Burstein HJ, Hurvitz SA, Johnston SRD and Vidal GA. A look at current and potential treatment approaches for hormone receptor-positive, HER2-negative early breast cancer. Cancer. 2022 Jun 1;128 Suppl 11:2209-2223. doi: 10.1002/cncr.34161.

Genomic signatures have been developed based on patterns of tumor RNA expression in key genes involved in pathogenesis and correlate well with ER and PgR expression, histologic grade, cell proliferation, and moreover provide important information on prognosis and ROR (see **Table 1**). The most widely used genomic test is the 21-gene assay (Oncotype Dx) that evaluates 16 cancer-related genes and 5 reference genes assigning a recurrence score (RS) of 0 to 100. Initial retrospective studies validated this assay as a prognostic tool in patients with node-negative, HR-positive EBC and investigated whether it could be a predictive tool for adjuvant chemotherapy benefit. Patients with low RS (<11) had an excellent 9-year prognosis (>90% chance of being free of recurrence) and no benefit from chemotherapy, whereas high RS (>25) was associated with a much higher ROR, which was reduced in those given adjuvant chemotherapy.[7,8] For those with an intermediate score (RS 11–25), it was unclear whether there was any benefit from chemotherapy.

The subsequent prospective TAILORx study randomly assigned patients with node-negative disease and an intermediate RS of 11 to 25 to either ET alone or chemotherapy plus ET.[9] Nine-year invasive disease-free survival (iDFS), distant recurrence-free survival (DRFS), and OS were similar in both treatment arms, suggesting no benefit for chemotherapy in patients with an intermediate RS; this was especially the case in postmenopausal women, whereas subgroup analyses according to age suggested potential chemotherapy benefit in younger patients (aged ≤ 50 years) with an RS of 16 to 25. Subsequent refinement of prognosis has been provided by integrating RS with tumor grade and size with patient age into the RSClin tool, providing more accurate risk of distant recurrence than either RS or clinical-pathological features alone.[10] As such, in postmenopausal patients it became clear that in node-negative disease RS could be used to identify those patients who do not need chemotherapy, reserving it for those with biologically more aggressive breast cancer (RS > 25) as estimated by the 21-gene assay.

More recently Oncotype Dx was also evaluated in node-positive patients (1 to 3 positive nodes) in the randomized phase 3 RxPONDER study, randomizing patients with an RS of less than or equal to 25 to adjuvant ET with or without chemotherapy.[11] After 5 years of median follow-up, postmenopausal patients with an RS less than or equal to 25 did not benefit from adjuvant chemotherapy, whereas in younger, premenopausal women chemotherapy was associated with a 46% reduction in iDFS events compared with adjuvant ET alone, although it is unclear whether these benefits relate to the ovarian suppressive effects of cytotoxic therapy. These prospective data from 2 large trials have been deemed practice changing, resulting in a significant evidence-based de-escalation of systemic chemotherapy use in postmenopausal women with HR+ EBC.

Several other genomic panels assessing between 5 and 70 genes have been developed and evaluated in HR+ EBC in both prospective and retrospective studies, and all of them provide prognostic information on 10-year recurrence risk.[12] The 70-gene signature (MammaPrint) divides patient dichotomously into low and high genomic risk and was prognostic for time to distant metastasis and OS in retrospective validation studies[13]; this led to the prospective MINDACT trial, in which patients with discordant clinical and genomic risk were assigned to receive chemotherapy or not based solely on either their clinical or genomic risk group. The 5-year distant metastasis-free survival (DMFS) rate was 94.7% in patients with high clinical risk and low genomic risk treated with ET alone, suggesting the 70-gene signature could identify a group of patients (both node-negative and node-positive) who may not need adjuvant chemotherapy.[14] In particular, for postmenopausal patients aged greater than 50 years, an unplanned exploratory analysis in the HR+, HER2-negative subset showed similar 8-year DMFS with or without chemotherapy (90.2% vs 90.0%).

In postmenopausal women with ER-positive EBC the PAM-50 (Prosigna) signature evaluates 50 classifier genes and 5 control genes, categorizing HR+ breast tumors into intrinsic subtypes (ie, luminal A, luminal B, HER2-enriched, basal, normal) and assigning an ROR score ranging from 0 to 100. The PAM50 ROR score was prognostic in postmenopausal women for 10-year distant recurrence risk in patients with node-negative and node-positive disease from the ATAC and ABCSG-8 studies,[15] adding significant prognostic information compared with the 21-gene RS or IHC-based analysis of ER, PgR, HER2, and proliferation (Ki-67).[16] Likewise in postmenopausal women with HR+ EBC, the Breast Cancer Index, which combines a 5-gene prognostic molecular grade index with a 2-gene predictive biomarker ratio of HoxB13 and interleukin-17B receptor, was prognostic for both early and late recurrences in the Trans-ATAC study,[17] and predictive for benefit from extended adjuvant therapy in patients with node-negative or node-positive HR+ EBC.[18]

In terms of clinical utility, although the available gene expression assays vary with respect to the information they provide and populations assessed in the validation studies, they all provide additional prognostic information compared with clinical-pathologic factors alone. International guidelines all recommend the use of gene expression assays in patients with HR+ HER2-negative EBC with 0 to 3 positive nodes to assess the ROR and inform decisions regarding the use of adjuvant chemotherapy (Table 2), while not recommending any 1 genomic assay over another.[19,20] Although all the available assays provide valuable prognostic information, the 21-gene assay is currently the only one with prospective data supporting its ability to predict for chemotherapy benefit,[19] and the St Gallen International Consensus Guidelines have since recommended against routine use of chemotherapy for postmenopausal women with stage I or II (including 1–3 positive lymph nodes) HR+ breast cancers that had a lower-risk genomic signature (ie, Oncotype RS < 25) (see Table 2).[21] The Prosigna and Breast Cancer Index assays are useful to assess risk for late recurrences in HR+ EBC, which may be useful in determining candidates for extended adjuvant ET.

Table 2
Adjuvant systemic therapy options for hormone receptor-positive human epidermal growth factor receptor-2-negative early breast cancer

Anatomic Stage	Tumor and Nodal Stage	Endocrine Therapy	Chemotherapy
Stage I	T1ab N0	AI or Tam, 5 years	No
	T1c N0	AI or Tam, 5 years	
Stage II	N0 (node negative)	Consider AI as extended therapy, especially after initial 2–5 years of Tam	Not indicated if favorable biology. Only indicated for those within high genomic risk signature or unfavorable biology
	N1 (1–3+ LN)	Extended AI therapy	
Stage III		Extended AI therapy	Yes

Abbreviations: AI, aromatase inhibitor; LN, lymph node; Tam, Tamoxifen; TN, tumour size, nodal status.

Historically, the St Gallen Panel has favored AI-based therapy in higher-risk tumors defined by T and N stage, grade, and Ki67 score.

Extended therapy implies 10 years of treatment, although some studies indicate that 10 years may not offer benefit beyond that seen with 7 to 8 years of endocrine therapy.

Favorable biology: Lower-risk genomic signature (eg, RS ≤25 [node-positive] or 16–25 [node-negative], or 70-gene signature "low"); strongly ER-positive with low to intermediate grade, and/or lower baseline Ki-67, or decrease in Ki-67 with preoperative exposure to endocrine therapy (dynamic Ki-67).

Unfavorable biology: Higher-risk genomic signature (eg, recurrence score >25 or 70-gene signature "high"); lower ER expression, intermediate to high grade, and/or higher baseline Ki-67, or lack of decline in Ki-67 with preoperative exposure to endocrine therapy (dynamic Ki-67).

Adapted from Burstein HJ, Curigliano G, Thurlimann B, et al. Customising local and systemic therapies for women with early breast cancer: the St Gallen International Consensus Guidelines for treatment of early breast cancer. Ann Oncol. 2021 Oct;32(10):1216-1235.021.

ADJUVANT ENDOCRINE THERAPY IN POSTMENOPAUSAL HORMONE RECEPTOR-POSITIVE EARLY BREAST CANCER

The Early Breast Cancer Trialists' Collaborative Group meta-analyses first showed that 5 years of adjuvant tamoxifen significantly reduced risk of disease recurrence and improved OS in HR+ EBC, even in tumors in which ER expression is low (ie, between 1% and 10%).[3] Tamoxifen provides equivalent benefit in luminal A and luminal B tumors and reduces local-regional recurrence, even in small breast cancers less than 1 cm in size.[22] The extent of ER expression determined by IHC together with coexpression of PgR strongly correlates with endocrine sensitivity and degree of benefit from adjuvant ET with tamoxifen.[23]

Approximately 20 years ago, new options for adjuvant endocrine treatment in postmenopausal women arose following trials that compared 5 years of aromatase inhibitors (AIs) with 5 years of tamoxifen in HR+ EBC.[24] The AIs letrozole, anastrozole, and exemestane all block conversion of androgens to estrogens in postmenopausal women, suppressing estrogen levels by 90% resulting in significant antiproliferative effects in HR+ breast cancer cells.[25] Long-term follow-up from the ATAC and BIG 1-98 adjuvant trials in postmenopausal HR+ EBC showed that 5 years of adjuvant anastrozole or letrozole significantly reduced distant recurrences compared with 5 years of tamoxifen.[26,27] Likewise, for premenopausal or perimenopausal women who initially start on tamoxifen but then are confirmed as postmenopausal and switch to an AI, this sequencing strategy is superior to tamoxifen alone.[25,27] However, for women with small stage I or IIA node-negative HR+ EBC (often detected by mammographic screening) the numerical advantage for AIs over tamoxifen is minimal (2%–3% reduction is ROR at 10 years), whereas the quantitative benefit is much greater for AIs

over tamoxifen in higher-risk disease as determined by anatomic stage or adverse biological features,[25,28] or by histologic type such as invasive lobular breast cancer.[29]
Given the overall improved efficacy results, most postmenopausal patients with
HR+ EBC are now treated with AIs as initial therapy, although in very-low-risk disease
tamoxifen is still a very reasonable option (see **Table 2**).

An equally important consideration to efficacy when deciding between AIs and
tamoxifen is their difference in side effects and patient tolerability. Both therapies can
enhance menopausal vasomotor symptoms such as hot flashes and night sweats
that can disturb sleep and contribute to fatigue. Tamoxifen can cause vaginal discharge,
increase the risk for deep vein thrombosis, and cause endometrial cancer, whereas AIs
commonly cause arthralgia, vaginal dryness, and hair thinning and may accelerate osteoporosis. These symptoms may affect patient compliance for patients required to take
these medications for a minimum of 5 years.[30] For women in whom an AI is associated
with an unacceptable side effect profile, switching to another class of AI (ie, from letrozole to exemestane) or to tamoxifen may be better tolerated, while exercise or acupuncture can also reduce musculoskeletal symptoms.[31] The reverse sequence of an AI-
tamoxifen is as effective as tamoxifen-AI sequence (distant recurrence-free interval at
8 years: 88.7% vs 88.1%),[32] suggesting it is a safe strategy to offer patients unable
to tolerate an AI long term. Likewise, data from the phase 3 SOLE trial also showed
that short treatment breaks after an initial 5 years of AI therapy in postmenopausal patients are feasible with similar benefit for intermittent (9 months on, 3 months off) versus
continuous dosing of letrozole, and will not compromise long-term benefit.[33] These
different treatment strategies and interventions to manage toxicities are important considerations to maximize patient compliance during adjuvant ET.

One important feature of HR+ EBC is the ongoing annual ROR beyond 5 years,
which although small is constant, such that recurrences up to 10 or even 20 years later
will occur, being more frequent in those with higher nodal and tumor stage or higher
grade,[34] or adverse biological features as determined by genomic signatures[35]; this
has led to several studies of extended adjuvant ET comparing 10 versus 5 years of
treatment. These studies have demonstrated improved disease-free survival when
extended AI therapy was given for 5 additional years following an initial 5 years of
tamoxifen, an AI, or sequential tamoxifen-AI therapy.[36] Whether 10 years is needed
in all patients is not clear, and the ABCSG-16 study showed a similar benefit for 2 additional years of AI therapy instead of 5 years, suggesting that therapy could be stopped
at 7 years without compromising outcomes.[37] A meta-analysis of almost 25,000 patients showed that extending ET beyond 5 years significantly reduced recurrence,
but it also reported differential benefit based on the degree of nodal involvement.
Five years of additional AI therapy reduced recurrence by 1.1% in node-negative patients, 3.8% in those with 1 to 3 positive nodes, and 7.7% in those with 4 or more positive nodes.[38] As such, International Consensus Guidelines[21] now recommend that
5 years of ET (tamoxifen or an AI) may be sufficient for stage I/IIA low-risk breast cancers, whereas patients with higher-stage disease and increased nodal involvement
should be strongly considered for extended-duration ET for a minimum of 7 to 8 years
that includes an AI for some or all of that period (see **Table 2**).

ADJUVANT CHEMOTHERAPY IN POSTMENOPAUSAL HORMONE RECEPTOR-POSITIVE EARLY BREAST CANCER

The true role of adjuvant chemotherapy in HR+ EBC has become better defined in
recent years, especially in postmenopausal women in whom there has been significant
de-escalation of use following the introduction of genomic signatures to define

chemotherapy benefit in patients with lower anatomic stage. Nodal status remains a strong prognostic factor and marker of risk, but importantly does not define that chemotherapy is required. Patients with HR+ breast cancer who have a higher clinical stage (ie, extensive nodal burden or stage III disease) do probably have significant risk to warrant adjuvant chemotherapy use regardless of their genomic signature,[21] albeit the absolute chemotherapy benefit in low genomic risk/high clinical stage may be minimal as shown in the MINDACT study.[14] Unlike other subtypes of breast cancer such as triple-negative or HER2-positive EBC, neoadjuvant (preoperative) chemotherapy has a low chance of inducing a complete pathologic response, but still may be warranted to improve surgical options by downstaging those with large T3 node-positive breast cancers.

Biological information in HR+ EBC is very likely to be a more powerful predictor than clinical stage for benefit from adjuvant therapies (both endocrine and cytotoxic). The European Society for Medical Oncology (ESMO) and St Gallen Consensus Guidelines recommend consideration of adjuvant chemotherapy for patients with luminal A tumors who also have a high disease burden ($\geq$4 lymph nodes, $\geq$T3) as well as those with luminal B proliferative tumors, whereas patients with low-grade luminal A tumors and low genomic risk likely derive minimal (if any) benefit from adjuvant chemotherapy and should be treated with adjuvant ET alone.[5,21] For those HR+ tumors that are either node-negative or have low nodal burden (1–3 nodes, N1) but have some increased clinical risk features (size, grade, vascular invasion), a gene expression profile is strongly considered to determine both the prognosis and whether chemotherapy is indicated.[5,21] The National Comprehensive Cancer Network guidelines list the Oncotype Dx 21-gene assay as the preferred testing option for node-negative disease and postmenopausal patients with node-positive disease, strongly recommending adjuvant chemotherapy in all patients with stage I or II HR+ disease with a high-risk genomic signature (RS $\geq$26).[19] In contrast, based on data from the TAILORx and RxPONDER trials in node-negative and node-positive HR+ disease, respectively, adjuvant chemotherapy does not provide significant benefit in postmenopausal patients with 3 or less positive nodes and a low-risk genomic signature (RS < 26) (see **Table 2**).[9,11]

Standard adjuvant chemotherapy regimens for breast cancer have historically included anthracyclines, alkylators, and in the last 20 years taxanes. There are geographic differences in the preferred regimens for HR+ breast cancer, and some parts of the world have seen a shift away from the use of anthracyclines. In patients with HR+, node-negative disease, docetaxel plus cyclophosphamide (TC) was more effective that a taxane plus doxorubicin/cyclophosphamide (TaxAC), whereas patients with HR+ disease with a high tumor burden showed benefit from the addition of anthra-cyclines.[39] Other studies have shown similar benefit for 4 cycles of epirubicin/cyclo-phosphamide followed by docetaxel (EC-T) versus 6 cycles of TC in patients with EBC, regardless of HR status.[40] As such, 4 cycles of a nonanthracycline-based regimen (ie, TC), 4 cycles of an anthracycline regimen (AC/EC), or 12 weeks of weekly paclitaxel are all common adjuvant choices for low- to intermediate-risk HR+ breast cancer, whereas a sequential anthracycline-taxane regimen, such as accelerated EC $\times$ 4 followed by weekly paclitaxel $\times$12, is commonly used for high-risk HR+ disease. Adverse events (AEs) associated with chemotherapy are always an important consideration when selecting adjuvant therapy. Both anthracyclines and taxanes are commonly associated with alopecia, and anthracyclines have a smaller risk for serious events such as cardiac damage, whereas taxanes can cause peripheral neuropathy. In older (>70 years) postmenopausal patients with higher-risk HR+ EBC, a balanced discussion of the quantitative adjuvant benefits versus any potential harms from chemotherapy is especially important in shared decision making with individual patients.

ADDITIONAL ADJUVANT SYSTEMIC THERAPIES IN HIGHER-RISK HORMONE RECEPTOR-POSITIVE EARLY BREAST CANCER

Despite current locoregional and systemic treatments for HR+ EBC, one-fifth of patients will still experience disease recurrence within the first 10 years.[24] For postmenopausal patients with HR+ EBC, additional therapy in the form of bisphosphonates such as zoledronic acid every 6 months for 3 years has been shown to not only mitigate the risk of osteoporosis from ET with AIs but also reduce the risk of disease recurrence.[41] Clinical and pathologic factors in HR+ EBC that are associated with recurrence risk include larger tumor size, extent of nodal involvement, and higher grade of tumor, which indicates more proliferative disease (ie, luminal B with a high Ki-67 index).[42] In patients with HR+ disease with more than 4 positive nodes, or if 1 to 3 nodes are involved additional risk factors such as grade 3 disease or large tumor size greater than 5 cm, the risk of early recurrence in the first 5 years can be up to 20% and as high as those with triple-negative EBC.[43] For this high-risk HR+ patient population, there is a need for more effective adjuvant treatment approaches.

Cyclin-dependent kinases (CDKs) are involved in cell cycle regulation in HR+ breast cancer, and in recent years orally active and potent inhibitors of CDK4 and CDK6 combined with ET have been approved as treatment of HR+ advanced breast cancer.[44] Three randomized trials of adjuvant CDK4/6 inhibitors added to ET in high-risk HR+ EBC have been undertaken and reported results. Palbociclib was investigated in the adjuvant setting in the phase 3 PALLAS study, which evaluated the addition of 2 years of palbociclib to tamoxifen or an AI versus ET alone in patients with stage II or III HR+, HER2-negative EBC.[45,46] The primary end point of iDFS was not improved in the investigational arm at the second interim analysis, and palbociclib treatment was discontinued for futility. The second trial to report was the double-blind, placebo-controlled, randomized phase 3 PENELOPE-B trial, which enrolled women with high-risk HR+ HER2-negative primary breast cancer with residual invasive disease after taxane-containing neoadjuvant chemotherapy.[47] At the final analysis, the addition of 1 year of palbociclib to adjuvant ET failed to demonstrate improved iDFS (hazard ratio, 0.93; 95% confidence interval, 0.74–1.17).

In contrast, the third randomized phase 3 trial monarchE demonstrated a significant benefit from the addition of adjuvant abemaciclib to ET in patients with HR+ HER2-negative, node-positive, high-risk EBC.[48] High-risk disease was defined as 4 or more positive nodes or 1 to 3 positive nodes with either a grade 3 tumor, a tumor greater than or equal to 5 cm in size, or high proliferation rate (Ki-67 level $\geq$20%). More than 95% of these high-risk patients had received chemotherapy and 56% were postmenopausal, and they received standard ET with or without 2 years of abemaciclib. A preplanned interim analysis after 15.5 months' follow-up demonstrated a statistically significant improvement in iDFS (primary endpoint) with the addition of abemaciclib,[48] and at the updated analysis after a median of 27 months' follow-up the hazard ratio had strengthened to 0.696 ($P < .0001$).[49] The benefit was consistent across patient subgroups (including the postmenopausal group), and abemaciclib reduced the risk of DRFS by 31.3%. A high Ki-67 (>20%) was clearly prognostic with a 3-year iDFS rate for the ET alone control arm of 79% for high Ki-67 and 87% for low Ki-67, with added benefit from abemaciclib in both high and low Ki-67 groups (Fig. 1).[49] Abemaciclib had a manageable safety profile, and the most common AEs were gastrointestinal (diarrhea, nausea, abdominal pain), fatigue, and measured cytopenias.[48,49] Most AEs started early, and for those who required therapy interruption/ dose reduction, thereafter they were able to remain on therapy. On the basis of these data, abemaciclib has recently been approved in many countries in combination with

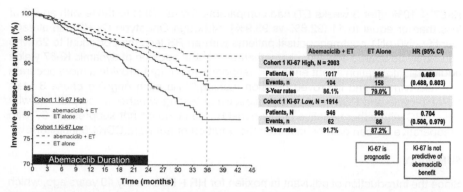

Fig. 1. Prognostic but not predictive effect of Ki-67 in Cohort 1 of monarchE trial. Figure depicts invasive disease-free survival according to treatment arm among patients enrolled into Cohort 1 in teh monarchE trial, subdivided by baseline tumor Ki-67 with high Ki-67 greater than 20%, low Ki-67 less than 20%. ET, endocrine therapy; HR, hazard ratio. (*Adapted from* Harbeck N, Burstein HJ, Hurvitz SA, et al. A look at current and potential treatment approaches for hormone receptor-positive, HER2-negative early breast cancer. Cancer 2022;128 Suppl 11:2209–23. doi:10.1002/cncr.34161.)

ET for the adjuvant treatment of high-risk HR+ EBC, and whereas in the United States approval has initially been restricted to those with node-positive disease and also high Ki-67,[50] in clinical practice updated ASCO guidelines have endorsed its use in the wider node-positive high-risk monarchE trial population.[51]

FUTURE DIRECTIONS FOR ADJUVANT SYSTEMIC THERAPIES IN HORMONE RECEPTOR-POSITIVE EARLY BREAST CANCER

Although there has been significant progress in applying knowledge about the biology of HR+ breast cancer to the estimation of risk and selection of appropriate adjuvant systemic therapies, the information on relative risk reduction from adding any given therapy is generated from clinical trials of hundreds of patients with HR+ breast cancer. This is a heterogeneous disease with a spectrum of biological features (see **Table 1**), and in clinical practice there remains limited ability to accurately predict response or resistance on an individual basis to any adjuvant therapy whether it be endocrine based, cytotoxic, or targeted such as CDK 4/6 inhibitors. Providing a more personalized prediction of benefit from adjuvant systemic therapies could further refine treatment selection and improve clinical outcomes.

One such approach in HR+ postmenopausal EBC is to use a short exposure for 2 to 4 weeks to ET with an AI, and measure change in cancer cell proliferation (dynamic Ki-67) before and after ET with the resulting 2-week Ki-67*post* score that integrates both predictive and prognostic information in HR+ EBC.[52] The predictive value of dynamic Ki-67 for postmenopausal women with HR+ EBC was demonstrated in the phase 3 POETIC trial in which those with a reduction in Ki-67 levels to less than 10% after 2 weeks of an AI had a 5-year recurrence risk of 8.4%, compared with 21.5% for those with persistently high Ki-67 after neoadjuvant therapy.[53] Likewise, complete cell cycle arrest with Ki-67*post* less than 2.7% has been shown as strongly prognostic for those patients with an excellent prognosis on adjuvant ET alone.[54] More recently the ADAPT trialists examined the integration of this biomarker with Oncotype Dx in postmenopausal patients with node-negative/1 to 3 node-positive (pN0/pN1) HR+ EBC.[55] Patients with an RS of 12 to 25 and response to preoperative ET (evidenced by post

Ki-67 $\leq$ 10% after 3 weeks ET) had comparable 5-year iDFS to those with an RS of less than or equal to 11 (92.6% vs 93.9%). Although Oncotype Dx RS can already identify pN0/pN1 postmenopausal patients with an RS less than or equal to 25 who can safely be spared adjuvant chemotherapy,[9,11] the addition of dynamic Ki-67 yields additional information about endocrine response that might provide a more accurate risk assessment and improved decision making.[52] As such ongoing phase 3 trials (APAPT-cycle and POETIC-A) are prospectively testing whether those patients with HR+ EBC with either negative or low nodal burden who do not suppress Ki-67 with preoperative ET can gain benefit from the addition of adjuvant CDK4/6 inhibitors.[12]

SUMMARY

Since the introduction of adjuvant tamoxifen for HR+ EBC nearly 40 years ago, which was the first adjuvant systemic therapy to significantly improve clinical outcome in this form of breast cancer,[3] substantial progress has been made in both a deeper understanding of the biology of HR+ EBC that is now used to inform assessment of risk and prognosis and more effective adjuvant systemic therapies. For postmenopausal HR+ EBC ET remains the mainstay of treatment, with extended duration for many and the addition of targeted CDK 4/6 inhibitors for those with node-positive high-risk disease, and de-escalation of chemotherapy for those in whom it is unlikely to be of benefit. As such, systemic adjuvant therapy is now highly tailored and individualized for this most common form of breast cancer.

CLINICS CARE POINTS

- Accurate assessment of risk in HR+ postmenopausal breast cancer should include clinical-pathologic staging, biological information from receptor status, and where indicated genomic profiling to ascertain both prognosis and predictive benefit from adjuvant therapy.
- ET with AIs or tamoxifen is used in all HR+ postmenopausal EBC for between 5 and 10 years depending on the level of risk and tolerability.
- Shared decision making about adjuvant chemotherapy should discuss relative risk reduction and toxicity, and for postmenopausal women with N0 or N1 disease and an Oncotype recurrence score of less than 25, chemotherapy is not indicated
- Adjuvant abemaciclib should be considered for high-risk node-positive HR+ EBC to further reduce risk

DISCLOSURE

Grants for laboratory/clinical research to institution from AstraZeneca, Pfizer, Eli Lilly, and Puma Biotechnology. Consulting/advisory personal fees from Eli Lilly, Pfizer, Novartis, AstraZeneca, and Sanofi Genzyme. Speaker fees Eisai, AstraZeneca, and Roche/Genentech.

ACKNOWLEDGEMENT

Support provided by National Institute for Health Research funding to the Royal Marsden and Institute of Cancer Research Biomedical Research Centre.Support also provided by National Institute for Health Research funding to the Royal Marsden and Institute of Cancer Research Biomedical Research Centre.

REFERENCES

1. Howlader N, Altekruse SF, Li CI, et al. US incidence of breast cancer subtypes defined by joint hormone receptor and HER2 status. J Natl Cancer Inst 2014; 106(5):dju055.
2. Burstein HJ. Systemic therapy for estrogen receptor-positive, HER2-negative breast cancer. N Engl J Med 2020;383:2557–70.
3. Early Breast Cancer Trialists' Collaborative Group. Relevance of breast cancer hormone receptors and other factors to the efficacy of adjuvant tamoxifen: patient level meta-analysis of randomised trials. Lancet 2011;378:771–84.
4. Giuliano AE, Edge SB, Hortobagyi GN. Eighth edition of the AJCC Cancer staging manual: breast cancer. Ann Surg Oncol 2018;25:1783–5.
5. Cardoso F, Kyriakides S, Ohno S, et al. Early breast cancer: ESMO clinical practice guidelines for diagnosis, treatment and follow-up. Ann Oncol 2019;30: 1194–220.
6. Allison KH, Hammond ME, Dowsett M, et al. Estrogen and progesterone receptor testing in breast cancer: ASCO/CAP Guideline Update. J Clin Oncol 2020;38: 1346–66.
7. Paik S, Shak S, Tang G, et al. A multigene assay to predict recurrence of tamoxifen-treated, node-negative breast cancer. N Engl J Med 2004;351: 2817–26.
8. Paik S, Tang G, Shak S, et al. Gene expression and benefit of chemotherapy in women with node-negative, estrogen receptor-positive breast cancer. J Clin Oncol 2006;24:3726–34.
9. Sparano JA, Gray RJ, Makower DF, et al. Adjuvant chemotherapy guided by a 21-gene expression assay in breast cancer. N Engl J Med 2018;379:111–21.
10. Sparano JA, Crager MR, Tang G, et al. Development and validation of a tool integrating the 21-gene recurrence score and clinical-pathological features to individualize prognosis and prediction of chemotherapy benefit in early breast cancer. J Clin Oncol 2021;39:557–64.
11. Kalinsky K, Barlow WE, Gralow JR, et al. 21-Gene Assay to Inform Chemotherapy Benefit in Node-Positive Breast Cancer. N Eng J Med 2021;385:2336–47.
12. Harbeck N, Burstein HJ, Hurvitz SA, et al. A look at current and potential treatment approaches for hormone receptor-positive, HER2-negative early breast cancer. Cancer 2022;128(Suppl 11):2209–23.
13. Buyse M, Loi S, van't Veer L, et al. Validation and clinical utility of a 70-gene prognostic signature for women with node-negative breast cancer. J Natl Cancer Inst 2006;98:1183–92.
14. Cardoso F, van't Veer LJ, Bogaerts J, et al. for the MINDACT Investigators. 70-gene signature as an aid to treatment decisions in early-stage breast cancer. N Engl J Med 2016;375:717–29.
15. Gnant M, Sestak I, Filipits M, et al. Identifying clinically relevant prognostic subgroups of postmenopausal women with node-positive hormone receptor-positive early-stage breast cancer treated with endocrine therapy: a combined analysis of ABCSG-8 and ATAC using the PAM50 risk of recurrence score and intrinsic subtype. Ann Oncol 2015;26:1685–91.
16. Dowsett M, Sestak I, Lopez-Knowles E, et al. Comparison of PAM50 risk of recurrence score with Oncotype DX and IHC4 for predicting risk of distant recurrence after endocrine therapy. J Clin Oncol 2013;31:2783–90.
17. Sgroi DC, Sestak I, Cuzick J, et al. Prediction of late distant recurrence in patients with oestrogen-receptor-positive breast cancer: a prospective comparison of the

breast-cancer index (BCI) assay, 21-gene recurrence score, and IHC4 in the TransATAC study population. Lancet Oncol 2013;14:1067–76.

18. Bartlett JMS, Sgroi DC, Treuner K, et al. Breast Cancer Index and prediction of benefit from extended endocrine therapy in breast cancer patients treated in the Adjuvant Tamoxifen-To Offer More? (aTTom) trial. Ann Oncol 2019;30: 1776–83.

19. National Comprehensive Cancer Network. Breast cancer (version 7.2021). https://www.nccn.org/professionals/physician_gls/pdf/breast.pdf. [Accessed 8 August 2022].

20. Andre F, Ismaila N, Henry NL, et al. Use of biomarkers to guide decisions on adjuvant systemic therapy for women with early-stage invasive breast cancer: ASCO clinical practice guideline update-integration of results from TAILORx. J Clin Oncol 2019;37:1956–64.

21. Burstein HJ, Curigliano G, Thurlimann B, et al. Customising local and systemic therapies for women with early breast cancer: the St Gallen International Consensus Guidelines for treatment of early breast cancer. Ann Oncol 2021; 32(10):1216–1235.021.

22. Fisher B, Bryant J, Dignam JJ, et al. Tamoxifen, radiation therapy, or both for prevention of ipsilateral breast tumor recurrence after lumpectomy in women with invasive breast cancers of one centimeter or less. J Clin Oncol 2002;20:4141–9.

23. Harvey JM, Clark GM, Osborne CK, et al. Estrogen receptor status by immunohistochemistry is superior to the ligand-binding assay for predicting response to adjuvant endocrine therapy in breast cancer. J Clin Oncol 1999;17:1474–81.

24. Early Breast Cancer Trialists' Collaborative Group (EBCTCG). Aromatase inhibitors versus tamoxifen in early breast cancer: patient-level meta-analysis of the randomised trials. Lancet 2015;386:1341–52.

25. Smith IE, Dowsett M. Aromatase inhibitors and breast cancer. N Engl J Med 2003; 348(24):2431–42.

26. Cusick J, Sestak I, Baum M, et al, on behalf of the ATAC/LATTE Investigators. Effect of anastrozole and tamoxifen as adjuvant treatment for early-stage breast cancer: 10-year analysis of the ATAC trial. Lancet Oncol 2010;11:1135–41.

27. Ruhstaller T, Giobbie-Hurder A, Colleoni M, et al. for the members of the BIG 1-98 Collaborative Group and the International Breast Cancer Study Group. Adjuvant letrozole and tamoxifen alone or sequentially for postmenopausal women with hormone receptor-positive breast cancer: long-term follow-up of the BIG 1-98 trial. J Clin Oncol 2019;37:105–14.

28. Viale G, Regan MM, Dell'Orto P, et al. Which patients benefit most from adjuvant aromatase inhibitors? Results using a composite measure of prognostic risk in the BIG 1-98 randomized trial. Ann Oncol 2011;22:2201–7.

29. Metzger Filho O, Giobbie-Hurder A, Mallon E, et al. Relative effectiveness of letrozole compared with tamoxifen for patients with lobular carcinoma in the BIG 1-98 trial. J Clin Oncol 2015;33:2772–9.

30. Chirgwin JH, Giobbie-Hurder A, Coates AS, et al. Treatment adherence and its impact on disease-free survival in the Breast International Group 1-98 trial of tamoxifen and letrozole, alone and in sequence. J Clin Oncol 2016;34:2452–9.

31. Gupta A, Henry NL, Loprinzi CL. Management of aromatase inhibitorinduced musculoskeletal symptoms. JCO Oncol Pract 2020;16:733–9.

32. Regan MM, Neven P, Giobbie-Hurder A, et al. Assessment of letrozole and tamoxifen alone and in sequence for postmenopausal women with steroid hormone receptor-positive breast cancer: the BIG 1-98 randomised clinical trial at 8·1 years median follow-up. Lancet Oncol 2011;12:1101–8.

33. Colleoni M, Luo W, Karlsson P, et al. on behalf of the SOLE Investigators. Extended adjuvant intermittent letrozole versus continuous letrozole in postmenopausal women with breast cancer (SOLE): a multicentre, open-label, randomised, phase 3 trial. Lancet Oncol 2018;19:127–38.

34. Pan H, Gray R, Braybrooke J, et al. 20- Year risks of breast-cancer recurrence after stopping endocrine therapy at 5 years. N Engl J Med 2017;377:1836–46.

35. Sestak I, Dowsett M, Zabaglo L, et al. Factors predicting late recurrence for estrogen receptor-positive breast cancer. J Natl Cancer Inst 2013;105:1504–11.

36. Burstein HJ, Lacchetti C, Anderson H, et al. Adjuvant endocrine therapy for women with hormone receptor–positive breast cancer: ASCO Clinical Practice Guideline focused update. J Clin Oncol 2019;37:423–38.

37. Gnant M, Fitzal F, Rinnerthaler G, et al. Duration of Adjuvant Aromatase-Inhibitor Therapy in Postmenopausal Breast Cancer. N Engl J Med 2021;385(5):395–405.

38. Gray R, Early Breast Cancer Trialists' Collaborative Group. Effects of prolonging adjuvant aromatase inhibitor therapy beyond five years on recurrence and cause-specific mortality: an EBCTCG meta-analysis of individual patient data from 12 randomised trials including 24,912 women. Cancer Res 2019;79(suppl). Abstract GS3-03.

39. Blum JL, Flynn PJ, Yothers G, et al. Anthracyclines in early breast cancer: the ABC trials-USOR 06-090, NSABP B-46-I/USOR 07132, and NSABP B-49 (NRG Oncology). J Clin Oncol 2017;35:2647–55.

40. Nitz U, Gluz O, Clemens M, et al. behalf of the West German Study Group PlanB Investigators. West German Study PlanB Trial: adjuvant four cycles of epirubicin and cyclophosphamide plus docetaxel versus six cycles of docetaxel and cyclophosphamide in HER2-negative early breast cancer. J Clin Oncol 2019;37:799–808.

41. Early Breast Cancer Trialists' Collaborative Group (EBCTCG). Adjuvant bisphosphonate treatment in early breast cancer: meta-analyses of individual patient data from randomised trials. Lancet 2015;386:1353–61.

42. Harbeck N, Penault-Llorca F, Cortes J, et al. Breast cancer. Nat Rev Dis Primers 2019;5:66.

43. Nelson DR, Brown J, Morikawa A, et al. Breast cancer-specific mortality in early breast cancer as defined by high-risk clinical and pathologic characteristics. PLoS ONE 2022;17(2):e0264637. https://doi.org/10.1371/journal.pone.0264637. Available at:.

44. Spring LM, Wander SA, Andre F, et al. Cyclin-dependent kinase 4 and 6 inhibitors for hormone receptor-positive breast cancer: past, present, and future. Lancet 2020;395:817–27.

45. Mayer EL, Dueck AC, Martin M, et al. Palbociclib with adjuvant endocrine therapy in early breast cancer (PALLAS): interim analysis of a multicentre, open-label, randomised, phase 3 study. Lancet Oncol 2021;22:212–22.

46. Gnant M, Dueck AC, Frantal S, et al. Adjuvant Palbociclib for Early Breast Cancer: The PALLAS Trial Results (ABCSG-42/AFT-05/BIG-14-03). J Clin Oncol 2022; 40(3):282–93.

47. Loibl S, Marmé F, Martin M, et al. Palbociclib for residual high-risk invasive HR-positive and HER2-negative early breast cancer—the Penelope-B trial. J Clin Oncol 2021;39:1518–30.

48. Johnston SRD, Harbeck N, Hegg R, et al. Abemaciclib Combined With Endocrine Therapy for the Adjuvant Treatment of HR+, HER2-, Node-Positive, High-Risk, Early Breast Cancer (monarchE). J Clin Oncol 2020;38(34):3987–98.

49. Harbeck N, Rastogi P, Martin M, et al. Adjuvant abemaciclib combined with endocrine therapy for high-risk early breast cancer: updated efficacy and Ki-67 analysis from the monarchE study. Ann Oncol 2021;32(12):1571–81.
50. Royce M, Osgood C, Mulkey F, et al. FDA Approval Summary: Abemaciclib with endocrine therapy for high-risk early breast cancer. J Clin Oncol 2022;40: 1155–62.
51. Giordano SH, Freedman RA, Somerfield MR, et al. Abemaciclib with endocrine therapy in the treatment of high-risk early breast cancer: ASCO optimal adjuvant chemotherapy and targeted therapy guideline rapid recommendation update. J Clin Oncol 2022;40(3):307–9.
52. Dowsett M. Testing endocrine response for managing primary estrogen receptor-positive breast cancer. J Clin Oncol 2022;40(23):2520–3.
53. Smith I, Robertson J, Kilburn L, et al. Long-term outcome and prognostic value of Ki67 after perioperative endocrine therapy in postmenopausal women with hormone-sensitive early breast cancer (POETIC): an open-label, multi-centre, parallel-group, randomised, phase 3 trial. Lancet Oncol 2020;21:1443–54.
54. Ellis MJ, Suman VJ, Hoog J, et al. Ki67 proliferation index as a tool for chemotherapy decisions during and after neoadjuvant aromatase inhibitor treatment of breast cancer; results from the American College of Surgeons Oncology Group Z1031 Trial (Alliance.) J Clin Oncol 2017;35(10):1061–9.
55. Nitz UA, Gluz O, Kümmel S, et al. Endocrine therapy response and 21-gene expression assay for therapy guidance in HR+/HER2- early breast cancer. J Clin Oncol 2022;40(23):2557–67.

Role of Immunotherapy in Early- and Late-Stage Triple-Negative Breast Cancer

Stefania Morganti, MD[a,b,c,d,e], Sara M. Tolaney, MD, MPH[a,b,c],*

KEYWORDS

- TNBC • Breast cancer • Immunotherapy • Biomarkers • PDL1
- Immune checkpoint inhibitors

KEY POINTS

- The combination of immune checkpoint inhibitors and chemotherapy is the new standard of care for triple-negative breast cancer in both the early-stage and first-line metastatic setting.
- Many open questions need to be solved—what is the ideal chemotherapy backbone, the optimal sequencing of treatments, the best endpoints, and biomarkers is unknown.
- Predictive biomarkers of immunotherapy benefit are lacking.
- New agents and strategies to expand the population that may derive a benefit from immunotherapy are warranted.

INTRODUCTION

The advent of immune checkpoint inhibitors (ICI) has revolutionized cancer treatment across several tumor types, with unprecedented durable responses in patients with late-stage tumors (**Fig. 1**). However, initial studies failed to demonstrate similar improvements in breast cancer (BC). The immune landscape of BC is very different from so-called hot tumors such as lung cancer or melanoma, in which immune escape plays a significant role in tumor progression and where tumor mutational burden (TMB) may be substantially different.[1]

This article previously appeared in *Hematology/Oncology* Clinics volume 37 issue 1 February 2023.

[a] Medical Oncology, Dana-Farber Cancer Institute, Boston, MA, USA; [b] Breast Oncology Program, Dana-Farber Brigham Cancer Center, Boston, MA, USA; [c] Harvard Medical School, Boston, MA, USA; [d] Broad Institute of MIT and Harvard, Boston, MA, USA; [e] Department of Oncology and Hemato-Oncology, University of Milan, Istituto Europeo di Oncologia, Milan, Italy
* Corresponding author. Dana-Farber Cancer Institute, 450 Brookline Ave., Boston, MA 02215.
E-mail address: Sara_Tolaney@dfci.harvard.edu

Clinics Collections 14 (2024) 323–340
https://doi.org/10.1016/j.ccol.2024.02.027
2352-7986/24/© 2024 Elsevier Inc. All rights reserved.

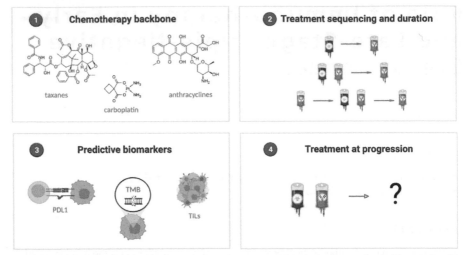

Fig. 1. Immunotherapy in triple-negative breast cancer: open questions (Created with BioRender.com).

Defined by the absence of actionable targets, triple-negative breast cancer (TNBC) is an aggressive BC subtype, and chemotherapy has represented the only available therapeutic option. However, TNBC is also the most immune-infiltrated among breast tumors, suggesting that the interaction between immune and tumor cells may play a role and that immunotherapy might be active.[2] Although single-agent ICIs proved largely ineffective,[3–6] subsequent studies showed that combining chemotherapy and ICI improved outcomes in both early[7] and advanced[8] TNBC. Despite this, many patients do not derive the expected benefit from immunotherapy, and we still do not know how to identify them.

Here, the authors review the data for immunotherapy in TNBC, along with questions and challenges that need to be faced.

DISCUSSION
Early-Stage Setting

Historically, treatment of early-stage TNBC (eTNBC) relied on chemotherapy administered as a sequence of multiple drugs before or after surgery. Although neoadjuvant chemotherapy was never shown to improve outcomes over adjuvant chemotherapy, administration of systemic treatment before surgery has clinical advantages, including assessment of tumor response in vivo and risk stratification and modulation of treatment after surgery.[9] Indeed, the achievement of a pathologic complete response (pCR) at surgery correlates with excellent long-term outcomes[10] and is now an established surrogate endpoint in this setting.

In 2021, results of the KEYNOTE 522 (KN522) trial[7] demonstrated the value of adding ICI to chemotherapy as neoadjuvant treatment of stage 2 and 3 eTNBC. KN522 was a phase III, randomized trial that compared pembrolizumab plus a 4-drug chemotherapy regimen (carboplatin-paclitaxel followed by epirubicin-cyclophosphamide [EC] or adriamycin-cyclophosphamide [AC]) to chemotherapy alone. After surgery, patients continued pembrolizumab to complete 1 year of treatment. Adding pembrolizumab increased the pCR rate (64.8% vs 51.2%, $P < 0.001$)[7] and improved the 3-year event-free survival (EFS) to 84.5% in the experimental arm versus 76.8% in the control arm (hazard ratio [HR] 0.63, $P = 0.0003$).[11]

Trials with other ICIs have yielded less straightforward results (**Table 1**). For instance, the phase II GeparNuevo trial, investigating nanoparticle albumin-bound paclitaxel (nab-paclitaxel) followed by EC with or without durvalumab, did improve the primary endpoint of pCR (53.4% vs 44.2%; odds ratio [OR]: 1.45; $P = 0.287$).[12] At the same time, it showed a benefit for adding the ICI in terms of invasive disease-free survival (iDFS), with a 3-year iDFS of 84.9% versus 76.9% (HR 0.54, $P = 0.0559$), and overall survival (OS), with a 3-year OS of 95.1% versus 83.1% (HR 0.26, $P = 0.0076$),[13] although it was not powered for survival analysis. Similarly, in the phase III NeoTRIP study, the combination of atezolizumab plus carboplatin and nab-paclitaxel did not improve pCR over carboplatin plus nab-paclitaxel only (48.6% vs 44.4%; OR: 1.18; $P = 0.48$).[14] So far, the primary study endpoint, EFS, has not been reported. On the other hand, the IMpassion031 study, investigating nab-paclitaxel followed by AC ± atezolizumab met its primary endpoint, showing a significantly higher pCR rate (57.6% vs 41.1%, $P = 0.0044$), and a trend toward longer EFS.[15] The phase III GeparDouze study (NCT03281954), testing the same regimen but with the addition of carboplatin in combination to nab-paclitaxel, is ongoing.

In summary, immunotherapy can be active in patients with eTNBC, but these conflicting results highlight how many questions remain.

Chemotherapy backbone
The KN522 regimen (pembrolizumab with sequential paclitaxel/carboplatin then anthracycline/cyclophosphamide) deployed a maximal number of chemotherapy agents; it remains unclear what the best chemotherapy backbone should be. Anthracyclines have traditionally been the cornerstone of (neo)adjuvant therapy for high-risk TNBC. However, these agents have been associated with potentially severe, long-term side effects, such as cardiac failure and secondary hematologic malignancies.[16] However, when combined with ICI, anthracyclines seem to be particularly effective. For instance, the phase II TONIC trial,[17] which compared different induction strategies in patients with metastatic TNBC (mTNBC), showed the highest objective response rate with doxorubicin (35%). In addition, indirect data favoring anthracyclines may be derived from studies that did not administer anthracyclines before surgery. The anthracycline-free regimen of the NeoTRIP study failed to show a pCR improvement, suggesting that anthracyclines might be needed to boost ICI activity.[14] In contrast, data from the Pembro8-noAC arm of the I-SPY2 study showed an equal estimated pCR rate for paclitaxel followed by AC and for pembrolizumab plus paclitaxel followed by pembrolizumab only, although low in both arms (27%).[18] Furthermore, the recently presented phase II NeoPACT trial showed an impressive pCR rate of 58% with carboplatin AUC 5 plus docetaxel and pembrolizumab, with a 2-year EFS of 89%.[19] Despite the limitations of both trials—the first closed prematurely due to lack of activity and the second being a small, single-arm study—these findings might suggest that not all patients do require anthracyclines. At present, administration of anthracyclines as part of the KN522 regimen is standard practice. Nevertheless, these data are reassuring for patients unable to tolerate anthracyclines or with contraindications.

KN522 notably included platinum chemotherapy as part of the regimen, even though platinum was not universally recommended to all patients before the KN522 trial owing to inconclusive neo/adjuvant data. Three major trials investigated adding platinum to various drugs.[20–22] Although all 3 studies demonstrated a pCR benefit, the DFS advantage observed in the BrighTNess and GeparSixto was not seen in the CALGB40603 study.[20–22] In addition, in the I-SPY2 trial, patients receiving

Table 1
Randomized trials investigating neoadjuvant chemo-immunotherapy for patients with early-stage triple-negative breast cancer

Trial	Study Design	Primary endpoint	n	Arms	Median Follow up	pCR	EFS (or iDFS) and OS	Comments
KEYNOTE-522[7,11]	Randomized 2:1, placebo-controlled phase III	pCR and EFS in ITT	1174	(TCb -> AC) + pembro or placebo, followed by adjuvant pembro or placebo	39.1 mo	ITT: 64.8% vs 51.2%; $P < 0.001$ / PDL1+: 68.9% vs 54.9% / PDL1-: 45.3% vs 30.3%	3-y EFS 84.5% vs 76.8% (HR 0.63, $P = 0.0003$) / 3-y OS 89.7% vs 86.9% (HR 0.72, $P = 0.032$)	The updated, unpublished analysis reports a lower pCR difference (63% vs 55.6%)
Impassion031[15]	Randomized 1:1, placebo-controlled phase III	pCR in ITT and PDL1+	333	(nabTCb -> ddAC) + atezo or placebo, followed by adjuvant atezo or placebo	Ex: 20.6 mo Co: 19.8 mo	ITT: 58% vs 41%; $P = 0.004$ / PDL1+: 68.8% vs 49.3% / PDL1-: 48% vs 34%	EFS HR 0.76 (95% CI 0.40-1.44) OS HR 0.69 (95% CI 0.25-1.87)	Capecitabine allowed; not powered for survival analyses
NeoTRIP[14]	Randomized 1:1, open-label, phase III	EFS in ITT	280	nabTCb ± atezo, followed by adjuvant AC or EC	N/A	ITT: 48.6% vs 44.4% OR 1.18; $P = 0.48$. / PDL1+: 59.5% vs 51.9% / PDL1-: 33.9% vs 35.4%	Not yet reported	Significantly higher TILs in the control arm
GeparDouze NCT03281954	Randomized 1:1, placebo-controlled phase III	pCR and EFS in ITT	1520	(TCb -> AC) + atezo or placebo, followed by adjuvant atezo or placebo	N/A	Not yet reported	Not yet reported	Estimated primary completion date: December 31, 2023

Gepar Nuevo[12]	Randomized 1:1, placebo-controlled, phase II	pCR in ITT	174	(nabT -> AC) + durva or placebo, followed by adjuvant TPC Window cohort: 2-wk durva before starting	42.2 mo	ITT: 53.4% vs 44.2%; P = 0.224 window cohort: 61.0% vs 41.4%; P = 0.035	3-y iDFS 84.9% vs 76.9% (HR 0.54, P = 0.0559); 3-y iDFS 91.4% vs 79.5% (HR 0.37, P = 0.015); 3-y OS 95.1% vs 83.1% (HR 0.26, P = 0.0076)	Randomization stratified by TILs; durva in the neoadjuvant setting only; not powered for survival analyses
I-SPY2[23]	Adaptively randomized, open-label, phase II	pCR in ITT	ITT: 250 (181 Co + 69 Ex) TNBC: 114 (85 Co + 29 Ex)	T ± pembro -> AC, followed by adjuvant TPC	Ex: 2.8 y; Co: 3.5 y	TNBC: 60% vs 22%	TNBC: EFS HR 0.6	Pembro administered with T only (4 cycles); SOC adjuvant therapy per NCCN guidelines recommended; not powered for survival analyses

Abbreviations: A, adriamycin; atezo, atezolizumab; C, cyclophosphamide; Cb, carboplatin; Co, control arm; D, docetaxel; dd, dose dense; iDFS, invasive disease-free survival; durva, durvalumab; EFS, event-free survival; Ex, experimental arm; ITT, intention to treat; N/A, not available; nabT, nab-paclitaxel; OS, overall survival; pCR, pathologic complete response; pembro, pembrolizumab; SOC, standard of care; T, paclitaxel; TILs, tumor-infiltrating lymphocytes; TNBC, triple-negative breast cancer; TPC, treatment of physician's choice.

pembrolizumab plus paclitaxel followed by EC/AC (hence the same as in the KN522 study, but without platinum and with lower pembrolizumab exposure) achieved a pCR rate of 60%, only slightly inferior to the 64.8% of the KN522 study.[23] Moreover, EFS observed in the GeparNuevo and KN522 were very similar, despite the fact that the first did not include platinum and administered ICI only before surgery.[7,12] Inclusion of platinum in the neoadjuvant therapy for patients with eTNBC is thus controversial. Although it is recommended for patients with high-risk (ie, node-positive, stage III) tumors, it is not standard practice for most stage II tumors, for which a case-by-case management is preferred. Moreover, platinum is frequently responsible for severe myelotoxicity, which may compromise dose intensity in this setting. Indeed, early withdrawal of platinum can be considered in patients with poor tolerance.

Setting and sequencing of treatments

Whether ICIs should be administered before or after surgery is unknown, and 3 large, phase III trials are currently investigating ICI in the adjuvant setting (**Table 2**). These trials differ in terms of setting (postneoadjuvant vs adjuvant), regimen administered, as well as population risk. None of these studies will answer the question of whether neoadjuvant ICI should be continued in the adjuvant setting, after surgery. Following the KN522 study, pembrolizumab is now routinely continued for an additional 27 weeks in all patients, although patients with pCR are likely to derive little benefit, given the excellent outcome of pCR patients in both arms.[11] Hence, whether or not pembrolizumab should be continued after a pCR is a matter of debate. Other studies suggest that omission of adjuvant ICI may have little impact on outcomes. In the GeparNuevo trial, durvalumab was administered in the neoadjuvant setting only and had similar long-term outcomes as KN522.[12] Similarly, the 2-year EFS in the NeoPACT study was 89%, despite the fact that only 4% of patients received adjuvant pembrolizumab.[19] A planned trial, OptimICE-pCR, led by Alliance, hopes to randomize patients after pCR following preoperative pembrolizumab/chemotherapy to adjuvant pembrolizumab or not.

Patients with residual disease seemed to derive the highest from pembrolizumab in the KN522 trial,[11,24] although this derives from an exploratory, post-hoc analysis not controlled for multiplicity.[24] In addition, administration of currently approved post-neoadjuvant agents, such as capecitabine or olaparib, was not allowed. In 2017, a few months after the KN522 trial was started, the CREATE-X[25] study showed a survival benefit with addition of capecitabine in the setting of residual disease after neoadjuvant therapy for eTNBC. More recently, the OlympiA[26] trial also proved that 1 year of adjuvant olaparib leads to an improvement in both DFS and OS in high-risk, germline BRCA carriers with eTNBC after both adjuvant and neoadjuvant chemotherapy.

Despite these controversies, pembrolizumab is generally continued after surgery in combination with either capecitabine or olaparib for patients with residual disease, as safety data from the metastatic setting showed that the combination therapy with checkpoint inhibition is safe.[27,28]

Finally, the optimal sequencing strategy between immunotherapy and chemotherapy remains unknown. In the GeparNuevo study, a subset of patients in the experimental arm received a 2-week run-in of durvalumab only. Notably, this was the only subset in which a pCR benefit was observed.[12] Although different patient and tumor characteristics between the window and nonwindow cohorts might justify the difference in response, a priming immunologic effect of durvalumab only cannot be excluded.

Biomarkers

Many correlative studies have investigated different biomarkers in patients receiving chemo-ICI, but none have identified which patients derive a significant benefit

Table 2
Randomized trials investigating adjuvant immunotherapy in patients with early-stage triple-negative breast cancer

Trial	Study Design	Primary Endpoint	Sample Size	Setting	Inclusion Criteria	Treatment
SWOG S1418 (NCT02954874)	Randomized, open-label, phase III	iDFS	1155	Postneoadjuvant	• TNBC (ER/PR ≤ 5%) • Residual disease ≥ 1 cm and/or positive lymph nodes	1-y pembro vs observation
IMpassion030/ ALEXANDRA (NCT03498716)	Randomized, open-label, phase III	iDFS	2300	Adjuvant	• Stage II–III TNBC	(wT → ddAC) +/-atezo, followed by maintenance atezo in the experimental arm
A-BRAVE (NCT02926196)	Randomized, open-label, phase III	DFS DFS in PDL1+ patients	474	Stratum A: postadjuvant Stratum B: postneoadjuvant	• TNBC (ER/PR ≤ 10%); • Stage IIB–III TNBC • After anthracycline- and taxane-based adjuvant CT • TNBC (ER/PR ≤ 10%); • Residual disease • Adjuvant chemotherapy <6 mo allowed	Avelumab vs observation

Abbreviations: A, adriamycin; atezo, atezolizumab; C, cyclophosphamide; dd, dose dense; DFS, disease-free survival; iDFS, invasive disease-free survival; pembro, pembrolizumab; TNBC, triple-negative breast cancer; wT, weekly paclitaxel.

specifically from the ICI component. In the KN522 study, programmed cell death-ligand 1-positive (PDL1+) tumors showed a higher pCR rate than PD-L1-negative (PDL1−) irrespective of arm of therapy, but the benefit of immunotherapy was consistent in both PDL1+ and PDL1− tumors.7 A similar finding emerged from the IMpassion031 study, where the benefit from the addition of atezolizumab was independent of PDL1 expression,[15] whereas the NeoTRIP trial showed a significantly higher benefit from ICI only in PDL1+ BC.[14] The reason for this discrepancy is unknown, but differences in the chemotherapy backbone—without anthracyclines in the NeoTRIP trial—or the proportion of immune cells 1+ versus 2+/3+ have been offered as potential explanations.

The prognostic and predictive role of tumor-infiltrating lymphocytes (TILs) has been also widely explored. High TILs have been shown to correlate with excellent long-term outcomes in patients with TNBC receiving chemotherapy only,[29] and even in patients treated with surgery alone,[30] highlighting the crucial role of the immunosurveillance in TNBC.

A correlation between TILs and higher pCR has also been observed across trials investigating chemo-ICI combinations, although findings about a predictive role for immunotherapy benefit have been conflicting. In the GeparNuevo study, stromal TILs (sTILs) were shown to independently predict pCR in both arms,[31] whereas baseline sTILs were found to correlate with higher pCR only in the atezolizumab arm of the NeoTRIP study.[32] In the NeoPACT study, an impressive pCR rate of 76% was observed in tumors with sTILs greater than or equal to 30%, which represented 48% of cases.[29] sTILs have also been assessed at cycle 2 in the NeoTRIP study, where they have been found to strongly correlate with pCR in both arms.[32] Of note, a significant arm imbalance of TILs in favor of the chemotherapy only arm was noticed in this trial, and investigators claimed that this difference was a potential reason for the lack of pCR benefit.[14]

Several other immune-related biomarkers have been investigated, including immune-associated signatures and TMB.[31,33,34] Most of them have proved to be highly intercorrelated, and none has been shown to specifically predict immunotherapy benefit.

Advanced Stage Setting

Phase I trials investigating ICIs in patients with pretreated mTNBC failed to show important benefit.[3,4,35,36] Nevertheless, signs of activity were seen in less pretreated patients with PDL1+ tumors, suggesting that different patient selection might define cohorts benefitting from immunotherapy. The use of concurrent ICI chemotherapy in first-line treatment of mTNBC has been shown to favorably affect outcomes. The KEYNOTE 355 study (KN355) was a randomized, phase III study investigating the addition of pembrolizumab to chemotherapy vs chemotherapy alone in patients with treatment-naïve mTNBC, with 3 chemotherapy options (ie, nab-paclitaxel, paclitaxel, and carboplatin-gemcitabine).[8] Patients were stratified according to PDL1 expression, as assessed by the composite positive score (CPS) with the 22C3 antibody. The trial had 2 primary endpoints: PFS and OS in the intent-to-treat (ITT) population and in patients with PDL1+ (a CPS $\geq$ 10 and a CPS $\geq$ 1) tumors. A statistically significant benefit was observed for PDL1+ (CPS>10) tumors in terms of both PFS (HR 0.65; $P = 0.0012$)[8] and OS (HR 0.73; $P = 0.0093$),[37] whereas there was no significant difference for PDL1− BC. No heterogeneity was observed for the 3 chemotherapy backbones, with a slightly higher benefit from taxanes emerging from the subgroup analysis[8]; however, one has to be cautious when interpreting these data, as patients were not randomized to the specific chemotherapy agent, and physicians were more likely to choose carboplatin plus gemcitabine in patients experiencing early relapse.

Data investigating atezolizumab in the same setting, however, have been controversial. The IMpassion130 was a phase III, randomized study investigating the addition of atezolizumab to first-line nab-paclitaxel.[38] The trial was positive for PFS in the ITT population, a co-primary endpoint, with a median PFS of 7.2 versus 5.5 months (HR 0.80, $P = 0.0025$), and in the PDL1+ subgroup (7.5 vs 5.0 months; HR 0.62, $P < 0.001$). A clinically meaningful benefit in OS in PDL1+ was also observed (25.4 vs 17.9 months; HR 0.67),[39] although owing to the analytical plan of the trial, this was not statistically significant. A very similar study, IMpassion131 phase III trial, investigated paclitaxel with or without atezolizumab and showed no benefit for adding ICI treatment even in PDL1+ patients.[40] Several reasons for these discrepancies have been hypothesized, including the need for steroids with paclitaxel, and the unprecedented OS outcome observed with paclitaxel alone in the control arm. Although atezolizumab was granted accelerated approval for mTNBC in 2019 based on IMpassion130 study, the negative findings from IMpassion131 led the company to withdraw the drug indication in the United States.

Duration, sequencing, and later lines

Duration of immunotherapy is an important consideration in mTNBC. As in other tumor types, there are some long-responders with mTNBC who derive a benefit from ICI lasting many years. Indeed, around 28% of patients with mTNBC with PDL1 CPS greater than 10 receiving ICI in the KN355 study were progression free at 2 years,[11] compared with the ~30% to 37% rate with first-line anti-PD1 monotherapy for melanoma[41,42] and ~20% with first-line chemo-immunotherapy for non–small cell lung cancer (NSCLC).[43,44] Evidence suggests that stopping treatment after 2 years should be safe in patients with melanoma and NSCLC,[45] but evidence in BC is lacking.

In parallel, trials are investigating whether a different sequence strategy of chemotherapy followed by maintenance ICIs might be beneficial. From a biological standpoint, a priming chemotherapy phase may promote tumor immunity through both the induction of immunogenic cell death (ICD) and the killing of suppressive immune cells. The SAFIR-02 trial, which investigated the administration of maintenance durvalumab after chemotherapy in human epidermal growth factor receptor 2 (HER2)-negative advanced BC, was negative in the ITT population but showed a significant advantage in TNBC (n = 82, 14.0 vs 21.2 months, HR 0.54; $P = 0.04$) and PDL1+ tumors (12.1 vs 25.8 months, HR 0.42; $P = 0.06$).[46] Alternative maintenance strategies combining ICI with targeted agents or chemotherapy after a chemotherapy-only phase are under investigation.

Little is known regarding the best second-line treatment of progression following the first-line ICI-based treatment. At present, there is no role for continuing ICI therapy beyond overt progression.

Biomarkers

Although expression of PDL1 by tumor and immune cells predicts ICI benefit for patients with mTNBC [8,35,38,40] PDL1 is far from a perfect biomarker for patient selection. Different studies relied on distinct assays to assess PDL1. The KEYNOTE trials used the Dako 22C3 assay and applied the CPS to define PDL1 positivity,[8] whereas the IMpassion trials used the Ventana SP142 assay and the immune score (IC).[38,40] The former assay counts the number of PDL1 staining cells (tumor cells, lymphocytes, macrophages) divided by the total number of tumor cells, whereas the PDL1 IC score is defined by the proportion of tumor area occupied by PDL1 staining immune cells of any intensity. Other assays and scoring criteria are also available.

A re-analysis of samples from the IMpassion130 study showed a poor inter-assay overlap, with only moderate concordance for the SP142, SP263 Ventana, and 22C3 Dako assays (r Spearman 0.57–0.69).[47] Nevertheless, correlation with clinical activity was similar (PFS HR 0.60–0.68; OS HR 0.74–0.79). Interestingly, the CPS cutoff that better reflected the PDL1+ population by SP142 was 10, which is the same cutoff that was shown to predict benefit from pembrolizumab in the KN355 study.[47]

Perhaps more critically, PDL1 is a dynamic biomarker, with expression that changes in time and across different metastatic sites. Higher rates of PDL1+ tumors are usually observed in primary versus metastatic samples, and PDL1+ positivity is especially low in particular metastatic sites such as liver, skin, and bone.[48,49] Of note, all samples for PDL1 assessment in the KN355 were metastatic, whereas the IMpassion130 allowed both primary and metastatic samples.

Finally, in contrast to what was observed for other tumor types, the level of expression in PDL1+ tumors did not seem to correlate with OS in trials where ICIs were given with chemotherapy.[8,49] Conversely, a trend toward an OS benefit was observed in patients receiving ICI alone, such as in the Keynote 119 (KN119) trial. Although KN119 failed to prove any OS difference between patients with pretreated TNBC receiving pembrolizumab single-agent or chemotherapy, patients with CPS greater than 20, who represented around 18% of the overall population, seemed to experience greater OS benefit from pembrolizumab (OS HR 0.58%, 95% 0.38–0.88).[34]

Additional biomarkers have been investigated in patients with mTNBC, including TILs, TMB, phosphatase and tensin homolog (PTEN) mutations, and other immune-related signatures. Both high TMB (>10) and PTEN wild-type status have been correlated with longer PFS in a retrospective study including 62 women with mTNBC who received different ICI-based regimens.[50] Efficacy of ICI monotherapy has been also investigated in small prospective trials of patients with high TMB, such as the NIMBUS[51] and TAPUR[52] studies. Although signal of activity was observed, most patients did not derive a benefit, and questions remain about assays and the cutoffs that should be used, as the most compelling responses were seen in tumors with TMB substantially higher than 10.

Evidence is conflicting about the role of TILs as a predictive biomarker of immunotherapy benefit. Although atezolizumab and pembrolizumab monotherapy studies showed that clinical activity was highest in sTILs + tumors,[6,35] correlative data from the IMpassion130 showed that benefit of ICI plus chemotherapy over chemotherapy alone was seen only in patients who are both sTILs+ and PDL1+.[49] Notably, the level of TILs is lower in metastatic sites than in primary tumors, in line with the described shift toward a more immune-evasive tumor microenvironment from primary to metastatic BC.

Toxicity

ICIs are well tolerated by most patients, without major differences in the incidence of both low- and high-grade adverse events (AEs) between patients receiving chemo-immunotherapy or chemotherapy alone.[11,14,15,37,38,40] However, ICIs may lead to unique, immune-related AEs (irAEs) that follow the hyperactivation of the immune system.

Most frequent irAEs observed in major clinical trials investigating ICIs in patients with TNBC include infusion reactions (3%–18%), skin rash (1%–49%), hypothyroidism (6%–18%), hyperthyroidism (3%–6%), and pneumonitis (1%–4%) (**Table 3**). Although rare, these toxicities can be both life-threatening and permanent; this is particularly

Table 3
Most frequent toxicities reported in phase III randomized trials investigating immunotherapy with or without chemotherapy in triple-negative breast cancer

	KEYNOTE-522[7]	Impassion031[15]	NeoTRIP[14]	KEYNOTE-355[8]	IMpassion130[38]	IMpassion131[40]	KEYNOTE-119[35]
Treatment regimen	(TCb -> AC) + pembro -> adjuvant pembro	(nabTCb -> ddAC) + atezo -> adjuvant atezo	NabTCb + atezo -> adjuvant AC or EC	(T or NabT or CbGem) + pembro	NabT + atezo	NabT + atezo	Pembro monotherapy
IRAEs, any grade[a]	Infusion reactions 18% Hypothyroidism 15.1% Severe skin reaction 5.7% Hyperthyroidism 5.2% Adrenal insufficiency 2.6% Pneumonitis 2.2% Thyroiditis 2.0%	Rash 49% Infusion reactions 10.4% Hypothyroidism 6.7% Hyperthyroidism 3.0% Pneumonitis 1.2% Hepatitis 1.2% Ocular toxicity 1.2%	Infusion reactions 8% Hypothyroidism 6% Thyroiditis 1.5% Colitis 1.5% Pancreatitis 1.5%	Hypothyroidism 15% Hyperthyroidism 5% Pneumonitis 2% Colitis 2% Severe skin reaction 2%	Rash 34% Hypothyroidism 17.3% Hyperthyroidism 4.4% Pneumonitis 3.1% Hepatitis 2.2% Meningoencephalitis 1% Colitis 1%	Rash 33% Hypothyroidism 14% Hyperthyroidism 6% Pneumonitis 4% Infusion reactions 3% Hepatitis 2% Pancreatitis 2% Diabetes 1%	Hypothyroidism 7% Hyperthyroidism 4% Pneumonitis 1% Severe ski[b] reaction 1% Adrenal insufficiency 1%
IRAEs, grade 3[b]	Severe skin reaction 4.7% Infusion reactions 2.6% Hypophysitis 1.3% Adrenal insufficiency 1% Pneumonitis 0.9% Hypothyroidism 0.5%	Rash 3.7% Pneumonitis 0.6% Colitis 0.6% Encephalitis 0.6% Diabetes 0.6% Infusion reactions 0.6%	Infusion reactions 1% Pancreatitis 1.5% Colitis 1%	Hypothyroidism <1% Hyperthyroidism <1% Pneumonitis 1% Colitis <1% Severe skin reaction 2%	Hepatitis 1.3% Rash 0.9%	Pancreatitis 2% Diabetes 0.9% Rash 0.9% Pneumonitis 0.7% Infusion reactions 0.7% Hepatitis 0.5%	Pneumonitis 1% Severe skin reaction 1% Myositis 1%

(continued on next page)

Table 3
(continued)

	KEYNOTE-522[7]	Impassion031[15]	NeoTRIP[14]	KEYNOTE-355[8]	IMpassion130[38]	IMpassion131[40]	KEYNOTE-119[35]
Discontinuation rate due to AE	27.7%	22.6%	25.4%	18.3%	15.9%	21%	3%
Grade 5 IRAEs (n of patients)	Autoimmune encephalitis (2) Pneumonitis (1)	None	Unknown causes (1)	None	Autoimmune hepatitis (1)	Polymyositis (1)	None

Abbreviations: A, adriamycin; atezo, atezolizumab; C, cyclophosphamide; Cb, carboplatin; D, docetaxel; dd, dose dense; E, epirubicin; Gem, gemcitabine; IRAEs, immune-related adverse events; n, number; NabT, nab-paclitaxel; pembro, pembrolizumab; T, paclitaxel.
[a] Events with frequency >1% here reported
[b] Events with frequency >0.5% here reported.

relevant in the early-stage setting, in which this may translate in long-life consequences such as the need of hormone replacement therapy that follows ICI-induced endocrinopathies.[53]

irAEs are more common in the first weeks of treatment but may potentially occur anytime during therapy and even after treatment discontinuation.[53] In the KN522 study, most of the ICI-related toxicities were observed during the neoadjuvant phase, although a few high-grade irAEs leading to treatment discontinuation or death were observed also in the adjuvant phase.[11]

SUMMARY

Although the combination of ICI plus chemotherapy is helping patients with both early and advanced TNBC, many questions are still unanswered. Pembrolizumab is the only Food and Drug Administration–approved ICI in TNBC, as none of the other ICIs have shown a statistically significant benefit in a phase III study. Although biological differences have not been proved and are unlikely to exist, it is possible that distinct ICIs may be responsible for the discrepancies observed across trials. We do not have head-to-head comparisons between ICIs, and it is unlikely that we will have them in the future.

Although different chemotherapy backbones have been evaluated, it remains controversial as to which, if any, is best. In the early-stage setting, patients are currently treated with a 5-drug regimen, which is likely to represent an overtreatment for many of them. New stratification tools are needed to select patients for treatment escalation and de-escalation beyond the established pCR. Circulating tumor DNA (ctDNA) monitoring is a promising tool in this direction. In the I-SPY2 trial, ctDNA clearance showed a strong correlation with pCR and long-term outcomes,[54] and ongoing trials are investigating whether ctDNA monitoring might be used as a dynamic biomarker for treatment escalation and de-escalation.

On the other hand, although pCR is still valuable at the individual level, pCR's role as surrogate biomarker is unclear. Notably, no pCR difference was observed in the GeparNuevo trial, despite a significant advantage in long-term outcomes.[13] EFS data from the NeoTRIP trial, not yet reported, might provide similar findings.

Many immune biomarkers have been investigated in patients with TNBC, but only PDL1 is approved, and only in the metastatic setting. All others immune-related biomarkers have proved to be highly intercorrelated and were mainly used to identify patients with a good prognosis, instead of those patients who might derive the highest benefit from immunotherapy.[12,49] Indeed, highly infiltrated tumors have optimal response to chemotherapy alone, and we still do not know which patients really need immunotherapy. ICIs are well tolerated by most patients but might lead to potentially severe and, frequently, permanent toxicities (see **Table 3**). It is thus crucial to determine how to best select those patients who are unlikely to derive benefit from ICIs, especially in the curative setting.

Finally, new strategies are needed to understand how to convert "cold" into "hot" tumors and thus increase the proportion of patients who might benefit from ICI. Some proof-of-concept studies showed that sequencing might matter, either by administering an immunotherapy-only run-in or oppositely by boosting the immune response through chemotherapy-induced ICD. Similarly, co-administration of radiation therapy might increase immune sensitivity through the so-called abscopal effect. Novel agents are also under investigation, such as ADCs and vaccines.[55] Preclinical data have shown a potential synergy between ADCs and immunotherapy, and many trials are investigating different ADC-ICI combinations.[56–58]

In conclusion, although several steps have been made since the beginning of the immunotherapy journey for TNBC, many others are needed to address several unsolved questions in this field.

CLINICS CARE POINTS

- Neoadjuvant pembrolizumab plus a 4-drug chemotherapy regimen (paclitaxel-carboplatin followed by doxorubicin [or epirubicin]-cyclophosphamide) followed by adjuvant pembrolizumab is the standard of care for high-risk, stage II/III eTNBC.
- The optimal chemotherapy backbone is not yet defined.
- Predictive biomarkers of immunotherapy benefit for eTNBC are lacking.
- Whether immunotherapy should be administered before or after surgery is unknown.
- Pembrolizumab plus chemotherapy (taxanes or carboplatin plus gemcitabine) is the standard of care for mTNBC with PDL1 CPS greater than 10.
- PDL1 expression is the only biomarker available in the advanced setting.
- The most effective second-line option for mTNBC is not established.
- ICIs are well tolerated by most patients, although potentially responsible for rare but severe or permanent toxicities.
- New drugs and strategies to expand the population of patients that can benefit from immunotherapy are warranted.

DISCLOSURE

S.M. Tolaney reports receiving institutional research funds and honoraria from AstraZeneca, Eli Lilly & Co, Merck, Nektar, Novartis, Pfizer, Genentech/Roche, Immunomedic/Gilead, Bristol-Myers Squibb, Eisai, Nanostring, Sanofi, Odonate, and Seattle Genetics; institutional research funds from Exelixis and Cyclacel; and honoraria from Puma, Daiichi Sankyo, Athenex, OncoPep, Kyowa Kirin Pharmaceuticals, Samsung Bioepsis Inc., CytomX, Certara, Mersana Therapeutics, Ellipses Pharma, 4D Pharm, OncoSec Medical Incorporated, Chugai Pharmaceuticals, BeyondSpring Pharmaceuticals, OncXerna, Zymeworks, Zentalis, Blueprint Medicines, Reveal Genomics, ARC Therapeutics and Myovant. Stefania Morganti has no conflicts of interest to declare.

FUNDING

S. Morganti is supported by the American-Italian Cancer Foundation Post-Doctoral Research Fellowship, year 2021 to 2022.

REFERENCES

1. Drake CG, Lipson EJ, Brahmer JR. Breathing new life into immunotherapy: review of melanoma, lung and kidney cancer. Nat Rev Clin Oncol 2014;11(1):24–37.
2. Bianchini G, De Angelis C, Licata L, et al. Treatment landscape of triple-negative breast cancer - expanded options, evolving needs. Nat Rev Clin Oncol 2022; 19(2):91–113.
3. Nanda R, Chow LQM, Dees EC, et al. Pembrolizumab in patients with advanced triple-negative breast cancer: Phase Ib KEYNOTE-012 study. J Clin Oncol 2016; 34(21):2460–7.

4. Adams S, Schmid P, Rugo HS, et al. Pembrolizumab monotherapy for previously treated metastatic triple-negative breast cancer: cohort A of the phase II KEYNOTE-086 study. Ann Oncol 2019;30(3):397–404.

5. Dirix LY, Takacs I, Jerusalem G, et al. Avelumab, an anti-PD-L1 antibody, in patients with locally advanced or metastatic breast cancer: a phase 1b JAVELIN Solid Tumor study. Breast Cancer Res Treat 2018;167(3):671–86.

6. Emens LA, Cruz C, Eder JP, et al. Long-term clinical outcomes and biomarker analyses of atezolizumab therapy for patients with metastatic triple-negative breast cancer: A phase 1 study. JAMA Oncol 2019;5(1):74–82.

7. Schmid P, Cortes J, Pusztai L, et al. Pembrolizumab for early triple-negative breast cancer. N Engl J Med 2020;382(9):810–21.

8. Cortes J, Cescon DW, Rugo HS, et al. Pembrolizumab plus chemotherapy versus placebo plus chemotherapy for previously untreated locally recurrent inoperable or metastatic triple-negative breast cancer (KEYNOTE-355): a randomised, placebo-controlled, double-blind, phase 3 clinical trial. Lancet 2020; 396(10265):1817–28.

9. Burstein HJ, Curigliano G, Thürlimann B, et al. Customizing local and systemic therapies for women with early breast cancer: the St. Gallen International Consensus Guidelines for treatment of early breast cancer 2021. Ann Oncol 2021;32(10):1216–35.

10. Cortazar P, Zhang L, Untch M, et al. Pathological complete response and long-term clinical benefit in breast cancer: the CTNeoBC pooled analysis. Lancet 2014;384(9938):164–72.

11. Schmid P, Cortes J, Dent R, et al. VP7-2021: KEYNOTE-522: Phase III study of neoadjuvant pembrolizumab + chemotherapy vs. placebo + chemotherapy, followed by adjuvant pembrolizumab vs. placebo for early-stage TNBC. Ann Oncol 2021;32(9):1198–200.

12. Loibl S, Untch M, Burchardi N, et al. A randomised phase II study investigating durvalumab in addition to an anthracycline taxane-based neoadjuvant therapy in early triple-negative breast cancer: clinical results and biomarker analysis of GeparNuevo study. Ann Oncol 2019;30(8):1279–88.

13. Loibl S, Schneeweiss A, Huober JB, et al. Durvalumab improves long-term outcome in TNBC: results from the phase II randomized GeparNUEVO study investigating neodjuvant durvalumab in addition to an anthracycline/taxane based neoadjuvant chemotherapy in early triple-negative breast cancer (TNBC). J Clin Oncol 2021;39(15_suppl):506.

14. Gianni L, Huang CS, Egle D, et al. Pathologic complete response (pCR) to neoadjuvant treatment with or without atezolizumab in triple-negative, early high-risk and locally advanced breast cancer: NeoTRIP Michelangelo randomized study. Ann Oncol 2022;33(5):534–43.

15. Mittendorf EA, Zhang H, Barrios CH, et al. Neoadjuvant atezolizumab in combination with sequential nab-paclitaxel and anthracycline-based chemotherapy versus placebo and chemotherapy in patients with early-stage triple-negative breast cancer (IMpassion031): a randomised, double-blind, phase 3 trial. Lancet 2020;396(10257):1090–100.

16. Hurvitz SA, McAndrew NP, Bardia A, et al. A careful reassessment of anthracycline use in curable breast cancer. NPJ Breast Cancer 2021;7(1):134.

17. Voorwerk L, Slagter M, Horlings HM, et al. Publisher Correction: Immune induction strategies in metastatic triple-negative breast cancer to enhance the sensitivity to PD-1 blockade: the TONIC trial. Nat Med 2019;25(7):1175.

18. Liu MC, Robinson PA, Yau C, et al. Abstract P3-09-02: Evaluation of a novel agent plus standard neoadjuvant therapy in early stage, high-risk HER2 negative breast cancer: Results from the I-SPY 2 TRIAL. In: Poster session abstracts. American Association for Cancer Research; 2020. https://doi.org/10.1158/1538-7445. sabcs19-p3-09-02.

19. Sharma P, Stecklein SR, Yoder R, et al. Clinical and biomarker results of neoadjuvant phase II study of pembrolizumab and carboplatin plus docetaxel in triple-negative breast cancer (TNBC) (NeoPACT). J Clin Orthod 2022; 40(16_suppl):513.

20. Loibl S, Weber KE, Timms KM, et al. Survival analysis of carboplatin added to an anthracycline/taxane-based neoadjuvant chemotherapy and HRD score as predictor of response-final results from GeparSixto. Ann Oncol 2018;29(12):2341–7.

21. Shepherd JH, Ballman K, Polley MYC, et al. CALGB 40603 (alliance): Long-term outcomes and genomic correlates of response and survival after neoadjuvant chemotherapy with or without carboplatin and bevacizumab in triple-negative breast cancer. J Clin Oncol 2022;40(12):1323–34.

22. Geyer CE, Sikov WM, Huober J, et al. Long-term efficacy and safety of addition of carboplatin with or without veliparib to standard neoadjuvant chemotherapy in triple-negative breast cancer: 4-year follow-up data from BrighTNess, a randomized phase III trial. Ann Oncol 2022;33(4):384–94.

23. Nanda R, Liu MC, Yau C, et al. Effect of pembrolizumab plus neoadjuvant chemotherapy on pathologic complete response in women with early-stage breast cancer: An analysis of the ongoing phase 2 adaptively randomized I-SPY2 trial. JAMA Oncol 2020;6(5):676–84.

24. Pusztai L, Denkert C, O'Shaughnessy J, et al. Event-free survival by residual cancer burden after neoadjuvant pembrolizumab + chemotherapy versus placebo + chemotherapy for early TNBC: Exploratory analysis from KEYNOTE-522. J Clin Oncol 2022;40(16_suppl):503.

25. Masuda N, Lee SJ, Ohtani S, et al. Adjuvant capecitabine for breast cancer after preoperative chemotherapy. N Engl J Med 2017;376(22):2147–59.

26. Tutt ANJ, Garber J, Gelber RD, et al. VP1-2022: Pre-specified event driven analysis of Overall Survival (OS) in the OlympiA phase III trial of adjuvant olaparib (OL) in germline BRCA1/2 mutation (gBRCAm) associated breast cancer. Ann Oncol 2022;33(5):566–8.

27. Vinayak S, Tolaney SM, Schwartzberg LS, et al. TOPACIO/Keynote-162: Niraparib + pembrolizumab in patients (pts) with metastatic triple-negative breast cancer (TNBC), a phase 2 trial. J Clin Oncol 2018;36(15_suppl):1011.

28. Domchek SM, Postel-Vinay S, Im SA, et al. Abstract OT3-05-03: MEDIOLA: An open-label, phase I/II basket study of olaparib (PARP inhibitor) and durvalumab (anti-PD-L1 antibody)–Additional breast cancer cohorts. In: Ongoing clinical trials. American Association for Cancer Research; 2019. https://doi.org/10.1158/ 1538-7445.sabcs18-ot3-05-03.

29. Denkert C, von Minckwitz G, Darb-Esfahani S, et al. Tumour-infiltrating lymphocytes and prognosis in different subtypes of breast cancer: a pooled analysis of 3771 patients treated with neoadjuvant therapy. Lancet Oncol 2018;19(1): 40–50.

30. de Jong VMT, Wang Y, Ter Hoeve ND, et al. Prognostic value of stromal tumor-infiltrating lymphocytes in young, node-negative, triple-negative breast cancer patients who did not receive (neo)adjuvant systemic therapy. J Clin Oncol 2022;40(21):2361–74.

31. Karn T, Denkert C, Weber KE, et al. Tumor mutational burden and immune infiltration as independent predictors of response to neoadjuvant immune checkpoint inhibition in early TNBC in GeparNuevo. Ann Oncol 2020;31(9):1216–22.

32. Bianchini G, Huang CS, Egle D, et al. LBA13 Tumour infiltrating lymphocytes (TILs), PD-L1 expression and their dynamics in the NeoTRIPaPDL1 trial. Ann Oncol 2020;31:S1145–6.

33. Dugo M, Huang CS, Egle D, et al. Abstract P2-07-12: Triple negative breast cancer subtypes and early dynamics of the 27-gene IO score predict pCR in the NeoTRIPaPDL1 trial. Cancer Res 2022;82(4_Supplement):07–12.

34. Sinn BV, Loibl S, Karn T, et al. Abstract PD5-05: Pre-therapeutic PD-L1 expression and dynamics of Ki-67 and gene expression during neoadjuvant immune-checkpoint blockade and chemotherapy to predict response within the Gepar-Nuevo trial. In: Poster discussion abstracts. American Association for Cancer Research; 2019. https://doi.org/10.1158/1538-7445.sabcs18-pd5-05.

35. Winer EP, Lipatov O, Im SA, et al. Pembrolizumab versus investigator-choice chemotherapy for metastatic triple-negative breast cancer (KEYNOTE-119): a randomised, open-label, phase 3 trial. Lancet Oncol 2021;22(4):499–511.

36. Tolaney SM, Kalinsky K, Kaklamani VG, et al. Eribulin plus pembrolizumab in patients with metastatic triple-negative breast cancer (ENHANCE 1): A phase Ib/II study. Clin Cancer Res 2021;27(11):3061–8.

37. Rugo HS, Schmid P, Cescon DW, et al. Abstract GS3-01: Additional efficacy endpoints from the phase 3 KEYNOTE-355 study of pembrolizumab plus chemotherapy vs placebo plus chemotherapy as first-line therapy for locally recurrent inoperable or metastatic triple-negative breast cancer. In: General session abstracts. American Association for Cancer Research; 2021. https://doi.org/10.1158/1538-7445.sabcs20-gs3-01.

38. Schmid P, Adams S, Rugo HS, et al. Atezolizumab and nab-paclitaxel in advanced triple-negative breast cancer. N Engl J Med 2018;379(22):2108–21.

39. Emens LA, Adams S, Barrios CH, et al. First-line atezolizumab plus nab-paclitaxel for unresectable, locally advanced, or metastatic triple-negative breast cancer: IMpassion130 final overall survival analysis. Ann Oncol 2021;32(8):983–93.

40. Miles D, Gligorov J, André F, et al. Primary results from IMpassion131, a double-blind, placebo-controlled, randomised phase III trial of first-line paclitaxel with or without atezolizumab for unresectable locally advanced/metastatic triple-negative breast cancer. Ann Oncol 2021;32(8):994–1004.

41. Wolchok JD, Rollin L, Larkin J. Nivolumab and ipilimumab in advanced melanoma. N Engl J Med 2017;377(25):2503–4.

42. Robert C, Ribas A, Schachter J, et al. Pembrolizumab versus ipilimumab in advanced melanoma (KEYNOTE-006): post-hoc 5-year results from an open-label, multicentre, randomised, controlled, phase 3 study. Lancet Oncol 2019;20(9):1239–51.

43. Gadgeel S, Rodríguez-Abreu D, Speranza G, et al. Updated analysis from KEYNOTE-189: Pembrolizumab or placebo plus pemetrexed and platinum for previously untreated metastatic nonsquamous non-small-cell lung cancer. J Clin Oncol 2020;38(14):1505–17.

44. Paz-Ares L, Vicente D, Tafreshi A, et al. A randomized, placebo-controlled trial of pembrolizumab plus chemotherapy in patients with metastatic squamous NSCLC: Protocol-specified final analysis of KEYNOTE-407. J Thorac Oncol 2020;15(10):1657–69.

45. Marron TU, Ryan AE, Reddy SM, et al. Considerations for treatment duration in responders to immune checkpoint inhibitors. J Immunother Cancer 2021;9(3): e001901.

46. Bachelot T, Filleron T, Bieche I, et al. Durvalumab compared to maintenance chemotherapy in metastatic breast cancer: the randomized phase II SAFIR02-BREAST IMMUNO trial. Nat Med 2021;27(2):250–5.

47. Rugo HS, Loi S, Adams S, et al. PD-L1 immunohistochemistry assay comparison in atezolizumab plus nab-paclitaxel-treated advanced triple-negative breast cancer. J Natl Cancer Inst 2021;113(12):1733–43.

48. Rozenblit M, Huang R, Danziger N, et al. Comparison of PD-L1 protein expression between primary tumors and metastatic lesions in triple negative breast cancers. J Immunother Cancer 2020;8(2):e001558.

49. Emens LA, Molinero L, Loi S, et al. Atezolizumab and nab-paclitaxel in advanced triple-negative breast cancer: Biomarker evaluation of the IMpassion130 study. J Natl Cancer Inst 2021;113(8):1005–16.

50. Barroso-Sousa R, Keenan TE, Pernas S, et al. Tumor mutational burden and PTEN alterations as molecular correlates of response to PD-1/L1 blockade in metastatic triple-negative breast cancer. Clin Cancer Res 2020;26(11):2565–72.

51. Barroso-Sousa R, Li T, Reddy S, et al. Abstract GS2-10: Nimbus: A phase 2 trial of nivolumab plus ipilimumab for patients with hypermutated her2-negative metastatic breast cancer (MBC). Cancer Res 2022;82(4_Supplement). GS2-10.

52. Alva AS, Mangat PK, Garrett-Mayer E, et al. Pembrolizumab in patients with metastatic breast cancer with high tumor mutational burden: Results from the targeted agent and profiling utilization registry (TAPUR) study. J Clin Oncol 2021; 39(22):2443–51.

53. Haanen JBAG, Carbonnel F, Robert C, et al. Management of toxicities from immunotherapy: ESMO Clinical Practice Guidelines for diagnosis, treatment and follow-up. Ann Oncol 2018;29(Suppl 4):iv264–6.

54. Magbanua MJM, Swigart LB, Wu HT, et al. Circulating tumor DNA in neoadjuvant-treated breast cancer reflects response and survival. Ann Oncol 2021;32(2): 229–39.

55. Isakoff SJ, Adams S, Soliman HH, et al. Abstract P3-09-15: A phase 1b study of PVX-410 (PVX) vaccine plus durvalumab (DUR) as adjuvant therapy in HLA-A2+ early stage triple negative breast cancer (eTNBC) to assess safety and immune response. In: Poster session abstracts. American Association for Cancer Research; 2020. https://doi.org/10.1158/1538-7445.sabcs19-p3-09-15.

56. Garrido-Castro AC, Keenan TE, Li T, et al. Saci-IO HR+: Randomized phase II trial of sacituzumab govitecan (SG) +/- pembrolizumab in PD-L1+ hormone receptor-positive (HR+)/HER2- metastatic breast cancer (MBC). J Clin Oncol 2021;39(15_suppl):TPS1102.

57. Garrido-Castro AC, Keenan TE, Li T, et al. Saci-IO TNBC: Randomized phase II trial of sacituzumab govitecan (SG) +/- pembrolizumab in PD-L1- metastatic triple-negative breast cancer (mTNBC). J Clin Oncol 2021;39(15_suppl): TPS1106.

58. Spring LM, Tolaney SM, Desai N, et al. Abstract OT-03-06: Phase 2 study of response-guided neoadjuvant sacituzumab govitecan (IMMU-132) in patients with localized triple-negative breast cancer (NeoSTAR). In: Ongoing clinical trials abstracts. American Association for Cancer Research; 2021. https://doi.org/10. 1158/1538-7445.sabcs20-ot-03-06.

Surgical Treatment

Postoperative Complications from Breast and Axillary Surgery

Sam Z. Thalji, MD[a], Chandler S. Cortina, MD, MS, FSSO[a],
Meng S. Guo, MD[b], Amanda L. Kong, MD, MS, FSSO[a],*

KEYWORDS

- Postoperative complications • Hematoma • Seroma • Nerve injury • Lymphedema

KEY POINTS

- Potential complications after breast and axillary surgery are numerous and vary in incidence and presentation.
- Risk profiles depend on the procedure performed, extent of axillary dissection, and the inclusion of various reconstructive techniques.
- Knowledge of potential complications and approaches for management are important components of the preoperative discussion with patients.
- Incidence, risk factors, presentation, implications to the patient, risk-reducing approaches, and management of postoperative complications after breast and axillary surgery (with or without reconstruction) are discussed herein.

INTRODUCTION

The prospective benefit of any operation must be weighed against the risk of its complications. Although surgery of the breast and axilla is generally well tolerated by patients, the breast surgeon recognizes that complications can occur even when operating with experience on the lowest risk patients. The operative repertoire ranges from breast conserving surgery (BCS), mastectomy (including skin-sparing and nipple-sparing types), to modified radical mastectomy (MRM), with each procedure carrying a different expected surgical morbidity. In the axilla, the majority of patients will only require a sentinel lymph biopsy (SLNB) with some for whom an axillary lymph node dissection (ALND) is still indicated. Select patients are candidates for omission of surgical nodal staging altogether. Each procedural component carries a unique risk

This article previously appeared in *Surgical Clinics* volume 103 issue 1 February 2023.
[a] Department of Surgery, Division of Surgical Oncology, Medical College of Wisconsin, Milwaukee, WI, USA; [b] Department of Plastic Surgery, Medical College of Wisconsin, Milwaukee, WI, USA
* Corresponding author. Department of Surgery/ Division of Surgical Oncology, 8701 Watertown Plank Road, Milwaukee, WI 53226.
E-mail address: akong@mcw.edu

Clinics Collections 14 (2024) 341–359
https://doi.org/10.1016/j.ccol.2024.02.028

profile that the surgeon must be well versed in explaining to patients in a practical format. Patients and families who are fully informed of potential complications before their operation describe greater trust in their surgeon and are better able to comanage complications with the surgical team, when they occur.[1]

EARLY COMPLICATIONS
Postoperative hematoma

Clinically significant hematoma formation after breast and axillary surgery is an uncommon complication that requires early recognition and urgent management. The incidence of postoperative hematoma requiring operative evacuation after breast surgery is estimated at less than 2% and seems to be higher among patients who receive mastectomy alone compared with patients who undergo immediate reconstruction or BCS.[2] Vessels arising from the pectoralis muscle are the most common primary source of postoperative bleeding while axillary hematomas are rare and are usually not associated with an identifiable source.[3] Postoperative hematomas generally accumulate within 12 to 24 hours after the initial operation and present as a palpable firm mass or fluid collection with spreading ecchymosis overlying the resection site and continued sanguineous output from surgical drains, when present. Skin tightness and eventually hemodynamic changes may occur if the hematoma is not recognized promptly and bleeding continues. The risk of postoperative hematoma after mastectomy is not altered by operative or oncologic factors and is higher among patients receiving anticoagulation.[4] Aside from sequelae of continued bleeding after surgery, hematomas may compromise the cosmetic outcome after reconstruction, threaten skin flaps or grafts, and are associated with the development of capsular contracture after implant-based reconstruction.[5]

Postoperative hematomas that present with jeopardized skin flaps, expansion, or hemodynamic instability must immediately return to the operating room for evacuation and exploration. Small minimally symptomatic hematomas are not uncommon and can be safely observed for evidence of stability and resolution. Vacuum-assisted percutaneous evacuation is being studied for delayed hematomas without the above alarm signs as a means to avoid reoperation.[6] Hematoma formation is minimized by practicing the fundamental surgical principle of diligent intraoperative hemostasis. Compressive dressings are commonly applied to decrease hematoma and seroma formation; however, this practice has not been definitively shown to reduce these unwanted complications.[7] Ancillary surgical techniques such as anchoring sutures and tissue sealants do not prevent hematoma formation.[8] Patients on anticoagulation should be managed following current guidelines (see "Venous Thromboembolism" section) and counseled regarding the increased risk of hematoma formation both immediately after surgery and on resuming anticoagulation.

SEROMA

Seroma formation is reported in up to 50% of patients after breast and axillary surgery.[9] Seromas consist of fluid accumulation in the postresection dead space and are more common after mastectomy and ALND than BCS and SLNB.[9] The exact cause of seroma formation is multifactorial, and lymph leak after the resection of axillary nodes is a known contributing factor for axillary seroma development.[10] Fluid output is highly variable between patients, although output typically declines in the first 48 hours after surgery.[11] Seromas can cause pain and discomfort, delay of subsequent treatments such as radiation therapy, impaired wound healing and dehiscence, flap ischemia, and poor cosmetic outcome. Seroma formation is associated with obesity, diabetes, increasing comorbidities, use of electrocautery, male sex, and vigorous postoperative shoulder exercise.[12–14]

Incidence of seroma after breast and axillary surgery is greatly reduced with the routine use of closed suction drains after mastectomy, large volume lumpectomies, and ALND.[15] There is no consensus criteria for optimal timing of drain removal after surgery based on duration or output; however, a recent meta-analysis found that drain removal within 24-48 hours after surgery was associated with a 50% increased risk of seroma development compared with drains removed more than 72 hours after surgery or after hospital discharge.[16] Axillary exclusion is a closure technique wherein the superior skin flap is sutured to the free edge of the pectoralis major and lateral chest wall to exclude the axillary fossa from the mastectomy cavity after MRM; small series have shown decreased overall fluid output and time to drain removal.[17] As is the case for postoperative hematoma, ancillary techniques including tissue sealants, fibrin glue, or sclerotherapy have not been shown to be effective in reducing seroma formation.[11] Seromas presenting after drain removal can be managed with percutaneous aspiration and/or drain replacement. When infection is suspected, fluid cultures should be sent before starting empiric antibiotics for accurate source determination. Ultrasound evaluation can visualize loculations, which may lead to incomplete percutaneous drainage, to assure that all fluid has been removed at the time of aspiration or that drains are located within the appropriate space. Operative drainage should be pursued in the case of multiple incomplete aspirations, concern for continued infection, or abscess.

INFECTION

Surgical site infections (SSIs) after breast and axillary surgery range in presentation from superficial cellulitis overlying the area of surgical incisions to deep abscesses accumulating in the dead-space, or implant, or tissue flap infection. Two large studies found the rate of SSI to be 3.2% to 3.3% after mastectomy and 1.3% to 1.4% after BCS.[18,19] SSIs occur in up to 10% to 15% of patients after mastectomy with immediate reconstruction, particularly when implants are placed.[20] Rates of SSI are neither different when comparing between various tissue flap techniques nor different when comparing between implant-based techniques.[21,22] The rate of uncomplicated cellulitis treated conservatively with outpatient antibiotics is often not captured in most studies and may be underreported. Risk factors for SSI after breast and axillary surgery include obesity, current smoking, diabetes, chronic obstructive pulmonary disease, and a hospital length of stay shorter than 1 day. A history of radiation treatment of previous breast cancer treatment is not associated with a significant increase in the rate of SSI in patients who undergo completion mastectomy with reconstruction for a local recurrence.[23,24] The rate of SSI is mildly increased among patients who receive ALND compared with SLNB.[25] Patients should be counseled to watch for local symptoms including spreading warmth/erythema of the skin, fullness in their resection site, incisional discharge, or a change in their drain output, as well as systemic symptoms including fever.

Management of SSIs after breast and axillary surgery depends on the severity of the infection. Superficial SSIs, including uncomplicated cellulitis, can be treated with outpatient oral antibiotics. Persistent infection or physical examination findings indicating an underlying fluid collection should prompt an ultrasound evaluation with aspiration and culture of fluid to direct antibiotic choice. Abscesses with loculations or those otherwise resistant to aspiration require operative drainage through the original incision. Suspicion of infection in the setting of a tissue expander or implant should be investigated promptly with ultrasound or cross-sectional imaging. Any fluid around the implant must be drained and cultured. Implant salvage is possible with inpatient intravenous antibiotics; however, if the infection progresses to dehiscence or fails to resolve within 48 hours, then operative exploration is necessary.[26] The presence of a biofilm makes implant salvage beyond 48 hours unlikely.

Perioperative prophylactic antibiotics have been shown in multiple clinical trials to reduce the incidence of SSIs after breast and axillary surgery.[27,28] The American Society of Breast Surgeons recommends the use of antibiotic prophylaxis before any type of mastectomy.[29] Although antibiotic prophylaxis before BCS and excisional biopsies should be considered for patients with risk factors for infection, there is no clear benefit among patients at low or average risk for SSI.[30–32] First-line antimicrobials include cefazolin or ampicillin-sulbactam. For beta-lactam allergies, clindamycin or vancomycin is appropriate. Perioperative prophylaxis should not extend beyond 24 hours, even with drains or implants in place.[33,34] The antibiotic choice must be made in the context of the local antibiogram and surgeons should consult with their institution's infectious disease service and pharmacy team to determine the most appropriate choice for antibiotic coverage at their location.

SKIN FLAP NECROSIS

The objective of performing a mastectomy is complete removal of the breast parenchyma, which inevitably leaves the overlying skin with a thin layer of subcutaneous tissue from which it receives vascular and nutritional support. The skin flaps are at risk of ischemia from overdissection that may progress to necrosis, which jeopardizes cosmesis and reconstruction. Extreme cases may require surgical debridement and skin grafting. The reported rates of skin necrosis after mastectomy with or without reconstruction vary considerably (5%–30%) owing to heterogeneity in defining necrosis, especially in minor cases.[35,36] Risk factors for skin flap necrosis after mastectomy include older age, obesity, large breasts, hypertension, active smoking, sarcopenia, prior radiation treatment, incision placement, and tissue expander volume.[36–38] Skin-sparing mastectomies are not associated with an increased risk of skin necrosis compared with conventional flat mastectomy. However, nipple-sparing mastectomies have been shown to be at increased risk of skin necrosis due the longer skin flaps that are created.[39]

Ultimately, the risk of skin flap necrosis depends on the technique of the breast surgeon to balance oncologic resection of all breast tissue while sparing appropriate subcutaneous fat. The thickness of the subcutaneous layer between the dermis and the breast parenchyma is highly variable between patients and does not correlate with age or obesity.[40] The presence of an investing fascia superficialis between breast parenchyma and subcutaneous fat is not macroscopically visible in all patients. In cases where the familiar avascular plane of dissection is not apparent, it has been shown that skin flaps with a thickness 5 mm or lesser are at increased risk of postoperative necrosis.[41] Newer technologies have emerged to aid in the evaluation of skin flap perfusion. Fluorescent angiography with indocyanine green allows the plastic surgeon to monitor tissue perfusion in real time and has been shown to decrease the incidence of postoperative necrosis.[42] Hyperspectral imaging of tissue oxygenation is a contrast-free method that allows for perfusion assessment during and after the operation to identify at risk skin before becoming clinically apparent.[43] When areas of skin do become ischemic or threatened, initial conservative management includes removing volume from tissue expanders, avoiding external pressure, and maintaining patient euthermia. Topical nitroglycerin ointment and dimethyl sulfoxide may be applied and have been shown to reduce postoperative skin necrosis when applied as part of the surgical dressing in a randomized controlled trial.[44] In the absence of superimposed infection or implant exposure, full thickness necrosis can be observed and allowed to heal and contract by secondary intention. Hyperbaric oxygen treatment may reduce the surface area threatened by ischemia and allow some patients to avoid additional operation.[45] Excisional debridement and skin grafting is reserved for large areas of necrosis and those refractory to conservative measures.

NIPPLE AND NIPPLE–AREOLAR COMPLEX NECROSIS

Nipple-sparing mastectomy with immediate reconstruction is an oncologically acceptable technique in carefully selected patients. Dissection of the glandular tissue under the nipple–areolar complex (NAC) disrupts the complex of vasculature, smooth muscle, and sensory nerves leading to denervation and ischemia.[46] Full-thickness nipple necrosis has been reported in up to 5% of patients and partial thickness necrosis in up to 24%.[47] As with skin necrosis, the true rate of nipple necrosis may be under-reported.[48] Risk factors for nipple necrosis include smoking, large ptotic breasts (due to a longer distance from the NAC to intact perforators), periareolar incisions, and certain direct-to-implant techniques.[39,48] When a periareolar incision is necessary, an inferior incision results in less vascular disruption than a superior incision. Although radiation is associated with higher odds of skin necrosis, a meta-analysis found no association between a prior history of radiotherapy or receipt of adjuvant radiotherapy and nipple necrosis.[49]

Management of nipple necrosis follows the same principles as with skin flap necrosis. Most cases are treated conservatively allowing the necrotic tissue to demarcate and to salvage the cosmetic outcome later. Negative pressure wound vacuums may help increase blood flow to a threatened NAC.[50]

VENOUS THROMBOEMBOLISM

The risk of venous thromboembolism (VTE), defined as deep vein thrombosis (DVT) and/or pulmonary embolism (PE), is inherently increased in the perioperative period. Malignancy itself is a thrombophilic condition and many of the cytotoxic and hormonal therapies for breast cancer treatment further increase the risk. The incidence of VTE after breast and axillary surgery is lower compared with operations within the chest and abdomen; however, patients with breast cancer still represent 14% of all cancer-related VTE.[51,52] Previous studies report DVT occurring in 0.2% to 4% and PE in 0.12% to 2% after breast and axillary surgery.[53–55] VTE is more common after mastectomy compared with BCS, and immediate autologous reconstruction techniques are associated with the highest risk.[53,56] The addition of ALND to the operation may increase the risk of VTE.[57] Further risk factors include malignancy (as opposed to in situ lesions or benign pathologic condition), age younger than 65 years, obesity, general anesthesia, increased operating time, longer hospitalization (>3 days), and prior history of VTE.[53,55,58]

The American Society of Breast Surgeons has published consensus guidelines for the use of VTE prophylaxis for breast and axillary operations.[59] As with all major operations, early ambulation and sequential compression devices are recommended for all patients. The decision to use preoperative chemoprophylaxis is made on an individualized basis. For patients without prior risk factors for VTE, preoperative chemoprophylaxis is recommended before mastectomy with immediate reconstruction and for those under general anesthesia for less than 3 hours. For those undergoing less extensive operations, risk of VTE may be stratified with the Caprini score.[60] The use of preoperative chemoprophylaxis is not associated with a difference in bleeding complications after breast surgery.[61] For patients on chronic anticoagulation, the American College of Chest Physicians guidelines provide recommendations on the timing of anticoagulation interruption and the use of bridging anticoagulation.[62–64] In the context of these guidelines, breast and axillary surgery is normally considered low-risk for major bleeding. Certain individual factors may raise the risk among some patients receiving more extensive resections (including ALND) into the high-risk category. Postoperative chemoprophylaxis is commonly used after surgery for other solid tumors (eg, colorectal) and has been explored after surgery for breast cancer because most instances of VTE occur after discharge.[54] Perioperative and post-operative VTE prophylaxis regimens have shown inconsistent efficacy after surgery for breast cancer and some studies associate a higher bleeding risk.[54,65] The use of postoperative prophylaxis is not supported by any guidelines at this time.

NERVE INJURY AND POSTOPERATIVE PAIN

Injury to major motor and sensory nerves in the axilla during dissection and clearance of the nodal tissue may lead to pain, paresthesia, and motor deficits with variable resolution over time. The incidence of nerve injury is higher among patients who receive ALND compared with SLNB; however, SLNB still carries a risk.[66] In one prospective trial, more than 30% of patients who underwent SLNB for breast cancer reported sensory deficits 6 months after surgery.[67]

The long thoracic nerve courses from its cervical origin posterior to the brachial plexus and axillary vasculature to run along the chest wall and terminates in the lower border of the serratus anterior muscle. The long thoracic nerve provides motor innervation to the serratus anterior, where dysfunction leads to an unstable winged scapula that inhibits shoulder abduction and overhead arm movement.[68] Although complete transection of the long thoracic nerve is uncommon, the incidence of scapular asymmetry is reportedly greater than 50% immediately after ALND and most patients recover quickly.[69] A prospective series examining scapular winging after ALND for breast cancer using electromyography found 11.3% of patients had long thoracic injury at 1 month from surgery but only 2.3% had evidence at 12 months.[69] Patients with low BMI may be more likely to notice and report mild scapular asymmetry, which may not be apparent in patients with higher BMI.[70]

The thoracodorsal nerve originates from the posterior cord of the brachial plexus and courses along the posterior wall of the axilla to innervate the latissimus dorsi muscle. Injury to the thoracodorsal nerve results in weakness of shoulder adduction and internal rotation. The medial pectoral nerve arises from the medial cord of the brachial plexus and crosses the axilla to pierce the pectoralis minor muscle before continuing to innervate the pectoralis major. The lateral pectoral nerve originates from the lateral cord of the brachial plexus and crosses the axilla superiorly to the medial pectoral nerve where it terminates on the deep surface of the pectoralis major.[71] Injury to the lateral pectoral nerve during ALND results in limited shoulder mobility and atrophy of the pectoralis major and minor. Isolated injuries to the lateral pectoral nerve typically do not result in significant disability and do not affect the cosmetic outcome of subpectoral implant-based reconstructions.[72]

Injury to the intercostobrachial nerve during ALND is the most common iatrogenic nerve injury among all surgical procedures.[73] The intercostobrachial nerve originates from the lateral cutaneous branch of the second intercostal nerve, and its pathway across the axilla into the posteromedial border of the upper arm frequently varies.[74] The intercostobrachial nerve provides cutaneous sensation to the skin of the upper half of the posterior and medial arm. Injury to the nerve can cause paresthesia to this area and is associated with increased postoperative pain and reduced quality of life.[75] The nerve is susceptible to traction injury and neuroma formation on intact but injured nerves and may cause delayed symptoms that have been reported as high as 80% to 100% in patients after ALND but is significantly lower after SLNB.[75–77] Moderate-to-severe pain is seen is 50% of patients after ALND beyond the first postoperative week but many report improvement with time.[78,79]

Nerve injury is primarily avoided with technical diligence and awareness of potential anatomic variations. Many surgeons avoid paralysis during MRM or ALND. For patients with persistent pain after mastectomy or axillary surgery, conservative treatment begins with physical and cognitive therapy as well as medications such as antidepressants and neuromodulators.[80] Targeted interventions including nerve blocks, radiofrequency neurolysis, and steroid injections have been shown to provide durable relief and improve quality of life.[81] Intraoperative nerve monitoring during MRM is currently being explored to determine efficacy.[82] Operative approaches, including nerve transfers, have been described for select patients with chronic pain secondary to intercostobrachial injury or palsy related to long thoracic injury.[83] Postmastectomy pain syndrome is a form of chronic neuropathic pain caused by direct injury in the operating room, from subsequent scar tissue, or from radiation therapy. Postmastectomy pain syndrome is further discussed in the "Quality of Life" article.

BRACHIAL PLEXOPATHY

Breast and axillary operations require the patient to lie supine with the ipsilateral arm extended. Malposition of the patient or inattentive repositioning of the arm during the operation can lead to overstretch and subsequent injury to the brachial plexus. Postoperative brachial plexopathies usually present as painless weakness along the distribution of the upper cords: proximally the deltoid and biceps may be weak while the distal hand may be relatively spared. Brachial plexopathy after breast and axillary surgery is uncommon and can be avoided largely with careful padding and ensuring the arm position is abducted no more than 90°.[84,85] Brachial plexopathy can also occur secondary to direct extension of the breast tumor and can also occur in 1% to 2% of patients after radiation treatment.[86,87] The majority of operative and radiation-induced cases of brachial plexopathy is due to demyelination of intact nerves and will resolve with conservative management such as occupational or physical therapy.

LONG-TERM COMPLICATIONS
Lymphedema

Oncologic clearance of the axillary lymph nodes can lead to clinically significant lymphedema. Interstitial fluid from the skin and subcutaneous tissue of the breast and arm is collected by superficial lymphatic capillaries, which drain into the deep lymphatics and eventually into the axillary lymph nodes.[88] Lymph drains first into 1 to 2 dominant sentinel nodes in the lateral axilla before distributing into 20 to 40 regional axillary nodes. Lymphedema develops gradually with mild swelling and asymptomatic volume increase of the affected upper arm. This swelling can progress to the ipsilateral chest and distal arm and will initially resolve with arm elevation and night rest. Eventually the swelling and edema may become refractory to positioning and significant disability can develop as the arm becomes more encumbered. In later stages, the fluid edema progresses to fat deposition and tissue fibrosis.[89]

More than 20% of patients will experience symptomatic lymphedema after an extensive ALND.[90–92] The incidence of lymphedema after SLNB is still 3% to 8%

despite the comparatively limited dissection.[93,94] Although advances in axillary surgery have allowed for less aggressive treatments while maintaining disease control, surgeons and radiation oncologists may still be overtreating the axilla resulting in increased rates of lymphedema.[95–100] Patients should be educated on the risk of lymphedema development before therapy and survey data has found variability in the risk of lymphedema quoted by surgeons and radiation oncologists when discussing lymphedema.[90] The onset of lymphedema after breast and axillary surgery is typically delayed, with symptoms beginning approximately 12 to 30 months after surgery; ALND is associated with early onset (<12 months) lymphedema while delayed onset is usually seen after regional radiotherapy.[93] Early asymptomatic increases in arm volume within 3 months of surgery may predict eventual lymphedema development.[101] Risk factors for lymphedema development include ALND, mastectomy (compared with BCS), greater number of nodes harvested (after both ALND and SLNB), age older than 65 years, obesity, postoperative cellulitis, regional lymph node radiation, and prolonged adjuvant chemotherapy (particularly taxanes).[92,102,103] Secondary ALND after positive SLNB does not increase the risk of lymphedema compared with primary ALND.[104]

Early recognition and application of conservative treatments are key in minimizing the morbidity associated with lymphedema. Risk assessment tools exist to stratify the risk profile of individual patients.[102] Patients should be counseled to monitor the ipsilateral limb. Although avoidance of venipuncture and blood pressure cuffs in the ipsilateral limb is commonly recommended, there is no data supporting their association with increased risk of lymphedema development, and they are not contraindicated in patients without lymphedema.[105] Surveillance programs that include limb circumference measurements at defined intervals have been shown to reduce and maintain limb volume and prevent lymphedema progression.[106] Conservative strategies are frequently effective in treating early stage lymphedema and patients should be referred to a certified lymphedema therapist when available. Initial management aims to reduce limb volume and consists of supervised manual lymphatic drainage and multiple layer compression bandaging over several weeks.[107] Once volume and symptom reduction is achieved, the maintenance phase transitions to self-drainage and compression garments.[93] Exercise (aerobic and resistance-based), skin care, and patient education are important during all phases.[108] Patients with refractory symptoms without significant tissue changes may be candidates for operative strategies that attempt to restore drainage of the accumulated lymph. Vascularized lymph node transplants and lymphovenous bypass are operations that have been demonstrated to effectively reduce limb volume and symptoms in select patients.[109] Once fatty and fibrous deposition occurs in late stages, operative strategies shift toward reducing fibrofatty tissue in the form of direct excision and liposuction. Selective sparing of key drainage routes during ALND using the axillary reverse mapping technique has shown promising initial results and further study and physician education aim to elucidate its ability to reduce rates of lymphedema.[110,111]

AXILLARY WEB SYNDROME

Axillary web syndrome (also known as cording) is a common condition after breast and axillary surgery wherein subcutaneous cord-like scarring develops in the axilla and may extend down the arm and chest wall. The cause of these cords, which can be painful and limit shoulder movement, is thought to be related to lymphatic injury.[112] Axillary webbing of any severity occurs in up to 50% of patients and often presents within the first 2 months after surgery although cords may also develop and relapse years afterward.[113] The incidence is highest after ALND but is also seen after SLNB. Risk factors include lower BMI, younger age, greater number of lymph nodes removed, and adjuvant chemotherapy and radiation.[113,114] It is imperative that surgeons can clinically distinguish cording of the chest wall from Mondor disease of the breast. Cording in the axilla is sometimes associated with nodules, which may mimic metastasis and should be promptly evaluated. Treatment of axillary web syndrome is primarily physiotherapy with gentle manual cord manipulating, stretching, and myofascial release.[115]

SECONDARY ANGIOSARCOMA

Radiation-associated angiosarcoma of the breast is a rare but devastating sequela of a commonly delivered treatment of breast cancer. Although the receipt of radiation to the breast, chest, and axilla raises the risk of angiosarcoma 26-fold, the incidence remains less than 0.1%.[116] Therefore, for most patients, the benefits of disease control with postoperative radiation far outweigh the risk of angiosarcoma. However, patients with certain heritable mutation syndromes who are at higher risk for radiation-induced tumors (eg, retinoblastoma) should be counseled regarding this risk of radiation and tailor the patient's treatment plan accordingly.[117] Radiation-associated angiosarcomas occur at a median 10 years after breast radiation, although cases have been reported as early as 14 months and as late as 54 years.[118–120] Cases usually present as skin changes that can be confused for infection, moderate or severe radiation skin changes, or recurrence of the primary breast cancer and any suspicion should prompt biopsy to differentiate the diagnosis. Treatment involves wide local excision and often chemotherapy given the metastatic propensity of angiosarcoma. Short-course hyperfractionated reirradiation in selected patients who previously received BCS and radiation is shown to improve local disease control and is well tolerated.[121]

Lymphangiosarcoma in the setting of longstanding lymphedema of the extremity (Stewart-Treves syndrome) is a very rare entity with less than 1000 cases reported in the literature, and the majority is associated with MRM.[122] This cutaneous malignancy progresses slowly and subtly, eventually leading to purpuric macules and extensive masses with a high rate of metastasis.[123] Radical resection is required while chemotherapy and radiation are minimally effective.

DELAYED BREAST RECONSTRUCTION-RELATED COMPLICATIONS

Although the various plastic reconstructive techniques for breast surgery are associated with their own specific complications to be comanaged by the patient and the plastic surgeon, certain delayed complications may present as a remote change in the shape of the breast and prompt presentation to the oncologic surgeon. Capsular contracture may occur after implant-based reconstruction where the normally thin fibrous capsule around the implant grows to become firm and calcified. This contracture can lead to pain and distortion of the breast.[124] Capsular contracture may develop years after implant placement and the cumulative risk increases the longer it is in place.[5] Radiation therapy may increase the risk of capsular contracture and submuscular and subfascial implants are associated with decreased risk.[125] Diagnosis and grading of the contracture is typically made clinically with physical examination, although concern for alternate diagnoses should trigger appropriate imaging. Correction requires the removal of the implant along with capsulectomy or capsulotomy. Incidentally discovered recurrence or second primary breast cancer is rare but has been reported, and excised capsules should be sent for pathologic evaluation.[126]

Breast implant-associated anaplastic large cell lymphoma (ALCL) is a rare T-cell lymphoma originating specifically around textured implants.[127] More than 500 cases have been reported since 2012 along with more than 30 deaths.[128] Implant associated ALCL typically presents as a malignant effusion around the implant causing swelling, asymmetry, and pain. The median time to occurrence is 11 years after implant surgery. ALCL should be suspected if a fluid collection develops more than 1 year after implant surgery. Workup of this condition requires ultrasound evaluation and aspiration of any fluid surrounding the implant to rule out infectious cause, and fluid should be sent for cytology. Fluid analysis yields positive staining for CD30 and negative for anaplastic lymphoma kinase expression in implant-associated ALCL.[129] For patients with localized disease, complete excision of the implant, capsule, and any associated masses completes treatment. Patients with unresectable chest wall invasion or regional lymphadenopathy require adjuvant chemotherapy with lymphoma regimens.

PSYCHOSOCIAL IMPACTS OF BREAST SURGERY

Changes in physical appearance and function related to surgery are a common source of psychological distress for patients with breast cancer. Aside from the morbidity related to postoperative complications described above, operations of the breast can lead to measurable changes in quality of life, self-esteem and body image, sexual function and satisfaction, and future perspective.[130,131] Factors associated with decreased psychosocial well-being after surgery include younger age at diagnosis, more extensive surgery, lower income, history of depression, and a lack of social support.[132–134] Compared with mastectomy, BCS is associated with higher self-reported body image and sexual function.[135,136] Nonetheless, many patients who undergo BCS experience breast asymmetry (sometimes delayed due to radiation changes) and changes to nipple sensation and function, and patients should be counseled accordingly.[137] Patients who receive prophylactic mastectomy report relatively higher ratings of satisfaction and quality of life, and low rates of decisional regret.[138,139] Discussing these potential outcomes with patients can help set expectations and facilitate informed treatment decisions.

For the majority of patients who receive an operation for breast cancer, self-evaluations of psychological and emotional well-being will improve with time and often return to preoperative levels.[132,137] Cognitive-behavioral and psychoeducational therapies are effective and becoming more accessible as psychologic support is increasingly recognized as an important component of the multidisciplinary oncology team.[140] There is a growing library of information technology to empower health literacy that is shown to improve quality of life for patients with breast cancer.[140] Early involvement of a breast reconstruction surgeon informs patients of an expanding array of techniques aimed at improving postoperative satisfaction. Nipple-sparing mastectomy, when feasible, is associated with improved body image and sexual well-being compared with other types of mastectomy.[141,142] Newer techniques that aim to reinnervate the NAC after nipple-sparing mastectomy in order to improve sensation are under investigation.[143]

CLINICS CARE POINTS

- The incidence of postoperative hematoma requiring operative evacuation after breast surgery is estimated at less than 2%. Expanding hematoma, jeopardized skin flaps, or hemodynamic instability require early recognition and return to the operating room.

- Seroma formation is reported in up to 50% of patients after breast and axillary surgery. Large or symptomatic seromas presenting after drain removal can be managed with percutaneous aspiration and/or drain replacement.

- The rate of surgical site infection is 1.3% to 1.4% after lumpectomy and 3.2% to3.3% after mastectomy, although certain reconstructive techniques are associated with rates of 10% to 15%. Preoperative antibiotic prophylaxis is recommended for all types of mastectomy. For average risk patients, preoperative antibiotics show no benefit for lumpectomy or excisional biopsy.

- Venous thromboembolism occurs in up to 4% of patients after breast and axillary surgery and is more common after mastectomy than lumpectomy especially in the setting of immediate autologous reconstruction. For patients without risk factors, preoperative chemoprophylaxis is recommended before mastectomy with immediate reconstruction, for general anesthesia less than 3 hours, and for those meeting criteria based on a risk stratification assessment.

- Injury to major motor and sensory nerves in the axilla may lead to pain, paresthesia, and motor deficits with variable resolution over time. Nerve injury is primarily avoided with technical diligence and awareness of potential anatomic variations. Many surgeons avoid paralysis during formal axillary dissection.

DISCLOSURE

No relevant disclosures.

REFERENCES

1. Bernat JL, Peterson LM. Patient-Centered Informed Consent in Surgical Practice. Arch Surg 2006;141(1):86–92.
2. Browne JP, Jeevan R, Gulliver-Clarke C, et al. The association between complications and quality of life after mastectomy and breast reconstruction for breast cancer. Cancer 2017;123(18):3460–7.
3. Barton MB, West CN, Liu ILA, et al. Complications following bilateral prophylactic mastectomy. J Natl Cancer Inst Monogr 2005;35:61–6.
4. Seth AK, Hirsch EM, Kim JYS, et al. Hematoma after mastectomy with immediate reconstruction: an analysis of risk factors in 883 patients. Ann Plast Surg 2013;71(1):20–3.
5. Handel N, Cordray T, Gutierrez J, et al. A long-term study of outcomes, complications, and patient satisfaction with breast implants. Plast Reconstr Surg 2006; 117(3):757–67.
6. Almasarweh S, Sudah M, Joukainen S, et al. The Feasibility of Ultrasound-guided Vacuum-assisted Evacuation of Large Breast Hematomas. Radiol Oncol 2020;54(3):311.
7. O'Hea BJ, Ho MN, Petrek JA. External compression dressing versus standard dressing after axillary lymphadenectomy. Am J Surg 1999;177(6):450–3.
8. Bullocks J, Basu CB, Hsu P, et al. Prevention of Hematomas and Seromas. Semin Plast Surg 2006;20(4):233.
9. Srivastava V, Basu S, Shukla VK. Seroma Formation after Breast Cancer Surgery: What We Have Learned in the Last Two Decades. J Breast Cancer 2012;15(4):373.
10. Montalto E, Mangraviti S, Costa G, et al. Seroma fluid subsequent to axillary lymph node dissection for breast cancer derives from an accumulation of afferent lymph. Immunol Lett 2010;131(1):67–72.

11. Van Bemmel AJM, Van De Velde CJH, Schmitz RF, et al. Prevention of seroma formation after axillary dissection in breast cancer: a systematic review. Eur J Surg Oncol 2011;37(10):829–35.

12. Unger J, Rutkowski R, Kohlmann T, et al. Potential risk factors influencing the formation of postoperative seroma after breast surgery - a prospective study. Anticancer Res 2021;41(2):859–67.

13. Shamley DR, Barker K, Simonite V, et al. Delayed versus immediate exercises following surgery for breast cancer: a systematic review. Breast Cancer Res Treat 2005;90(3):263–71.

14. de Oliveira LL, de Aguiar SS, Bender PFM, et al. Men have a higher incidence of seroma after breast cancer surgery. Asian Pac J Cancer Prev 2017;18(5):1423–7.

15. He XD, Guo ZH, Tian JH, et al. Whether drainage should be used after surgery for breast cancer? A systematic review of randomized controlled trials. Med Oncol 2011;28(SUPPL. 1):22–30.

16. Shima H, Kutomi G, Sato K, et al. An optimal timing for removing a drain after breast surgery: a systematic review and meta-analysis. J Surg Res 2021;267:267–73.

17. Faisal M, Abu-Elela ST, Mostafa W, et al. Efficacy of axillary exclusion on seroma formation after modified radical mastectomy. World J Surg Oncol 2016;14(1):1–5.

18. De Blacam C, Ogunleye AA, Momoh AO, et al. High body mass index and smoking predict morbidity in breast cancer surgery: a multivariate analysis of 26,988 patients from the national surgical quality improvement program database. Ann Surg 2012;255(3):551–5.

19. Pastoriza J, McNelis J, Parsikia A, et al. Predictive factors for surgical site infections in patients undergoing surgery for breast carcinoma. Am Surg 2021;87(1):68–76.

20. McCullough MC, Chu CK, Duggal CS, et al. Antibiotic prophylaxis and resistance in surgical site infection after immediate tissue expander reconstruction of the breast. Ann Plast Surg 2016;77(5):501–5.

21. Chen CM, Halvorson EG, Disa JJ, et al. Immediate postoperative complications in DIEP versus free/muscle-sparing TRAM flaps. Plast Reconstr Surg 2007;120(6):1477–82.

22. Sbitany H, Serletti JM. Acellular dermis-assisted prosthetic breast reconstruction: a systematic and critical review of efficacy and associated morbidity. Plast Reconstr Surg 2011;128(6):1162–9.

23. Chang DW, Barnea Y, Robb GL. Effects of an autologous flap combined with an implant for breast reconstruction: an evaluation of 1000 consecutive reconstructions of previously irradiated breasts. Plast Reconstr Surg 2008;122(2):356–62.

24. Thiruchelvam PTR, Leff DR, Godden AR, et al. Primary radiotherapy and deep inferior epigastric perforator flap reconstruction for patients with breast cancer (PRADA): a multicentre, prospective, non-randomised, feasibility study. Lancet Oncol 2022;23(5):682–90.

25. Degnim AC, Throckmorton AD, Boostrom SY, et al. Surgical site infection (SSI) after breast surgery: impact of 2010 CDC Reporting Guidelines. Ann Surg Oncol 2012;19(13):4099.

26. Viola GM, Selber JC, Crosby M, et al. Salvaging the infected breast tissue expander: a standardized multidisciplinary approach. Plast Reconstr Surg Glob Open 2016;4(6). https://doi.org/10.1097/GOX.0000000000000676.

27. Gallagher M, Jones DJ, Bell-Syer SV. Prophylactic antibiotics to prevent surgical site infection after breast cancer surgery. Cochrane Database Syst Rev 2019; 9(9). https://doi.org/10.1002/14651858.CD005360.PUB5.

28. Bold RJ, Mansfield PF, Berger DH, et al. Prospective, randomized, double-blind study of prophylactic antibiotics in axillary lymph node dissection. Am J Surg 1998;176(3):239–43.

29. American Society of Breast Surgeons T. Consensus Guideline on Preoperative Antibiotics and Surgical Site Infection in Breast Surgery. Available from: https://www.breastsurgeons.org/docs/statements/Consensus-Guideline-on-Preoperative-Antibiotics-and-Surgical-Site-Infection-in-Breast-Surgery.pdf.

30. Giguère GB, Poirier B, Provencher L, et al. Do preoperative prophylactic antibiotics reduce surgical site infection following wire-localized lumpectomy? A single-blind randomized clinical trial. Ann Surg Oncol 2022;29(4):2202–8.

31. Petersen L, Carlson K, Kopkash K, et al. Preoperative antibiotics do not reduce postoperative infections following needle-localized lumpectomy. Breast J 2017; 23(1):49–51.

32. Kong A, Tartter PI, Zappetti D. The Significance of Risk Factors for Infection in Patients Undergoing Lumpectomy and Axillary Dissection. Breast J 1997; 3(2):81–4.

33. Alderman A, Gutowski K, Ahuja A, et al. ASPS clinical practice guideline summary on breast reconstruction with expanders and implants. Plast Reconstr Surg 2014;134(4):648e–55e.

34. Bağhaki S, Soybir GR, Soran A. Guideline for antimicrobial prophylaxis in breast surgery. J Breast Heal 2014;10(2):79.

35. Robertson SA, Jeevaratnam JA, Agrawal A, et al. Mastectomy skin flap necrosis: challenges and solutions. Breast Cancer (Dove Med Press) 2017. https://doi.org/10.2147/BCTT.S81712.

36. Matsen CB, Mehrara B, Eaton A, et al. Skin flap necrosis after mastectomy with reconstruction: a prospective study. Ann Surg Oncol 2016;23(1):257–64.

37. Yabe S, Nakagawa T, Oda G, et al. Association between skin flap necrosis and sarcopenia in patients who underwent total mastectomy. Asian J Surg 2021; 44(2):465–70.

38. Chun YS, Verma K, Rosen H, et al. Use of tumescent mastectomy technique as a risk factor for native breast skin flap necrosis following immediate breast reconstruction. Am J Surg 2011;201(2):160–5.

39. Galimberti V, Vicini E, Corso G, et al. Nipple-sparing and skin-sparing mastectomy: Review of aims, oncological safety and contraindications. The Breast 2017;34:S82–4.

40. Robertson SA, Rusby JE, Cutress RI. Determinants of optimal mastectomy skin flap thickness. Br J Surg 2014;101(8):899–911.

41. Wiberg R, Andersson MN, Svensson J, et al. Prophylactic mastectomy: postoperative skin flap thickness evaluated by MRT, ultrasound and clinical examination. Ann Surg Oncol 2020;27(7):2221–8.

42. Ogawa A, Nakagawa T, Oda G, et al. Study of the protocol used to evaluate skin-flap perfusion in mastectomy based on the characteristics of indocyanine green. Photodiagnosis Photodyn Ther 2021;35:102401, 1.

43. Pruimboom T, Lindelauf AAMA, Felli E, et al. Perioperative hyperspectral imaging to assess mastectomy skin flap and DIEP flap perfusion in immediate autologous breast reconstruction: a pilot study. Diagnostics (Basel, Switzerland) 2022;12(1). https://doi.org/10.3390/DIAGNOSTICS12010184.

44. Gdalevitch P, Van Laeken N, Bahng S, et al. Effects of nitroglycerin ointment on mastectomy flap necrosis in immediate breast reconstruction: a randomized controlled trial. Plast Reconstr Surg 2015;135(6):1530–9.

45. Spruijt NE, Hoekstra LT, Wilmink J, et al. Hyperbaric oxygen treatment for mastectomy flap ischaemia: a case series of 50 breasts. Diving Hyperb Med 2021; 51(1):2.

46. Nicholson BT, Harvey JA, Cohen MA. Nipple-areolar complex: normal anatomy and benign and malignant processes. Radiographics 2009;29(2):509–23.

47. Mallon P, Feron JG, Couturaud B, et al. The role of nipple-sparing mastectomy in breast cancer: a comprehensive review of the literature. Plast Reconstr Surg 2013;131(5):969–84.

48. Ahn SJ, Woo TY, Lee DW, et al. Nipple-areolar complex ischemia and necrosis in nipple-sparing mastectomy. Eur J Surg Oncol 2018;44(8):1170–6.

49. Zheng Y, Zhong M, Ni C, et al. Radiotherapy and nipple–areolar complex necrosis after nipple-sparing mastectomy: a systematic review and meta-analysis. Radiol Med 2017;122(3):171–8.

50. Chicco M, Huang TCT, Cheng HT. Negative-pressure wound therapy in the prevention and management of complications from prosthetic breast reconstruction: a systematic review and meta-analysis. Ann Plast Surg 2021;87(4):478–83.

51. De Martino RR, Goodney PP, Spangler EL, et al. Variation in thromboembolic complications among patients undergoing commonly performed cancer operations. J Vasc Surg 2012;55(4):1035–40.e4.

52. Tafur A, Fuentes H, Caprini J, et al. Predictors of early mortality in cancer-associated thrombosis: analysis of the RIETE database. TH Open Companion J Thromb Haemost 2018;2(2):e158–66.

53. Castaldi M, George G, Stoller C, et al. Independent predictors of venous thromboembolism in patients undergoing reconstructive breast cancer surgery. Plast Surg (Oakville, Ont) 2021;29(3):160–8.

54. Rochlin DH, Sheckter CC, Pannucci C, et al. Venous thromboembolism following microsurgical breast reconstruction: a longitudinal analysis of 12,778 patients. Plast Reconstr Surg 2020;146(3):465–73.

55. Londero AP, Bertozzi S, Cedolini C, et al. Incidence and risk factors for venous thromboembolism in female patients undergoing breast surgery. Cancers (Basel) 2022;14(4). https://doi.org/10.3390/CANCERS14040988/S1.

56. Konoeda H, Yamaki T, Hamahata A, et al. Incidence of deep vein thrombosis in patients undergoing breast reconstruction with autologous tissue transfer. Phlebology 2017;32(4):282–8.

57. Lovely JK, Nehring SA, Boughey JC, et al. Balancing venous thromboembolism and hematoma after breast surgery. Ann Surg Oncol 2012;19(10):3230–5.

58. Nwaogu I, Yan Y, Margenthaler JA, et al. Venous thromboembolism after breast reconstruction in patients undergoing breast surgery: an american college of surgeons NSQIP analysis. J Am Coll Surg 2015;220(5):886–93.

59. American Society of Breast Surgeons T. Consensus Guideline on Venous Thromboembolism (VTE) Prophylaxis for Patients Undergoing Breast Operations. Available from: https://www.breastsurgeons.org/docs/statements/Consensus-Guideline-on-Venous-Thromboembolism-VTE-Prophylaxis-for-Patients-Undergoing-Breast-Operations.pdf.

60. Pannucci CJ, Swistun L, MacDonald JK, et al. Individualized venous thromboembolism risk stratification using the 2005 caprini score to identify the benefits and harms of chemoprophylaxis in surgical patients: a meta-analysis. Ann Surg 2017;265(6):1094–103.

61. Keith JN, Chong TW, Davar D, et al. The timing of preoperative prophylactic low-molecular-weight heparin administration in breast reconstruction. Plast Reconstr Surg 2013;132(2):279–84.

62. Stevens SM, Woller SC, Baumann Kreuziger L, et al. Executive summary: antithrombotic therapy for VTE disease: second update of the CHEST guideline and expert panel report. Chest 2021;160(6):2247–59.

63. Kearon C, Akl EA, Ornelas J, et al. Antithrombotic therapy for VTE disease: CHEST guideline and expert panel report. Chest 2016;149(2):315–52.

64. Douketis JD, Spyropoulos AC, Spencer FA, et al. Perioperative management of antithrombotic therapy: antithrombotic therapy and prevention of thrombosis, 9th ed: american college of chest physicians evidence-based clinical practice guidelines. Chest 2012;141(2):e326S–50S.

65. Klifto KM, Gurno CF, Major M, et al. Pre-, intra-, and/or postoperative arterial and venous thromboembolism prophylaxis for breast surgery: Systematic review and meta-analysis. J Plast Reconstr Aesthet Surg 2020;73(1):1–18.

66. Lucci A, McCall LM, Beitsch PD, et al. Surgical complications associated with sentinel lymph node dissection (SLND) plus axillary lymph node dissection compared with SLND alone in the American College of Surgeons Oncology Group trial Z0011. J Clin Oncol 2007;25(24):3657–63.

67. Kozak D, Głowacka-Mrotek I, Nowikiewicz T, et al. Analysis of undesirable sequelae of sentinel node surgery in breast cancer patients – a prospective cohort study. Pathol Oncol Res 2018;24(4):891.

68. Meininger AK, Figuerres BF, Goldberg BA. Scapular winging: an update. J Am Acad Orthop Surg 2011;19(8):453–62.

69. Flávia De Oliveira J, Bezerra T, Carolina A, et al. Incidence and risk factors of winged scapula after axillary lymph node dissection in breast cancer surgery. Appl Cancer Res 2009;29(2):69–73.

70. Adriaenssens N, De Ridder M, Lievens P, et al. Scapula alata in early breast cancer patients enrolled in a randomized clinical trial of post-surgery short-course image-guided radiotherapy. World J Surg Oncol 2012;10. https://doi.org/10.1186/1477-7819-10-86.

71. Macchi V, Tiengo C, Porzionato A, et al. Medial and lateral pectoral nerves: course and branches. Clin Anat 2007;20(2):157–62.

72. Prakash KG, Saniya K. Anatomical study of pectoral nerves and its implications in surgery. J Clin Diagn Res 2014;8(7). https://doi.org/10.7860/JCDR/2014/8631.4545.

73. Sharp E, Roberts M, Żurada-Zielińska A, et al. The most commonly injured nerves at surgery: a comprehensive review. Clin Anat 2021;34(2):244–62.

74. Zhu JJ, Liu XF, Zhang PL, et al. Anatomical information for intercostobrachial nerve preservation in axillary lymph node dissection for breast cancer. Genet Mol Res 2014;13(4):9315–23.

75. Henry BM, Graves MJ, Pękala JR, et al. Origin, Branching, and Communications of the Intercostobrachial Nerve: a Meta-Analysis with Implications for Mastectomy and Axillary Lymph Node Dissection in Breast Cancer. Cureus 2017; 9(3). https://doi.org/10.7759/CUREUS.1101.

76. Vadivelu N, Schreck M, Lopez J, et al. Pain after mastectomy and breast reconstruction. Am Surg 2008;74(4):285–96.

77. Mansel RE, Fallowfield L, Kissin M, et al. Randomized multicenter trial of sentinel node biopsy versus standard axillary treatment in operable breast cancer: the ALMANAC Trial. J Natl Cancer Inst 2006;98(9):599–609.

78. Andersen KG, Aasvang EK, Kroman N, et al. Intercostobrachial nerve handling and pain after axillary lymph node dissection for breast cancer. Acta Anaesthesiol Scand 2014;58(10):1240–8.

79. Gärtner R, Jensen MB, Nielsen J, et al. Prevalence of and factors associated with persistent pain following breast cancer surgery. JAMA 2009;302(18): 1985–92.

80. Chappell AG, Yuksel S, Sasson DC, et al. Post-mastectomy pain syndrome: an up-to-date review of treatment outcomes. JPRAS Open 2021;30:97–109.

81. Yang A, Nadav D, Legler A, et al. An interventional pain algorithm for the treatment of postmastectomy pain syndrome: a single-center retrospective review. Pain Med 2021;22(3):677–86.

82. Tokgöz S, Karaca Umay E, Yilmaz KB, et al. Role of intraoperative nerve monitoring in postoperative muscle and nerve function of patients undergoing modified radical mastectomy. J Investig Surg 2021;34(7):703–10.

83. Noland SS, Krauss EM, Felder JM, et al. Surgical and clinical decision making in isolated long thoracic nerve palsy. Hand (N Y) 2018;13(6):689.

84. Warner MA, Blitt CD, Butterworth JF, et al. Practice advisory for the prevention of perioperative peripheral neuropathies: a report by the American Society of Anesthesiologists Task Force on Prevention of Perioperative Peripheral Neuropathies. Anesthesiology 2000;92(4):1168–82.

85. Zhang J, Moore AE, Stringer MD, et al. Iatrogenic upper limb nerve injuries: a systematic review. ANZ J Surg 2011;81(4):227–36.

86. Rudra S, Roy A, Brenneman R, et al. Radiation-Induced Brachial Plexopathy in Patients With Breast Cancer Treated With Comprehensive Adjuvant Radiation Therapy. Adv Radiat Oncol 2020;6(1). https://doi.org/10.1016/J.ADRO.2020. 10.015.

87. Jack MM, Smith BW, Capek S, et al. The spectrum of brachial plexopathy from perineural spread of breast cancer. J Neurosurg 2022;1–10. https://doi.org/10. 3171/2021.12.JNS211882.

88. Suami H, Scaglioni MF. Lymphedema Management: Anatomy of the Lymphatic System and the Lymphosome Concept with Reference to Lymphedema. Semin Plast Surg 2018;32(1):5.

89. Campisi CC, Molinari L, Campisi CS, et al. Surgical research, staging-guided technical procedures and long-term clinical outcomes for the treatment of peripheral lymphedema: the Genoa Protocol. J Surg Surg Res 2020;6(1):041–50.

90. Cortina CS, Yen TWF, Bergom C, et al. Breast cancer-related lymphedema rates after modern axillary treatments: How accurate are our estimates? Surgery 2022;171(3):682–6.

91. Naoum GE, Roberts S, Brunelle CL, et al. Quantifying the impact of axillary surgery and nodal irradiation on breast cancer-related lymphedema and local tumor control: Long-term results from a prospective screening trial. J Clin Oncol 2020;38(29):3430–8.

92. DiSipio T, Rye S, Newman B, et al. Incidence of unilateral arm lymphoedema after breast cancer: a systematic review and meta-analysis. Lancet Oncol 2013; 14(6):500–15.

93. McLaughlin SA, Brunelle CL, Taghian A. Breast cancer–related lymphedema: risk factors, screening, management, and the impact of locoregional treatment. J Clin Oncol 2020;38(20):2341.

94. Galimberti V, Cole BF, Zurrida S, et al. Axillary dissection versus no axillary dissection in patients with sentinel-node micrometastases (IBCSG 23-01): a phase 3 randomised controlled trial. Lancet Oncol 2013;14(4):297–305.

95. Cortina CS, Kong AL. ASO author reflections: the evolving multidisciplinary management of the axilla in mastectomy patients. Ann Surg Oncol 2021;1–2. https://doi.org/10.1245/S10434-021-10585-Y.

96. Cortina CS, Bergom C, Craft MA, et al. A national survey of breast surgeons and radiation oncologists on contemporary axillary management in mastectomy patients. Ann Surg Oncol 2021;28(10):5568–79.

97. Cortina CS, Kong AL. Comment on "women could avoid axillary lymph node dissection by choosing breast-conserving therapy instead of mastectomy. Ann Surg Oncol 2021;28(3):772–3.

98. Morrow M, Jagsi R, Chandler M, et al. Surgeon attitudes toward the omission of axillary dissection in early breast cancer. JAMA Oncol 2018;4(11):1511–6.

99. Donker M, van Tienhoven G, Straver ME, et al. Radiotherapy or surgery of the axilla after a positive sentinel node in breast cancer (EORTC 10981-22023 AMAROS): a randomised, multicentre, open-label, phase 3 non-inferiority trial. Lancet Oncol 2014;15(12):1303–10.

100. Giuliano AE, Ballman KV, McCall L, et al. Effect of axillary dissection vs no axillary dissection on 10-year overall survival among women with invasive breast cancer and sentinel node metastasis: the ACOSOG Z0011 (Alliance) randomized clinical trial. JAMA 2017;318(10):918–26.

101. McDuff SGR, Mina AI, Brunelle CL, et al. Timing of lymphedema after treatment for breast cancer: when are patients most at risk? Int J Radiat Oncol 2019; 103(1):62–70.

102. Basta MN, Wu LC, Kanchwala SK, et al. Reliable prediction of postmastectomy lymphedema: the risk assessment tool evaluating lymphedema. Am J Surg 2017;213(6):1125–33.e1.

103. Armer JM, Ballman KV, McCall L, et al. Factors associated with lymphedema in women with node-positive breast cancer treated with neoadjuvant chemotherapy and axillary dissection. JAMA Surg 2019;154(9):800–9.

104. Husted Madsen A, Haugaard K, Soerensen J, et al. Arm morbidity following sentinel lymph node biopsy or axillary lymph node dissection: a study from the Danish Breast Cancer Cooperative Group. Breast 2008;17(2):138–47.

105. McLaughlin SA, DeSnyder SM, Klimberg S, et al. Considerations for clinicians in the diagnosis, prevention, and treatment of breast cancer-related lymphedema, recommendations from an expert panel: part 2: preventive and therapeutic options. Ann Surg Oncol 2017;24(10):2827–35.

106. Stout Gergich NL, Pfalzer LA, McGarvey C, et al. Preoperative assessment enables the early diagnosis and successful treatment of lymphedema. Cancer 2008;112(12):2809–19.

107. McNeely ML, Magee DJ, Lees AW, et al. The addition of manual lymph drainage to compression therapy for breast cancer related lymphedema: a randomized controlled trial. Breast Cancer Res Treat 2004;86(2):95–106.

108. Schmitz KH, Ahmed RL, Troxel A, et al. Weight lifting in women with breast-cancer-related lymphedema. N Engl J Med 2009;361(7):664–73.

109. Schaverien MV, Asaad M, Selber JC, et al. Outcomes of vascularized lymph node transplantation for treatment of lymphedema. J Am Coll Surg 2021; 232(6):982–94.

110. Tummel E, Ochoa D, Korourian S, et al. Does axillary reverse mapping prevent lymphedema after lymphadenectomy? Ann Surg 2017;265(5):987–92.

111. DeSnyder SM, Yi M, Boccardo F, et al. American society of breast surgeons' practice patterns for patients at risk and affected by breast cancer-related lymphedema. Ann Surg Oncol 2021;28(10):5742–51.

112. YANG E, LI X, LONG X. Diagnosis and treatment of axillary web syndrome: an overview. Chin J Plast Reconstr Surg 2020;2(2):128–36.

113. Koehler LA, Haddad TC, Hunter DW, et al. Axillary web syndrome following breast cancer surgery: symptoms, complications, and management strategies. Breast Cancer (London) 2019;11:13.

114. O'Toole J, Miller CL, Specht MC, et al. Cording following treatment for breast cancer. Breast Cancer Res Treat 2013;140(1):105–11.

115. Fourie WJ, Robb KA. Physiotherapy management of axillary web syndrome following breast cancer treatment: discussing the use of soft tissue techniques. Physiotherapy 2009;95(4):314–20.

116. Cohen-Hallaleh RB, Smith HG, Smith RC, et al. Radiation induced angiosarcoma of the breast: outcomes from a retrospective case series. Clin Sarcoma Res 2017;7(1):15.

117. Kleinerman RA, Tucker MA, Tarone RE, et al. Risk of new cancers after radiotherapy in long-term survivors of retinoblastoma: an extended follow-up. J Clin Oncol 2005;23(10):2272–9.

118. Mito JK, Mitra D, Barysauskas CM, et al. A Comparison of outcomes and prognostic features for radiation-associated angiosarcoma of the breast and other radiation-associated sarcomas. Int J Radiat Oncol Biol Phys 2019;104(2):425–35.

119. Deutsch M, Safyan E. Angiosarcoma of the breast occurring soon after lumpectomy and breast irradiation for infiltrating ductal carcinoma: a case report. Am J Clin Oncol 2003;26(5):471–2.

120. De Smet S, Vandermeeren L, Christiaens MR, et al. Radiation-induced sarcoma: analysis of 46 cases. Acta Chir Belg 2008;108(5):574–9.

121. Smith TL, Morris CG, Mendenhall NP. Angiosarcoma after breast-conserving therapy: Long-term disease control and late effects with hyperfractionated accelerated re-irradiation (HART) 2014;53(2):235–41. https://doi.org/10.3109/0284186X.2013.819117.

122. Sharma A, Schwartz RA. Stewart-treves syndrome: pathogenesis and management. J Am Acad Dermatol 2012;67(6):1342–8.

123. Bernia E, Rios-Viñuela E, Requena C. Stewart-treves syndrome. JAMA Dermatol 2021;157(6):721.

124. Araco A, Caruso R, Araco F, et al. Capsular contractures: a systematic review. Plast Reconstr Surg 2009;124(6):1808–19.

125. Namnoum JD, Largent J, Kaplan HM, et al. Primary breast augmentation clinical trial outcomes stratified by surgical incision, anatomical placement and implant device type. J Plast Reconstr Aesthet Surg 2013;66(9):1165–72.

126. Lapid O., Noels E.C., Meijer S.L., et al., Pathologic findings in primary capsulectomy specimens: analysis of 2531 patients, Aesthet Surg J, 34 (5), 2014, 714-718.

127. Doren EL, Miranda RN, Selber JC, et al. U.S. epidemiology of breast implant-associated anaplastic large cell lymphoma. Plast Reconstr Surg 2017;139(5):1042–50.

128. McCarthy CM, Loyo-Berríos N, Qureshi AA, et al. Patient registry and outcomes for breast implants and anaplastic large cell lymphoma etiology and epidemiology (PROFILE): initial report of findings, 2012-2018. Plast Reconstr Surg 2019;143:65S–73S (3S A Review of Breast Implant-Associated Anaplastic Large Cell Lymphoma).

129. Clemens MW, Jacobsen ED, Horwitz SM. 2019 NCCN Consensus guidelines on the diagnosis and treatment of breast implant-associated anaplastic large cell lymphoma (BIA-ALCL). Aesthet Surg J 2019;39(Supplement_1):S3–13.
130. Helms RL, O'Hea EL, Corso M. Body image issues in women with breast cancer 2008;13(3):313–25. https://doi.org/10.1080/13548500701405509.
131. Cornell LF, Mussallem DM, Gibson TC, et al. Trends in sexual function after breast cancer surgery. Ann Surg Oncol 2017;24(9):2526–38.
132. Rosenberg SM, Dominici LS, Gelber S, et al. Association of breast cancer surgery with quality of life and psychosocial well-being in young breast cancer survivors. JAMA Surg 2020;155(11):1035–42.
133. Campbell-Enns H, Woodgate R. The psychosocial experiences of women with breast cancer across the lifespan: a systematic review protocol. JBI Database Syst Rev Implement Reports 2015;13(1):112–21.
134. Janowski K, Tatala M, Jedynak T, et al. Social support and psychosocial functioning in women after mastectomy. Palliat Support Care 2020;18(3):314–21.
135. Ng ET, Ang RZ, Tran BX, et al. Comparing quality of life in breast cancer patients who underwent mastectomy versus breast-conserving surgery: a meta-analysis. Int J Environ Res Public Health 2019;16(24):4970.
136. Aerts L, Christiaens MR, Enzlin P, et al. Sexual functioning in women after mastectomy versus breast conserving therapy for early-stage breast cancer: a prospective controlled study. Breast 2014;23(5):629–36.
137. Parker PA, Youssef A, Walker S, et al. Short-term and long-term psychosocial adjustment and quality of life in women undergoing different surgical procedures for breast cancer. Ann Surg Oncol 2007;14(11):3078–89.
138. Anderson C, Islam JY, Elizabeth Hodgson M, et al. Long-term satisfaction and body image after contralateral prophylactic mastectomy. Ann Surg Oncol 2017;24(6):1499–506.
139. Parker PA, Peterson SK, Shen Y, et al. Prospective study of psychosocial outcomes of having contralateral prophylactic mastectomy among women with nonhereditary breast cancer. J Clin Oncol 2018;36(25):2630–8.
140. Guarino A, Polini C, Forte G, et al. The Effectiveness of Psychological Treatments in Women with Breast Cancer: A Systematic Review and Meta-Analysis. J Clin Med 2020;9(1). https://doi.org/10.3390/JCM9010209.
141. Didier F, Radice D, Gandini S, et al. Does nipple preservation in mastectomy improve satisfaction with cosmetic results, psychological adjustment, body image and sexuality? Breast Cancer Res Treat 2009;118(3):623–33.
142. Wei CH, Scott AM, Price AN, et al. Psychosocial and sexual well-being following nipple-sparing mastectomy and reconstruction. Breast J 2016;22(1):10–7.
143. Tevlin R, Brazio P, Tran N, et al. Immediate targeted nipple-areolar complex re-innervation: Improving outcomes in immediate autologous breast reconstruction. J Plast Reconstr Aesthet Surg 2021;74(7):1503–7.

Novel Approaches to Breast Reconstruction

Anne Warren Peled, MD[a],*, Nicholas W. Clavin, MD[b]

KEYWORDS

- Mastectomy • Oncoplastic surgery • Autologous reconstruction
- Breast neurotization

KEY POINTS

- Option of nipple-sparing mastectomy can be offered to patients with macromastia or significant ptosis through a staged approach.
- Advanced oncoplastic reconstruction techniques can expand possibilities for breast conservation even with larger tumors.
- Newer reconstructive options allow for preserving and restoring sensation after mastectomy.

INTRODUCTION

As breast oncologic surgical procedures and approaches have evolved in recent years, so have breast reconstruction techniques. Newer advances focus on expanding the options of reconstructive approaches and patient selection, optimizing quality of life, and helping improve postsurgical survivorship. These advances span from techniques to expand criteria for nipple-sparing mastectomies, optimizing and enhancing oncoplastic surgery, evolving autologous reconstruction options, and preserving and restoring sensation after mastectomy.

Expanding the Option of Nipple-Sparing Mastectomy

During the past 2 decades as nipple-sparing mastectomy (NSM) has become more widely adopted, oncologic indications have expanded to now include nearly all patients from an oncologic standpoint other than those with gross involvement of the nipple–areolar complex or other contraindications to preserving the breast skin envelope. However, many people are still not considered good candidates for NSM because of large or ptotic breasts, which can significantly increase the chance of

This article previously appeared in *Surgical Clinics* volume 103 issue 1 February 2023.
[a] Sutter Health California Pacific Medical Center Breast Cancer Program, 2100 Webster Street, Suite 222, San Francisco, CA 94115, USA; [b] Department of Plastic Surgery, Atrium Health, 1025 Morehead Medical Drive, #200; Charlotte, NC 28204, USA
* Corresponding author.
E-mail address: Drpeled@apeledmd.com

surgical complications and be challenging from a reconstructive standpoint.[1,2] These patients are typically recommended to have skin-sparing mastectomies as an alternative,[3] which prevents them from getting the known esthetic and psychological benefits of preservation of the entire breast skin envelope.[4]

Multiple alternatives to skin-sparing mastectomies in patients with large or ptotic breasts have been described, including simultaneous mastopexy/reduction of the skin envelope using a dermal pedicle at the time of NSM[5,6] or the use of free nipple grafting.[7,8] One of the most popular approaches is a staged NSM, with an initial breast reduction/mastopexy to act as a vascular delay before subsequent NSM. This approach was pioneered by Spear and colleagues,[9] who reported performing staged NSM through the mastopexy incisions a minimum of 4 weeks following mastopexy/reduction, with low rates of ischemic complications. Other authors have published subsequent large case series using this approach for both therapeutic and prophylactic indications in combination with implant-based and autologous reconstructions, showing excellent outcomes concerning nipple–areolar complex viability and reconstructive success.[10–12]

We offer a staged approach to NSM for any patient with larger than D/DD-cup sized-breasts or moderate Grade II ptosis or greater, both in prophylactic and therapeutic settings. For patients with diagnosed cancer, the initial procedure involves lumpectomy with/without axillary surgery as indicated and bilateral oncoplastic reduction mastopexy/mammoplasty. The staged NSM is then done approximately 2.5 to 3 months after the lumpectomy, or earlier if thought to be necessary from an oncology perspective. Immediate reconstruction with either direct-to-implant, immediate autologous, or 2-stage reconstruction with initial tissue expander placement is performed at the time of mastectomy (**Fig. 1**). If adjuvant chemotherapy is recommended, this is

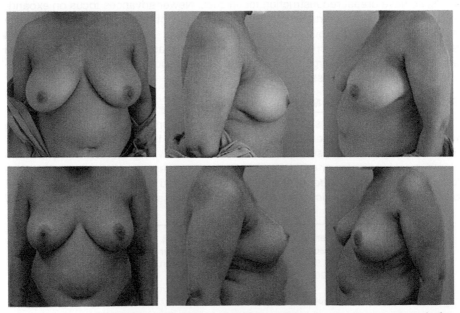

Fig. 1. A 39-year-old woman with BRCA1 mutation and left Stage I breast cancer before (*above*) and after (*below*) initial lumpectomy and bilateral oncoplastic reduction mammoplasty followed by staged NSM and prepectoral implant reconstruction.

done before mastectomy. Additionally, if surgical pathologic condition from the lumpectomy/axillary surgery leads to a recommendation for postmastectomy radiation therapy, further discussion regarding the true "need" for the mastectomy is had as part of a shared decision-making conversation with the patient. Given the increased risk of complications following postmastectomy radiation therapy in patients having implant-based (and to a lesser extent, autologous) reconstruction and the improved safety profile with lumpectomy and oncoplastic reconstruction,[13,14] these patients are encouraged to consider going on to postlumpectomy radiation rather than proceeding with the staged mastectomy if mastectomy is not truly medically indicated.

For prophylactic mastectomies, staged NSM is typically done a minimum of 3 months following initial reduction mastopexy/mammoplasty to optimize healing and minimize the chance of complications. Reconstructive options at the staged mastectomy are similar to those for therapeutic cases. Our preference is to do a superior/superior-medial pedicle for the initial reduction mastopexy/mammoplasty and then do the staged NSM through the inferior vertical portion of the reduction incision, thus completely avoiding the dermal pedicle created during the reduction and ideally optimizing the vascularity to the rest of the mastectomy skin flap (**Fig. 2**).

Optimizing and Enhancing Oncoplastic Surgery

The term oncoplastic surgery typically describes reconstruction of lumpectomy defects, usually involving immediate reconstruction done at the time of lumpectomy. The spectrum of oncoplastic surgery includes everything from esthetic scar placement for lumpectomy with limited local tissue rearrangement to more complex reconstruction involving oncoplastic mastopexies or reduction mammoplasties. Several classification systems based on the volume of resection and anticipated reconstructive technique have been developed to help guide clinical management.[15–17]

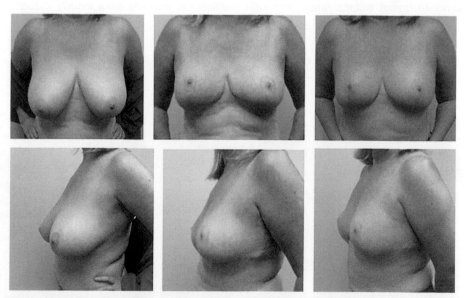

Fig. 2. A 55-year-old woman with BRCA2 mutation before (*left*) and after (*center*) initial reduction mammoplasty followed by staged NSM and prepectoral implant reconstruction (*right*).

More advanced oncoplastic techniques can be especially helpful for patients with large breasts or macromastia, particularly given the potential challenges of performing postmastectomy reconstruction in this patient population. Studies have shown numerous benefits from oncoplastic reduction mammoplasty for these patients. First, many patients with macromastia have significant baseline functional symptoms from their large breasts, which are known to be well relieved through reduction mammoplasty.[18] Offering large-breasted patients newly diagnosed with breast cancer a simultaneous breast reduction at the time of lumpectomy has been shown to provide a number of quality-of-life benefits and high levels of patient satisfaction.[19–21] We have found in our practices that these patients are some of our happiest patients who undergo breast reconstruction, with many patients feeling and looking much better than they did before their diagnosis (**Fig. 3**). Of note, oncoplastic reduction mammoplasty can be offered to any patient who can safely undergo the procedure from a medical standpoint and would like to reduce the size of their breasts, whether they truly require it from a reconstructive standpoint based on tumor size/extent of lumpectomy reconstruction or not.[22] In addition to the quality-of-life and functional benefits, oncoplastic reduction mastopexy/mammoplasty is thought to improve radiation delivery given the known increase in dose inhomogeneity seen in patients with larger, more ptotic breasts.[23,24] It has also been shown to improve margin control as compared with standard lumpectomy due to the ability to take more generous resection specimens, leading to lower rates of unplanned return to the OR for re-excision or completion mastectomy.[25,26] Finally, for patients with large breasts who might otherwise consider mastectomy, oncoplastic reduction has been shown to significantly lower the risk of complications as compared with mastectomy and reconstruction, including the need for additional operative procedures and complications leading to delays in adjuvant therapy.[13,27,28]

Other indications for more advanced oncoplastic reconstruction techniques include reconstruction of multifocal/multicentric lumpectomy defects and patients with large tumor-to-breast volume ratios. Although multicentric cancers were initially thought

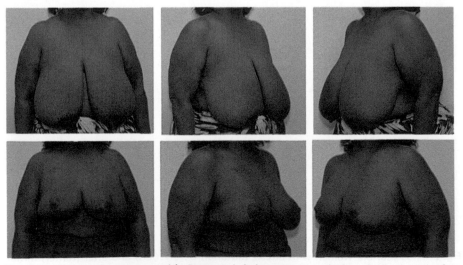

Fig. 3. A 52-year-old woman with Stage II left breast cancer before (*above*) and after (*below*) lumpectomy and bilateral oncoplastic reduction mammoplasty.

of as a contraindication to breast conservation,[29] more recent studies have reconsidered this recommendation and shown it to be oncologically equivalent if clear margins can be achieved.[30–32] Reconstruction, however, can be more challenging, particularly with multicentric disease where resection is required from multiple quadrants. In these cases, more advanced approaches such as round block, circumvertical, or Wise pattern reduction/mastopexy can be helpful both to allow for access to all of the area of resection and to allow for more extensive soft tissue reconstruction. Using extended pedicles or secondary pedicles for additional reconstructive volume may be necessary if reconstruction of multiple defects is required.[33,34] Additionally, patients with smaller breasts and larger tumor-to-breast volume ratios as well as patients of any breast size requiring extensive resection may be able to avoid mastectomy if more advanced oncoplastic approaches are offered. The concept of "extreme oncoplasty" was coined by Dr Mel Silverstein and colleagues in 2015,[35] which describes approaches to breast conservation through oncoplastic reconstruction in these more complex scenarios. Their workhorses for reconstruction of larger lumpectomy defects include Wise pattern reductions and split reduction procedures, which entail reconfiguring the Wise pattern design to allow for skin removal over the tumor.[36] Other surgeons have taken these principles and expanded indications for breast conservation and oncoplastic reconstruction in their practices as well, demonstrating good oncologic outcomes even in scenarios traditionally managed with mastectomy.[37,38]

Advancements in Autologous Reconstruction

Breast reconstruction using autologous flaps was first described in 1906 by Tanzini,[39] who reported using a myocutaneous latissimus dorsi flap to reconstruct a mastectomy defect. Earlier approaches such as this and flap reconstruction options throughout much of the twentieth century required complete muscle sacrifice harvest typically with either latissimus dorsi or transverse rectus abdominis myocutaneous (TRAM) flap reconstruction. As the concept of perforator flaps was introduced and techniques were optimized,[40] flap reconstruction evolved to allow for muscle-sparing options, with the deep inferior epigastric perforator flap being the most commonly described and utilized perforator flap option.[41] At many centers, deep inferior epigastric perforator (DIEP) flaps are the workhorse of their flap reconstruction programs, allowing patients the benefits of decreased abdominal donor site morbidity including lower rates of abdominal wall hernias as well as lower rates of fat necrosis.[42,43]

Although the abdomen is usually the preferred donor site for autologous reconstruction, some patients may not be candidates due to insufficient tissue or prior abdominal surgery affecting the vascular supply to the flaps.[44] In these cases, other perforator flaps can be considered, typically either the superior or inferior gluteal artery perforator (SGAP/IGAP) or profunda artery perforator (PAP) flaps. Some centers routinely use gluteal artery perforator flaps when abdominal flaps are not available or even as a first choice for reconstruction, describing the benefits of safe and reliable harvest with low rates of complications.[45] Limitations of the flap include the need for harvest in the prone position, which can add significant time to the procedure and precludes simultaneous flap harvest during the mastectomy in immediate reconstruction cases, as well as some concerns for donor site morbidity, particularly with IGAP flaps.[46,47] PAP flaps have been described more frequently in the literature recently, likely due to the reliable vascular anatomy,[48] minimal donor site morbidity and low complication rates,[49,50] and the ability to harvest the flap in the supine position potentially concurrently with the mastectomy, as well as the ability to shape the flap to achieve good esthetic outcomes (**Fig. 4**).[51]

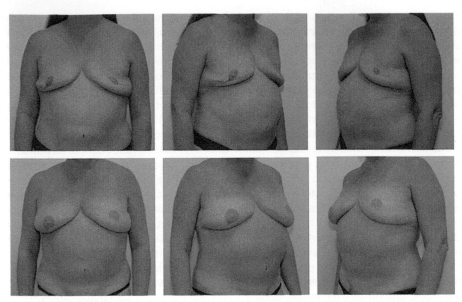

Fig. 4. A 47-year-old woman with a history of bilateral mastectomies and failed implant reconstruction as well as abdominoplasty before (*above*) and after (*below*) bilateral PAP flap reconstruction.

Other options for flap reconstruction when there is insufficient donor site tissue are stacked flaps, where more than one flap is used to reconstruct the breast, or hybrid flap reconstruction, where an implant is placed deep to the flap to add more volume. For stacked flaps, typical combinations included stacked combination DIEP/PAP flaps, stacked PAP flaps,[44] and stacked DIEP flaps for unilateral reconstruction.[52–54] These combinations allow for more volume than a single flap could provide, although still allowing patients a fully autologous reconstruction (**Fig. 5**). Although operative times are significantly longer with stacked flaps, studies comparing complication profiles following stacked flap reconstruction to single flap reconstruction have not shown increased risk of complications including flap loss or donor site complications.[55]

Another option for patients who need more volume than a single flap can provide is hybrid reconstruction, which combines autologous and implant-based reconstruction.[56] The technique has been described as either delayed or simultaneous placement of a prepectoral implant at the time of flap (typically DIEP flap or latissimus dorsi) reconstruction in order to achieve patients' desired size goals.[57] This approach has shown a favorable safety profile[58,59] and high rates of patient satisfaction.[60]

Preserving and Restoring Sensation After Mastectomy

Although so many advances have been made over time to improve the esthetics of postmastectomy reconstruction, one of the major limitations of mastectomy has been the loss of sensation following surgery. Prior studies have shown the loss of sensation to be very common in people undergoing mastectomy, with rates of return of breast skin and nipple sensation reported in the range of 2% to 26% following NSM,[61–63] indicating the vast majority of patients do not have meaningful sensation following mastectomy. The loss of sensation not only affects erogenous sensation and intimacy following mastectomy[64] but the loss of protective sensation can also

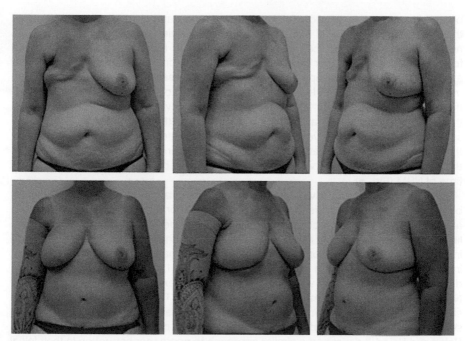

Fig. 5. A 43-year-old woman with a history of Stage II right breast cancer treated with simple mastectomy before (*above*) and after (*below*) stacked DIEP flap reconstruction.

lead to burns and other injuries, which can have devastating reconstructive consequences.[65,66] For some patients the loss of sensation can be very distressing and can significantly affect patient satisfaction as well as quality of life.[63,67]

Although there has been a more recent focus on preserving and restoring sensation after mastectomy, sensation restoration has actually been described with autologous reconstruction since the early 1990s. Early reports by Slezak and colleagues in 1992[68] involved intercostal nerve reconstruction at the time of delayed TRAM flap reconstruction for patients who had undergone prior mastectomy, with improved sensation seen in reinnervated reconstructed breasts compared with controls. Subsequent studies describing nerve reconstruction using either nerve conduits or nerve autografts at the time of flap reconstruction have shown improved objective return of sensation as well as better patient-reported overall and erogenous sensation with reinnervated flaps.[69–71] More recent data have come out of the Sensation-NOW trial, which is a multisite prospective case-control registry study assessing outcomes following autologous reconstruction and flap neurotization.[72] Momeni and colleagues[73] described outcomes from 22 patients who had abdominally based autologous reconstruction with or without neurotization at a minimum of 1-year follow-up. Patients who underwent neurotization were significantly more likely to have return of protective sensation on cutaneous pressure threshold evaluation compared to controls.

Although the majority of studies describing neurotization and autologous reconstruction are focused on restoring sensation after mastectomy has already been completed, more recent advances have focused on trying to preserve sensation at the time of mastectomy. This is done through a combination of nerve preservation (when oncologically feasible) and nerve reconstruction with either autografts or allografts. Ducic[74] and Djohan[75] have significantly contributed to our understanding of breast nerve anatomy to allow for nerve preservation and immediate reconstruction through cadaver studies of dissections of mastectomies and abdominal flaps with nerve harvest. Based on their dissections, they have recommended consideration for use of nerve allograft for reconstruction to ensure complete sensory nerve repair as well as delineated anticipated nerve anatomy to assist with identification during mastectomy. Peled and Peled described their approach to preserving sensation at the time of mastectomy in 2019,[76] reporting that they carefully identify the lateral thoracic intercostal nerves at the time of mastectomy (typically T4 and T5, although sometimes T3) and preserve them if oncologically safe, wherein the nerves run in the subcutaneous tissue rather than the breast parenchyma itself. In their study, they combine nerve preservation with nipple–areolar complex neurotization at the time of NSM (**Fig. 6**).

With the technological advancements of nerve allografts, nerve reconstruction can be done not only with flap reconstruction, where donor site nerves can be used but also with implant-based reconstruction. A small number of studies have been published to date describing nerve reconstruction at the time of mastectomy and implant-based reconstruction but more data are anticipated with the growing interest in the procedure from both surgeons and patients.[77] Djohan and colleagues[78] first described their experience with nipple–areolar complex neurotization at the time of NSM and immediate implant reconstruction in 2020. They performed nerve reconstruction with allografts from the lateral fourth intercostal nerves to carefully identified subareolar nerves and reported on the improvement in objective sensation over time. Peled and Peled[76] described a similar approach to nerve reconstruction in their initial study, with 91% of patients achieving return to baseline sensation of their nipple–areolar complex by a mean follow-up of 13 months. Neurotization at the time of immediate autologous reconstruction has also been described, with a similar approach concerning preservation of as much length of the native intercostal nerve as possible at coaptation to a subareolar nerve. Tevlin and colleagues[79] reported sensory outcomes in their case-control study of nipple reinnervation during immediate autologous reconstruction, demonstrating full return to baseline sensation in the group undergoing neurotization.

Outcomes research around sensation preservation and restoration after mastectomy continues to evolve as well, with an increased focus on determining the optimal patient-reported outcomes tools and metrics to assess sensation,[67,80] as well as more

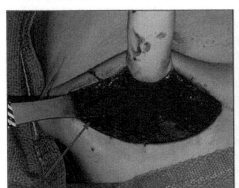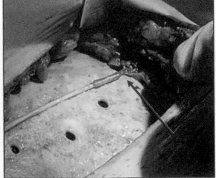

Fig. 6. Example of nerve preservation during NSM (*left*) and intercostal nerve reconstruction using a nerve allograft coapted to a subareolar nerve (*right*).

objective sensory outcomes assessment.[81,82] Advances in outcomes measures as well as more outcomes data from these procedures will be essential in helping determine best practices and selection criteria, as well as ensuring insurance coverage for patients.

CLINICS CARE POINTS

- Nerve preservation and reconstruction at the time of mastectomy can safely and effectively provide patients with sensation after mastectomy.
- Use of initial reduction mammoplasty or mastopexy can extend the option of nipple-sparing mastectomy in therapeutic and prophylactic situations.

DISCLOSURE

Dr A.W. Peled is a consultant/speaker for Axogen, Allergan, Sientra, and Stryker. Dr N.W. Clavin is a consultant/speaker for Allergan and Stryker.

REFERENCES

1. Stolier AJ, Levine EA. Reducing the risk of nipple necrosis: technical observations in 340 nipple-sparing mastectomies. Breast J 2013;19:173–9.
2. McCarthy CM, Mehrara BJ, Riedel E, al at. Predicting complications following expander/implant breast reconstruction: an outcomes analysis based on preoperative clinical risk. Plast Reconstr Surg 2008;121:1886–92.
3. Nava MB, Cortinovis U, Ottolenghi J, et al. Skin-reducing mastectomy. Plast Reconstr Surg 2006;118:603–10.
4. Howard MA, Sisco M, Yao K, et al. Patient satisfaction with nipple-sparing mastectomy: a prospective study of patient reported outcomes using the BREAST-Q. J Surg Oncol 2016;114:416–22.
5. Salibian AH, Harness JK, Mowlds DS. Primary buttonhole mastopexy and nipple-sparing mastectomy: a preliminary report. Ann Plast Surg 2016;77:388–95.
6. Aliotta RE, Scomacao I, Duraes EFR, et al. Pushing the envelope: skin-only mastopexy in single-stage nipple-sparing mastectomy with direct-to-implant breast reconstruction. Plast Reconstr Surg 2021;147:38–45.
7. Doren EL, Kuykendall LVE, Lopez JJ, et al. Free nipple grafting: an alternative for patients ineligible for nipple-sparing mastectomy? Ann Plast Surg 2014;72:S112–5.
8. Kim EK, Cho JM, Lee JW. Skin-sparing mastectomy and immediate nipple graft for large, ptotic breast. J Breast Cancer 2019;22:641–6.
9. Spear SL, Rottman SJ, Seiboth LA, et al. Breast reconstruction using a staged nipple-sparing mastectomy following mastopexy or reduction. Plast Reconstr Surg 2012;129:572–81.
10. Momeni A, Kanchwala S, Sbitany H. Oncoplastic procedures in preparation for nipple-sparing mastectomy and autologous breast reconstruction: controlling the breast envelope. Plast Reconstr Surg 2020;145:914–20.
11. Salibian AA, Frey JD, Karp NS, et al. Does staged breast reduction before nipple-sparing mastectomy decrease complications? A matched cohort study between staged and nonstaged techniques. Plast Reconstr Surg 2019;144:1023–32.
12. Economides JM, Graziano F, Tousimis E, et al. Expanded algorithm and updated experience with breast reconstruction using a staged nipple-sparing mastectomy

following mastopexy or reduction mammaplasty in the large or ptotic breast. Plast Reconstr Surg 2019;143:688e, 97e.

13. Peled AW, Sbitany H, Foster RD, et al. Oncoplastic mammoplasty as a strategy for reducing reconstructive complications associated with postmastectomy radiation therapy. Breast J 2014;20:302–7.

14. Stein MJ, Karir A, Arnaout A, et al. Quality-of-life and surgical outcomes for breast cancer patients treated with therapeutic reduction mammoplasty versus mastectomy with immediate reconstruction. Ann Surg Oncol 2020;27:4502–12.

15. Clough KB, Kaufman GJ, Nos C, et al. Improving breast cancer surgery: a classification and quadrant per quadrant atlas for oncoplastic surgery. Ann Surg Oncol 2010;17:1375–91.

16. Chatterjee A, Gass J, Patel K, et al. A consensus definition and classification system of oncoplastic surgery developed by the American Society of Breast Surgeons. Ann Surg Oncol 2019;26:3436–44.

17. Patel K, Bloom J, Nardello S, et al. An oncoplastic surgery primer: common indications, techniques, and complications in Level I and 2 volume displacement oncoplastic surgery. Ann Surg Oncol 2019;26:3063–70.

18. Strong B, Hall-Findlay EJ. How does volume of resection relate to symptom relief for reduction mammaplasty patients? Ann Plast Surg 2015;75:376–82.

19. Acea-Nebril B, Cereijo-Garea C, Garcia-Novoa A, et al. The role of oncoplastic breast reduction in the conservative management of breast cancer: complications, survival, and quality of life. J Surg Oncol 2017;115:679–86.

20. Denis-Katz HS, Ghaedi BB, Fitzpatrick A, et al. Oncological safety, surgical outcome, and patient satisfaction of oncoplastic breast-conserving surgery with contralateral balancing reduction mammoplasty. Plast Surg (Oakv) 2021;29:235–42.

21. Patel K, Hannah CM, Gatti ME, et al. A head-to-head comparison of quality of life and aesthetic outcomes following immediate, staged-immediate, and delayed oncoplastic reduction mammaplasty. Plast Reconstr Surg 2011;127:2167–75.

22. Di Micco R, O'Connell RL, Barry PA, et al. Standard wide local excision or bilateral reduction mammoplasty in large-breasted women with small tumours: surgical and patient-reported outcomes. Eur J Surg Oncol 2017;43:636–41.

23. Prabhakar R, Rath GK, Julka PK, et al. Breast dose heterogeneity in CT-based radiotherapy treatment planning. J Med Phys 2008;33:43–8.

24. Fernando IN, Ford HT, Powles TJ, et al. Factors affecting acute skin toxicity in patients having breast irradiation after conservative surgery: a prospective study of treatment practice at the Royal Marsden Hospital. Clin Oncol (R Coll Radiol) 1996;8:226–33.

25. Losken A, Pinell-White X, Hart AM, et al. The oncoplastic reduction approach to breast conservation therapy: benefits for margin control. Aesthet Surg J 2014;34:1185–91.

26. Piper ML, Esserman LJ, Sbitany H, et al. Outcomes following oncoplastic reduction mammoplasty: a systematic review. Ann Plast Surg 2016;76:S222–6.

27. Losken A, Pinell XA, Eskenazi BR. The benefits of partial versus total breast reconstruction for women with macromastia. Plast Reconstr Surg 2010;125:1051–6.

28. Tong WMY, Baumann DP, Villa MT, et al. Obese women experience fewer complications after oncoplastic breast repair following partial mastectomy than after immediate total breast reconstruction. Plast Reconstr Surg 2016;137:777–91.

29. Morrow M, Strom EA, Bassett LW, et al. Standard for breast conservation therapy in the management of invasive breast carcinoma. CA Cancer J Clin 2002;52: 277–300.
30. Masannat YA, Agrawal A, Maraqa L, et al. Multifocal and multicentric breast cancer, is it time to think again? Ann R Coll Surg Engl 2020;102:62–6.
31. Tan MP, Sitoh NY, Sim AS. Breast conservation treatment for multifocal and multicentric breast cancers in women with small-volume breast tissue. ANZ J Surg 2017;87:E5–10.
32. Kadioglu H, Yucel S, Yildiz S, et al. Feasibility of breast conserving surgery in multifocal breast cancers. Am J Surg 2014;208:457–64.
33. Losken A, Hart AM, Dutton JW, et al. The expanded use of autoaugmentation techniques in oncoplastic breast surgery. Plast Reconstr Surg 2018;141:10–9.
34. Bellizzi A, Vella Baldacchino R, Kazzazi F, et al. The successful use of disparate pedicle types for bilateral therapeutic mammaplasties during breast conservation surgery. J Surg Case Rep 2021;3:rjab064.
35. Silverstein MJ, Savalia N, Khan S, et al. Extreme oncoplasty: breast conservation for patients who need mastectomy. Breast J 2015;21:52–9.
36. Silverstein MJ, Savalia NB, Khan S, et al. Oncoplastic split reduction with intraoperative radiation therapy. Ann Surg Oncol 2015;22:3405–6.
37. Savioli F, Seth S, Morrow E, et al. Extreme oncoplasty: breast conservation in patients with large, multifocal, and multicentric breast cancer. Breast Cancer 2021; 13:353–9. Dove Med Press.
38. Koppiker CB, Noor AU, Dixit S, et al. Extreme oncoplastic surgery for multifocal/multicentric and locally advanced breast cancer. Int J Breast Cancer 2019;4262589.
39. Tanzini I. Spora il mio nuova processo di amputazione della mammella. Riforma Med 1906;22:757.
40. Koshima I, Soeda S. Inferior epigastric artery skin flap without rectus abdominis muscle. Br J Plast Surg 1989;42:645.
41. Healy C, Allen RJ Sr. The evolution of perforator flap breast reconstruction: twenty years after the first DIEP flap. J Reconstr Microsurg 2014;30:121–5.
42. Garvey PB, Buchel EW, Pockaj BA, et al. DIEP and pedicled TRAM flaps: a comparison of outcomes. Plast Reconstr Surg 2006;117:1711–9.
43. Knox ADC, Ho AL, Leung L, et al. Comparison of outcomes following autologous breast reconstruction using the DIEP and pedicled TRAM flaps: a 12-year clinical retrospective study and literature review. Plast Reconstr Surg 2016;138:16–28.
44. Haddock NT, Cho MJ, Gassman A, et al. Stacked profunda artery perforator flap for breast reconstruction in failed or unavailable deep inferior epigastric perforator flap. Plast Reconstr Surg 2019;143:488e, 94e.
45. Granzow JW, Levine JL, Chiu ES, et al. Breast reconstruction with gluteal artery perforator flaps. J Plast Reconstr Aesthet Surg 2006;59:614–21.
46. Godbout E, Farmer L, Bortoluzzi P, et al. Donor-site morbidity of the inferior gluteal artery perforator flap for breast reconstruction in teenagers. Can J Plast Surg 2013;21:19–22.
47. Mirzabeigi M, Au A, Jandali S, et al. Trials and tribulations with the inferior gluteal artery perforator flap in autologous breast reconstruction. Plast Reconstr Surg 2011;128:614e, 24e.
48. Largo RD, Chu CK, Chang EI, et al. Perforator mapping of the profunda artery perforator flap: anatomy and clinical experience. Plast Reconstr Surg 2020; 146:1135–45.

49. Qian B, Xiong L, Li J, et al. A systematic review and meta-analysis on microsurgical safety and efficacy of profunda artery perforator flap in breast reconstruction. J Oncol 2019;29:9506720.
50. Allen RJ Jr, Lee Z, Mayo JL, et al. The profunda artery perforator flap experience for breast reconstruction. Plast Reconstr Surg 2016;138:968–75.
51. Atzeni M, Salzillo R, Haywood R, et al. Breast reconstruction using the profunda artery perforator (PAP) flap: technical refinements and evolution, outcomes, and patient satisfaction based on 116 consecutive flaps. J Plast Reconstr Aesthet Surg 2022;75:1617–24.
52. Martinez CA, Fairchild B, Secchi-Del Rio R, et al. Bilateral outpatient breast reconstruction with stacked DIEP and vertical PAP flaps. Plast Reconstr Surg Glob Open 2021;9:e3878.
53. Haddock NT, Suszynski TM, Teotia SS. Consecutive bilateral breast reconstruction using stacked abdominally based and posterior thigh free flaps. Plast Reconstr Surg 2021;147:294–303.
54. DellaCroce FJ, Sullivan SK, Trahan C. Stacked deep inferior epigastric perforator flap breast reconstruction: a review of 110 flaps in 55 cases over 3 years. Plast Reconstr Surg 2011;127:1093–9.
55. Haddock NT, Cho MJ, Teotia SS. Comparative analysis of single versus stacked free flap breast reconstruction: a single center experience. Plast Reconstr Surg 2019;144:369e, 77e.
56. Kanchwala S, Momeni A. Hybrid breast reconstruction- the best of both worlds. Gland Surg 2019;8:82–9.
57. Scafati ST, Cavaliere A, Aceto B, et al. Combining autologous and prosthetic techniques: the breast reconstruction scale principle. Plast Reconstr Surg Glob Open 2017;5:e1602.
58. Momeni A, Kanchwala S. Hybrid prepectoral breast reconstruction: a surgical approach that combines the benefits of autologous and implant-based reconstruction. Plast Reconstr Surg 2018;142:1109–15.
59. Lee HC, Lee J, Park SH, et al. The hybrid latissimus dorsi flap in immediate breast reconstruction: a comparative study with the abdominal-based flap. Ann Plast Surg 2021;86:394–9.
60. Bach AD, Morgenstern IH, Horch RE. Secondary "hybrid reconstruction" concept with silicone implants after autologous breast reconstruction: is it safe and reasonable? Med Sci Monit 2020;26:e921329.
61. Chirappapha P, Srichan P, Lertsithichai P, et al. Nipple-areola complex sensation after nipple-sparing mastectomy. Plast Reconstr Surg Glob Open 2018;6:e1716.
62. Dossett LA, Lowe J, Sun W, et al. Prospective evaluation of skin and nipple-areola sensation and patient satisfaction after nipple-sparing mastectomy. J Surg Oncol 2016;114:11–6.
63. Djohan R, Gage E, Gatherwright J, et al. Patient satisfaction following nipple-sparing mastectomy and immediate breast reconstruction: an 8-year outcome study. Plast Reconstr Surg 2010;125:818–29.
64. Boswell EN, Dizon DS. Breast cancer and sexual function. Transl Androl Urol 2015;4:160–8.
65. Faulkner HR, Colwell AS, Liao EC, et al. Thermal injury to reconstructed breasts from commonly used warming devices: a risk for reconstructive failure. Plast Reconstr Surg Glob Open 2016;4:e1033.
66. Seth R, Lamyman MJ, Athanassopoulos A, et al. Too close for comfort: accidental burn following subcutaneous mastectomy and immediate implant reconstruction. J R Soc Med 2008;101:39–40.

67. Peled AW, Amara D, Piper ML, et al. Development and validation of a nipple-specific scale for the BREAST-Q to assess patient-reported outcomes following nipple-sparing mastectomy. Plast Reconstr Surg 2019;143:1010–7.

68. Slezak S, McGibbon B, Dellon AL. The sensational transverse rectus abdominis musculocutaneous (TRAM) flap: return of sensibility after TRAM breast reconstruction. Ann Plast Surg 1992;28:210–7.

69. Blondeel PN, Demuynck M, Mete D, et al. Sensory nerve repair in perforator flaps for autologous breast reconstruction: sensational or senseless? Br J Plast Surg 1999;52:37–44.

70. Spiegel AJ, Menn ZK, Eldor L, et al. Breast reinnervation: DIEP neurotization using the third anterior intercostal nerve. Plast Reconstr Surg Glob Open 2013; 1:e72.

71. Beugels J, Bijkerk E, Lataster A, et al. Nerve coaptation improves the sensory recovery of the breast in DIEP flap breast reconstruction. Plast Reconstr Surg 2021; 148:273–84.

72. Available at: https://clinicaltrials.gov/ct2/show/NCT01526681 -. Accessed 6.1.22.

73. Momeni A, Meyer S, Shefren K, et al. Flap neurotization in breast reconstruction with nerve allografts: 1-year clinical outcomes. Plast Reconstr Surg Glob Open 2021;9:e3328.

74. Ducic I, Yoon J, Momeni A, et al. Anatomical considerations to optimize sensory recovery in breast neurotization with allograft. Plast Reconstr Surg Glob Open 2018;6:e1985.

75. Gatherwright J, Knackstedt R, Djohan R. Anatomic targets for breast reconstruction neurotization: past results and future possibilities. Ann Plast Surg 2019;82: 207–12.

76. Peled AW, Peled ZM. Nerve preservation and allografting for sensory innervation following immediate implant breast reconstruction. Plast Reconstr Surg Glob Open 2019;7:e2332.

77. Peled AW, Peled ZM. Sensory reinnervation after mastectomy with implant-based reconstruction. Ann Breast Surg. Submitted for publication.

78. Djohan R, Scomacao I, Knackstedt R, et al. Neurotization of the nipple-areola complex during implant-based reconstruction: evaluation of early sensation recovery. Plast Reconstr Surg 2020;146:250–4.

79. Tevlin R, Brazio P, Tran N, et al. Immediate targeted nipple-areolar complex reinnervation: improving outcomes in immediate autologous breast reconstruction. J Plast Reconstr Aesthet Surg 2021;74:1503–7.

80. Tsangaris E, Klassen AF, Kaur MN, et al. Development and psychometric validation of the BREAST-Q sensation module for women undergoing post-mastectomy breast reconstruction. Ann Surg Oncol 2021;28:7842–53.

81. Vartanian ED, Lo AY, Hershenhouse KS, et al. The role of neurotization in autologous breast reconstruction: can reconstruction restore breast sensation? J Surg Oncol 2021;123:1215–31.

82. Weissler JM, Koltz PF, Carney MJ, et al. Sifting through the evidence: a comprehensive review and analysis of neurotization in breast reconstruction. Plast Reconstr Surg 2018;141:550–65.

Modern Approaches to Implant-Based Breast Reconstruction

Ara A. Salibian, MD[a], Nolan S. Karp, MD[b],*

KEYWORDS

- Breast reconstruction • Nipple-sparing mastectomy • Cohesive implant
- Acellular dermal matrix

KEY POINTS

- Successful implant-based breast reconstruction requires a team approach between the breast surgeon and plastic surgeon.
- Patient selection, mastectomy flap quality, and surgical technique are critical in nipple-sparing mastectomy.
- Modern highly cohesive implants have esthetic benefits in breast reconstruction though preoperative discussion of all implant-related risks is paramount.
- Support materials including acellular dermal matrix have both risks and benefits in breast reconstruction and their use should be individualized.

INTRODUCTION

Implant-based reconstruction remains the most common form of breast reconstruction today.[1] Although many of the basic principles of implant-based reconstruction have not changed, several core components of these procedures have evolved toward what can be considered the "modern" approach. This approach is focused on a team-based paradigm,[2] in which the breast and plastic surgeons work together with the patient throughout all phases of care to optimize both oncologic and reconstructive outcomes.

Specific advances in this field include the evolution of mastectomy techniques, which allow for preservation of the skin envelope and nipple, when indicated to optimize esthetic results without compromising oncologic safety through nipple-sparing mastectomy (NSM).[3,4] The implant technology improved to offer more cohesive and form-stable implants[5] that are particularly beneficial in the reconstructive setting.

This article previously appeared in *Clinics in Plastic Surgery* volume 50 issue 2 April 2023.
[a] Division of Plastic and Reconstructive Surgery, University of California, Davis, 2335 Stockton Blvd., NAOB 6th floor, Sacramento, CA 95817, USA; [b] Hansjörg Wyss Department of Plastic Surgery, New York University Langone Health, 305 East 47th Street, Suite 1A, New York, NY 10017, USA
* Corresponding author.
E-mail address: nolan.karp@nyulangone.org

On the other hand, the association of textured implants with breast implant-associated anaplastic large cell lymphoma (BIA-ALCL)[6,7] changed considerations with implant selection and resulted in the introduction of smooth, tabbed tissue expanders. The use of support materials such as acellular dermal matrix (ADM) helped minimize complications such as capsular contracture[8] and introduced new techniques such as immediate implant[9] and prepectoral reconstruction.[10] Moreover, evidence-based reporting in breast reconstruction has been incorporated within a greater, critical focus on patient-reported outcomes[11] and shared decision-making.[12,13]

The modern approach to implant-breast reconstruction encompasses the evolution in all of these techniques and considerations. In this article, the authors focus specifically on modern mastectomy considerations and how they impact implant-based breast reconstruction, current prosthesis choices and their impact on outcomes, and our current understanding of support materials in implant-based breast reconstruction.

MODERN APPROACH TO MASTECTOMY
Mastectomy Flap Quality

The success of implant-based breast reconstruction is tied to the preceding mastectomy. The ablative and reconstructive surgeries, however, should not be considered as sequential events, but instead as interdependent components of the same procedure. The transition to this approach is dictated by the teamwork between the breast surgeon and the plastic surgeon, with proactive communication throughout the preoperative, intraoperative, and postoperative treatment of patients.[2]

A thorough understanding of the lamellar structure of the breast and its fascial system[14] is paramount in interpreting mastectomy flap quality. The corpus mammae are held within an irregular pseudocapsule from the surrounding adipose tissue. A distinct superficial layer of the superficial fascia, also referred to as the anterior lamina fascia, separates a thinner layer of subcutaneous fat from deeper, lobular anterior lamellar fat.[15] These fascial layers, along with the thickness of the subcutaneous tissue, can be visualized on preoperative breast MRI (**Fig. 1**) as well as ultrasound. Preoperative imaging can serve as a useful guide for both the breast and plastic surgeons to estimate the thickness of mastectomy flaps and their implications for implant-based reconstructive choices.

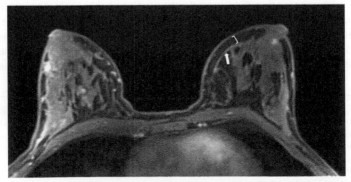

Fig. 1. Preoperative breast MRI can be useful in understanding the fascial layers of the breast and subcutaneous tissue thickness. The white arrow denotes the level of the breast pseudocapsule and the white brackets the thickness of the adipose tissue superficial to the mastectomy plane.

The thickness of the subcutaneous layer of the breast varies significantly among different patients, with an increased body mass index (BMI) correlating with a thicker layer of subcutaneous tissue.[16] Therefore, thick flaps do not necessarily equal well-perfused flaps and vice versa. Instead, the relative thickness of the preoperative subcutaneous layer of the breast to the thickness of the mastectomy flap plays a more important role in predicting perfusion, with ratios less than around 70% associated with ischemic complications of the skin envelope.[17]

The thickness of the subcutaneous layer also varies significantly within each breast, with breast tissue reaching the dermis at the vertical Cooper's ligaments. In this regard, surgical dissection along the appropriate anatomic planes is significantly more important than the absolute thickness of a flap with regard to perfusion. Overall flap thickness can have important implications for esthetic results, especially in prepectoral reconstruction where implant edges and rippling are more visible in thin patients. Aside from relative flap thickness, several other factors are important in assessment of mastectomy flap quality and can be used to predict potential ischemic complications of the skin envelope (**Box 1**).[18] Clinical assessment of incision edge bleeding, preservation of subcutaneous tissue, and the extent of visible dermis and cautery burns are all important variables. Adjunctive imaging modalities such as indocyanine green angiography can be useful tools for perfusion assessment.[19]

Nipple-Sparing Mastectomy

Mastectomy flap quality is particularly important in NSM as perfusion becomes an even more critical factor given the preservation of the entire skin envelope and nipple-areola complex (NAC). NSM has demonstrated equivalent oncologic outcomes[3] and superior esthetic and patient-reported outcomes[4] compared with its traditional mastectomy counterpart. Criteria for oncologic indications for NSM based on tumor-to-nipple distance continue to evolve. Although a 2-cm cutoff was traditionally used, more recent studies have demonstrated similar rates of pathologic nipple involvement[20] and locoregional recurrence[21] with tumor-to-nipple distances (TNDs) less than or equal to 1 cm, whereas other studies have found an increased locoregional recurrence rate below 1 cm.[22] Long-term recurrence rates with different cutoffs and consideration of other tumor characteristics are still needed.

Box 1
Important factors in evaluating mastectomy flap quality

Preservation of subcutaneous tissue on underside of mastectomy flap

Extent of visible dermis

Bleeding at incision edges[a]

Relative mastectomy flap thickness[b]

Extent of electrocautery burns

Visible skin mottling

Adjunctive imaging modalities[a]

[a]Interpretation difficult if epinephrine-containing infiltration utilized. [b]Ratio of preoperative subcutaneous tissue thickness to postmastectomy flap thickness.

Incision planning is a critical component of NSM given its significant implications for esthetic results, perfusion of the skin envelope, and access for oncologic extirpation. Although multiple choices exist, certain trends have become readily apparent with the abundance of literature on this topic. A recent meta-analysis of 9975 NSMs confirmed the increased risk of nipple necrosis with periareolar incisions.[23] Similarly, inverted-T or wise-pattern incisions have also been associated with ischemic complications of the skin envelope[24,25] likely because of more significant disruption of the subdermal plexus and creation of a T-point. The inframammary fold (IMF) incision has become the most widely used NSM incision[23] given its esthetic location and low risk of ischemic skin envelope complications (**Fig. 2**).[25–27]

Patient selection, and therefore proper assessment of risk factors for complications, also plays an important role in NSM outcomes. Well-known risk factors for postoperative complications include elevated BMI,[26] tobacco use,[28] radiation,[26] and diabetes.[29] Other variables include mastectomy indication, as therapeutic NSMs have also been found to have a higher complication rate than prophylactic NSM[30] as well as reconstructive modality with immediate implant and autologous reconstruction associated with increased complication rates compared with two-stage tissue expander reconstruction.[31] Different risk calculators for complications after mastectomy and reconstruction are available[32,33] and can be particularly useful for preoperative patient counseling.

Increasing breast size as correlated by greater mastectomy weights[34] and ptosis[35] have also been found to be predictors of postoperative complications. NSM has been demonstrated to be safe after breast reduction and mastopexy.[36] Furthermore, staged breast reduction before NSM, originally described by Spear and colleagues,[37]

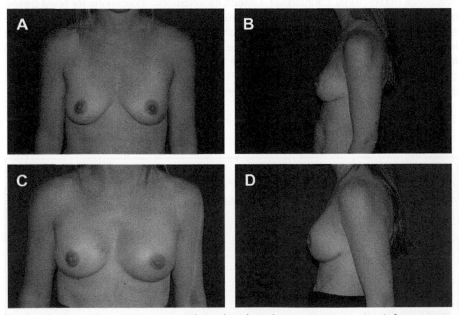

Fig. 2. Nipple-sparing mastectomy with implant-based reconstruction using inframammary fold incisions. Preoperative (*A,B*) and postoperative (*C,D*) photos of a 40-year-old woman with staged breast reconstruction with tissue expanders replaced with smooth round moderate profile 265-mL gel implants.

has been found to decrease rates of major mastectomy flap necrosis in these patients (**Fig. 3**).[38] Immediate reconstruction and concomitant mastopexy has also been described in implant-based reconstruction. Several techniques can be used including the button-hole mastopexy[39,40] and wise and skin reduction patterns[41–44] with the NAC either pedicled on the dermal plexus or transposed as a free graft. Excellent mastectomy flap quality is paramount in these cases to maintain already-compromised perfusion to the NAC that is now being transposed.

MODERN IMPLANT CHOICES

The breast implant technology has undergone a significant evolution since its introduction. Today's line of breast implants are characterized by improved gel-fill ratios, better implant shell design, and increased gel-crosslinking aimed to decrease

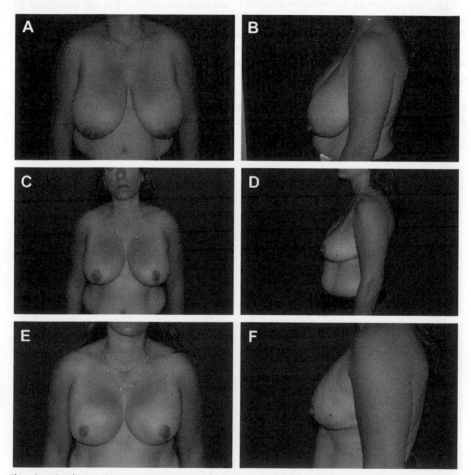

Fig. 3. Nipple-sparing mastectomy with breast reduction before implant-based breast reconstruction. A 38-year-old woman presented for breast reduction (*A, B*). Breast reduction with 380 gm removed on the right and 410 gm removed on the left (*C,D*). The patient subsequently underwent dual-plane NSM and immediate implant reconstruction using smooth high-profile silicone implants (*E,F*).

complications such as rippling, malposition, and gel bleed while improving form stability of implants and subsequently breast esthetics.[45] Several implant characteristics are variable within, and among different manufacturers, including implant cohesivity, texturing, shape, size, and projection.

Implant cohesivity is related to the degree of gel cross-linking and has important implications for shape, form, fill, firmness, and feel.[46] More cohesive implants will have greater form stability and upper pole projection but can feel firmer to patients which may be undesirable.[47] Modern highly cohesive, form-stable implants have been particularly useful in prepectoral breast reconstruction to minimize rippling and improve upper pole fill (**Fig. 4**),[48] both of which can be more challenging in thinner patients without the additional coverage provided by the pectoralis major. The degree of implant cohesivity should be individualized to each patient and mastectomy defect, importantly discussing all options and involving patients in the selection preoperatively.

The introduction of form-stable implants has also allowed for the development of anatomic, shaped implants that are suggested to provide a more natural appearance. Studies, however, have demonstrated similar postoperative patient satisfaction and quality-of-life metrics between round and shaped implants after breast reconstruction.[49,50] In addition, the association of macrotextured implants with BIA-ALCL[6] has had significant implications for implant choices, favoring the use of smooth, round implants, especially in the breast cancer population. Recent US Food and Drug Administration (FDA) safety requirements for breast implants were also implemented which include a required patient decision checklist and a "black box" warning on all breast

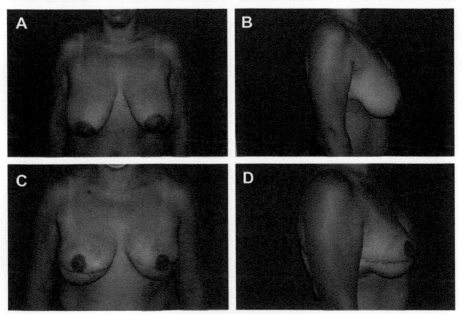

Fig. 4. Breast reconstruction with highly cohesive formal stable implants. Preoperative (*A, B*) and postoperative (*C, D*) photos of a 40-year-old woman with bilateral skin-sparing mastectomy (SSM) and prepectoral immediate implant reconstruction with ADM and vicryl mesh using highly cohesive gel implants: 605 mL. She subsequently had three-dimensional nipple-areola tattoos.

implants describing increasing lifetime risks of complications as well as associations with BIA-ALCL and symptoms of breast implant illness.[51] These changes further reinforce the importance of preoperative patient counseling and education for informed, shared decision-making.

SUPPORT MATERIALS IN IMPLANT RECONSTRUCTION
Acellular Dermal Matrix

The introduction of ADM for use in breast reconstruction by Breuing and colleagues ushered in a rapid adoption of ADM-assisted techniques in implant-based reconstructive procedures. "Dual-plane", or partial submuscular reconstruction, remains a widely used technique,[1] in which the ADM is typically used for inferolateral prosthesis coverage after being sutured to the cut edge of the pectoralis major muscle superiorly, and the IMF and anteriorly axillary line inferolaterally (**Fig. 5**).

In comparison to traditional total submuscular coverage, dual-plane ADM techniques have less morbidity as well as the ability to perform immediate implant reconstructions.[9] Esthetic results have also been suggested to be superior to total submuscular coverage[52,53] given improved control and expansion of the lower pole (**Fig. 6**). Although several studies have cited faster tissue expander filling with dual-plane reconstruction,[54,55] these data, in addition to pain outcomes, are conflicting.[56]

The additional benefits of ADM use have also been described including decreasing periprosthetic fibrosis[57–59] and a subsequent association with lower rates of capsular contracture,[8] in addition to a potential protective effect against rippling[60] and radiation fibrosis.[61,62] With the "resurgence" of prepectoral reconstruction, ADM use has further been advocated as a means of defining the breast pocket, supporting the implant, and decreasing the inflammatory processes leading to capsular contracture.[10]

However, the complication profile of ADM cannot be ignored.[63] Certain initial concerns of significantly increased major complication rates with ADM[64] were improved with modifications to ADM processing from aseptic to sterile manufacturing that decreased rates of infection.[65] However, more recent meta-analyses still suggest an increased risk of certain complications with ADM-assisted reconstructions, particularly infection and seroma.[66,67] The significant cost of ADM use must also be considered,[63,68] especially when multiple sheets are needed as with certain prepectoral techniques.

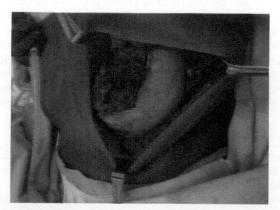

Fig. 5. Intraoperative photograph of dual-plane breast reconstruction with acellular dermal matrix sutured to pectoralis major border.

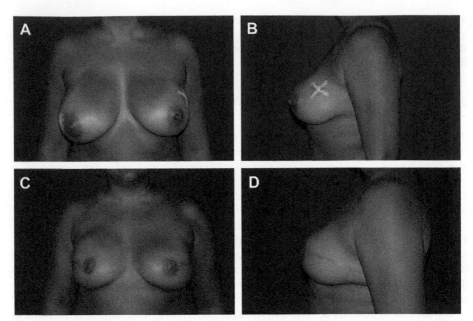

Fig. 6. Implant-based breast reconstruction with dual-plane technique. Preoperative (*A, B*) and postoperative (*C, D*) photos of a 42-year-old woman with staged dual-plane skin-sparing mastectomy with smooth round gel implants: 700 cc on the right and 750 cc on the left.

Synthetic Mesh

The use of synthetic mesh in breast reconstruction has stemmed from an effort to decrease cost associated with biologic support materials. Retrospective series using polyglactin 910 in a dual-plane technique have demonstrated low complication rates[69,70] as well as a cost-benefit compared with ADM-assisted reconstruction.[71] Other types of synthetic mesh such as titanium-coated polypropylene have also been extensively studied[72] and demonstrated to have improved complication profiles to ADM in prospective trials.[73]

Synthetic mesh can also be used in conjunction with ADM to decrease cost. This is particularly useful in prepectoral immediate implant reconstruction that can require multiple sheets of ADM. Techniques include laying of ADM within synthetic mesh along the inferolateral border[74] or splitting ADM and synthetic mesh along the inferior and superior aspects of the implant, respectively (**Fig. 7**).[75] These studies have importantly demonstrated the short-term safety profile of synthetic mesh as well as decreased material costs.[75] Long-term data on capsular contracture will be needed to determine the true utility of synthetic mesh in implant-based reconstruction.

Implant-Based Reconstruction Without Mesh

Since the introduction of biologic and synthetic meshes and the utilization of the prepectoral plane in breast reconstruction, reports of implant placement without support materials have also been described (**Fig. 8**). A recent 10-year series of 250 two-stage prepectoral reconstruction after NSM demonstrated a low short-term complication rate and a 4.0% rate of grade III/IV capsular contracture at an average of 55.5 months of follow-up.[76] The introduction of tabbed tissue expanders and the concept of

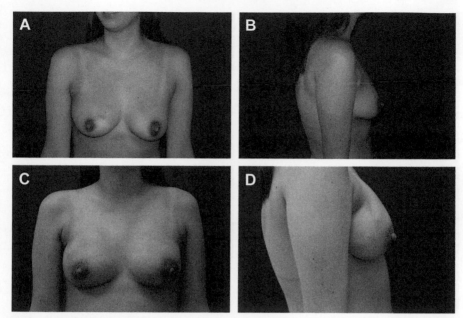

Fig. 7. Immediate implant breast reconstruction in the prepectoral plane with split mesh technique. Preoperative (*A, B*) and postoperative (*C, D*) photos of a 35 year old with right breast cancer and BRCA1 gene mutation who had NSM with prepectoral DTI using ADM and vicryl mesh and highly cohesive 325 mL implants.

mastectomy pocket tailoring has further brought into question the need for ADM solely as means of implant support. Recent comparative studies in two-stage pectoral reconstruction with and without ADM have demonstrated comparable short-term complication rates[77,78] as well as similar esthetic results and patient satisfaction with decreased cost.[78]

Immediate implant reconstruction without mesh support has also been described,[79] though much less frequently, likely due to concerns of implant support and control. The use of adipodermal flaps in wise-pattern skin reduction patterns has been suggested as a means of addressing these issues to offload the weight of the implant and define the pocket.[41,42] Excellent perfusion of the mastectomy flaps with adequate tissue thickness is paramount in such cases, however, to avoid potentially significant complications. A 2021 systematic review of prepectoral reconstruction suggested similar rates of complications between mesh and no-mesh reconstructions, though data were inconclusive given the lack of comparative studies.[80]

Modern Approach to Support Materials

The use of support materials in breast reconstruction has changed significantly over the last 15 years. An initial surge in the use of these materials since their introduction may now be followed by a trend toward more selective usage. This can be attributed to increasing published data on outcomes and complications as well as newer prosthetic devices such as tabbed expanders. Furthermore, in March of 2019, the US FDA Medical Devices Advisory Committee reinforced that surgical mesh, including human-derived ADM, in breast reconstruction was considered nonhomologous use and not cleared or approved by the FDA with a need for further clinical evaluation.[81] This

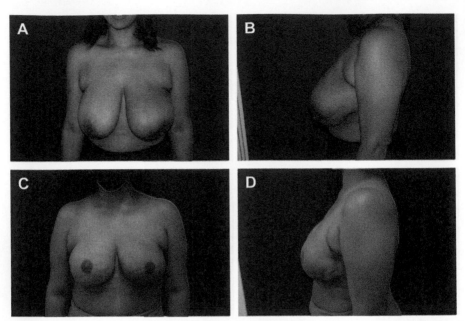

Fig. 8. Two-staged prepectoral breast reconstruction without ADM. Preoperative (*A, B*) and postoperative (*C, D*), photos of a 46 year old with left breast DCIS. The patient underwent skin-sparing mastectomies immediate tissue expander placement in the prepectoral plane without ADM. She subsequently underwent implant exchange to highly cohesive 750 smooth round gel implants. She had nipple reconstruction and tattoos.

has prompted the use of ADM and synthetic mesh in breast reconstruction to fall under further scrutiny.

The modern approach to support materials in implant-based reconstruction requires an individualized protocol for each patient and mastectomy defect. Multiple variables are taken into account including patient desires, NAC preservation, current and desired breast size, and intraoperative mastectomy flap thickness and quality. A spectrum of techniques can then be used based on the particular scenario including (1) total submuscular reconstruction, (2) dual-plane reconstruction with ADM, or (3) prepectoral reconstruction with anterior ADM coverage, combined ADM and synthetic mesh, or no support material.

Total submuscular reconstruction confers the most vascularized prosthesis protection in cases of mastectomy flap viability concern, though some may prefer to delay reconstruction all together if submuscular techniques are not preferred by the surgeon or patient. Dual-plane reconstruction allows for immediate implant placement in thinner patients that may otherwise have undesirable esthetic sequelae of prepectoral implants. The use of support material in prepectoral reconstruction often falls to surgeon preference, particularly with the advent of tabbed tissue expanders,[77] though most reports of prepectoral immediate implant placement use some form of biologic or synthetic mesh for immediate support.[82–85] Eventually, long-term capsular contracture data on prepectoral reconstruction with and without support will be needed. In the end, the ability to comfortably use any of these techniques and appropriately counsel patients on the risks and benefits of each option will afford the plastic surgeon the greatest ability to individualize results and optimize outcomes.

SUMMARY

The modern approach to implant-based breast reconstruction is a synthesis of evolution in surgical techniques, advancement in material technologies and focus on the patient-centered delivery of care through a team-oriented approach. Successful reconstructive outcomes are intimately tied to mastectomy quality in both skin- and nipple-sparing cases which requires close collaboration with the oncologic surgeon. Current implant models offer a wide selection of choices to optimize esthetic outcomes but continue to have inherent risks that must be thoroughly discussed with patients preoperatively. The use of support materials in breast reconstruction, such as ADM, is evolving as modern tabbed expanders may not require the same degree of prosthesis support, though further research is necessary to refine indications. Optimizing outcomes requires knowledge of all current techniques and the flexibility to adapt surgical plans to individualize care for each patient undergoing implant-based breast reconstruction.

CLINICS CARE POINTS

- Successful implant-based reconstruction requires close collaboration between the plastic surgeon and breast surgeon with regard to mastectomy and reconstruction planning.
- Relative mastectomy flap thickness and mastectomy flap quality are critical factors in reconstructive outcomes.
- Inframammary fold Incisions have the lowest complication rates in nipple-sparing mastectomy and immediate implant-based reconstruction.
- Highly cohesive implants may be particularly beneficial in prepectoral reconstruction to minimize rippling and improve upper pole fill at a tradeoff for increased implant firmness
- Acellular dermal matrix-assisted breast reconstruction has demonstrated low rates of capsular contracture but has also been associated with higher rates of infection and seroma. Further research is needed to refine indications and selective use may be warranted.

DISCLOSURE

Dr Karp owns shares in Surgical Innovations Associates.

REFERENCES

1. ASPS National Clearinghouse of Plastic Surgery Procedural Statistics. Plastic surgery statistics report. 2020. Available at: https://www.plasticsurgery.org/documents/News/Statistics/2020/plastic-surgery-statistics-full-report-2020.pdf. Accessed February 20, 2022.
2. Storm-Dickerson T, Sigalove N. Prepectoral breast reconstruction: the breast surgeon's perspective. Plast Reconstr Surg 2017;140(6S Prepectoral Breast Reconstruction):43S–8S.
3. Adam H, Bygdeson M, de Boniface J. The oncological safety of nipple-sparing mastectomy - a Swedish matched cohort study. Eur J Surg Oncol 2014;40(10): 1209–15.
4. Rossi C, Mingozzi M, Curcio A, et al. Nipple areola complex sparing mastectomy. Gland Surg 2015;4(6):528–40.
5. Calobrace MB, Capizzi PJ. The biology and evolution of cohesive gel and shaped implants. Plast Reconstr Surg 2014;134(1 Suppl):6S–11S.

6. Clemens MW, Brody GS, Mahabir RC, et al. How to diagnose and treat breast implant-associated anaplastic large cell lymphoma. Plast Reconstr Surg 2018; 141(4):586e–99e.

7. Rastogi P, Riordan E, Moon D, et al. Theories of etiopathogenesis of breast implant-associated anaplastic large cell lymphoma. Plast Reconstr Surg 2019; 143(3S A Review of Breast Implant-Associated Anaplastic Large Cell Lymphoma):23S–9S.

8. Salzberg CA, Ashikari AY, Koch RM, et al. An 8-year experience of direct-to-implant immediate breast reconstruction using human acellular dermal matrix (AlloDerm). Plast Reconstr Surg 2011;127(2):514–24.

9. Choi M, Frey JD, Alperovich M, et al. Breast in a day": examining single-stage immediate, permanent implant reconstruction in nipple-sparing mastectomy. Plast Reconstr Surg 2016;138(2):184e–91e.

10. Sbitany H. Important considerations for performing prepectoral breast reconstruction. Plast Reconstr Surg 2017;140(6S Prepectoral Breast Reconstruction): 7S–13S.

11. Pfob A, Mehrara BJ, Nelson JA, et al. Towards patient-centered decision-making in breast cancer surgery: machine learning to predict individual patient-reported outcomes at 1-year follow-up. Ann Surg 2021. https://doi.org/10.1097/SLA. 0000000000004862. Online ahead of print.

12. Momoh AO, Griffith KA, Hawley ST, et al. Patterns and correlates of knowledge, communication, and receipt of breast reconstruction in a modern population-based cohort of patients with breast cancer. Plast Reconstr Surg 2019;144(2): 303–13.

13. Lee CN, Ubel PA, Deal AM, et al. How informed is the decision about breast reconstruction after mastectomy?: a prospective, cross-sectional study. Ann Surg 2016;264(6):1103–9.

14. Duncan AM, Al Youha S, Joukhadar N, et al. Anatomy of the breast fascial system: a systematic review of the literature. Plast Reconstr Surg 2022;149(1):28–40.

15. Rehnke RD, Groening RM, Van Buskirk ER, et al. Anatomy of the superficial fascia system of the breast: a comprehensive theory of breast fascial anatomy. Plast Reconstr Surg 2018;142(5):1135–44.

16. Frey JD, Salibian AA, Choi M, et al. Optimizing outcomes in nipple-sparing mastectomy: mastectomy flap thickness is not one size fits all. Plast Reconstr Surg Glob Open 2019;7(1):e2103.

17. Frey JD, Salibian AA, Choi M, et al. Mastectomy flap thickness and complications in nipple-sparing mastectomy: objective evaluation using magnetic resonance imaging. Plast Reconstr Surg Glob Open 2017;5(8):e1439.

18. Frey JD, Salibian AA, Bekisz JM, et al. What is in a number? Evaluating a risk assessment tool in immediate breast reconstruction. Plast Reconstr Surg Glob Open 2019;7(12):e2585.

19. Diep GK, Hui JY, Marmor S, et al. Postmastectomy reconstruction outcomes after intraoperative evaluation with indocyanine green angiography versus clinical assessment. Ann Surg Oncol 2016;23(12):4080–5.

20. Dent BL, Miller JA, Eden DJ, et al. Tumor-to-Nipple distance as a predictor of nipple involvement: expanding the inclusion criteria for nipple-sparing mastectomy. Plast Reconstr Surg 2017;140(1):1e–8e.

21. Wu ZY, Kim HJ, Lee J, et al. Recurrence outcomes after nipple-sparing mastectomy and immediate breast reconstruction in patients with pure ductal carcinoma in situ. Ann Surg Oncol 2020;27(5):1627–35.

22. Frey JD, Salibian AA, Lee J, et al. Oncologic trends, outcomes, and risk factors for locoregional recurrence: an analysis of tumor-to-nipple distance and critical factors in therapeutic nipple-sparing mastectomy. Plast Reconstr Surg 2019; 143(6):1575–85.

23. Daar DA, Abdou SA, Rosario L, et al. Is there a preferred incision location for nipple-sparing mastectomy? A systematic review and meta-analysis. Plast Reconstr Surg 2019;143(5):906e–19e.

24. Munhoz AM, Aldrighi CM, Montag E, et al. Clinical outcomes following nipple-areola-sparing mastectomy with immediate implant-based breast reconstruction: a 12-year experience with an analysis of patient and breast-related factors for complications. Breast Cancer Res Treat 2013;140(3):545–55.

25. Frey JD, Salibian AA, Levine JP, et al. Incision choices in nipple-sparing mastectomy: a comparative analysis of outcomes and evolution of a clinical algorithm. Plast Reconstr Surg 2018;142(6):826e–35e.

26. Colwell AS, Tessler O, Lin AM, et al. Breast reconstruction following nipple-sparing mastectomy: predictors of complications, reconstruction outcomes, and 5-year trends. Plast Reconstr Surg 2014;133(3):496–506.

27. Donovan CA, Harit AP, Chung A, et al. Oncological and surgical outcomes after nipple-sparing mastectomy: do incisions matter? Ann Surg Oncol 2016;23(10): 3226–31.

28. McCarthy CM, Mehrara BJ, Riedel E, et al. Predicting complications following expander/implant breast reconstruction: an outcomes analysis based on preoperative clinical risk. Plast Reconstr Surg 2008;121(6):1886–92.

29. Matsen CB, Mehrara B, Eaton A, et al. Skin flap necrosis after mastectomy with reconstruction: a prospective study. Ann Surg Oncol 2016;23(1):257–64.

30. Frey JD, Salibian AA, Karp NS, et al. Comparing therapeutic versus prophylactic nipple-sparing mastectomy: does indication inform oncologic and reconstructive outcomes? Plast Reconstr Surg 2018;142(2):306–15.

31. Frey JD, Choi M, Salibian AA, et al. Comparison of outcomes with tissue expander, immediate implant, and autologous breast reconstruction in greater than 1000 nipple-sparing mastectomies. Plast Reconstr Surg 2017;139(6): 1300–10.

32. Frey JD, Salibian AA, Choi M, et al. Putting together the pieces: development and validation of a risk-assessment model for nipple-sparing mastectomy. Plast Reconstr Surg 2020;145(2):273e–83e.

33. Naoum GE, Ho AY, Shui A, et al. Risk of developing breast reconstruction complications: a machine-learning nomogram for individualized risk estimation with and without postmastectomy radiation therapy. Plast Reconstr Surg 2022; 149(1):1e–12e.

34. Frey JD, Salibian AA, Karp NS, et al. The impact of mastectomy weight on reconstructive trends and outcomes in nipple-sparing mastectomy: progressively greater complications with larger breast size. Plast Reconstr Surg 2018;141(6): 795e–804e.

35. De Vita R, Zoccali G, Buccheri EM, et al. Outcome evaluation after 2023 nipple-sparing mastectomies: our experience. Plast Reconstr Surg 2017;139(2): 335e–47e.

36. Alperovich M, Tanna N, Samra F, et al. Nipple-sparing mastectomy in patients with a history of reduction mammaplasty or mastopexy: how safe is it? Plast Reconstr Surg 2013;131(5):962–7.

37. Spear SL, Rottman SJ, Seiboth LA, et al. Breast reconstruction using a staged nipple-sparing mastectomy following mastopexy or reduction. Plast Reconstr Surg 2012;129(3):572–81.
38. Salibian AA, Frey JD, Karp NS, et al. Does staged breast reduction before nipple-sparing mastectomy decrease complications? A matched cohort study between staged and nonstaged techniques. Plast Reconstr Surg 2019;144(5):1023–32.
39. Salibian AH, Harness JK, Mowlds DS. Primary buttonhole mastopexy and nipple-sparing mastectomy: a preliminary report. Ann Plast Surg 2016;77(4):388–95.
40. Movassaghi K, Stewart CN. The "smile mastopexy": a novel technique to aesthetically address the excess skin envelope in large, ptotic breasts while preserving nipple areolar complex during prosthetic breast reconstruction. Aesthet Surg J 2022;42(6):NP393–403.
41. Safran T, Al-Halabi B, Viezel-Mathieu A, et al. Skin-reducing mastectomy with immediate prepectoral reconstruction: surgical, aesthetic, and patient-reported outcomes with and without dermal matrices. Plast Reconstr Surg 2021;147(5):1046–57.
42. Mosharrafa AM, Mosharrafa TM, Zannis VJ. Direct-to-Implant breast reconstruction with simultaneous nipple-sparing mastopexy utilizing an inferiorly based adipodermal flap: our experience with prepectoral and subpectoral techniques. Plast Reconstr Surg 2020;145(5):1125–33.
43. Manrique OJ, Banuelos J, Abu-Ghname A, et al. Surgical outcomes of prepectoral versus subpectoral implant-based breast reconstruction in young women. Plast Reconstr Surg Glob Open 2019;7(3):e2119.
44. Aliotta RE, Scomacao I, Duraes EFR, et al. Pushing the envelope: skin-only mastopexy in single-stage nipple-sparing mastectomy with direct-to-implant breast reconstruction. Plast Reconstr Surg 2021;147(1):38–45.
45. Chang EI, Hammond DC. Clinical results on innovation in breast implant design. Plast Reconstr Surg 2018;142(4S The Science of Breast Implants):31S–8S.
46. Salibian AA, Karp NS. Cohesive implants in revisionary breast reconstruction: strategies for optimizing aesthetic outcomes. Ann Breast Surg 2020;4.
47. Ram E, Lavee J, Freimark D, et al. Improved long-term outcomes after heart transplantation utilizing donors with a traumatic mode of brain death. J Cardiothorac Surg 2019;14(1):138.
48. Sbitany H, Lee KR. Optimizing outcomes in 2-stage prepectoral breast reconstruction utilizing round form-stable implants. Plast Reconstr Surg 2019;144(1S Utilizing a Spectrum of Cohesive Implants in Aesthetic and Reconstructive Breast Surgery):43S–50S.
49. Khavanin N, Clemens MW, Pusic AL, et al. Shaped versus round implants in breast reconstruction: a multi-institutional comparison of surgical and patient-reported outcomes. Plast Reconstr Surg 2017;139(5):1063–70.
50. Macadam SA, Ho AL, Lennox PA, et al. Patient-reported satisfaction and health-related quality of life following breast reconstruction: a comparison of shaped cohesive gel and round cohesive gel implant recipients. Plast Reconstr Surg 2013;131(3):431–41.
51. U.S. Food and Drug Administration. Breast implants. 2021. Available at: https://www.fda.gov/medical-devices/implants-and-prosthetics/breast-implants. Accessed March 12, 2022.
52. Vardanian AJ, Clayton JL, Roostaeian J, et al. Comparison of implant-based immediate breast reconstruction with and without acellular dermal matrix. Plast Reconstr Surg 2011;128(5):403e–10e.

53. DeLong MR, Tandon VJ, Farajzadeh M, et al. Systematic review of the impact of acellular dermal matrix on aesthetics and patient satisfaction in tissue expander-to-implant breast reconstructions. Plast Reconstr Surg 2019;144(6):967e–74e.

54. Sbitany H, Sandeen SN, Amalfi AN, et al. Acellular dermis-assisted prosthetic breast reconstruction versus complete submuscular coverage; a head-to-head comparison of outcomes. Plast Reconstr Surg 2009;124(6):1735–40.

55. Sbitany H, Serletti JM. Acellular dermis-assisted prosthetic breast reconstruction: a systematic and critical review of efficacy and associated morbidity. Plast Reconstr Surg 2011;128(6):1162–9.

56. McCarthy CM, Lee CN, Halvorson EG, et al. The use of acellular dermal matrices in two-stage expander/implant reconstruction: a multicenter, blinded, randomized controlled trial. Plast Reconstr Surg 2012;130(5 Suppl 2):57S–66S.

57. Stump A, Holton LH 3rd, Connor J, et al. The use of acellular dermal matrix to prevent capsule formation around implants in a primate model. Plast Reconstr Surg 2009;124(1):82–91.

58. Basu CB, Leong M, Hicks MJ. Acellular cadaveric dermis decreases the inflammatory response in capsule formation in reconstructive breast surgery. Plast Reconstr Surg 2010;126(6):1842–7.

59. Tevlin R, Borrelli MR, Irizarry D, et al. Acellular dermal matrix reduces myofibroblast presence in the breast capsule. Plast Reconstr Surg Glob Open 2019; 7(5):e2213.

60. Nahabedian MY, Glasberg SB, Maxwell GP. Introduction to "prepectoral breast reconstruction. Plast Reconstr Surg 2017;140(6S Prepectoral Breast Reconstruction):4S–5S.

61. Komorowska-Timek E, Oberg KC, Timek TA, et al. The effect of AlloDerm envelopes on periprosthetic capsule formation with and without radiation. Plast Reconstr Surg 2009;123(3):807–16.

62. Sbitany H, Wang F, Peled AW, et al. Immediate implant-based breast reconstruction following total skin-sparing mastectomy: defining the risk of preoperative and postoperative radiation therapy for surgical outcomes. Plast Reconstr Surg 2014; 134(3):396–404.

63. Ivey JS, Abdollahi H, Herrera FA, et al. Total muscle coverage versus AlloDerm human dermal matrix for implant-based breast reconstruction. Plast Reconstr Surg 2019;143(1):1–6.

64. Weichman KE, Wilson SC, Weinstein AL, et al. The use of acellular dermal matrix in immediate two-stage tissue expander breast reconstruction. Plast Reconstr Surg 2012;129(5):1049–58.

65. Weichman KE, Wilson SC, Saadeh PB, et al. Sterile "ready-to-use" AlloDerm decreases postoperative infectious complications in patients undergoing immediate implant-based breast reconstruction with acellular dermal matrix. Plast Reconstr Surg 2013;132(4):725–36.

66. Zhao X, Wu X, Dong J, et al. A meta-analysis of postoperative complications of tissue expander/implant breast reconstruction using acellular dermal matrix. Aesthet Plast Surg 2015;39(6):892–901.

67. Lee KT, Mun GH. Updated evidence of acellular dermal matrix use for implant-based breast reconstruction: a meta-analysis. Ann Surg Oncol 2016;23(2): 600–10.

68. de Blacam C, Momoh AO, Colakoglu S, et al. Cost analysis of implant-based breast reconstruction with acellular dermal matrix. Ann Plast Surg 2012;69(5): 516–20.

69. Haynes DF, Kreithen JC. Vicryl mesh in expander/implant breast reconstruction: long-term follow-up in 38 patients. Plast Reconstr Surg 2014;134(5):892–9.
70. Meyer Ganz O, Tobalem M, Perneger T, et al. Risks and benefits of using an absorbable mesh in one-stage immediate breast reconstruction: a comparative study. Plast Reconstr Surg 2015;135(3):498e–507e.
71. Tessler O, Reish RG, Maman DY, et al. Beyond biologics: absorbable mesh as a low-cost, low-complication sling for implant-based breast reconstruction. Plast Reconstr Surg 2014;133(2):90e–9e.
72. Dieterich M, Paepke S, Zwiefel K, et al. Implant-based breast reconstruction using a titanium-coated polypropylene mesh (TiLOOP Bra): a multicenter study of 231 cases. Plast Reconstr Surg 2013;132(1):8e–19e.
73. Gschwantler-Kaulich D, Schrenk P, Bjelic-Radisic V, et al. Mesh versus acellular dermal matrix in immediate implant-based breast reconstruction - a prospective randomized trial. Eur J Surg Oncol 2016;42(5):665–71.
74. Gfrerer L, Liao EC. Technique refinement in prepectoral implant breast reconstruction with vicryl mesh pocket and acellular dermal matrix support. Plast Reconstr Surg Glob Open 2018;6(4):e1749.
75. Karp NS, Salibian AA. Splitting the difference: using synthetic and biologic mesh to decrease cost in prepectoral immediate implant breast reconstruction. Plast Reconstr Surg 2021;147(3):580–4.
76. Salibian AH, Harness JK, Mowlds DS. Staged suprapectoral expander/implant reconstruction without acellular dermal matrix following nipple-sparing mastectomy. Plast Reconstr Surg 2017;139(1):30–9.
77. Salibian AA, Bekisz JM, Kussie HC, et al. Do we need support in prepectoral breast reconstruction? Comparing outcomes with and without ADM. Plast Reconstr Surg Glob Open 2021;9(8):e3745.
78. Manrique OJ, Huang TC, Martinez-Jorge J, et al. Prepectoral two-stage implant-based breast reconstruction with and without acellular dermal matrix: do we see a difference? Plast Reconstr Surg 2020;145(2):263e–72e.
79. Viezel-Mathieu A, Alnaif N, Aljerian A, et al. Acellular dermal matrix-sparing direct-to-implant prepectoral breast reconstruction: a comparative study including cost analysis. Ann Plast Surg 2020;84(2):139–43.
80. DeLong MR, Tandon VJ, Bertrand AA, et al. Review of outcomes in prepectoral prosthetic breast reconstruction with and without surgical mesh assistance. Plast Reconstr Surg 2021;147(2):305–15.
81. Committee USFaDAGaPSDPotMDA. Available at: https://www.fda.gov/media/122962/download. Accessed February 20, 2022.
82. Jafferbhoy S, Chandarana M, Houlihan M, et al. Early multicentre experience of pre-pectoral implant based immediate breast reconstruction using Braxon((R)). Gland Surg 2017;6(6):682–8.
83. Jones G, Yoo A, King V, et al. Prepectoral immediate direct-to-implant breast reconstruction with anterior AlloDerm coverage. Plast Reconstr Surg 2017;140(6S):31S–8S. Prepectoral Breast Reconstruction).
84. Reitsamer R, Peintinger F. Prepectoral implant placement and complete coverage with porcine acellular dermal matrix: a new technique for direct-to-implant breast reconstruction after nipple-sparing mastectomy. J Plast Reconstr Aesthet Surg 2015;68(2):162–7.
85. Becker H, Lind JG 2nd, Hopkins EG. Immediate implant-based prepectoral breast reconstruction using a vertical incision. Plast Reconstr Surg Glob Open 2015;3(6):e412.

Prepectoral Breast Reconstruction

Francis D. Graziano, MD, Jocelyn Lu, MD, Hani Sbitany, MD*

KEYWORDS

- Prepectoral breast reconstruction • Breast reconstruction • Acellular dermal matrix
- Implant-based reconstruction

KEY POINTS

- Prepectoral breast reconstruction has become a popular method of postmastectomy breast reconstruction due to its numerous benefits in properly selected patients.
- Prepectoral reconstruction, as compared with retropectoral position, provides the benefit of leaving the pectoralis major muscle in its anatomic position, resulting in decreased acute and chronic pain, avoidance of animation deformity, and improved upper extremity strength.
- Careful patient selection and intraoperative mastectomy flap evaluation are critical to obtaining optimal results in prepectoral breast reconstruction.
- Acellular dermal matrices allow for control of the breast envelope and implant position, resulting in high levels of patient satisfaction and esthetic outcomes.

INTRODUCTION

Implant-based reconstruction continues to be the most commonly performed procedure for postmastectomy breast reconstruction in the United States, with over 103,000 cases performed in 2020.[1,2] Traditional methods of submuscular or partial submuscular/partial acellular dermal matrix (ADM) (dual-plane) are still commonly used.[3] Although the submuscular implant reconstruction technique offers the benefit of reliable vascularized coverage, it disrupts the native anatomy of the chest wall. This is due to the elevation and often disinsertion of the pectoralis major muscle during implant pocket creation. Prepectoral breast reconstruction involves placement of the breast implant or tissue expander above the pectoralis and serratus muscles, thus leaving the chest wall muscles in their original positions.[4] The reported benefits of the prepectoral breast reconstruction technique include decreased acute and chronic postoperative pain, avoidance of animation deformity, precise control of the implant pocket, and high levels of patient satisfaction.[5,6] Also, prepectoral reconstruction technique avoids enveloping the implant in the pectoralis muscle, which

This article previously appeared in Clinics in Plastic Surgery volume 50 issue 2 April 2023.
Division of Plastic and Reconstructive Surgery, Department of Surgery, Icahn School of Medicine at Mount Sinai, New York, NY, USA
* Corresponding author. 425 West 59th Street, 7th Floor, New York, NY 10019.
E-mail address: Hani.Sbitany@mountsinai.org

Clinics Collections 14 (2024) 391–401
https://doi.org/10.1016/j.ccol.2024.02.022
2352-7986/24/© 2024 Elsevier Inc. All rights reserved.

can become fibrotic and tight, especially in the setting of postmastectomy radiation.[7] The fibrotic pectoralis muscle can cause translational force on the implant leading to malposition and capsular contracture.[7] As the prosthesis is placed closer to the skin with less vascularized soft tissue coverage, it is critical for the surgeon to assess preoperative and perioperative factors to ensure optimal outcomes. Through proper patient selection and ideal surgical technique, prepectoral breast reconstruction can be performed with high esthetic and patient satisfaction while also minimizing patient morbidity.

PREOPERATIVE CONSIDERATIONS
Patient Selection

As with any operation, patient selection is critical for optimal results. A full assessment of the patient's past medical and surgical history should be performed with particular attention to conditions that can affect wound healing and mastectomy vascular supply. Conditions that can impair mastectomy flap perfusion include peripheral vascular disease, diabetes, preoperative radiation, smoking, and obesity. Conditions that may cause delayed wound healing include immunosuppression, steroid use, and connective tissue disorders (ie, Ehlers-Danlos). Poorly controlled diabetes (hemoglobin A1c > 7.0), obesity (body mass index [BMI] greater than 35), and active/recent smoking are considered contraindications to prepectoral breast reconstruction and are associated with an increased risk of mastectomy flap necrosis and implant infection or extrusion.[8]

Although prepectoral breast reconstruction is typically used in the immediate setting after mastectomy, prepectoral technique can also be considered in a delayed fashion. Most commonly, this is seen in the group of patients who underwent a prior mastectomy and submuscular implant reconstruction, and now present with complaints of chronic pain, capsular contracture, and/or animation deformity. In these patients, the implant can be converted from subpectoral to prepectoral position, often with the aid of ADM for implant support. These patients largely have immediate relief of animation deformity and improved pain.[6] Lastly, patients who underwent no reconstruction at the time of mastectomy can be candidates for prepectoral reconstruction. In this group of patients, the mastectomy flaps have undergone the delay phenomena, and therefore raising these mastectomy flaps with placement of prepectoral tissue expander or implant can be performed relatively reliably.

Radiation status
Another important consideration is the radiation status of the patient. Patients who underwent preoperative radiation therapy have an increased risk of dehiscence and wound healing complications due to impaired microcirculation.[9] In our opinion, these patients typically benefit from autologous rather than prepectoral implant-based reconstruction. However, in contrast, patients who are planning to receive postmastectomy radiation therapy (PMRT) can be considered for prepectoral breast reconstruction. Although rates of complications are increased in patients who undergo PMRT after prepectoral reconstruction, they are similar to complication rates in patients undergoing submuscular implant reconstruction with PMRT.[10,11] In fact, some authors have suggested that prepectoral breast reconstruction in the setting of PMRT significantly decreases the rate of capsular contracture and implant migration when compared with submuscular reconstruction.[12,13] As such, prepectoral breast reconstruction can be considered in this subset of patients who require PMRT, as prepectoral reconstruction allows for potentially more predictable esthetic outcomes following radiation.

Oncologic considerations

In addition to assessing patient-specific comorbidities, oncologic considerations should be analyzed preoperatively. From a tumor-specific standpoint, patients with tumors that invade the chest wall fascia or come within 0.5 cm of the chest wall are contraindicated for prepectoral breast reconstruction.[14] Given the location of the tumor, these patients have a higher chance of chest wall recurrence.[15] If prepectoral reconstruction was to be performed in patients with chest wall tumors, recurrence would be difficult to detect due to the overlying breast implant. Therefore, patients with chest wall tumors or tumors within 0.5 cm of the chest wall should be considered for submuscular reconstruction. Submuscular implant-based reconstruction allows for the chest wall to be more easily palpated by self-exam or on clinical exam.

Additional oncologic considerations include inflammatory breast cancer, patients with stage IV breast cancer, or patients with the aggressive axillary disease. These disease processes are relative contraindications to prepectoral breast reconstruction given their needs for aggressive adjuvant therapy.[16] Lastly, although not a contraindication to prepectoral breast reconstruction, superficial tumors can lead to varying amounts of skin resection, which can lead to distortion of the mastectomy skin envelope and subsequent abnormal implant positioning. Planned skin pattern resection and resultant esthetic outcomes should be discussed with the patient preoperatively to set expectations.

Infection control

Special attention should be given to preventing postoperative infections in prepectoral breast reconstruction. Without vascularized muscle coverage over the implant, postoperative infection can threaten implant loss. Patients should have nasal swabs for Methicillin-resistant *Staphylococcus aureus* (MRSA), and if positive, topical mupirocin is recommended for decolonization.[17] All patients, regardless of MRSA status, are recommended to perform Hibilcens showers the night before surgery. On the day of surgery, intravenous Ancef (or Clindamycin for patients with allergies) should be injected within 60 minutes of incision to decrease the rate of surgical site infections.

INTRAOPERATIVE TECHNIQUES
Intraoperative Mastectomy Flap Assessment

It is critical to examine the soft tissue of the mastectomy skin following completion of the mastectomy before proceeding with prepectoral reconstruction. Mastectomy flaps must be assessed for adequate perfusion and viability. This process starts with a clinical examination of the mastectomy, assessing for dermal bleeding at the mastectomy flap margin and the presence of subcutaneous tissue along the underside of the mastectomy flap. Presence of subcutaneous tissue on the mastectomy flap indicates the preservation of the subdermal plexus, and is more likely to be well perfused. Areas with exposed dermis on the underside require caution and careful clinical consideration, depending on the area. If near the mastectomy flap margin then the authors opt to excise these portions. However, if areas of exposed dermis are not easily amenable to excision, then the authors typically prefer to delay the reconstruction to allow for the mastectomy flaps to revascularize and recover. Delayed prepectoral breast reconstruction can then take place typically at a minimum of 3 weeks after the mastectomy. Another option in the setting of exposed dermis on the underside of the skin flap is subpectoral reconstruction if this is deemed safe and aligns with the patient's goals.

Although thicker mastectomy flaps can often signify improved vascularity, thin flaps do not necessarily mean a poorly perfused flap. Patients with thinner body habitus and lower BMI often have a thinner layer of subcutaneous tissue before the breast capsule.[18] Therefore, in this patient population, thin mastectomy flaps are expected and often have adequate perfusion.

In cases where patients have thin but viable mastectomy flaps, the senior author suggests performing two-stage breast reconstruction with tissue expanders. In these cases, tissue expanders are placed with minimal to no fill, therefore decreasing the amount of tension and stretch on the skin. This can result in less venous congestion relative to aggressive tissue expander fill or large direct to implant placement.[19]

In addition, perfusion assessment devices can provide useful information regarding mastectomy skin flap perfusion.[20–22] Most commonly used perfusion devices often use indocyanine green angiography and allow for real-time assessment of mastectomy flap perfusion. These devices allow for the assessment of nonviable areas which allows for direct excision at the time of immediate reconstruction.[23] The perfusion data can also be used to inform the decision to proceed with either prepectoral or subpectoral reconstruction. These devices can be useful adjuncts to clinical examination.

Acellular Dermal Matrices Use

Proper utilization of ADMs for implant support and breast pocket control has become an essential aspect of successful prepectoral breast reconstruction.[24] Advocates for using ADM in prepectoral reconstruction cite higher rates of implant exposure and capsular contracture in cases where implants are placed subcutaneously without ADM support.[25] The advent of ADM use has made prepectoral breast reconstruction safer with a decreased inflammatory response to implant placement, thus improving esthetic results.[26] Prior studies have shown that prepectoral breast reconstruction with ADM is equally safe as subpectoral reconstruction.[27,28]

Various ADM products exist on the market with different qualities including meshing and thickness. The senior author of this study prefers thin ADM for prepectoral reconstruction due to improved engraftment with the mastectomy skin flaps. Studies have found that the use of thicker ADMs can lead to higher rates of seroma, longer need for drains, and decreased rates of engraftment.[29,30] For this reason, we recommend using ADM sheets with a maximal thickness of 2 mm, or thinner, for soft tissue support in prepectoral reconstruction.

ADM allows for precise control of the boundaries of the reconstruction and therefore it is critical to identify anatomic borders of the breast. Although it is the breast surgeon's primary objective to provide oncologic safety, it can be common for the breast surgeon to remove soft tissue beyond the borders of the breast. In these cases, it is important to use preoperative markings along with manual palpation to identify the original inframammary fold (IMF), medial, lateral, and superior borders of the breast. After borders of the breast have been identified, then ADM can be used to reestablish these borders of the reconstructed breast.

ADM is used to cover the entire anterior surface and varying amounts of the posterior surface based on the surgeon's preferred technique.[31–33] The senior author recommends using a two-layer cuff technique at the inferior aspect of the implant to bolster the recreated IMF (**Fig. 1**). This technique is performed by placing the most inferior portion of the ADM posterior to the inferior aspect of the implant and suturing the ADM to the chest wall. Then as the ADM transitions from the posterior to the anterior aspect of the implant, the most inferior portion of the sling is sutured to the chest wall. This double cuff at the IMF helps ensure long-term support at the IMF and decreases the risk of implant descent.[8] In the case of nipple-sparing mastectomy through an inframammary approach, the superior and lateral/medial aspects of the ADM are inset in place, followed by implant placement and two-layer cuff creation (**Figs. 2–6**). In the case of skin-sparing mastectomy, the two-layer cuff is created first,

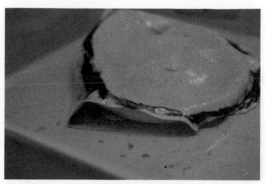

Fig. 1. Senior author's preferred method of ADM inset for anterior implant coverage, showing the two-layer cuff technique at the inferior aspect of the implant.

then the lateral, medial, and superior borders of the ADM are fixated in place after implant placement. In both ADM inset techniques, the whole anterior aspect of the implant is covered with ADM. ADM inset allows for precise control of the reconstructed breast pocket and can result in long-term esthetic results (**Fig. 7**A and B).

Larger amounts of ADM are used in prepectoral reconstruction when compared with dual-plane reconstruction. This is of particular importance as ADM has been found to have higher rates of seroma postoperatively.[34,35] Consideration must be given to proper drain management to prevent seromas and allow for incorporation of ADM with surrounding soft tissues. The senior recommends leaving at least one drain in place for 2 to 3 weeks. In the case of larger breasts, two drains can be placed, one drain in the potential space between the mastectomy flap and the ADM and one drain in the breast pocket. It may be beneficial to use ADM with fenestrations to allow for fluid egress and prevention of seroma formation.[36]

Preventing and Addressing Postoperative Rippling

An issue that can arise postoperatively in implant-based reconstruction is the occurrence of rippling.[37] This can be an issue in prepectoral reconstruction, where the upper pole cannot be buffered underneath the pectoralis muscle. Placement of ADM itself can help provide additional soft tissue coverage and potentially prevent implant rippling, especially in low BMI patients with thin mastectomy flaps.[38] The senior author has three main techniques to both address and prevent implant rippling. First, in the setting of

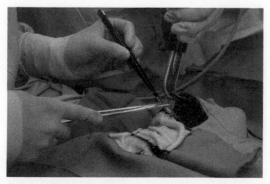

Fig. 2. Superior, medial, and lateral aspects of the ADM are inset first in the case of a nipple sparing mastectomy.

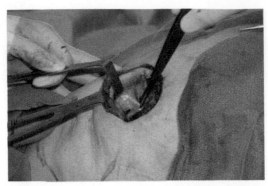

Fig. 3. After the implant is placed in the ADM pocket, the two-layer cuff is created by placing the most inferior portion of the ADM posterior to the inferior aspect of the implant and suturing the ADM to the chest wall. Roughly a 2 to 3 cm cuff of ADM is placed posterior to the implant.

two-stage breast reconstruction, it is advisable to underfill the tissue expander relative to the anticipated final implant size. In the senior author's practice, the final volume of the tissue expander is, on average, 150 to 200 cc less than the estimated implant volume. This technique is performed so that the permanent implant is placed in a tight breast envelope, therefore minimizing rippling in the final reconstruction.

Second, implant selection with regard to implant cohesivity and base width is critical for preventing implant rippling. The senior author's preference is to use a smooth, round, filled to capacity silicone implant with high cohesivity. High-capacity fill decreases the amount of rippling on the implant surface which translates to decrease visible rippling externally in the final reconstruction. It is also important to select an implant with a base width that closely matches the base width dimension of the ADM pocket. Implants that have base widths that are narrower than the ADM base width pocket are more susceptible to rippling. Choosing an implant with high cohesivity can also mitigate the potential for postoperative rippling.

Third and lastly, fat grafting can be used as an adjunctive procedure in prepectoral breast reconstruction. Fat grafting can help increase mastectomy flap thickness, especially in the upper pole, and subsequently decrease visible rippling.[39,40] This technique also has the benefit of improving upper pole contour, which may be an issue in prepectoral reconstruction. As the pectoralis muscle is not draping over the superior aspect of the implant, patients can develop an abrupt, unnatural transition from the

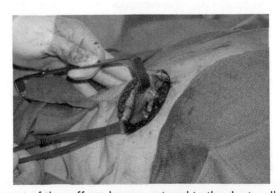

Fig. 4. Superior aspect of the cuff can be seen sutured to the chest wall.

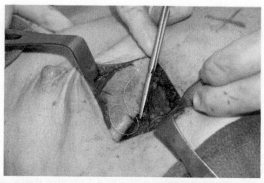

Fig. 5. Most inferior aspect of the ADM is then sutured in place.

chest wall to implant. Fat grafting to the area can improve this transition between the chest wall and implant while also reducing any rippling that may be present. In the senior author's experience, fat grafting can typically be performed at the time of tissue expander to implant exchange. These three techniques can be used to both prevent and address potential postoperative rippling in prepectoral reconstruction.

POSTOPERATIVE CONSIDERATIONS AND COMPLICATIONS
Postoperative Dressings

Postoperative dressings are typically based on surgeon preference. The senior author recommends reinforcing the skin closure with a water-tight dressing, either surgical skin glue or steri-strips. This can be further reinforced with a nonadherent gauze bandage and semiocclusive dressing. Drain site dressings have been a topic of debate, with a recent study showing no decrease in infectious complications in immediate tissue expander reconstruction with use of Biopatch drain cover (Ethicon, Somerville, NJ).[41] Whether to use a drain dressing or not is a surgeon-dependent issue.

Infections

As with any implant-based reconstruction, surgical site infections require immediate attention. This is especially true in prepectoral breast reconstruction. With no pectoralis muscle, any breakdown of the skin can lead to ADM and implant exposure. Patients with suspected surgical site infections should be given oral antibiotics and followed closely as an outpatient. If a patient develops any systematic symptoms or

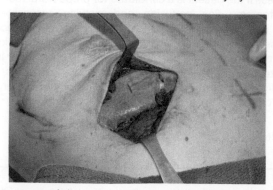

Fig. 6. Most inferior aspect of the ADM can been seen sutured to chest wall. At this point, the ADM is fully inset to the chest wall.

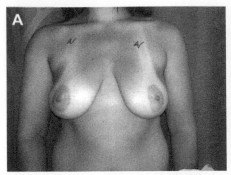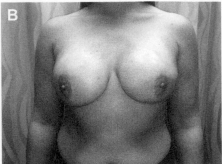

Fig. 7. (*A*) A 38-year-old woman presented with BRCA 1 positive status, and made a decision to undergo bilateral nipple-sparing mastectomies. She desired a large size postoperatively, and thus underwent bilateral prepectoral tissue expander placement. Mastectomies were done through an inframammary approach, and with a wedge excision of lower pole skin to alleviate her pseudoptosis in each breast. At the second stage, the expanders were exchanged for round cohesive silicone gel implants. (*B*) At 2 years postoperatively, she maintains a stable, soft breast reconstruction on each side.

has signs of a threatened implant exposure then the patient requires immediate surgical debridement, threatened skin excision, implant exchange, and intravenous antibiotics. It is critical to treat possible implant infections early and aggressively due to the risk of biofilm formation. Biofilms are difficult to eradicate and often lead to persistent infections, even with long-term intravenous antibiotic use. Prior studies have shown infection rates for implant-based reconstruction to range between 10% and 15% after two-stage reconstruction and direct to implant; however, no differences in infection rate were seen between prepectoral and subpectoral reconstruction.[42,43]

SUMMARY

Prepectoral breast reconstruction has become a popular technique for postmastectomy breast reconstruction due to its numerous benefits. Prepectoral reconstruction provides the benefit of decreased acute and chronic pain, avoidance of animation deformity, improved upper extremity strength, high patient satisfaction, and esthetic outcomes. Preoperatively, patient selection is key to minimize the risk of postoperative complications and optimize outcomes. Oncologic factors should be considered preoperatively to assess if the patient is a candidate for prepectoral reconstruction. Intraoperatively, mastectomy flap perfusion and viability assessment with clinical examination and perfusion devices are critical for successful reconstructive outcomes. ADM is used to re-establish natural breast borders, provide long-term implant support and minimize capsular contracture. Fat grafting and proper implant selection can help minimize or prevent rippling. Reconstructive surgeons should critically assess preoperative patient characteristics and intraoperative surgical techniques to obtain optimal outcomes in prepectoral breast reconstruction.

CLINICS CARE POINTS

Pearls:
- Intraoperative mastectomy skin flap assessment is crucial for successful outcomes. Both clinical examination (assessing for dermal bleeding at skin edges, presence of

subcutaneous tissue present on the underside of the mastectomy flap) and indocyanine green angiography perfusion devices can help determine the viability of the skin flaps.

- ADM provides an important adjunctive role in recreating the breast borders, allowing for precise control of the breast pocket while also providing long-term support of the implant. It is important to use drains and to leave them in place for 2 to 3 weeks to minimize the potential for seroma formation.

Pitfalls:

- Do not perform prepectoral breast reconstruction in patients with preoperative radiation therapy, recent/active smoking, uncontrolled diabetes (hemoglobin A1c > 7), or obesity (BMI > 35). However, patients who are receiving PMRT can be considered for prepectoral reconstruction.
- Patients with tumors that invade the chest wall or are within 5 mm of the chest wall are not candidates for prepectoral breast reconstruction.
- If performing two-stage reconstruction, do not fill the tissue expander to the same size as the intended final implant as this can lead to postoperative rippling. Instead aim to fill to 150 to 200 cc less than the planned permanent implant size.

FINANCIAL DISCLOSURE STATEMENT

Dr Sbitany is a consultant for Allergan, Inc. He received no compensation or support for this article. The remaining authors have no disclosures related to the content of this article.

REFERENCES

1. American Society of Plastic Surgeons. 2020 plastic surgery procedural statistics. https://www.plasticsurgery.org/documents/News/Statistics/2020/plastic-surgery-statistics-full-report-2020.pdf. [Accessed 27 July 2022].
2. Sbitany H, Amalfi AN, Langstein HN. Preferences in choosing between breast reconstruction options: a survey of female plastic surgeons. Plast Reconstr Surg 2009;124(6):1781–9.
3. Wang F, Peled AW, Garwood E, et al. Total skin-sparing mastectomy and immediate breast reconstruction: an evolution of technique and assessment of outcomes. Ann Surg Oncol 2014;21(10):3223–30.
4. Becker H, Lind JG 2nd, Hopkins EG. Immediate implant-based prepectoral breast reconstruction using a vertical incision. Plast Reconstr Surg Glob Open 2015;3(6):e412.
5. Sigalove S, Maxwell GP, Sigalove NM, et al. Prepectoral implant-based breast reconstruction: rationale, indications, and preliminary results. Plast Reconstr Surg 2017;139(2):287–94.
6. Sbitany H, Piper M, Lentz R. Prepectoral breast reconstruction: a safe alternative to submuscular prosthetic reconstruction following nipple-sparing mastectomy. Plast Reconstr Surg 2017;140(3):432–43.
7. Srinivasa DR, Holland M, Sbitany H. Optimizing perioperative strategies to maximize success with prepectoral breast reconstruction. Gland Surg 2019;8(1):19–26.
8. Sbitany H. Important considerations for performing prepectoral breast reconstruction. Plast Reconstr Surg 2017;140(6S Prepectoral Breast Reconstruction):7s–13s.
9. Bettinger LN, Waters LM, Reese SW, et al. Comparative study of prepectoral and subpectoral expander-based breast reconstruction and clavien IIIb score outcomes. Plast Reconstr Surg Glob Open 2017;5(7):e1433.

10. Graziano FD, Shay PL, Sanati-Mehrizy P, et al. Prepectoral implant reconstruction in the setting of post- mastectomy radiation. Gland Surg 2020;10(1):411–6.
11. Sbitany H, Gomez-Sanchez C, Piper M, et al. Prepectoral breast reconstruction in the setting of postmastectomy radiation therapy: an assessment of clinical outcomes and benefits. Plast Reconstr Surg 2019;143(1):10–20.
12. Sigalove S. Prepectoral breast reconstruction and radiotherapy-a closer look. Gland Surg 2019;8(1):67–74.
13. Sinnott CJ, Persing SM, Pronovost M, et al. Impact of postmastectomy radiation therapy in prepectoral versus subpectoral implant-based breast reconstruction. Ann Surg Oncol 2018;25(10):2899–908.
14. Vidya R, Berna G, Sbitany H, et al. Prepectoral implant-based breast reconstruction: a joint consensus guide from UK, European and USA breast and plastic reconstructive surgeons. Ecancermedicalscience 2019;13:927.
15. Buchanan CL, Dorn PL, Fey J, et al. Locoregional recurrence after mastectomy: incidence and outcomes. J Am Coll Surg 2006;203(4):469–74.
16. Mohamed MM, Al-Raawi D, Sabet SF, et al. Inflammatory breast cancer: new factors contribute to disease etiology: a review. J Adv Res 2014;5(5):525–36.
17. Hart A, Desai K, Yoo J, et al. Incidence of methicillin-resistant staphylococcus aureus (MRSA) carrier status in patients undergoing post-mastectomy breast reconstruction. Aesthet Surg J 2017;37(1):35–43.
18. Robertson SA, Rusby JE, Cutress RI. Determinants of optimal mastectomy skin flap thickness. Br J Surg 2014;101(8):899–911.
19. Sbitany H, Wang F, Peled AW, et al. Tissue expander reconstruction after total skin-sparing mastectomy: defining the effects of coverage technique on nipple/areola preservation. Ann Plast Surg 2016;77(1):17–24.
20. Phillips BT, Lanier ST, Conkling N, et al. Intraoperative perfusion techniques can accurately predict mastectomy skin flap necrosis in breast reconstruction: results of a prospective trial. Plast Reconstr Surg 2012;129(5):778e–88e.
21. Mazdeyasna S, Huang C, Bonaroti AR, et al. Intraoperative optical and fluorescence imaging of blood flow distributions in mastectomy skin flaps for identifying ischemic tissues. Plast Reconstr Surg 2022;150(2):282–7.
22. Pruimboom T, Schols RM, Van Kuijk SM, et al. Indocyanine green angiography for preventing postoperative mastectomy skin flap necrosis in immediate breast reconstruction. Cochrane Database Syst Rev 2020;4(4):Cd013280.
23. Mattison GL, Lewis PG, Gupta SC, et al. SPY imaging use in postmastectomy breast reconstruction patients: preventative or overly conservative? Plast Reconstr Surg 2016;138(1):15e–21e.
24. Johnson AC, Colakoglu S, Siddikoglu D, et al. Impact of dermal matrix brand in implant-based breast reconstruction outcomes. Plast Reconstr Surg 2022;150(1):17–25.
25. Snyderman RK, Guthrie RH. Reconstruction of the female breast following radical mastectomy. Plast Reconstr Surg 1971;47(6):565–7.
26. Basu CB, Jeffers L. The role of acellular dermal matrices in capsular contracture: a review of the evidence. Plast Reconstr Surg 2012;130(5 Suppl 2):118s–24s.
27. Sbitany H, Sandeen SN, Amalfi AN, et al. Acellular dermis-assisted prosthetic breast reconstruction versus complete submuscular coverage: a head-to-head comparison of outcomes. Plast Reconstr Surg 2009;124(6):1735–40.
28. Colwell AS, Damjanovic B, Zahedi B, et al. Retrospective review of 331 consecutive immediate single-stage implant reconstructions with acellular dermal matrix: indications, complications, trends, and costs. Plast Reconstr Surg 2011;128(6):1170–8.

29. Rose JF, Zafar SN, Ellsworth Iv WA. Does acellular dermal matrix thickness affect complication rate in tissue expander based breast reconstruction? Plast Surg Int 2016;2016:2867097.

30. Hur J, Han HH. Outcome assessment according to the thickness and direction of the acellular dermal matrix after implant-based breast reconstruction. Biomed Res Int 2021;2021:8101009.

31. Gui G, Gui M, Gui A, et al. Physical characteristics of surgimend meshed biological ADM in immediate prepectoral implant breast reconstruction. Plast Reconstr Surg Glob Open 2022;10(6):e4369.

32. Tierney BP, De La Garza M, Jennings GR, et al. Clinical outcomes of acellular dermal matrix (simpliderm and alloderm ready-to-use) in immediate breast reconstruction. Cureus 2022;14(2):e22371.

33. Khan A, Tasoulis MK, Teoh V, et al. Pre-pectoral one-stage breast reconstruction with anterior biological acellular dermal matrix coverage. Gland Surg 2021;10(3):1002–9.

34. Ho G, Nguyen TJ, Shahabi A, et al. A systematic review and meta-analysis of complications associated with acellular dermal matrix-assisted breast reconstruction. Ann Plast Surg 2012;68(4):346–56.

35. Lee KT, Mun GH. A meta-analysis of studies comparing outcomes of diverse acellular dermal matrices for implant-based breast reconstruction. Ann Plast Surg 2017;79(1):115–23.

36. Maisel Lotan A, Ben Yehuda D, Allweis TM, et al. Comparative study of meshed and nonmeshed acellular dermal matrix in immediate breast reconstruction. Plast Reconstr Surg 2019;144(5):1045–53.

37. Safran T, Al-Badarin F, Al-Halabi B, et al. Aesthetic limitations in direct-to-implant prepectoral breast reconstruction. Plast Reconstr Surg 2022;150(1):22e–31e.

38. Nahabedian MY, Glasberg SB, Maxwell GP. Introduction to "prepectoral breast reconstruction". Plast Reconstr Surg 2017;140(6S Prepectoral Breast Reconstruction):4s–5s.

39. Spear SL, Coles CN, Leung BK, et al. The safety, effectiveness, and efficiency of autologous fat grafting in breast surgery. Plast Reconstr Surg Glob Open 2016;4(8):e827.

40. Goodreau AM, Driscoll CR, Nye A, et al. Revising prepectoral breast reconstruction. Plast Reconstr Surg 2022;149(3):579–84.

41. Weichman KE, Clavin NW, Miller HC, et al. Does the use of biopatch devices at drain sites reduce perioperative infectious complications in patients undergoing immediate tissue expander breast reconstruction? Plast Reconstr Surg 2015;135(1):9e–17e.

42. Baker BG, Irri R, MacCallum V, et al. A prospective comparison of short-term outcomes of subpectoral and prepectoral strattice-based immediate breast reconstruction. Plast Reconstr Surg 2018;141(5):1077–84.

43. Bennett KG, Qi J, Kim HM, et al. Comparison of 2-year complication rates among common techniques for postmastectomy breast reconstruction. JAMA Surg 2018;153(10):901–8.

Modern Approaches to Pedicled Latissimus Dorsi Flap Breast Reconstruction with Immediate Fat Transfer

Salma A. Abdou, MD, Karina Charipova, MD,
David H. Song, MD, MBA*

KEYWORDS

- Autologous breast reconstruction • Latissimus dorsi pedicled flap • Fat grafting
- Lipotransfer

KEY POINTS

- One of the main limitations of the latissimus dorsi pedicled flap for breast reconstruction is insufficient volume. This often requires supplementation with an implant, predisposing patients to risks inherent to introducing a prosthesis that includes implant exposure, capsular contracture, infection, and need for reoperation.
- The latissimus dorsi flap with immediate fat transfer (LIFT) offers a single-stage breast reconstruction with high-volume fat transfer to provide sufficient volume with the patient's own tissue.
- The LIFT procedure is a viable breast reconstruction option for patients who desire autologous breast reconstruction but are not candidates for free tissue transfer, as well as a salvage option for women in whom a prior reconstruction has failed or produced unsatisfactory outcomes.

INTRODUCTION

Several studies have shown that autologous breast reconstruction provides superior esthetic and patient-reported outcomes as compared with implant-based reconstruction.[1-3] Analysis of breast questionnaire (BREAST-Q) responses of over 2,000 women showed that at 2-year follow-up, women who underwent autologous reconstruction were more satisfied with their reconstructive outcome and had better psychosocial

This article previously appeared in *Clinics in Plastic Surgery* volume 50 issue 2 April 2023.
Department of Plastic Surgery, MedStar Plastic and Reconstructive Surgery, Washington, DC, USA
* Corresponding author. 3800 Reservoir Road Northwest, PHC Building First Floor, Washington, DC 20007.
E-mail address: David.H.Song@medstar.net

Clinics Collections 14 (2024) 403–413
https://doi.org/10.1016/j.ccol.2024.02.023
2352-7986/24/Published by Elsevier Inc.

and sexual well-being than those who underwent implant-based reconstruction.[1] Furthermore, total 2-year health care costs associated with autologous reconstruction have also been shown to be lower than those of implant-based surgery despite the lower index cost of implant-based reconstruction.[3] Microsurgical abdominal-based free flaps are considered the gold standard for autologous breast reconstruction; however, not all patients are candidates (eg, patients with significant comorbidities that preclude them from prolonged anesthesia, history of abdominoplasty, or inadequate donor site volume). If this is the case in a patient who desires autologous breast reconstruction, the pedicled latissimus dorsi (LD) flap is commonly used as an alternative.

One of the main limitations of the LD pedicled flap for breast reconstruction is insufficient volume.[4] A variation of the LD flap, the extended LD flap, initially described by Hokin in 1983, sought to address this by incorporating lumbar fat extensions.[5] The extended LD flap has since evolved to include the parascapular and scapula "fat fascia."[5] Although they address the issue of insufficient volume, these technical modifications have had limited applications due to risk of increased donor site morbidity, which largely include increased seroma rates, wound dehiscence, and contour deformity.[5]

The use of an implant to supplement LD flap reconstruction is a popular breast reconstruction modality, but brings with it additional risk factors, including infection, extrusion, capsular contracture, and need for exchange in the future.[6,7] In a study of late results of LD flap with implant reconstruction at 10-year follow-up, 50% of patients required late reoperation for revision or removal of the implant with a total failure rate of 10%, reflecting those patients who required definitive implant removal.[6] Within the same study, formal measurements of breast position, patient questionnaires, and photographic assessments indicated that symmetry and overall esthetic outcomes of LD flap and implant reconstruction trended toward poor, suggesting that even those patients for whom surgery is successful are dissatisfied and frequently seek further revision with fat grafting to improve volume and contour.[6,8,9] Fat grafting as a method of augmenting volume in patients with prior LD flap reconstruction has been shown to significantly improve patient satisfaction (ie, 20% satisfied and 80% very satisfied) with minimal complications (eg, minor local infection, fat necrosis).[9]

Although the majority of the existing literature has focused on the use of lipotransfer as a secondary revision procedure following both autologous and implant-based reconstruction, fat grafting as the primary modality for volume enhancement of the LD flap at the time of reconstruction (LD and immediate fat transfer, ie, latissimus dorsi flap with immediate fat transfer [LIFT]) has been recently introduced as a viable option to address the volume limitations of the LD flap.[8,9] This approach not only mitigates many of the historical issues seen with the use of a prosthesis, but also allows for a single-stage reconstruction using all the patient's own tissue, making it a highly valuable technique in the plastic surgeon's armamentarium for breast reconstruction. Importantly, the LIFT procedure can also be offered to patients as a salvage option after either failed microsurgical or implant-based reconstructive efforts.

PATIENT SELECTION AND PREOPERATIVE COUNSELING

Several factors and patient characteristics must be considered during the initial discussion of and evaluation for autologous breast reconstruction including oncologic treatment plan, medical comorbidities, current breast volume/contour, body habitus, reconstructive goals, and patient preference. The abdomen is frequently the preferred donor site in microsurgical autologous reconstruction. Several abdominal-based free flaps for breast reconstruction have been described, which differ in the amount of abdominal muscle incorporated, for example, muscle-sparing transverse rectus abdominis flap (MS-TRAM), and deep inferior epigastric perforator (DIEP) flap. However, eligible patients must have sufficient abdominal fat to create the desired breast size. Furthermore, patients with a history of abdominal surgery that may have damaged or sacrificed source vessels, angiosomes, and perforators may not be eligible.[10,11] Patient comorbidities, including hypercoagulable state and tobacco use, must be considered before surgery and patients must be advised accordingly. A candid conversation should be had with each patient and her support system regarding complications to set expectations early. Patients should be made aware that certain comorbidities, such as hypercoagulable state, diabetes mellitus, and obesity inherently predispose them to increased risk of specific complications (eg, microvascular failure, delayed wound healing, infection). When discussing various options for autologous reconstruction, flap- and donor site-specific complications should also be noted given, for instance, the known associations between abdominal flaps and hernia risk (0% to 10%) and LD flaps and seroma formation (5% to 25%).[10]

When the patient desires autologous breast reconstruction, we offer the LIFT procedure in addition to the gold standard option of microsurgical reconstruction. The LIFT is preferred for patients who cannot safely receive prolonged anesthesia, have hypercoagulable disorders, or have a history of previous abdominal surgery, which makes their inferior epigastric system unreliable (**Box 1**). We do offer it as a fully autologous alternative with faster recovery, less anesthesia time, and no flap monitoring.[10,11] There exists a single study comparing the LIFT to abdominally based microsurgical breast reconstruction.[12] Patients who undergo the LIFT procedure for breast reconstruction have significantly shorter operative times and significantly shorter lengths of hospital stay than microsurgical breast reconstruction.

SURGICAL TECHNIQUE
Preoperative Markings

The LD flap is marked over the thoracolumbar fat pad with the patient upright in the preoperative area, considering patient preferences regarding the esthetic position of donor-site scars. Care is taken to orient the skin paddle along the natural creases of the back while allowing a gentle arch of rotation at the time of flap inset. The pinch test confirms no undue tension with closure of the donor site. Fat harvest sites vary

---

Box 1
Indications for a latissimus flap with immediate fat transfer (LIFT)

Indications for LIFT
- Patient desires autologous reconstruction
- Patient is a poor microvascular reconstruction candidate due to comorbidities (active smoking, hypercoagulable state, and obesity)
- Patient cannot undergo prolonged anesthesia
- Patient does not have alternative donor sites due to lack of adequate volume or previous surgery (eg, abdominal liposuction)
- Patient desires reduced recovery time and hospital length of stay

depending on patient body habitus but commonly include the abdomen, thighs, and flanks. Fat harvest sites are similarly marked in the preoperative area. The orientation of the skin paddle is carefully reassessed in the operating room as adjustments may be indicated based on need for soft tissue coverage, especially in instances of concurrent mastectomy.

Fat Harvest

Fat is harvested and processed according to the manufacturer's instructions. We use a mixture of 50 mL of lidocaine 1% with epinephrine 1:100,000 diluted into 1 L of normal saline for tumescence and hemostasis. The fat is aspirated with a 3-mm liposuction cannula directly into a REVOLVE fat processing system (LifeCell, Co., Bridgewater, NJ). The fat is rinsed and processed according to manufacturer's instructions and then divided into 10-mL aliquots for the final transfer.

Immediate Fat Transfer

The LD flap is harvested in the lateral decubitus position. Although some authors describe performing both flap and fat harvest simultaneously, using a two-team approach to decrease operative time, this may not always be possible. Importantly, the LD flap is not immediately released from its bony attachments at the spinous processes. Performing the fat grafting with the LD in situ serves the important purpose of providing stabilization to increase efficiency of the lipotransfer. This allows for a high-volume fat transfer; nearly a twofold increase in the volume of fat that can be safely transferred.

There are four primary locations for injecting the harvested fat: the LD skin paddle, the LD muscle, the mastectomy skin flaps, and the chest wall muscles (ie, pectoralis muscle, serratus muscle). Within the LD muscle and subcutaneous tissue, the fat is preferentially distributed in the portion that will ultimately form the lower breast pole upon final inset. Fat injection is done in a retrograde and fanlike fashion to allow for even distribution and smooth contour. Fat grafting directly into the LD muscle is safe given the absence of a large venous plexus. Furthermore, animal and clinical studies have shown that muscle is an appropriate recipient for lipotransfer owing to its robust blood supply.

Care is taken to avoid injection surrounding the vascular pedicle and the skin paddle is monitored closely for any signs of congestion. When the flap has been sufficiently augmented, the LD muscle is dis-originated from its bony attachments, denervated, and tunneled through the lateral thoracic tunnel to the anterior chest where it is inset to create the breast. Fat grafting before disinserting the flap is an important modification championed by the senior author to increase efficiency of the lipotransfer. In our experience, this technique results in an average of 66% fat take at 3 months follow-up. The most frequent complications following the LIFT procedure include donor-site seroma and delayed wound healing.

Postoperative Care

As patients undergoing LIFT do not require flap monitoring, patients have the option of leaving the same day or choosing to stay overnight in the hospital. In the senior author's practice, most patients who chose postoperative admission are discharged home within 24 to 48 h, making the LIFT a potentially more cost-effective option of reconstruction when compared with free tissue transfer. As all patients leave with at least one drain, follow-up is scheduled within one week of surgery to monitor incisional healing and drain outputs. Given the intrinsic increased risk of donor site seroma associated with the LD flap, the LIFT procedure is associated with longer time to drain removal compared with abdominally based flaps. Seromas are a known complication following the LD flap. There are reports on use of quilting sutures to decrease dead space, thus reducing drain output. However, the literature on this topic is largely composed of small case series. Furthermore, in the senior author's experience, use of quilting sutures may increase risk of hematoma without significantly reducing risk of seroma. We have not found that all patients who undergo LIFT require physical therapy, but all patients are monitored for ipsilateral upper extremity weakness or limited range of motion throughout follow-up and have the option of referral to outpatient therapy if they choose.

DISCUSSION

In 2009, the American Society of Plastic Surgeons reversed the moratorium on fat grafting. Since then, this technique has been widely used by plastic surgeons for both reconstructive and esthetic purposes. With regard to breast reconstruction, fat grafting is useful for revision to improve contour and symmetry after both autologous and implant baes reconstruction. High-volume fat grafting at the time of LD flap reconstruction has made the LIFT an attractive option for autologous breast reconstruction in patients who may not be candidates for microsurgical breast reconstruction. The senior author's technical modifications, which include performing lipotransfer before disorigination and denervation of the flap increases the speed and efficiency of fat grafting.[4]

Zhu and colleagues[13] provided an algorithm for the recommended recipient sites in fat grafted, volume-enhanced LD flap based on timing (immediate versus delayed) and indication (breast cancer versus prophylactic mastectomy) of reconstruction. In cases of immediate reconstruction after breast cancer removal, the chest wall muscles are not grafted to avoid dissemination of any residual tumor tissues. Furthermore, fat is not injected into the mastectomy skin flaps following mastectomy for breast cancer to avoid vascular compromise of the skin flaps.[13] In instances of immediate breast reconstruction following prophylactic mastectomy, residual fat may be further injected into the mastectomy flaps or chest wall for additional volume. Despite early concerns that fat transfer following breast cancer treatment may play a role in promoting tumorigenesis and angiogenesis, this has not been corroborated with clinical data.[14]

Compared with the 10-case series presented by Zhu and colleagues[13] in which the mean volume of fat grafting was 176 mL per breast, the senior author has shown that a nearly twofold increase in fat volume can be safely transferred in cases of immediate reconstruction without risk of flap loss. This increased graft take may indeed result from injection directly into a well-vascularized recipient site (ie, the LD muscle) as well as meticulous technique to ensure that fat is spread evenly within and across all injection sites.

The senior author's experience showcases that using the aforementioned techniques, especially maximization of volume enhancement using fat grafting, the LIFT procedure is now considered interchangeable with the DIEP flap in patients who have both options available to them.[12] As noted, patients with elevated body mass index and those who prefer to avoid prolonged hospitalization may be more inclined to pursue LIFT over abdominally based microsurgical reconstruction. In fact, the senior author's practice highlights that patients with prior history of unilateral DIEP flap can undergo subsequent contralateral LIFT with comparable results. This significantly supplements the armamentarium of non-microsurgeons to offer fully autologous options for breast reconstruction and in doing so, greatly increases accessibility for patients.

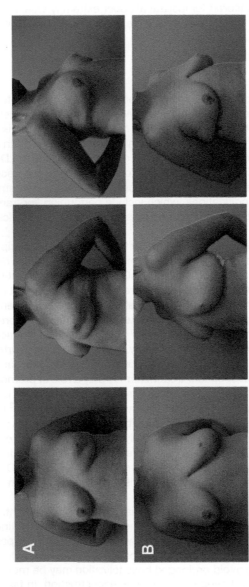

Fig. 1. A 46-year-old woman who presents 4 years following right nipple-sparing mastectomy and left skin-sparing mastectomy. The patient is unhappy with her implant-based reconstruction, mainly scar retraction and nipple asymmetry, and desires autologous breast reconstruction (A). The patient underwent latissimus dorsi flap reconstruction with immediate fat grafted from her abdomen. Photos above are 4 weeks postoperatively (B). *From* Allen R, Chen C, LoTiempo M. Deep Inferior Epigastric Artery Perforator Flap for Breast Reconstruction. In: Levine K, Vasile J, Chen C Allen R Sr, eds. Perforator Flaps for Breast Reconstruction. Edition 1, 2016, Thieme.

CASE DEMONSTRATION
Case 1

A 46-year-old woman with a history of breast cancer gene 2 (BRCA 2) mutation underwent right prophylactic mastectomy followed by implant-based reconstruction. Four years later, she presented to the senior author's practice to discuss options for breast revision due to dissatisfaction with her reconstruction. Her major concerns stemmed from multiple deformities, including scar retraction most notable at the inferior pole of the left breast, as well as nipple asymmetry. She underwent bilateral implant removal with anterior capsulectomy and bilateral LIFT with fat grafting from her abdomen (**Fig. 1**). Denervation of the flap ensures no animation deformities (**Fig. 2**).

Case 2

A 54-year-old woman with a history of left invasive ductal carcinoma with associated ductal carcinoma in situ underwent left lumpectomy and axillary dissection. Approximately 27 years later, patient was diagnosed with a new metaplastic carcinoma of the left breast and presented to the senior author's practice to discuss autologous options for immediate reconstruction. She underwent bilateral skin-sparing mastectomy with left sentinel lymph node biopsy and immediate bilateral LIFT with fat grafting from her abdomen (**Fig. 3**). Of note, patient was very active preoperatively and was able to return to return to her baseline level of activity including an intensive weight-lifting regimen less than 2 months after breast reconstruction.

Case 3

A 46-year-old woman with a history of Factor V Leiden mutation complicated by provoked saddle pulmonary embolus on Xarelto presented to the senior author's practice to discuss reconstructive options in the setting of newly diagnosed left node-positive multicentric breast cancer. Patient primarily expressed interest in autologous options as she desired to avoid prosthetic devices and the need for replacement procedures. Patient was recommended for LIFT due to her extensive history of hypercoagulable state. She underwent bilateral skin-sparing mastectomy with left axillary node dissection and immediate bilateral LIFT with fat grafting from her abdomen (**Fig. 4**). She was treated with Lovenox in the immediate postoperative period and more recently underwent bilateral nipple reconstruction with additional fat grafting to left breast.

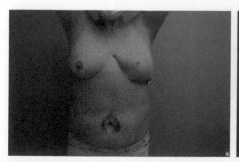
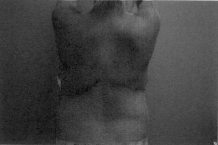

Fig. 2. Denervation of the flap ensures no animation deformities (*left*). Marking the skin paddle in preop with the patient standing up ensures scars are camouflaged in natural skin creases of the back.

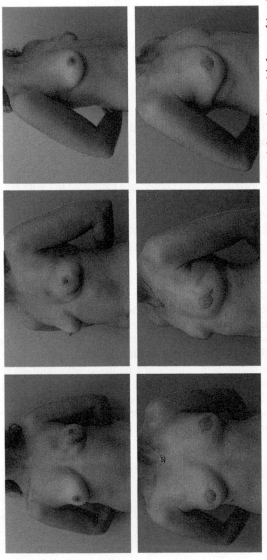

Fig. 3. A 54-year-old woman underwent a bilateral skin-sparing mastectomy followed by immediate bilateral LIFT with fat grafting from her abdomen.

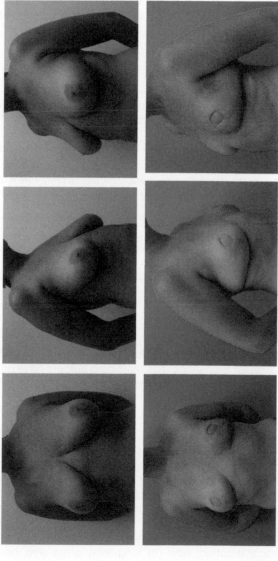

Fig. 4. A 46-year-old woman with left node-positive multicentric breast cancer and Factor V Leiden mutation underwent a bilateral skin-sparing mastectomy followed by bilateral LIFT for breast reconstruction.

SUMMARY

The pedicled LIFT is an excellent option for breast reconstruction in patients who desire autologous breast reconstruction but are not candidates for microsurgical reconstruction. Furthermore, use of fat grafting to augment the LD flap mitigates the complications associated with use of implant. Technical modifications such as performing lipotransfer before disinsertion of the muscle allow for safe, efficient, and high-volume fat grafting. As compared with the gold standard abdominally based microsurgical breast reconstruction, LD flap with immediate transfer offers patients shorter operative times and recovery.

CLINICS CARE POINTS

- Harvesting an extended latissimus dorsi flap and injecting fat in situ before release of the muscle from the spinous processes maximizes the surgeon's control while injecting fat into the flap.

- Preferentially injecting fat into the aspect of the flap that will form the inferior breast pole allows for a more natural contour to the flap.

- In immediate breast reconstruction following therapeutic mastectomy, care is taken to avoid fat transfer directly into the pectoralis major muscle, serratus muscle, and mastectomy skin flaps to avoid dissemination of residual tumor cells and vascular compromise, respectively; these sites can be injected in cases of prophylactic mastectomy and delayed reconstruction.

- Patients who undergo the latissimus dorsi flap with immediate fat transfer procedure for breast reconstruction have significantly shorter operative times and significantly shorter length of hospital stay than microsurgical breast reconstruction

DISCLOSURE

Dr D.H. Song receives royalties from Elsevier for Plastic Surgery, 3rd and 4th Editions, and Biomet Microfixation for Sternalock. The remaining authors have no financial disclosures, commercial associations, or any other conditions posing a conflict of interest to report.

REFERENCES

1. Santosa K, Qi J, Kim H, et al. Long-term patient-reported outcomes in postmastectomy breast reconstruction. JAMA Surg 2018;153(10):891–9.
2. Toyserkani N, Jorgensen M, Tabatabaeifar S, et al. Autologous versus Autologous versus implant-based breast reconstruction: a systematic review and meta-analysis of Breast-Q patient-reported outcomes-nbased bre. J Plast Reconstr Aesthet Surg 2020;73(2):278–85.
3. Lemaine V, Schilz S, Van Houten H, et al. Autologous breast reconstruction versus implant-based reconstruction: how do long-term costs and health care use compare? Plast Reconstr Surg 2020;145(2):303–11.
4. Economides JM, Song DH. Latissimus dorsi and immediate fat transfer (LIFT) for complete autologous breast reconstruction. Plast Reconstr Surg Glob Open 2018;6(1):1–6.
5. Chang D, Youssef A, Cha S, et al. Autologous breast reconstruction with the extended latissimus dorsi flap. Plast Reconstr Surg 2002;110(3):751–9.

6. Tarantino I, Banic A, Fischer T. Evaluation of late results in breast reconstruction by latissimus dorsi flap and prosthesis implantation. Plast Reconstr Surg 2006; 117(5):1387–94.
7. Chang DW, Barnea Y, Robb GL. Effects of an autologous flap combined with an implant for breast reconstruction: an evaluation of 1000 consecutive reconstructions of previously irradiated breasts. Plast Reconstr Surg 2008;122(2):356–62.
8. Thekkinkattil DK, Salhab M, McManus PL. Feasibility of autologous fat transfer for replacement of implant volume in complicated implant-assisted latissimus dorsi flap breast reconstruction. Ann Plast Surg 2015;74(4):397–402.
9. Sinna R, Delay E, Garson S, et al. Breast fat grafting (lipomodelling) after extended latissimus dorsi flap breast reconstruction: a preliminary report of 200 consecutive cases. J Plast Reconstr Aesthet Surg 2010;63(11):1769–77.
10. Nahabedian MY, Patel K. Autologous flap breast reconstruction: surgical algorithm and patient selection. J Surg Oncol 2016;113(8):865–74.
11. Rozen W, Garcia-Tutor E, Alonso-Burgos A, et al. The effect of anterior abdominal wall scars on the vascular anatomy of the abdominal wall: a cadaveric and clinical study with clinical implications. Clin Anat 2009;22(7):815–22.
12. Black CK, Zolper EG, Economides JM, et al. Comparison of the pedicled latissimus dorsi flap with immediate fat transfer versus abdominally based free tissue transfer for breast reconstruction. Plast Reconstr Surg 2020;146(2):137e–46e.
13. Zhu L, Mohan AT, Vijayasekaran A, et al. Maximizing the volume of latissimus dorsi flap in autologous breast reconstruction with simultaneous multisite fat grafting. Aesthet Surg J 2016;36(2):169–78.
14. Petit JY, Lohsiriwat V, Clough KB, et al. The oncologic outcome and immediate surgical complications of lipofilling in breast cancer patients: a multicenter study-milan-paris-lyon experience of 646 lipofilling procedures. Plast Surg Complet Clin Masters PRS- Breast Reconstr 2015;14–9. https://doi.org/10.1097/PRS.0b013e31821e713c.

Modern Approaches to Abdominal-Based Breast Reconstruction

Michael Borrero, MD, Hugo St. Hilaire, MD, Robert Allen, MD*

KEYWORDS

- Deep inferior epigastric perforator • DIEP • SIEA • DCIA
- Autologous breast reconstruction

KEY POINTS

- Abdominal-based reconstruction remains at the forefront of autologous breast reconstruction.
- Preoperative imaging and proper patient selection reduces complexity and expedites surgery.
- Muscle-sparing flaps including the deep inferior epigastric perforator (DIEP) and superficial inferior epigastric artery (SIEA) have increasingly high success rates and less abdominal wall morbidity.
- The deep circumflex iliac artery flap provides either additional abdominal soft tissue to augment the DIEP/SIEA flaps or its own flap when these flaps are unavailable.
- Surgeons should be familiar with delay phenomenon and its role in abdominal-based flaps.

INTRODUCTION

Breast reconstruction has evolved over the last few decades but one thing is for certain: the lower abdomen remains the preferred donor site for autologous breast reconstruction (ABR). Tissue volume is often robust and emulates healthy breast tissue. Perforator-based flaps have decreased abdominal wall morbidity. The patient is left with a single, low transverse scar as the only evidence of their surgery. Innovation has favored the field over the last 3 decades, including extended abdominal flaps, stacked flaps, delay procedures, neurotization, and perforator exchange techniques. Modern approaches to abdominal-based breast reconstruction need to be delineated to ensure excellent patient outcomes and professional success.

This article previously appeared in Clinics in Plastic Surgery volume 50 issue 2 April 2023.
LSU Department of Surgery, 1542 Tulane Avenue, New Orleans, LA 70112, USA
* Corresponding author.
E-mail address: boballen@diepflap.com

Clinics Collections 14 (2024) 415–432
https://doi.org/10.1016/j.ccol.2024.02.014
2352-7986/24/

Today, it is estimated that about 1 in 8 US women will develope invasive breast cancer, and this year alone, it is estimated that there will be 287,850 and 51,400 new cases of invasive and noninvasive (in situ) breast cancer, respectively.[1] Although implant-based reconstruction has surpassed autologous in the past, a recent study has shown that ABRs are increasing.[2]

The history of abdominal-based breast reconstruction dates to the early 1980s. It is during this time that Dr Carl Hartrampf pioneered the transverse rectus abdominus myocutaneous flap, colloquially known as the transverse rectus abdominis myocutaneous (TRAM) flap.[3] To his credit, and that of his team, the 1982 article detailing the TRAM flap procedure gained notoriety and sparked innovation within the realm of breast reconstruction. Moreover, although the TRAM flap remains a viable and successful reconstruction option to-date, the drawbacks soon became apparent, notably in the form of abdominal wall morbidity—hernias and bulging.

It was not long after that the senior author, Dr Allen, developed a solution—the deep inferior epigastric perforator (DIEP) flap. This was introduced in 1992 after thorough investigation of abdominal wall perforator anatomy. This was a major step in muscle-sparing breast reconstruction, and its innovation stimulated microsurgical advances. The benefits were apparent—equivocal success rates, inconspicuous scar, and complete avoidance of muscle harvest.

As the paradigm shifted toward muscle-sparing techniques, the superficial inferior epigastric flap also came to the forefront. The origin of this flap was well established for soft tissue reconstruction of the head and neck. The first published article regarding its use by Antia and Buch was in 1971.[4] Anatomic studies were published thereafter.[5] The flap was first used for free tissue transfer in breast reconstruction by the senior author in 1989.[6] This flap shares the same soft tissue components of the DIEP flap; however, the primary benefit is that it does not require abdominal fascial incision. Unfortunately, due the unreliable presence and caliber of the artery, a significant number of patients are not candidates for the flap, and those that undergo reconstruction with the SIEA flap are at an increased risk for arterial compromise and partial or total flap loss.[7] With that being said, the SIEA is the least invasive abdominal-based flap for breast reconstruction, and advances in imaging as well at using the delay phenomenon have increased SIEA utility and success.

To add to the abdominal-based flaps, the deep circumflex iliac artery (DCIA) flap has gained attention. This was initially described in 1979 by Taylor and colleagues[8] as the dominant supply for the groin flap. This pedicle perfuses the abdominal wall lateral and superior to the anterior superior iliac spine (ASIS), notably the flanks or "love handle." This area is often rich with soft tissue and underutilized.[9] It is also not reliably perfused by the DIEP or SIEA alone. It has the potential to provide ample soft tissue when the abdominal wall is inaccessible or does not provide enough volume for reconstruction.

PATIENT SELECTION AND CONSIDERATIONS

Recent trends have shown that ABR seems to be increasing. Indications for using abdominal-based flaps for breast reconstruction often include patient preference, severe soft tissue damage secondary to radiation therapy, and even failed implant reconstruction. Contraindications are few but include previous abdominoplasty or any procedure that has disrupted the inferior epigastric vascular supply to the abdominal wall. Considerations should always be made regarding the patient's known comorbidities. Nicotine products greatly influence flap outcomes, and therefore, all patients are counseled on smoking cessation for at least 1 month before and after surgery. This can be confirmed with a preoperative nicotinine test.

After determining that the patient is a surgical candidate for flap reconstruction, a thorough assessment of donor sites follows. There are multiple options but the priority flap is the DIEP flap. Assessing breast and donor volume concordance is critical. This depends on unilateral or bilateral reconstruction. If there is a significant discrepancy between the breast and abdominal donor sites, consideration for extended (eg, DCIA), stacked or hybrid flap reconstruction should be made and discussed with the patient. Fat grafting is often performed in the second stage. Stacked and extended abdominal flaps will be discussed briefly; however, they are beyond the purview of this article.

Of note, history of radiation therapy, or anticipation thereof, affects the decision-making process. Most commonly, in anticipation for adjuvant radiation therapy, flap reconstruction is delayed until the therapy is completed. A temporary or "bridge" expander if often considered to maintain as much of the skin envelope as possible until time of reconstruction.

Anatomy

Deep inferior epigastric

Abdominal wall anatomy including both the deep and superficial inferior epigastric systems are well described and have been corroborated in numerous studies, many of which by the senior author. The abdominal zones of arterial perfusion were initially described by Hartrampf.[10]

The deep inferior epigastric artery originates off the terminal aspect of the external iliac artery deep to the inguinal ligament. The artery courses superomedially through the abdominal wall and enters the rectus abdominis muscle, mostly commonly at the mid-rectus.[11,12] The branching pattern is variable, with perforators often originating within 6 cm caudal to the umbilicus.[13] Most perforators are musculocutaneous. Rarely, septocutaneous perforator wrapping around the medial edge of the rectus muscle may be encountered. A pedicle length of 10 cm can be easily achieved, artery diameter being 3 to 3.5 mm at its origin[14] (**Fig. 1**).

Superficial inferior epigastric

The superficial inferior epigastric flap is based off the named vessel. This artery most commonly originates from the common femoral artery approximately 2 to 3 cm inferior to the inguinal ligament such as the deep inferior epigastric. The origin can be variable, and it may also share a common trunk with the superficial circumflex iliac. The artery runs superiorly and will pierce the superficial fascia before branching and irrigating the anterior abdominal wall. Arterial presence and diameter are variable. Traditionally, the SIEA was recognized as being present in less than 50% of patients, and of adequate caliber for microvascular transfer is only ~50% of these patients.[5,15] Adequate caliber is typically defined as 1.5 mm in diameter or greater.

The superficial venous system is also important to recognize. The superficial inferior epigastric artery is often accompanied by venae comitantes. This is distinct from the superficial inferior epigastric vein, which drains the same soft tissues but courses separately and often medially away from the artery before draining into the common femoral vein.[15] SIEA pedicle length can be up to 8 cm and diameter ranges typically from 1.1 to 1.9 mm.

Deep circumflex iliac

The DCIA originates from the external iliac near the deep inferior epigastric artery. Similarly, there are 2 venae that accompany the artery. The artery travels laterally toward the ilium before piercing the transversalis fascia and giving off musculocutaneous perforators.[16] Immediately superior and lateral to the ASIS, the DCIA gives off

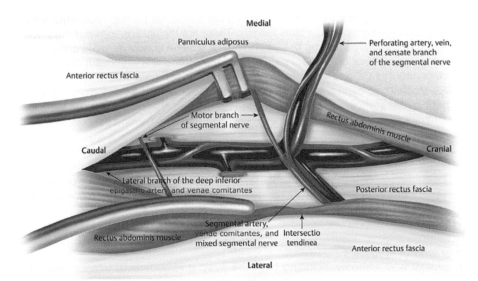

Fig. 1. Anatomy of abdominal wall, deep inferior epigastric pedicle, motor nerves perforating vessels (*From* Allen R, Chen C, LoTiempo M. Deep Inferior Epigastric Artery Perforator Flap for Breast Reconstruction. In: Levine K, Vasile J, Chen C Allen R Sr, eds. Perforator Flaps for Breast Reconstruction.)

and ascending branch, providing blood supply to the abdominal wall.[17] A lateral branch is also given off by the pedicle. This pedicle pierces the abdominal wall muscles to supply the overlying skin and subcutaneous tissues. Anatomic studies have shown that on average, there are less than 2 DCIA perforators and they are found 5 to 11 cm posterior to the ASIS and 1 to 35 mm superior to the iliac crest, establishing a zone of perfusion approximately 10 to 15 cm longitudinal by 20 to 30 cm transverse.[16,18]

Imaging

Preoperative imaging includes computed tomographic angiography (CTA), magnetic resonance angiography (MRA), and duplex ultrasonography. Preoperative imaging is performed routinely at our institution in the form of CTA with thin cuts (1 mm or less) for evaluation of the perforators. Vascular 3-dimensional reconstruction may be beneficial in some cases but is usually unnecessary.

Imaging aids the surgeon in the perforator selection process, which expedites the surgery and decreases complexity. Perforator location is confirmed at the time of surgery with preoperative Doppler localization on the abdominal skin (**Fig. 2**).

Surgical techniques

Deep inferior epigastric perforator flap. At the time of surgery, the patient's abdomen is marked preoperatively in the standing position similar to that of a traditional abdominoplasty. Landmarks include low transverse incision in the abdominal fold or 7 to8 cm above the introitus, and curvilinear extension to the anterior superior iliac spine. Based on abdominal wall volume, laxity, skin pinch assessment and location of the perforators, the superior incisional marking is made at or above the umbilicus. Preoperative imaging is routinely used to map perforators for selection, and the perforators are marked on the skin surface using a Doppler ultrasound probe before incision while

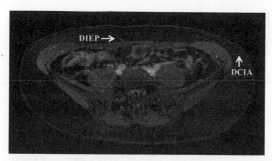

Fig. 2. Preoperative MRA with flap protocol (thin 1 mm cuts). Arrows denote right DIEA and left DCIA perforators. (*From* Allen RJ et al. The Stacked Hemiabdominal Extended Perforator Flap for Autologous Breast Reconstruction. Plast Reconstr Surg. 2018;142(6):1424-34.)

the patient is in the supine position. The present or anticipated breast footprint is marked on the chest wall also in the standing position.

The patient is positioned supine in the operating room with capability to flex the bed at the hip for abdominal closure if necessary. The arms are tucked, if possible, otherwise they are draped sterilely with access to manipulate the arm boards intraoperatively, especially during microsurgical anastomosis.

A 2-team approach is preferred so that chest recipient vessels can be exposed simultaneously with flap elevation. This especially expedites the surgery in delayed reconstruction.

Flap elevation begins with the low transverse incision. The surgery is performed under loupe magnification. Careful dissection 6 to 8 cm lateral to the midline is performed to identify the superficial venous system. The superficial veins are routinely identified and dissected distally below the superficial fascia until an adequate length and caliber vessel is achieved, typically 6 cm and 2 mm, respectively.

After the superficial vein has been isolated and ligated, flap elevation proceeds, usually from lateral to medial. Dissection is carried down to the abdominal wall muscular fascia, at which time careful dissection proceeds with bipolar electrocautery and Westcott microsurgical scissors. Target perforator(s) are identified and dissected circumferentially. If multiple perforators are being selected, it is beneficial to identify all perforators before fascial incision so that the incision can be properly oriented.

Once the perforators have been selected, the anterior rectus fascia is opened sharply, being mindful that the perforator may run immediately under the fascia. The fascia is opened longitudinally, connecting multiple perforators, if necessary, with gentle curve laterally in anticipation of the trajectory of the inferior epigastric pedicle. Most perforators are musculocutaneous, and their muscular courses are variable. The rectus muscle is split parallel to their axis of orientation (**Fig. 3**). Circumferential dissection of the pedicle is performed, and side branches are ligated. Preservation of motor nerve branches is critical to reduce abdominal wall morbidity.

The deep inferior epigastric vessels are dissected distally toward the origin until an adequate length and caliber is achieved. Typically, there are 2 veins. The remaining flap is elevated off the abdominal wall, and the midline incision is completed. At this time, the flap is completely perfused by the pedicle. The pedicle is ligated after the recipient vessels have been exposed and prepared. This limits ischemia time of the flap. Each vessel should be ligated separately. Often, the veins are marked with a surgical pen to establish orientation and prevent kinking or twisting after transfer to the recipient site. The flap is weighed, transferred to the chest, and secured in place.

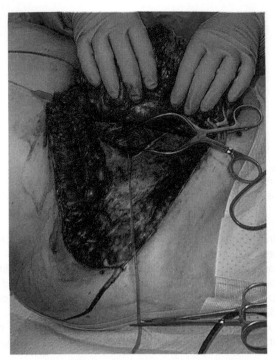

Fig. 3. Elevation of right hemiabdomen DIEP flap after intramuscular perforator dissection.

Superficial inferior epigastric artery flap

The beauty of the SIEA flap is the ease of dissection. The same principles of flap elevation apply, except there is no fascial incision or muscular dissection. The flap is elevated in a similar manner, beginning with the inferior incision. The superficial vein and inferior epigastric artery are identified, and careful microsurgical dissection is performed craniocaudal until adequate length and caliber of the vessels have been achieved. The preferred length is 6 to 8 cm and a diameter greater than 1.5 mm. After circumferential dissection of the vessels has been performed, the flap is elevated off the abdominal wall, ligating all perforators from the deep system. The flap is harvested, weighed, transferred, and inset in the same manner as previously discussed.

Deep circumflex iliac artery flap

The DCIA flap is often combined with the DIEP and SIEA flaps, what is colloquially known as a "stacked flap." The term "stacked" describes the use of multiple flaps, either conjoined, placed side-to-side, or on top of each other. The combination of flaps creates additional volume for reconstruction. Stacked flaps will be described in detail in a separate article; however, it is important to note their role in abdominal-based breast reconstruction.

DCIA flap markings differ if the flap is isolated or combined with the DIEP or SIEA.

An isolated DCIA flap is marked with the patient in the standing position. Preoperative imaging of the perforator location is reviewed and confirmed on the skin over the flanks, which is superior and lateral to the ASIS. The inferior mark is made first. It is inferior and lateral to the ASIS and begins in the midaxial line. It is drawn transversely posteriorly to incorporate as much soft tissue as possible above the superolateral buttocks. The distance from the perforator to the end point is roughly between 10 and

15 cm. The line is brought onto the anterior abdominal wall for another 10 to 15 cm. A skin pinch is performed to determine maximal width to provide a tension-free closure.

When combined, the DIEP or SIEA flap is marked first, then extended into the zone of perfusion of the DCIA perforator with lateral markings as described above (**Fig. 4**).

Elevation of the flap begins with the anterior incision, whether in isolation or combination with the DIEP/SIEA flap. Incision is carried down to musculofascial wall and proceeds laterally. Careful dissection is performed around the ASIS, the location of the perforator based on skin Doppler mark. Perforators are identified and circumferential dissection is performed at the muscle level. The posterior incision is then made, and the flap is elevated medially. The external abdominal oblique is incised parallel to the axis of muscle orientation such as the DIEP flap. Careful intramuscular dissection is performed because the pedicle tends to take a tortuous course through each muscle layer. Self-retaining retractors are placed, and pedicle course is traced to the location it pierces the internal abdominal oblique. The muscle is incised, and the pedicle traced medially to the transversalis fascia. The transversalis fascia marks the end point of dissection. Care is taken to identify lateral nerve branches that run in the plane between the internal abdominal oblique and the transversus abdominis. Pedicle length at this point is on average 6 cm with arterial diameter greater than 1.5 mm.[16]

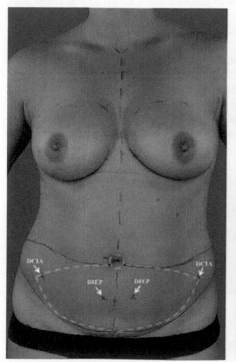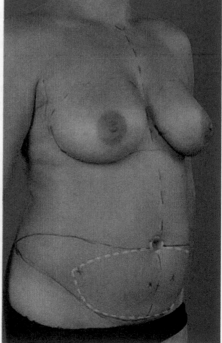

Fig. 4. Preoperative markings for an extended abdominal flap including DIEP (*dotted light blue*) and addition of DCIA flap (*solid dark blue*). (*From* Allen RJ et al. The Stacked Hemiabdominal Extended Perforator Flap for Autologous Breast Reconstruction. Plast Reconstr Surg. 2018;142(6):1424-34.)

Stacked, hemiabdominal extended perforator flap

The stacked, hemiabdominal extended perforator flap (SHAEP) was introduced as a novel approach in 2018.[19] This included the standard DIEP flap with addition to a more laterally based blood supply—DCIA, SCIA, SIEA, lumbar artery perforator—to enhance perfusion and augment volume. This was previously described by Buchel with combinations of the DIEP, SIEA, and DCIA.[16]

Flap elevation is described as above. Occasionally a lumbar artery perforator is the source vessel to perfuse the lateral abdominal tissue. Regardless, the lateral pedicle (ie, DCIA perforator) is dissected through the abdominal wall for approximately 6 to 8 cm to the ASIS. The pedicle is ligated and then an intraflap anastomosis is performed under the microscope on a sterile back table (**Fig. 5**). The lateral pedicle, often DCIA perforator, is anastomosed either to the cephalic continuation of the deep inferior epigastric, or to a sizeable lateral branch. This creates a stacked hemiabdominal extended flap that can be inset as a single, conjoined unit.

Chest vessel exposure and anastomosis

The recipient vessels for microsurgical anastomosis are the internal mammary artery and vein. Exposure begins first with creation of the breast pocket. Based on preoperative markings, skin flaps are elevated until the desired pocket is achieved. If tissue expanders are present, the expander is removed with complete capsulectomy. This prevents internal scar and deformation of the breast pocket from capsular contracture. If the expander is in the subpectoral or dual-plane position, the pectoralis major muscle is delaminated from the skin flap and sutured back down to the chest wall before exposure of the vessels.

After the pocket is recreated, a closed suction drain is placed and pectoralis muscle blocks are performed.

The internal mammary vessels are exposed under loupe magnification. The second intercostal is the optimal space for vessel diameter and preferred location for microsurgical anastomosis. In nipple-sparing mastectomies, this space may be difficult or impossible to obtain, at which point the third intercostal space is usually accessible.

The pectoralis muscle is incised parallel to the fibers. The subpectoral plane is developed over the second intercostal space as well as over the second and third

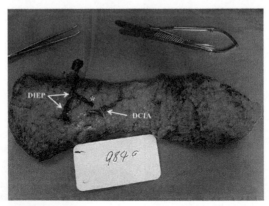

Fig. 5. Back table intra-flap anastomosis between DCIA and cephalic continuation of the DIEP. Asterisk denotes cephalic continuation of the deep inferior epigastric artery and vein. (*From* Allen RJ et al. The Stacked Hemiabdominal Extended Perforator Flap for Autologous Breast Reconstruction. Plast Reconstr Surg. 2018;142(6):1424-34.)

rib costal cartilage. At this point, a decision is made regarding the amount of costo-chrondral rib resection. With a large interspace, the vessels may be accessible without removing any rib cartilage. More often, a portion of the cartilage is removed. Our preference is to remove half of the width of the cartilage. This leaves half of the sternal articulation and maintains some stability to the chest wall.

Internal mammary perforator arteries and veins may be encountered during recipient vessel exposure. These should be evaluated to determine if they can be used as the recipient vessels, or at the very least if the perforating vein can be anastomosed to the flap superficial vein. The only caveat is that in nipple-sparing mastectomies, these perforators may be vital to nipple–areolar complex perfusion and, therefore, should be preserved (**Fig. 6**).

The fatty plane between the intercostals and the pleura is developed. This houses the internal mammary vessels, which lie within 2 to 3 cm of the sternal border. Venous anastomoses are performed with the venous coupler. Arterial anastomoses are performed with handsewn 9-0 nylon. If a superficial vein is being used, options are to perform a venous anastomosis at this time to the retrograde internal mammary vein, or to an intercostal perforating vein at the time of flap inset.

Internal Doppler implants are used in all buried flaps, and occasionally in flaps that have skin paddles for postoperative monitoring. The internal Doppler is placed around the postanastomotic artery (**Fig. 7**).

Superficial inferior epigastric artery flap—delaying the flap
Despite having a lower donor site morbidity, the SIEA flap remains less popular. This is because studies have shown higher complication rates, as high as 14% overall, with

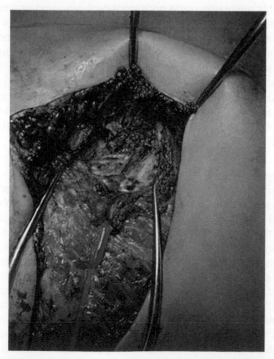

Fig. 6. Internal mammary vessel exposure with perforator in the second intercostal space.

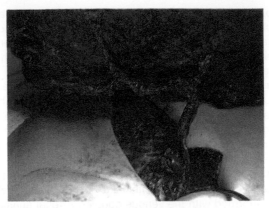

Fig. 7. DIEP flap anastomosis to internal mammary vessels.

arterial insufficiency, thrombosis or spasms being the most common causes, and reoperation rates between 6% and 20%.[7,20,21] The delay phenomenon, in which vessels surrounding the main pedicles are ligated to augment the pedicle's blood supply, has been well-acknowledged and recently applied and described by the senior author and his colleagues.[22] The delay procedure, which was primarily performed for the SIEA flap, requires subtotal elevation of the flap. The flap is elevated in the standard fashion, the superficial inferior epigastric vessels are identified and dissected circumferentially for several centimeters. The remaining flap is elevated, ligating all deep perforators. The caveat is that the flap is kept in continuity inferiorly and laterally via skin bridges (**Fig. 8**). This maintains some additional perfusion and drainage because the choke vessels open and the SIEA adapts to perfuse the flap. A recent study by the senior author and his team showed that mean cross-sectional diameter of the SIEA increased by an average of 0.9 mm after delay, from 1.37 to 2.26 mm.[22] The time interval between the delay procedure and reconstruction ranged from 6 days to 14 months, depending on the oncologic management. At least 6 days between delay and flap reconstruction is recommended. The delay procedure is performed on an outpatient basis, and the complications rates among the 24 flaps were comparable to the literature, with an overall 12% complication rate and no anastomotic revisions or flap loss (**Fig. 9**).

Perforator exchange
Yet another advancement in modern abdominal-based flap reconstruction is the perforator-to-perforator anastomosis or "perforator exchange" technique. This was introduced in 2019 by DellaCroce and colleagues.[23] Occasionally multiple perforators are selected per flap. Often, there is intervening muscle between the perforators. Perforator exchange is intraoperative technique that further reduces abdominal muscle morbidity eliminating any muscle transection when multiple perforators are being selected. The flap is elevated, and the perforators are carefully dissected to their fullest extent until limited by the intervening muscle. At this point, the dominant perforator and pedicle are dissected in the standard fashion, and any additional perforators are ligated or "disassembled" from the pedicle. Afterward, the flap is brought to a sterile back-table and the perforator is reanastomosed to either its branch or a comparable branch off the pedicle. This reestablishes perforator perfusion to the flap and obviates muscle sacrifice.

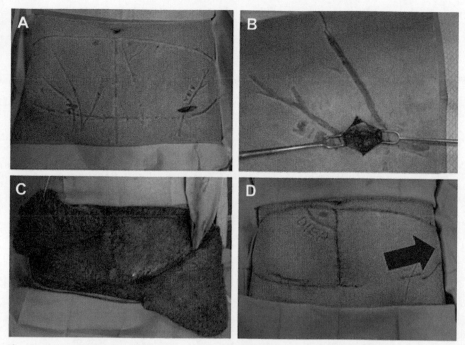

Fig. 8. Flap creation procedure for surgical delay of left SIEA flap and right DIEP flap. (*A*) Preoperative markings of abdominal flap design including the location and course of the SIEA, SIEV, and DIEA perforators bilaterally. (*B*) Incision over SIEA to verify arterial size intraoperatively. (*C*) Elevated left SIEA and right DIEP flaps. (*D*) Skin closure of delayed flaps, note the lateral skin and fascial attachment left during the delay procedure. (*From* Hoffman RD, Allen RJ et al. Surgical Delay-Induced Hemodynamic Alterations of the Superficial Inferior Epigastric Artery Flap for Autologous Breast Reconstruction. Ann Plast Surg. 2022;88(5 Suppl 5):S414-S21.)

Neurotization

Flap neurotization results remain elusive. Blondeel and colleagues[24] reported early on their experience with neurotization of breast flaps. Since then, there seems to be a trend toward both flap neurotization procedures, and several studies have demonstrated efficacy at 12 months.[25,26] Neurotization is not routinely performed at the senior author's institution, instead they are considered on a case-by-case basis. The preferred technique for neurotization is to use an interposition allograft between the anterior intercostal nerve in the second or third intercostal space. The donor nerve is identified with the pedicle and preserved during flap elevation. The nerve is harvested at the level exiting the fascia at which point it is strictly sensory. Under the microscope on the backtable, a neurorrhaphy is performed between the donor nerve and a processed nerve allograft of equivalent caliber. A 9-0 Nylon is used for epineurial repair. The flap is transferred to the recipient site. The anterior intercostal nerve is easily identified crossing over the internal mammary vessels from medial to lateral at the inferior border of the costal cartilage. After arterial and venous anastomosis, neurorrhaphy is performed from the intercostal nerve to the allograft in a similar fashion.

Flap contouring and inset

In standard bilateral breast reconstruction with DIEP flaps, each hemiabdomen reconstructs the contralateral breast. The flap is oriented such that the lateral tail of the

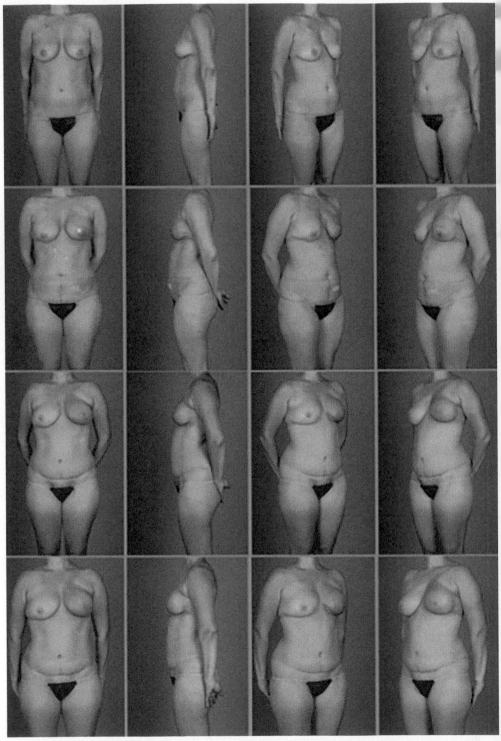

Fig. 9. Bilateral delayed SIEA reconstruction. First row: Preoperative images of 36-year-old woman with BRCA gene mutation and invasive ductal carcinoma of the left breast. Second row: images

abdominal flap is the superior point of the breast at time of inset. This point is the most distal point of perfusion and often causes troublesome fat necrosis. Once the anastomosis has been performed, the entire flap is inspected for healthy dermal bleeding. Usually, this superior tail is resected before inset, weighing less than 50 g.

With immediate flap reconstruction, a thorough inspection and assessment of the mastectomy skin flaps is important. Indocyanine green angiography can aid microsurgeons in determining mastectomy flap viability. Skin deficits should be identified and transposed to the flap. This is often necessary in irradiated breasts. The remaining skin of the flap is deepithelialized, with preference to remove all the dermis to prevent contracture at the superficial surface of the flap. Any further debulking is performed to contour the breast. The ability to contour or cone the breast depends on fat thickness and quality. The flap is inset, secured with absorbable suture from the superficial fascia to the chest wall. The superficial vein is anastomosed to an internal mammary vein perforator during the inset. Alternatively, it can be anastomosed to the retrograde internal mammary vein before inset.

Donor site management
With a 2-team approach, the abdominal wall closure can be performed after the flaps have been transferred to the recipient sites. The abdominal skin flap is elevated such as in a traditional abdominoplasty. Undermining is confined to the medial rectus above the umbilicus. The fascial incisions are closed with a 2-layer running 0-PDS or barbed equivalent suture. The patient is placed in a reflex or "beach-chair" position to facilitate closure. One or 2 closed suction drains are placed above the fascia. Progressive retention sutures are used to reduce tension at the skin closure and help prevent seroma formation. The abdomen is closed in a layered fashion including 2-0 polydioxanone suture (PDS) or barbed suture for Scarpa fascia and running 2-0 barbed suture for the deep dermal and subcuticular layers. Before closure, the umbilical stalk is identified, transposed to the skin surface, and retrieved through an elliptical excision with circumferential defatting prior. The umbilicus is inset with absorbable deep dermal and skin sutures.

If the DCIA flap has been harvested, the internal and external oblique musculofascial units are repaired with a PDS or equivalent barbed suture. Abdominal flap closure is the same. Incisions are dressed with an adhesive surgical tape (eg, Prineo, Ethicon, LLC USA). An abdominal binder or compression girdle is placed at the end of surgery.

Postoperative monitoring and care
The patient is transferred to the postanesthesia care unit. On receiving the patient, the nurse is shown the location of skin paddle perforator signals, which are marked intraoperatively with a prolene suture. Internal implantable Dopplers are also checked for signals (**Fig. 10**). The nurse performs flap checks every 15 minutes for the first hour, then every 30 minutes for the second hour. By this time, the patient is transferred to

---

take 70 postoperatively after surgical delayed of bilateral SIEA flaps with concurrent bilateral nipple-sparing mastectomy and tissue expander placement. Third row: images 160 days after SIEA-based autologous breast reconstruction. Fourth row: Images 54 days after second stage with the removal of skin islands at inframammary fold and dog-ear excision. (*From* Hoffman RD, Allen RJ et al. Surgical Delay-Induced Hemodynamic Alterations of the Superficial Inferior Epigastric Artery Flap for Autologous Breast Reconstruction. Ann Plast Surg. 2022;88(5 Suppl 5):S414-S21.)

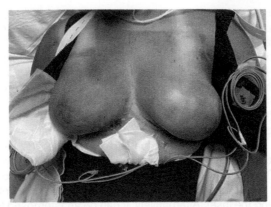

Fig. 10. Postoperative bilateral buried DIEP flaps monitored with internal Doppler. The internal Dopplers are placed around the post-anastomotic artery.

one of the medical-surgical floors that routinely cares for postsurgical free flap patients.

Flaps checks are then performed every 4 hours. A foley catheter is left in place overnight. Arterial lines are not used during surgery. Sequential compressive devices stay in place throughout the hospital stay and deep veinous thrombosis (DVT) chemoprophylaxis is initiated after surgery.

Postoperative day one the foley catheter is removed, the diet is advanced to regular, intravenous fluids are discontinued, and the patient is mobilized up into a chair. Flap checks are performed every 4 hours. On average patients remain in the hospital for 3 nights. Internal Doppler devices are cut flush with the skin before discharge. Patients follow-up on a weekly basis until their drains are removed. By week 6, they may perform rigorous activities without restrictions. Second-stage revisions are routinely performed at 3 months after reconstruction. This typically includes balancing procedures, mastopexy, scar revisions of the breast and donor sites, fat grafting, and nipple creation.

Complications

Complications can generally be categorized as related to either the flap or the donor site.

Flap-related complications include venous insufficiency, arterial thrombosis, and fat necrosis. Venous complications are more common than arterial complications and more commonly result from extrinsic factors such as hematoma, kinking, or twisting of the vein. Arterial thrombosis is less common and can be a result of technical error, severe mismatch, intrinsic damage from radiation or extrinsic factors such as compression.

The most common flap-related complication following autologous reconstruction is fat necrosis.[6] This is attributed to flap mal-perfusion and varies in predictability and extent of involvement. Many studies have demonstrated rates of fat necrosis between 6% and 40%.[6,27–30] Retrospective studies performed by the senior author and his institution have shown early complication rates including venous occlusion (3%), arterial occlusion (1%), and fat necrosis rates (12%) to be low and favorable when compared with alternative methods of reconstruction.[31–36]

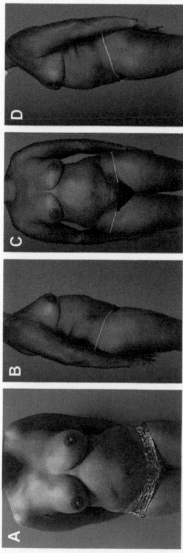

Fig. 11. (*A*) Preoperative image of a 63-year-old woman with history of BRCA gene mutation. (*B–D*) Images 12 months after bilateral prophylactic nipple sparing mastectomies with immediate DIEP reconstruction followed by second-stage revision including scar revisions and fat grafting.

Other complications following abdominal-based breast reconstruction include abdominal wall bulge/hernia, dehiscence, delayed wound healing, infection, hematoma, seroma. When compared with pedicled TRAM reconstruction, postoperative bulge following DIEP flap is reportedly lower (0.5% vs 9%).[31] Increased overall complication rates are associated with active smoking and postoperative radiation therapy. Uncontrolled hypertension, diabetes, and patient BMI greater than 40 are also associated with increased incidence in wound healing and infection complications.[31]

DISCUSSION

ABR has made great strides since the introduction of the DIEP flap in the early 1990s. Its adoption has been widespread and remarkable. Since then, advancements in microsurgical technique and preoperative imaging have helped to reduce surgical complexity and expedite flap reconstruction. Operating times, flap complications, and overall length of stay continue to decline. Surgical candidacy has increased. Emphasis is placed on immediate restoration of total breast volume that can be performed safely and with minimal abdominal wall morbidity. Therefore, modern abdominal-based breast reconstruction has evolved in the form of extended flaps (eg, DCIA), stacked flaps, and even delay procedures of the DIEP and SIEA flaps. Additionally, the field continues to experience innovation by flap neurotization and perforator exchange techniques to optimize sensory restoration and further minimize abdominal muscle morbidity. Immediate, completely buried bilateral ABR is no longer uncommon and represents the pinnacle of breast reconstruction.

SUMMARY

Now, more than ever, plastic surgeons are faced with increased demand in terms of bilateral and nipple-sparing reconstruction. The DIEP and SIEA flaps continue to produce excellent esthetic results with high patient satisfaction. The DCIA flap also has a niche in enhancing volume or acting as a secondary donor site when the DIEP is unavailable. Abdominal flaps are especially indicated for failure of prosthetic reconstruction and restoration of healthy, natural tissue in an irradiated breast. Autologous breast reconstruction requires the plastic surgeon to be well versed and adaptable in all aspects of abdominal-based breast reconstruction, applying multiple techniques to restore the breast to its natural shape and volume (**Fig. 11**).

CLINICS CARE POINTS

- Preoperative imaging (CTA or MRA) facilitates perforator mapping and surgical efficiency
- Volume disparities between breast and donor site may require extended or stacked flaps (eg, DCIA or PAP flaps)
- Supercharging with a superficial vein augments venous outflow and decreases risk of congestion and fat necrosis
- Consider a delay procedure in SIEA flap candidates when the artery is present but less than 1.5 mm
- ICG angiography can show intraoperative flap perfusion and aid in surgical decision-making
- Perform a perforator exchange to avoid sacrificing significant interposing rectus muscle
- Preserve motor nerves and limit abdominal flap undermining to reduce donor site morbidity and complications

DISCLOSURE

The authors declare that they have no relevant or material financial interests that relate to the information described in this article.

REFERENCES

1. Key statistics for breast cancer. American cancer society. 2022 [updated January 2022; cited 2022 1 July 2022]; Available at: cancer.org/cancer/breast-cancer.
2. Masoomi H, Hanson SE, Clemens MW, et al. Autologous breast reconstruction trends in the United States: using the nationwide inpatient sample database. Ann Plast Surg 2021;87(3):242–7.
3. Hartrampf CR, Scheflan M, Black PW. Breast reconstruction with a transverse abdominal island flap. Plast Reconstr Surg 1982;69(2):216–25.
4. Antia NH, Buch VI. Transfer of an abdominal dermo-fat graft by direct anastomosis of blood vessels. Br J Plast Surg 1971;24(1):15–9.
5. Taylor GI, Daniel RK. The anatomy of several free flap donor sites. Plast Reconstr Surg 1975;56(3):243–53.
6. Allen RJ, Treece P. Deep inferior epigastric perforator flap for breast reconstruction. Ann Plast Surg 1994;32(1):32–8.
7. Coroneos CJ, Heller AM, Voineskos SH, et al. SIEA versus DIEP arterial complications: a cohort study. Plast Reconstr Surg 2015;135(5):802e-7e.
8. Taylor GI, Townsend P, Corlett R. Superiority of the deep circumflex iliac vessels as the supply for free groin flaps. Plast Reconstr Surg 1979;64(5):595–604.
9. Elzinga K, Buchel E. The Deep Circumflex Iliac Artery Perforator Flap for Breast Reconstruction: un lambeau perforateur de l'artere iliaque circonflexe profonde pour la reconstruction mammaire. Plast Surg (Oakv) 2018;26(4):229–37.
10. Hutcheson HA, Hartrampf CR Jr. Breast reconstruction using abdominal tissue. Plast Surg Nurs 1986;6(3):97–104.
11. Milloy FJ, Anson BJ, McAfee DK. The rectus abdominis muscle and the epigastric arteries. Surg Gynecol Obstet 1960;110:293–302.
12. Hamdi H, Rebecca A. The deep inferior epigastric artery perforator flap (DIEAP) in breast reconstruction. Semin Plast Surg 2006;20:95–102.
13. Allen R, Chen C, LoTiempo M. Deep inferior epigastric artery perforator flap for breast reconstruction. In: Levine K, Vasile J, Chen C, et al, editors. Perforator flaps for breast reconstruction. New York: Thieme; 2016. p. 30–9.
14. Gagnon AB and Blondeell PN. Deep and superficial inferior epigastric artery perforator flaps and reconstructive surgery, Cirugia Plastica, 32 (4), 2006. p. 7-13.
15. Spiegel AJ. Superficial inferior epigastric artery flap for breast reconstruction. New York: Thieme: Perforator Flaps for Breast Reconstruction; 2016.
16. Buchel E. Deep circumflex iliac artery perforator flap for breast reconstruction. New York: Thieme: Perforator Flaps for Breast Reconstruction; 2016. p. 126–32.
17. Hendricks H, Ingianni G, Bohm E, et al. A microvascular peritoneal flap based on the deep circumflex iliac artery. Eur J Plast Surg 1995;18:88–90.
18. Bergeron L, Tang M, Morris SF. The anatomical basis of the deep circumflex iliac artery perforator flap with iliac crest. Plast Reconstr Surg 2007;120(1):252–8.
19. Beugels J, Vasile JV, Tuinder SMH, et al. The stacked hemiabdominal extended perforator flap for autologous breast reconstruction. Plast Reconstr Surg 2018; 142(6):1424–34.

20. Park JE, Shenaq DS, Silva AK, et al. Breast reconstruction with SIEA flaps: a single-institution experience with 145 free flaps. Plast Reconstr Surg 2016; 137(6):1682–9.
21. Selber JC, Samra F, Bristol M, et al. A head-to-head comparison between the muscle-sparing free TRAM and the SIEA flaps: is the rate of flap loss worth the gain in abdominal wall function? Plast Reconstr Surg 2008;122(2):348–55.
22. Hoffman RD, Maddox SS, Meade AE, et al. Surgical delay-induced hemodynamic Alterations of the superficial inferior epigastric artery flap for autologous breast reconstruction. Ann Plast Surg 2022;88(5 Suppl 5):S414–21.
23. DellaCroce FJ, DellaCroce HC, Blum CA, et al. Myth-busting the DIEP flap and an introduction to the abdominal perforator exchange (APEX) breast reconstruction technique: a single-surgeon retrospective review. Plast Reconstr Surg 2019; 143(4):992–1008.
24. Blondeel PN, Demuynck M, Mete D, et al. Sensory nerve repair in perforator flaps for autologous breast reconstruction: sensational or senseless? Br J Plast Surg 1999;52(1):37–44.
25. Momeni A, Meyer S, Shefren K, et al. Flap neurotization in breast reconstruction with nerve allografts: 1-year clinical outcomes. Plast Reconstr Surg Glob Open 2021;9(1):e3328.
26. Spiegel AJ, Menn ZK, Eldor L, et al. Breast reinnervation: DIEP neurotization using the third anterior intercostal nerve. Plast Reconstr Surg Glob Open 2013; 1(8):e72.
27. Nahabedian MY, Tsangaris T, Momen B. Breast reconstruction with the DIEP flap or the muscle- sparing (MS-2) free TRAM flap: is there a difference? Plast Reconstr Surg 2005;115(2):436–44 [discussion: 45-6].
28. Chen CM, Halvorson EG, Disa JJ, et al. Immediate postoperative complications in DIEP versus free/muscle-sparing TRAM flaps. Plast Reconstr Surg 2007;120(6): 1477–82.
29. Kroll SS. Fat necrosis in free transverse rectus abdominis myocutaneous and deep inferior epigastric perforator flaps. Plast Reconstr Surg 2000;106(3): 576–83.
30. Wu LC, Bajaj A, Chang DW, et al. Comparison of donor-site morbidity of SIEA, DIEP, and muscle-sparing TRAM flaps for breast reconstruction. Plast Reconstr Surg 2008;122(3):702–9.
31. Gill PS, Hunt JP, Guerra AB, et al. A 10-year retrospective review of 758 DIEP flaps for breast reconstruction. Plast Reconstr Surg 2004;113(4):1153–60.
32. Weichman KE, Tanna N, Broer PN, et al. Microsurgical breast reconstruction in thin patients: the impact of low body mass indices. J Reconstr Microsurg 2015; 31(1):20–5.
33. Levine SM, Snider C, Gerald G, et al. Buried flap reconhhstruction after nipple0sparing mastectomy: advancing toward single-stage breast reconstruction. Plast Reconstr Surg 2013;132(4). 489e-297e.
34. Broer PN, Weichman K, Tanna N, et al. Venous coupler size in autologous breast reconstruction–does it matter? Microsurgery 2013;33(7):514–8.
35. Weichman KE, Broer PN, Tanna N, et al. The role of autologous fat grafting in secondary microsurgical breast reconstruction. Ann Plast Surg 2013;71(1):24–30.
36. Tanna N, Broer PN, Weichman KE, et al. Microsurgical breast reconstruction for nipple-sparing mastectomy. Plast Reconstr Surg 2013;131(2):139e–47e.

Radiation Treatment

Radiation Treatment for Breast Cancer

Anderson Bauer, MD

KEYWORDS

- Radiation • Breast conservation • Whole breast radiation
- Accelerated partial breast radiation • Postmastectomy • Regional nodes
- Hypofractionation

KEY POINTS

- Knowledge of the fundamentals of radiation allows for a better understanding of breast cancer treatment.
- There are a variety of acceptable treatment techniques and dose-fractionation schedules for adjuvant breast radiation.
- Radiation treatment plays an important adjuvant role in breast conservation and also in the postmastectomy setting.
- Careful assessment of individual patient risk factors and treatment goals is essential in identifying the appropriate radiation treatment.

INTRODUCTION

Radiation is a well-established component of breast cancer treatment. This is primarily in the adjuvant setting in both breast conservation and also for many patients who have had mastectomy. The objective of radiation is to eradicate any microscopic tumor deposits remaining after surgery. It is important to understand the various techniques that are utilized in breast radiation. A multitude of factors can help to determine an ideal combination and sequence of surgery, radiation treatment, and systemic therapy for each patient. In addition to the curative setting, radiation can also have an important palliative role.

RADIATION TREATMENT OVERVIEW AND TECHNIQUES
Radiation Treatment Overview

The first radiation treatment of cancer is claimed to have occurred in 1896.[1] The technology of radiation treatment has changed dramatically since this time. Radiation is

This article previously appeared in *Surgical Clinics* volume 103 issue 1 February 2023.
Radiation Oncology Department, Marshfield Clinic Health System, 1001 North Oak Avenue, Marshfield, WI 54449, USA
E-mail address: bauer.anderson@marshfieldclinic.org

Clinics Collections 14 (2024) 433–445
https://doi.org/10.1016/j.ccol.2024.03.001

energy deposited in tissue that kills dividing cancer cells while preferentially allowing normal tissue cells to survive. In general, lower doses of radiation are required to treat postoperative microscopic disease compared to doses for macroscopic deposits of cancer.

The modern era of radiation began in the 1990s, when radiation oncologists began to regularly use CT-based planning. CT imaging is performed on the patient in the treatment position. Customized immobilization devices are used. Certain techniques can be used to minimize doses to specific normal tissues. For individuals with breast cancer, a deep inspiratory breath hold (DIBH) technique increases the distance between the heart and the breast/chest wall to minimize cardiac radiation dose.[2] A prone setup technique can be conducted for patients with larger, pendulous breasts to limit skin reactions while also potentially minimizing dose to the lung and heart.[3]

The CT image sets are sent to the treatment planning system computer. The radiation oncologist delineates the target volumes, which may include the whole breast, lumpectomy cavity, chest wall, and/or at-risk regional lymphatics for breast cancer. Avoidance structures anticipated to be in the treatment field are also drawn, including the heart, lungs, contralateral breast, brachial plexus, and/or thyroid gland. The computer planning software allows for the creation of a virtual treatment plan. **Fig. 1** shows a whole breast radiation treatment plan with tangent fields.

The radiation oncologist determines the treatment technique and prescribes a dose of radiation to be delivered to a specific target in a specified number of treatments. The dose is prescribed in Gray (Gy), and treatments are called fractions. Standard fractionation is typically recognized as 1.8–2.0 Gy per day to a total dose of 50–60 Gy. Hypofractionation schedules include doses of greater than 2.0 Gy per fraction to radiobiologically equivalent total doses (ie, 16 fractions of 2.66 Gy per day to a total of 42.56 Gy). The virtual plan is approved once appropriate target dose coverage and normal tissue sparing are achieved. The plan is transferred to the radiation treatment machine. Appropriate quality assurance is done on treatment plans to ensure accuracy and safety.

Techniques

A vast array of radiation techniques have been developed for cancer treatment, including for individuals with breast cancer. Different types of radiation used in these

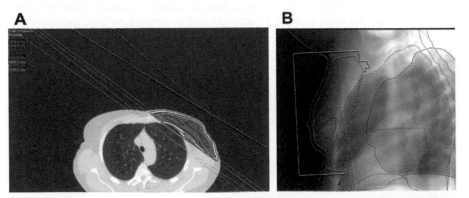

Fig. 1. (*A*). Planning CT axial view of whole breast tangent field arrangement designed to encompass the target volume while minimizing dose to the heart, lung, and contralateral breast. (*B*). Whole breast radiation tangent port corresponding to CT image (*A*). Field minimizes dose to the ipsilateral lung (*green*) and heart (*magenta*).

techniques include: photons, electrons, gamma rays (ie, iridium-192), and protons. Photon radiation is used for most external beam treatments and is the most common type of radiation. Iridium-192 is a radioactive isotope that is commonly used in brachytherapy. Proton therapy is not currently routinely used for breast cancer treatment, but there is an ongoing study for its potential expanded indications.[4]

External beam radiation is the most common type of treatment, including 3-dimensional conformal radiation treatment (3DCRT) and intensity-modulated radiation treatment (IMRT). Brachytherapy is a technique that involves placing a radiation source inside or next to an area requiring treatment; it is typically subdivided into intracavitary and interstitial techniques. Intraoperative radiation treatment (IORT) can be performed with an intraoperative beam (electron or photon) or as high-dose rate brachytherapy. Different techniques can be utilized to deliver doses to different targets. For example, brachytherapy is very effective at delivering a higher dose to a smaller volume, hence it is a technique used in partial breast radiation. The radiation is confined to the lumpectomy cavity with a small margin. The dosimetry for a brachytherapy plan is shown in **Fig. 2**. Partial breast treatment is typically done over ≤1 week, which is why it is called accelerated partial breast irradiation (APBI).

RADIATION TREATMENT IN THE NONMETASTATIC SETTING
Breast Conservation-Invasive Cancer

For women who have breast-conserving surgery, adjuvant radiation is a well-established treatment for both invasive breast cancers and ductal carcinoma in situ (DCIS). For invasive breast cancer, a large meta-analysis of 17 trials published in 2011 by the Early Breast Cancer Trialists' Collaborative Group (EBCTCG) showed the benefit of adjuvant whole breast radiation treatment (WBRT).[5] Ten-year risk of locoregional recurrence (LRR) was decreased by approximately half from 35 to 19 percent. Fifteen-year risk of breast cancer death was reduced from 25 to 21 percent. **Fig. 3** illustrates these curves.[5]

More modern studies have evaluated the benefit in low-risk patients, which are more commonly seen as screening continues to improve early detection. Cancer and Leukemia Group B (CALGB) 9343 evaluated women ≥70 years of age with T1N0, estrogen-receptor positive invasive ductal carcinoma treated by lumpectomy

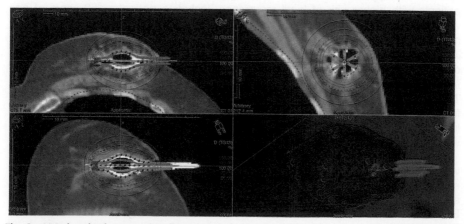

Fig. 2. APBI brachytherapy plan using SAVI multicatheter device. Rapid falloff of dose can be seen from 150% isodose line to 50% isodose line.

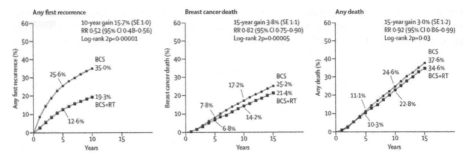

Fig. 3. This figure was published in Lancet, Vol. 378, Issue 9804; EBCTCG (Early Breast Cancer Trialists' Collaborative Group). "Effect of radiotherapy after breast-conserving surgery on 10-year recurrence and 15-year breast cancer death: meta-analysis of individual patient data for 10,801 women in 17 randomized trails" pp 1707-1716, Copyright Elsevier (2011), with permission.

to receive tamoxifen plus adjuvant radiation or tamoxifen alone. The adjuvant radiation had a statistically significant 10-year local recurrence reduction from 10 to 2 percent, but this did not impact breast cancer-specific survival or overall survival.[6] PRIME II evaluated women ≥65 years of age with invasive ductal carcinoma up to 3 cm in size treated by lumpectomy to receive adjuvant endocrine treatment plus whole breast radiation or adjuvant endocrine treatment only. This also showed that adjuvant radiation had a statistically significant 10-year local recurrence reduction from 9.8 to 0.9 percent, but no difference in overall and breast cancer-specific survival.[7] OncotypeDX may offer additional information on local recurrence risk in these low-risk patients, and the NRG Oncology study BR007 is further investigating this question.

WBRT with a hypofractionated regimen of 40–42.5 Gy in 15–16 fractions with or without a lumpectomy cavity boost of 10 Gy in 4–5 fractions has become the standard approach as studies have shown no significant differences in tumor control nor adverse effects when comparing the prior standard 5–6 week regimen to this shortened hypofractionated approach.[8–10] The 2018 American Society for Therapeutic Radiology and Oncology (ASTRO) Radiation Therapy for the Whole Breast Guidelines strongly recommended hypofractionated WBRT regardless of tumor grade, laterality, systemic therapy, and breast size. These guidelines also recommend a boost for all patients with higher risk of local recurrence, including patients ≤50 years of age with any grade disease, age 51–70 years of age with high-grade disease, or a positive margin.[11]

In regards to further hypofractionation, newer data also suggest the future potential of ultrashort whole breast radiation options from the FAST (28.5 Gy in 5 once-weekly fractions) and FAST-Forward (26 Gy in 5 fractions in 1 week) trials.[12–14] NRG/Radiation Therapy Oncology Group (RTOG) 1005 has been evaluating the option of 40 Gy in 15 fractions with a simultaneous integrated boost (SIB) of 48 Gy in 15 fractions to the lumpectomy cavity. This study was closed to accrual in 2014 and outcomes are still unpublished.[15]

APBI can be utilized to treat only the lumpectomy cavity with an appropriate margin, which is the area at highest risk of recurrence. This has been studied primarily using external beam radiation (typically 38.5 Gy in 10 fractions, twice daily) and brachytherapy (34 Gy in 10 fractions, twice daily) techniques. The National Surgical Adjuvant Breast and Bowel Project (NSABP) B-39/RTOG 0413 is a large phase 3 randomized trial of WBRT compared to APBI, which showed a 10-year cumulative incidence of ipsilateral breast tumor recurrence of 3.9 percent for WBRT versus 4.6 percent for

APBI.[16] There was no difference in cosmesis. The ASTRO consensus statement on APBI states that "suitable" candidates are $\geq$50 years of age, $\leq$2 cm invasive ductal carcinoma with at least 2 mm margins, no lymphvascular invasion, estrogen receptor positive, and gBRCA negative.[17] Additional partial breast fractionation schedules include a 5 fraction partial breast IMRT plan to 30 Gy delivered every other day, which was studied in the Florence trial (10-year Ipsilateral breast tumor recurrence of 2.5% for WBRT and 3.7% for APBI).[18] In addition, 40 Gy in 15 fractions partial breast radiation was found to be noninferior to WBRT in the UK IMPORT LOW trial.[19]

Intraoperative radiation treatment is a unique option as it is delivered at the time of breast-conserving surgery. This can be delivered with low-energy photons or electrons using an intraoperative applicator. The TARGIT trial used a mobile machine delivering approximately 20 Gy to the surface using 50 kV photons. The intraoperative radiation could be supplemented by EBRT when postoperative pathology revealed higher risk factors. Compared to standard WBRT, the intraoperative approach showed no statistically significant difference for local recurrence-free survival, mastectomy-free survival, distant disease-free survival, overall survival, and breast cancer mortality at a median follow-up of 8.6 years.[20] TARGIT was associated with improved breast cosmesis. The ELIOT trial used intraoperative electron treatment to deliver a dose of 21 Gy and was compared to WBRT. At a median follow-up of 12.4 years, there was an increase in 15-year ipsilateral breast tumor recurrence of 12.6 percent compared to 2.4 percent.[21]

Key Points-Invasive Breast Cancer

- Adjuvant radiation with a boost is recommended for patients $\leq$50 years of age with any grade disease, age 51–70 years of age with high-grade disease, or a positive margin.
- Individualized shared decision-making with provider and patient is important to decide which individuals may elect the de-escalation of radiation (no radiation lumpectomy boost or completely omit adjuvant WBRT).
- There is increasing use of hypofractionation for patients that have adjuvant radiation.
- APBI is a well-studied adjuvant radiation treatment option for selected patients.
- Genomic assays may become increasingly important to select appropriate low-risk patients who can forego adjuvant radiation.

Breast Conservation-Ductal Carcinoma In Situ

For DCIS, there is also a large meta-analysis by the EBCTG published in 2010 showing the reduction of local recurrence with adjuvant WBRT after breast-conserving surgery. 10-year risk of any ipsilateral breast event (either recurrent DCIS or invasive cancer) was decreased by approximately half from 28.1 to 12.9 percent.[22] However, there was no significant impact on overall survival. NSABP B-17 and NSABP B-24 further evaluated adjuvant radiation with tamoxifen. These trials demonstrated that radiation had a relatively greater impact on preventing local recurrence than tamoxifen. A combined analysis of these trials showed a 15-year cumulative incidence of ipsilateral breast tumor recurrence of 19.4 percent for lumpectomy alone, 8.9 percent for lumpectomy with radiation, 10 percent for lumpectomy with radiation + placebo, and 8.5 percent for lumpectomy with radiation + tamoxifen.[23] These results can be seen in **Fig. 4**.[23]

More modern studies have further evaluated adjuvant radiation for low-risk DCIS. NRG/RTOG 9804 evaluated patients with mammographically detected DCIS, $\leq$2.5 cm, final margins $\geq$3 mm, and low or intermediate nuclear grade. Adjuvant radiation significantly reduced the 15-year cumulative incidence of ipsilateral breast

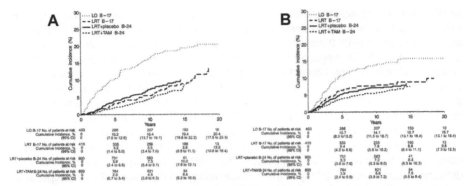

Fig. 4. Effects of radiation and tarnoxifen on the cumulative incidence of breast cancer events. (*A*) Invasive ipsilateral breast tumor recurrences (I-ISTR), (*B*) ductual carcinoma in situ-ipsilateral breast tumor recurrences (DCIS-IBTR). (Wapnir IL, Dignam JJ, Fisher B, et al. Long-term Outcomes of Invasive Ipsilateral Breast Tumor Recurrences After Lumpectomy in NSABP B-17 and B-24 Randomized Clinical Trials for DCIS. J Natl Cancer Inst. 2011; 103(6):478-88 by permission of Oxford University Press.)

recurrence from 15.1 to 7.1 percent; invasive local recurrence was reduced from 9.5 to 5.4 percent.[24] There was no significant difference in overall survival. ECOG 5194 followed 2 cohorts of women with DCIS treated with lumpectomy alone. 12-year rates of ipsilateral breast events were 14.4 percent for cohort 1 (low- or intermediate-grade DCIS with tumors ≤2.5 cm, negative margins ≥3 mm) and 24.6 percent for cohort 2 (high-grade DCIS, tumor size ≤1 cm, negative margins ≥3 mm), respectively.[25] These studies show that there is still significant recurrence even in women with favorable pathology. Genomic assays such as DCIS Score and DCISion RT can provide additional guidance on recurrence risk.[26,27]

In regards to the specifics of radiation treatment of DCIS, the 2018 ASTRO Radiation Therapy for the Whole Breast Guidelines recommend hypofractionated WBRT as an alternative to conventional fractionation in patients with DCIS.[11] It also stated that a tumor bed boost may be used for patients with any of the following criteria: ≤50 years of age, high grade, or margins <2 mm. In addition, ASTRO would consider patients ≥50 years of age with screening-detected DCIS, low or intermediate grade, and with margins ≥3 mm as "suitable" candidates for APBI.[17]

Key Points-Ductal Carcinoma In Situ

- Adjuvant radiation with a boost is recommended for high-grade DCIS, premenopausal patients, patients <50 years of age, tumors >2.5 cm, or margins <2 mm.
- Individualized shared decision-making with provider and patient is important to decide which individuals may elect the de-escalation of radiation (no radiation lumpectomy boost or completely omit adjuvant WBRT).
- There is increasing use of hypofractionation for patients that have adjuvant radiation.
- Genomic assays may become increasingly important to select appropriate low-risk patients who can forego adjuvant radiation.

Radiation for Locally Advanced Breast Cancer

Adjuvant radiation treatment of T2 lesions with high-risk features, T3/T4 lesions, and node-positive patients is typically more extensive than for early-stage breast cancers.

Historically, radiation for patients with locally advanced disease would comprehensively include the breast/chest wall and all regional nodes (dissected and undissected axilla, supraclavicular region, and internal mammary chain nodes).

A meta-analysis by the EBCTG of 22 trials published in 2014 showed an improvement in 10-year recurrence and 20-year breast cancer mortality in women with 4 or more positive nodes who received adjuvant radiation to the chest wall and regional lymphatics.[28] 10-year risk of local recurrence was decreased from 32.1 to 13.0 percent. The 20-year breast cancer mortality was decreased from 80 to 70.7 percent. These results can be seen in **Fig. 5**.[28]

Over time, there have been significant changes in systemic therapy, as well as diagnostic procedures. Multiple studies have continued to help refine the role of regional lymph node radiation treatment. National Cancer Institute of Canada (NCIC) MA.20 is a randomized trial that evaluated adding regional nodal radiation to whole breast radiation in patients with 1–3 positive axillary lymph nodes or negative nodes with high-risk features. High-risk features were defined as primary tumor measuring ≥5 cm or ≥2 cm with fewer than 10 axillary nodes removed with at least one additional high-risk feature (grade 3, estrogen-receptor negativity, or lymphvascular invasion).

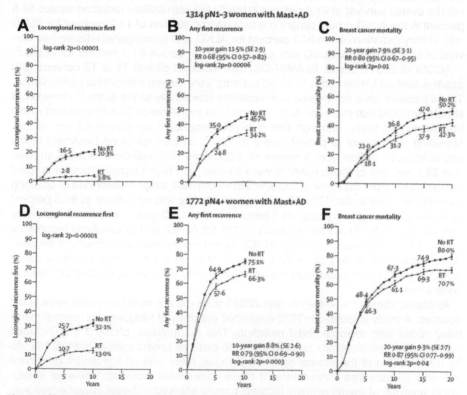

Fig. 5. Effect of radiotherapy (RT) after mastectomy and axillary dissection (Mast AD) on 10-year risks of locoregional and overall recurrence and on 20-year risk of breast cancer mortality in 1314 women with 1 to 3 pathologically positive nodes (pN1-3) and in 1772 women with 4 or more pathologically positive nodes (pN4+). (The Lancet, 2014, 383 (9935), p.2127-2135. EBCTG (Early Breast Cancer Trialists' Collaborative Group), "Effect of radiotherapy after mastectomy and axillary surgery on 10-year recurrence and 20-year breast cancer mortality: meta-analysis of individual patient data for 8135 women in 22 randomised trials".)

The regional nodal radiation significantly improved isolated local recurrence-free survival (95.2 versus 92.2 percent, p = 0.009), distant recurrence-free survival (86.3 versus 82.4 percent, p = 0.03) and overall disease-free survival (82 versus 77 percent, p = 0.01) at 10 years.[29]

EORTC 22922 is also a randomized trial that showed benefit to regional nodal radiation in patients with involved axillary nodes or central or medially located primary tumors. At a median follow-up of 15.7 years, regional nodal radiation was associated with a significant reduction in breast cancer mortality from 19.8 to 16.0 percent (p = 0.0055) and any breast cancer recurrence from 27.1 to 24.5 percent (p = 0.024).[30] At a median follow-up of 10.9 years, EORTC 22922 had shown a significant benefit with radiation to disease-free survival (72.1 versus 69.1%), distant disease-free survival (78 versus 75%), breast cancer mortality (12.5 versus 14.4%), and overall survival (82.3 versus 80.7%).

AMAROS evaluated the use of axillary radiation treatment in lieu of full axillary lymph node dissection (ALND) in patients with T1 or T2 disease with a positive sentinel lymph node dissection (SLND). This study included both breast conservation as well as patients with mastectomy (17%). The axillary radiation included all 3 levels of the axilla and the medial part of the supraclavicular fossa. At 10 years, AMAROS showed noninferior overall survival of 81.4 percent in the SLND with axillary radiation versus 84.6 percent in the ALND group, distant metastasis-free survival of 78.2 percent for SLND with axillary radiation versus 81.7 percent for ALND, and locoregional relapse-free survival of 83.0 percent for SLND with axillary radiation versus 81.2 percent for ALND.[31]

ACOSOG Z0011, similar to AMAROS, also included clinical T1 or T2 cancers with positive sentinel lymph nodes (1–2). All patients were treated with breast conservation. These patients were not treated with radiation specifically to the axilla.[32] However, it should be noted that there can be incidental dose to the low axilla with standard whole breast tangent fields, although this is highly dependent on patient's body shape. Moreover, 15 percent of patients were recorded as also receiving treatment in the supraclavicular region, and a review of 142 cases with sufficient records showed that 51.4 percent of those patients were treated with high tangents (cranial tangent border ≤2 cm from the humeral head) which would have a higher likelihood of covering more of the upper axilla.[33] The 10-year overall survival was noninferior at 86.3 percent in the SLND alone group versus 83.6 percent in the ALND group, as were disease-free survival (80.2% for SLND alone versus 78.2% for ALND) and locoregional recurrence (4.07% for SLND versus 3.59% for ALND). Given the decreased morbidity of lymphedema without the axillary dissection, these studies do not support the routine use of ALND in this patient population with limited axillary disease as defined by sentinel node excision.[32]

As stated above, the AMAROS and Z0011 trials did not treat comprehensive nodal volumes. A study published in 2022 evaluated the utility of including the internal mammary nodes with regional nodal radiation. This randomized, phase 3 trial included women with pathologically confirmed, node-positive breast cancer with ALND. As for the inclusion of the internal mammary nodes, there was no significant difference in 7-year disease-free survival rates if these nodes were included. However, a subgroup analysis of mediocentrally located tumors showed a 7-year disease-free survival rate improvement with internal mammary nodal radiation of 91.8 v. 81.6 percent and a breast cancer mortality reduction from 10.2 to 4.9 percent. There were no differences between the 2 groups in the incidence of adverse effects, including cardiac toxic effects and radiation pneumonitis.[34]

For node-positive patients who have had neoadjuvant chemotherapy, most patients receive postmastectomy radiation treatment, especially if there is any residual disease. There are 2 major ongoing trials that will help to define the role of adjuvant radiation treatment after the assessment of response to neoadjuvant chemotherapy. Alliance A011202 is a randomized phase 3 trial comparing axillary lymph node dissection to axillary radiation in patients with breast cancer (cT1-3 N1) who have positive sentinel lymph node disease after neoadjuvant chemotherapy. NSABP B-51/RTOG 1304 is a randomized phase 3 trial evaluating the role of postmastectomy chest wall/regional nodal radiation and postlumpectomy whole breast/regional nodal radiation in patients with documented positive axillary nodes before neoadjuvant chemotherapy who convert to pathologically negative axillary nodes after neoadjuvant chemotherapy.

As with early-stage invasive breast cancer and DCIS, there is also investigation into using a genomic-based assay to assess the risk of locoregional recurrence in patients with node-positive disease. The TAILOR RT trial (Canadian Cancer Trials Group MA 39) is currently accruing breast cancer patients with the following: ER positive, HER2 negative, 1–3 positive lymph nodes, and oncotype DX test recurrence scores <18. Patients are randomized to receive or omit adjuvant regional nodal radiation.

Key Points for Locally Advanced Breast Cancer

- Adjuvant radiation is recommended in patients with $\geq$4 axillary lymph nodes.
- Adjuvant radiation is recommended for patients with residual disease after neoadjuvant chemotherapy and/or patients with clinically node positive disease prior to neoadjuvant chemotherapy. There are 2 major ongoing trials that will help to clarify the role of adjuvant treatment in this setting.
- Individualized shared decision-making is important to decide which patients should have adjuvant radiation for patients with T2 tumors and 1–3 positive lymph nodes.
- Genomic assays may become increasingly important to select appropriate low-risk patients who can forego adjuvant radiation.

Radiation for Metastatic Breast Cancer

Although systemic therapy is the main treatment option for stage IV breast cancer, radiation can be an important local treatment for a specific site of cancer. This can include tumors compressing the spinal cord, tumors blocking an airway, painful chest wall lesions, bone metastases, and brain metastases. These courses of palliative radiation tend to be short in duration (1–10 fractions). Treatments can range from a very simple beam arrangement for bone metastasis to a complex stereotactic radiosurgery treatment of brain oligometastasis.

TOXICITIES/CONTRAINDICATIONS
Toxicities

Radiation toxicities will be less with lower doses and smaller treatment volumes. Therefore, these can vary based on techniques. Other treatments can also affect the extent of toxicities, including chemotherapy and extent of surgery. Overall, modern radiation treatment machines/techniques have contributed to a great reduction in the severity of toxicities compared to older studies. Skin reactions are still common, including erythema, hyperpigmentation, and peeling. Mild fatigue can also occur during the course of radiation treatment. Generally, these side effects resolve within 2–4 weeks after the completion of treatment.

Long-term complications are much less common and more difficult to calculate given the multifactorial nature of these side effects (such as age, genetic predisposition, medical comorbidities, other treatments, smoking history, and radiation techniques). Some representative estimates of these include cardiotoxicity (0.3% absolute increase in cardiac mortality in nonsmokers, 1.2% in smokers),[35] ≥ grade 2 pneumonitis (<2%),[29] secondary malignancy (generally low increased absolute risk of approximately 1:1000),[36] and lymphedema (increase after regional nodal radiation from 13% to 24% compared to ALND alone and from 2% to 6.1% after SLND).[37] In regards to the potential complications with breast reconstruction, there are many factors including radiation field size/dose of radiation, immediate versus delayed reconstruction, autologous versus implant-based reconstruction, and individual patient characteristics.[38]

Contraindications to Radiation Treatment

Relative contraindications to radiation treatment include active connective tissue disease involving the skin (ie, scleroderma) and prior radiation therapy at/near the chest wall or breast. Absolute contraindications include radiation treatment during pregnancy and being homozygous for ATM mutation.[39]

SUMMARY

Radiation is an important component of breast cancer treatment. The role of radiation will continue to be refined with advancing radiation technology as well as improvements in diagnostics, surgery, systemic therapies, and tumor biology assessment. Multidisciplinary management and addressing individual patient factors remain critical for excellent breast cancer patient care.

CLINICS CARE POINTS

- Radiation oncology should be included in decisions regarding adjuvant radiation for local control in breast conservation and locally advanced disease.

DISCLOSURE

The author has nothing to disclose.

REFERENCES

1. Grubbe EH. Priority in the therapeutic use of X-rays. Radiology 1933;21(2): 156–62.
2. Bergom C, Currey A, Desai N, et al. Deep inspiration breath hold: techniques and advantages for cardiac sparing during breast cancer irradiation. Front Oncol 2018;8:87.
3. Bergom C, Kelly T, Morrow N, et al. Prone whole-breast irradiation using three-dimensional conformal radiotherapy in women undergoing breast conservation for early disease yields high rates of excellent to good cosmetic outcomes in patients with large and/or pendulous breasts. Int J Radiat Oncol Biol Phys 2012; 83:3.
4. Mutter RW, Choi JI, Jimenez RB, et al. Proton therapy for breast cancer: a consensus statement from the particle therapy cooperative group bresat cancer subdommittee. Int J Radiat Oncol Biol Phys 2021;111(2):337–59.

5. EBCTG. Effect of radiotherapy after breast-conserving surgery on 10-year recurrence and 15-year breast cancer death: meta-analysis of individual patient data for 10801 women in 17 randomised trials. Lancet 2011;378:1707–16.
6. Hughes KS, Schnaper LA, Bellon JR, et al. Lumpectomy plus tamoxifen with or without irradiation in women age 70 years or older with early breast cancer: long-term follow-up of CALGB 9343. J Clin Oncol 2013;31(19):2382–7.
7. Kunkler IH, Williams LJ, Jack W, et al. Prime 2 Randomised trial (postoperative radiotherapy in minimum-risk elderly): wide local excision and adjuvant hormonal therapy +/- whole breast irradiation in women =/> 65 years with early invasive breast cancer: 10 year results. Cancer Res 2021;81(4_Supplement):GS2-03.
8. Whelan TJ, Pignol JP, Levine MN, et al. Long-term results of hypofractionated radiation therapy for breast cancer. N Engl J Med 2010;362(6):513–20.
9. Haviland JS, Owen JR, Dewar JA, et al. The UK standardisation of breast radiotherapy (START) trials of radiotherapy hypofractionation for treatment of early breast cancer: 10-year follow-up results of two randomised controlled trials. Lancet Oncol 2013;14:1086–94.
10. Shah C, Al-Hilli Z, Vicini F. Advances in breast cancer radiotherapy: implications for current and future practice. JCO Oncol Pract 2021;17(12):697–706.
11. Smith BD, Bellon JR, Blitzblau R, et al. Radiation therapy for the whole breast: executive summary of an american society for radiation oncology (ASTRO) evidence-based guideline. Pracital Radiat Oncol 2018;8:145–52.
12. Brunt AM, Haviland JS, Wheatley D, et al. Hypofractionated breast radiotherapy for 1 week versus 3 weeks (FAST-Forward): 5-year efficacy and late normal tissue effects results from a multicentre, non-inferiority, randomised, phase 3 trial. Lancet 2020;395(10237):1613–26.
13. Brunt AM, Haviland JS, Syndenham M, et al. Ten-year results of FAST: a randomized controlled trial of 5-fraction whole-breast radiotherapy for early breast cancer. J Clin Oncol 2020;38(28):3261–72.
14. Krug D, Baumann R, Combs SE, et al. Moderate hypofractionation remains the standard of care for whole-breast radiotherapy in breast cancer: considerations regarding FAST and FAST-forward. Strahlenther Onkol 2021;197:269–80.
15. ClinicalTrials.gov 2022;. https://clinicaltrials.gov/ct2/show/results/NCT01349322.
16. Vicini FA, Cecchini RS, White JR, et al. Long-term Primary results of accelerated partial breast irradiation after breast-conserving surgery for early-stage breast cancer: a radndomised, phase 3, equivalence trial. Lancet 2019;394(10215):2155–64.
17. Correa C, Harris EE, Leonardi MC, et al. Accelerated partial breast irradiation: executive summary for the update of an ASTRO evidence-based consensus statement. Pract Radiat Oncol 2017;7:73–9.
18. Meattini I, Marrazzo L, Calogero S, et al. Accelerated partial-breast irradiation compared with whole-breast irradiation for early breast cancer: long-term results of the randomized phase III APBI-IMRT-florence trial. J Clin Oncol 2020;38(35):4175–83.
19. Coles CE, Griffin CL, Kirby AM, et al. Partial-breast radiotherapy after breast conservation surgery for patients with early breast cancer (UK IMPORT LOW trial): 5-year Results from a multicentre, randomised, controlled, phase 3, non-inferiority trial. Lancet 2017;390:1048–60.
20. Vaidya JS, Bulsara M, Baum M, et al. Long term survival and local control outocomes from a single dose targeted intraoperative radiotherapy durin gLumpectomy (TARGIT_IORT) for early breast cancer: TARGIT-A randomised clinical trial. BMJ 2020;370:m2836. https://doi.org/10.1136/bmj.m2836.

21. Orecchia R, Veronesi U, Maisonneuve P, et al. Intraoperative irradiation for early breast cancer (ELIOT): long-term recurrence and survival outcomes from a single-centre, randomised, phase 3 equivalence trial. Lancet Oncol 2021;22: 597–608.

22. EBCTG. Overview of the randomized trials of radiotherapy in ductal carcinoma in situ of the breast. J Natl Cancer Inst Monographs 2010;41:162–77.

23. Wapnir IL, Dignam JJ, Fisher B, et al. Long-term outcomes of invasive ipsilateral breast tumor recurrences after lumpectomy in NSABP B-17 and B-24 randomized clinical trials for DCIS. J Natl Cancer Inst 2011;103(6):478–88.

24. McCormick B, Winter KA, Woodward W, et al. Randomized phase III trial evaluating radiation following surgical excision for good-risk ductal carcinoma in situ: long-term report from NRG oncology/RTOG 0984. J Clin Oncol 2021; 39(32):3574–82.

25. Solin LJ, Gray R, Hughes LL, et al. Surgical excision without radiation for ductal carcinoma in situ of the breast: 12-year results from the ECOG-ACRIN E5194 study. J Clin Oncol 2015;33(33):2938–44.

26. Solin LJ, Gray R, Baehner FL, et al. A multigene expression assay to predict local recurrence risk for ductal carcinoma in situ of the breast. J Natl Cancer Inst 2013; 105(10):701–10.

27. Weinmann S, Leo MC, Francisco M, et al. Validation of a ductal carcinoma in situ biomarker profile for risk of recurrence after breast-conserving surgery with and without radiotherapy. Clin Cancer Res 2020;26(15):4054–63.

28. EBCTG. Effect of radiotherapy after mastectomy and axillary surgery on 10-year recurrence and 20-year breast cancer mortality: meta-analysis of individual patient data for 8135 women in 22 randomized trials. Lancet 2014;383:2127–35.

29. Whelan TJ, Olivotto IA, Parulekar WR, et al. Regional nodal irradiation in early-stage breast cancer. N Engl J Med 2015;373(4):307–16.

30. Poortmans PM, Weltens C, Fortpied C, et al. Internal mammary and medial supraclavicular lymph node chain irradiation in stage I-III breast cancer (EORTC22922/ 10925): 15-year results of a randomised, phase 3 trial. Lancet Oncol 2020;21(12): 1602–10.

31. Rutgers E, Donker M, Poncet C, et al. Radiotherapy or surgery of the axilla after a positive sentinel node in breast cancer patients: 10 year follow up results of the EORTC AMAROS trial (EORTC 10981/22023). Cancer Res 2019;79(4). GS4–01.

32. Giuliano AE, Ballman KV, McCall L, et al. Effect of axillary dissection vs no axillary dissection on 10-year overall survival among women with invasive breast cancer and sentinel node metastasis the ACOSOG Z0011 (Alliance) randomized clinical trial. JAMA 2017;318(10):918–26.

33. Jagsi R, Chadha M, Moni J, et al. Radiation field design in the ACOSOG Z0011 (Alliance) trial. J Clin Oncol 2014;32(32):3600–6.

34. Kim YB, Byun HK, Kim DY, et al. Effect of elective internal mammary node irradiation on disease-free survival in women with node-positive breast cancer. JAMA Oncol 2022;8(1):96–105.

35. Taylor C, Correa C, Duane FK, et al. Estimating the risks of breast cancer radiotherapy: evidence from modern radiation doses to the lungs and heart and from previous randomized trials. J Clin Oncol 2017;35(15):1641–9.

36. Clarke M, Collins R, Darby S, et al. Effects of radiotherapy and of differences in the extent of surgery for early breast cancer on local recurrence and 15-year survival: an overview of the randomised trials. Lancet 2005;366:2087–106.

37. Warren LE, Miller CL, Horick N, et al. The impact of radiation therapy on the risk of lymphedema after treatment for breast cancer: a prospective cohort study. Int J Radiat Oncol Biol Phys 2014;88(3):565–71.
38. Ho A, Hu Z, Mehrara B, et al. Radiotherapy in the setting of breast reconstruction: types, techniques, and timing. Lancet Oncol 2017;18:e742–53.
39. Jordan RM, Oxenberg J. Breast cancer conservation therapy. [Updated 2021 Sep 22]. In: StatPearls [Internet]. Treasure Island (FL). StatPearls Publishing; 2022. Available at: https://www.ncbi.nlm.nih.gov/books/NBK547708.

Quality of Life

Quality of Life Issues Following Breast Cancer Treatment

James Abdo, MD*, Holly Ortman, MD, Natalia Rodriguez, MD,
Rachel Tillman, MD, Elizabeth O. Riordan, MD, Anna Seydel, MD

KEYWORDS

- Breast cancer • Survivorship • Lymphedema • Side effects • Quality of life
- Cancer-related cognitive deficit • Hormone therapy • Radiation therapy

KEY POINTS

- As more women develop and survive breast cancer with the increasing length of survival, we review the effects of therapy on their quality of life.
- Provide a patient viewpoint of life with breast cancer and side effects of treatment as well as common topics not often discussed.
- Identify common side effects of therapy, the risk factors leading to side effects, as well as their management.
- Understanding that as breast cancer survival continues to improve, survivorship and quality of life become increasingly important, and may influence cancer treatment, or guide care of common side effects.

INTRODUCTION

With an estimated 5 million breast cancer survivors in 2030,[1] it is important for the breast specialist to understand the impact recommended treatments have on patients to lessen the unwanted effects and improve the overall quality of life. This article explores what patients need beyond good outcomes to maintain a satisfactory quality of life. Quality of Life scoring systems cannot fully describe the subjective effects of cancer and its treatment. These metrics instead reflect the degree of patients' social support and lend evidence to patients' resilience. Subjective scores are minimally affected by measurable morbidities as patients adjust to their new baseline tolerating the side effects of treatment and minimizing the impact on their daily life. Instead of discussing the quality of life scores, this article aims to review the intangible effects of breast cancer treatment, the more concrete side effects of systemic and local therapy, and offer strategies to mitigate them.

This article previously appeared in *Surgical Clinics* volume 103 issue 1 February 2023.
No authors have financial disclosures.
Marshfield Medical Center, 1000 North Oak Street, Marshfield, WI 54449, USA
* Corresponding author.
E-mail address: abdo.james@marshfieldclinic.org

Clinics Collections 14 (2024) 447–459
https://doi.org/10.1016/j.ccol.2024.02.020
2352-7986/24/

Dr O'Riordan, a breast cancer surgeon who is also a breast cancer survivor, offers her insights from the patient's perspective, discussing those aspects of patient care that aren't easily measured or often discussed—that is, sex, intimacy, and fear of recurrence. This is followed by a more didactic review of the commonly investigated side effects of systemic and local treatment. We hope to arm the clinician with the tools necessary to discuss strategies that support behavior modifications and interventions to improve the quality of life for our patients with breast cancer.

Intangible Effects of Treatment

Social media
Patients with breast cancer are talking among themselves on multiple forums about the topics of self-esteem, diet, exercise, sex, intimacy, and anxiety regarding recurrence. Surgeons and oncologists should be potential participants in these conversations. Once a patient with a new diagnosis of breast cancer leaves the office, one of the first things s/he may do is scour the internet for information. It is worth spending a couple of hours walking in your patients' shoes to see what is available to them via social media and the internet. Are you familiar with any breast cancer patient forums, apps, or websites? Have you read any books or blogs written by a patient? Do you know what questions your patients are asking each other and what they really need? Questions they are too scared to ask their breast cancer specialist such as "Is it safe to have sex during chemo? I'm afraid my husband's hair will fall out." These are the issues beyond our evidence-based treatment that affect their everyday lives. Tell your patients that you know they are going to open their phones and computers and give them safe and useful resources to start their journey. This small gesture will make a huge difference to the quality of care you provide for your patients.

Diet
Wellness and nutrition experts on social media claim that various diets and supplements can cure or reduce the risk of getting cancer. Our patients are vulnerable, possibly scared, and quite willing to do anything to stop their cancer from coming back. It is imperative that the clinician talks to them about what they should be eating and drinking as they move forward with their life. The WHO recommends that patients with cancer simply eat a healthy, balanced diet including 6 servings of fruit and vegetables daily. That's it. There is no robust evidence at the moment to prove that any food group can increase or decrease its their risk of recurrence.

Obesity increases the risk of breast cancer recurrence and even death by 35% to 40%.[2] Despite eating normally, many women gain more weight during breast cancer treatment, especially once hormonal manipulation begins. For many women, this information is empowering—getting to and maintaining normal body weight is something patients can do to take control of their future. This is also true for patients who do not have an existing diagnosis of breast cancer. Postmenopausal weight loss reduces the risk of developing breast cancer—a 5% weight reduction lowers the risk of postmenopausal breast cancer by 12%. Conversely, greater than 5% weight gain in the postmenopausal period is associated with a 54% higher incidence of triple-negative disease.[3]

Patients may ask whether it is safe to take supplements they have read about online. Patients with cancer are a captive market, and many are spending hundreds of dollars each month on things they believe they need. All they need is a general multivitamin on top of any bone health supplement. For less common supplements, you can direct patients to a website[4] run by the Memorial Sloan Kettering Cancer Center which will provide current information on the supplement and data regarding its relationship to cancer.

Another important piece of advice to provide patients regarding behavior modifications is to reduce alcohol intake to less than five units per week. According to the National Institutes of Health, one "standard" drink contains roughly 14 g of pure alcohol, which is found in one of the following: 12 fL oz of regular beer, 9 oz of malt liquor, 5 ox of table wine, and 1.5 oz of hard liquor. In addition to postmenopausal weight gain, regular alcohol consumption can also increase the risk of breast cancer recurrence.[5]

Exercise

Exercise should be one of the first treatments you prescribe to every patient. It is effective at reducing side effects[6] such as fatigue, anxiety, and depression, as well as improving quality of life, sleep, and bone health. Exercise can be associated with a decrease in overall mortality for patients with breast cancer and is specifically recommended for patients with bony metastases as it improves physical function and reduces psychosocial morbidity.[7] Every patient should be "prescribed" 75 to 150 weekly minutes of vigorous aerobic activity and twice-weekly progressive resistance exercise targeting all major muscle groups.[7] A good starting place to educate yourself and your patients is the website and book created by Dr Kathryn Schmitz[8] https://www.movingthroughcancer.com. It explains why exercise is so important for patients and gives clear instructions for a resistance program that patients can do at home using simple equipment.

Sex and intimacy

Breast cancer treatment will affect a patient's sex life and it is important to ensure that someone on the treatment team opens the door to these conversations and is available to discuss patient concerns and review options. Challenges with sex and intimacy following treatment of breast cancer start with body image and how patients see themselves after surgery. Some patients grieve for their femininity and sexuality—taken away at a moment's notice following an operation for breast cancer. Breast reconstructions can look realistic, but many women don't realize until they have undergone the initial operation that their reconstructed breast mound is nothing more than that—a mound of tissue or silicone, often under numb skin, without sensation. Postoperative pain and scarring can make patients avoid physical contact with their partners. The added hair loss associated with chemotherapy and burned skin from radiotherapy take their toll on any woman's body image. Additionally, the side effects of hormonal manipulation push women into menopause overnight. Night sweats can cause unbroken sleep and separate bed covers. Vaginal dryness can make intercourse painful, cause bleeding and tearing, and lack of lubrication. Providing patients with information about vaginal dryness and lubricants (used during intercourse) and moisturizers (daily use) is an important component of a patient's cancer care. It is recommended that individuals use a natural lubricant with no parabens or preservatives. Start the conversation by asking patients what lubricant they use, so it seems like a normal part of sex. Have an "intimacy bag" in your clinic with samples of items that women could explore after talking to you and plan follow-up discussions as part of the routine cancer surveillance office visit.

The loss of libido can be damaging to relationships. Some women never feel the urge to have sex after their diagnosis of cancer. Two medications, Vyleesi and Addyi, have been approved by the Food & Drug Administration (FDA) for low sexual drive in premenopausal women, along with one over-the-counter supplement, Ristela, that benefit women of any age.[9,10] These medications have been shown to improve arousal, orgasm, satisfaction, and desire and can be considered for patients undergoing breast cancer treatment.[11]

Also important when counseling patients about sexual intercourse after breast cancer treatment is to remember to talk about the importance of contraception for any premenopausal woman having chemotherapy, HER2 treatment, or tamoxifen as these treatments are all teratogenic.

Vaginal estrogen does not increase the risk of recurrence for women taking Tamoxifen and aromatase inhibitors and should be offered to patients who need more help with lubrication. Vaginal estrogen may need to be used daily for severe symptoms. Dilators may also need to be used with a lubricant to gently stretch the vaginal walls and make intercourse less painful. Advocate for a sexual psychotherapist or advanced practice provider who has been trained in sexual health to be a part of the cancer treatment team and can see your patients in consultation from the time of diagnosis and throughout treatment into survivorship.

Mental health

The fear of recurrence is real for many patients with breast cancer. It can cause extreme anxiety, or "scanxiety" and "labxiety," whenever a patient has a routine mammogram, scan, or laboratories. Alternatively, some women do not realize that their cancer can come back, either locally or as a Stage IV disease. Indeed, a large number of women don't know what symptoms to look for, and more importantly, what to do if they're worried. It is important to provide clear instructions at surveillance visits about the signs and symptoms of a recurrence and who to call should symptoms develop or questions arise.

While nearly all patients with cancer exhibit depressive symptoms at the time of a new breast cancer diagnosis, approximately 25% of patients suffer from a major depressive episode following initial diagnosis.[12] Major depression is not uncommon after breast cancer[13] and can occur months or even years after treatment, often when patients need the most support. It is important that clinicians involved in breast cancer care have a mental health team or referral source to provide patients with options for both situational as well as prolonged depression.

Effects of Systemic Treatment

Cancer-related cognitive impairment

One of the most significant side effects of breast cancer and its treatment is the associated cognitive impairment, often referred to as "chemo-brain." Cancer-related cognitive impairment (CRCI) is a well-identified pattern of cognitive deficits reflecting the CNS toxic effects of not only chemotherapy, but of a systemic malignancy.[1] While most commonly the acquired cognitive deficits are found in verbal memory, sustained attention, executive function, and processing speed, additional domains can be affected such as visual memory, verbal fluency, and upper extremity fine motor dexterity. Even though these effects are well studied, the reported prevalence varies greatly, ranging from 12% to 82% of women with breast cancer.[1] Patients are very aware of these symptoms and discuss them routinely within patient support groups. Living with these cognitive deficits and developing coping strategies is a frequent topic in Facebook groups and other social media outlets. It is the connectivity of patients that have advanced the awareness of the systemic effects of cancer and its treatments among physicians and investigators and helped push the research into these fields.

Despite the frequent occurrence of these symptoms, obtaining objective evidence of cognitive dysfunction has been difficult.[14] Initial cross-sectional studies showed patients performed lower than expected on the neuropsychological testing for cognitive impairment. Subsequent prospective studies challenged the concept of "chemo brain" with some reporting no cognitive impairment and others limiting their effects to a few cognitive domains which are discordant with the patient's experience. Additionally, studies showed that CRCI was independent of chemotherapy, with deficits seen before receiving chemotherapy and in patients that did not receive chemotherapy.[14–16] Additional studies have added objective evidence with neuroimaging showing structural and functional changes In those patients who underwent chemotherapy raising further questions about the impact of cognitive decline on patients.[14,15] Several possibilities could explain these discrepancies—patient's abilities to compensate for the cognitive impairment in the affected domains, inability of testing to accurately capture the cognitive deficits, overlap of effects of depression and anxiety on cognitive function, or the possibility of small deficits having a large effect on patient's perception.

One suggested model for the conceptualization of the interaction between cancer, treatment, and cognitive function is the "soil, seed, and pesticides model," referring to the patient's predisposing factors, the disease-related factors of cancer, and the systemic treatments used to eradicate the cancer. While chemotherapy has been an obvious culprit, there is evidence that hormonal treatments and radiation therapy can also affect cognition.[1] While early age-related cognitive decline may put patients at risk of CRCI, cancer-related cognitive impairment does not seem to increase the risk of dementia.[17,18]

While patient risk factors such as age, diabetes, and hypertension may have an important role in determining chemotherapy regimens in the future,[16] the best predictor of the effects of CRCI is a patient's cognitive reserve (CR). Defined as innate and developed cognitive capacity, the cognitive reserve may be one of our most reliable predictors of severity. CR, which is influenced by education, occupational attainment, and lifestyle has been used as a measurement in studies evaluating brain pathology in disease states such as Alzheimer's, Parkinson's, traumatic brain injury, and multiple sclerosis. CR is influenced by both mentally or physically stimulating activities and it may be of use to identify those at risk of CRCI to guide resources available to attenuate the functional decline. Cognitive rehab training, meditation, and exercise are lifestyle modifications that have been shown to improve recovery from CRCI. In addition to comprehensive therapy, medications can also be used to mitigate the development and severity of cognitive impairment for our patients, including modafinil, antidepressants, cotinine, donepezil, and antioxidants.[18]

Peripheral neuropathy

Patients with breast cancer have some of the highest rates of chemotherapy-induced peripheral neuropathy (CIPN), with effects so severe it may affect oncologic outcomes by forcing dose modifications. The mechanism is through the demyelination of the dorsal root ganglion and peripheral nerves, causing numbness, paresthesias, or pain.[19,20] Common complaints include tingling, cold sensitivity, a feeling of wearing gloves or stockings, burning, freezing, shock-like, or electric pain.[21,22] While sensory and not motor nerves are often affected, patients have loss of proprioception and touch which lead to decreased dexterity and mobility impairing the patient's ability to perform activities of daily living. While neuropathy itself is distressing, these effects are compounded by worsening mental health for patients as they experience frustration, loss of purpose, and depression because they can no longer participate in activities of daily living.[23] Patients adjust to their degree of impairment due to CIPN and the impact of peripheral neuropathy on their daily life is not accurately reflected in the routine quality of life scores.[20] Introduction of more standardized scales such as the total neuropathy score, CIPN 20, and the FACT/GOG-NTX may help generalize findings amongst future studies to adequately measure the impact on quality of life.

Recognition of CIPN's effect on the quality of life has led to the search for treatments and prevention. Strategies to prevent peripheral neuropathy, which are being developed and include nutritional supplements and cryotherapy, have yet to show definitive benefits.[24] Pharmacologic treatment of neuropathy is limited, with duloxetine and pregabalin being the few medications shown to have an effect. Exercise has been shown to have some benefits as well. Presently, the only proven practice to manage peripheral neuropathy is to implement dose reductions to reduce the risk of developing permanent disabling neuropathy.

Hormone therapy

Approximately 75% of all patients with breast cancer are eligible to receive adjuvant endocrine therapy, such as a selective estrogen receptor modulator (SERM) like tamoxifen or an aromatase inhibitor like anastrozole.[25] When these medications are taken as directed, these therapies can reduce the risk of recurrence by 40% and reduce mortality by 33%.[26] However, side effects can be so severe that often patients choose to discontinue this essential therapy. Side effects of endocrine therapy include alopecia, anxiety, cognitive dysfunction, fatigue, hot flashes, sleep disturbances, loss of sexual interest, musculoskeletal pain, nausea, osteoporosis, dyspareunia, vaginal dryness, weight gain, and many more. In younger patients, the effects can be amplified due to the abrupt suppression of estrogen which pushes patients into menopause.[27]

Some studies have looked into the patient quality of life and how the medication's side effects correlate to medication adherence.[26] Multiple factors were assessed, most notably the daily impact of hormone therapy side effects. Patients report side effects as "excruciating," and many states that these side effects have limited their ability to do household maintenance, perform their work duties, or even do things as simple as getting out of bed. Effects can also exacerbate others; for example, hot flashes can cause sleep disturbances which then lead to fatigue, and can then result in cognitive decline or "brain fog."

Management strategies to combat hot flashes include pharmacologic options, such as gabapentin, venlafaxine, clonidine, oxybutynin, and progesterone analogs.[27] Offering support and recommending patients wear layers have a fan at their desk and air conditioning nearby, can help patients navigate their inevitable symptoms of hormonal treatment and improve compliance. Other side effects that play a key role in the quality of life for many patients taking hormone therapy are sexual dysfunction due to associated vulvovaginal changes, decreased libido, and psychosocial effects which can contribute to poor communication between partners. It has been shown that 79% of patients on an aromatase inhibitor report sexual dysfunction, and 24% of patients have stopped having sex with their partners.[28] As previously discussed, it is important to review vaginal lubricants and moisturizers with your patients as they embark on hormone therapy.

During follow-up appointments the focus is often on disease recurrence and side effects are downplayed or overlooked.[27] However, with the emergence of therapies to counteract these potentially debilitating side effects inclusive exercise; improved diet, additional medications, it is important to discuss these interventions as well as signs of recurrence in order to improve the patient's quality of life.

Effects of Local Treatment

Breast/chest wall pain

Postmastectomy pain syndrome (PMPS) is localized to the axilla, medial upper arm, breast, and chest wall, is described as neuropathic in nature, and persists more than 3 to 18 months after surgery.[29] Pain can be severe enough to not only interfere with sleep and daily activities but also lead to decreased use of the arm and the development of a frozen shoulder or complex regional pain syndrome. PMPS is caused by direct nerve injury or subsequent formation of a traumatic neuroma or scar tissue and presents with tingling, burning, and numbness. Often the anterior and lateral cutaneous branches are injured. Treatment often starts with pharmacotherapy with drugs targeting neuropathic pain such as gabapentin, carbamazepine, venlafaxine, and duloxetine which have been shown to be effective. If this is ineffective, surgical treatment such as axillary scar release or autologous fat grafting may be appropriate, along with physical therapy, to improve symptoms.[30]

Chronic breast/chest wall pain after surgery affects 25% to 60% of patients.[29] The prevalence of chronic pain varies by treatment and has been found to be 25% for patients treated with mastectomy without adjuvant therapy, and 60% for patients treated with breast-conserving therapy, axillary lymph node dissection, and radiation.[31] As in lymphedema, obesity is an independent risk factor for the development of breast pain. Age is also a significant risk factor with several studies showing young age to be a predictive factor for the development of chronic breast pain. In fact, increasing age is associated with a decrease in postoperative pain.[29] High-quality evidence and review of the literature—30 studies involving 19,813 patients—showed a significant association between persistent pain after breast cancer surgery and 2 nonmodifiable factors: younger age and radiotherapy.[32] The most significant associated modifiable factor is ALND, regardless of whether lumpectomy or mastectomy was performed. Women who underwent ALND experienced a 21% increase in the absolute risk of chronic postoperative pain. In addition to modifying the risk of lymphedema, efforts to omit ALND will also have a favorable impact on reducing the incidence of chronic postoperative pain. Other potentially modifiable associated risk factors for persistent pain are the degree of acute postoperative pain and presence of preoperative pain. Despite this, the use of regional anesthesia has not shown any improvement in reducing chronic pain or improving the overall quality of life.[32]

Lymphedema

Lymphedema is one of the most common and yet underestimated complications of breast cancer treatment. It is caused by the disruption of the lymphatics of the axillary system by cancer and its treatment. It is one of the most significant complications of breast cancer treatment and additionally can add a significant financial burden to patients affected. Lymphedema is progressive and debilitating and requires proactive diagnosis, surveillance, and therapy to reverse early stages and prevent progressing to later stages. Management has been modernized, and new techniques in limiting risk as well as managing lymphedema have been developed.

The risk of developing lymphedema is dependent on the extent of surgery or radiation performed in the axilla. As each additional therapy seems to have synergistic effects that increase the risk of lymphedema, limiting therapies to either one adjuvant therapy or no adjuvant therapy will be essential in limiting the incidence of lymphedema in breast cancer survivors.

Treatment of lymphedema should start at diagnosis as it is a progressive disease and in later stages is irreversible. Classically lymphedema was identified by symptoms such as swelling of the affected limb, pain, weakness, fatigue, impaired mobility, skin changes with "brawny edema," and recurrent infections.[33] But, waiting for patients to become symptomatic leads to later presentations with irreversible changes. Early diagnosis requires proactive surveillance with adequate follow-up. Developing a protocol for determining limb measurement and standardizing this within a practice is essential. Multiple studies have shown that objectively measured lymphedema may have little to no effect on patients' quality of life (QoL), while self-reported or symptomatic lymphedema has a severe effect on QoL. Factors affecting QoL include increased financial burden, restricted lifestyles and activities, and potential negative career impact with missed days at work and hospitalizations.[34–37] It is important to note that most reported incidences of lymphedema are likely to be low as many studies have inadequate follow-up periods of only 1 to 2 years.[34] Even though approximately 75% of lymphedema patients will present within 3 years of their operation,[38] a recent meta-analysis has shown the cumulative incidence of lymphedema increases to 40% at 10 years after treatment.[34,39]

In a review by Eaton and colleagues, upper extremity pain and decreased limb function were found to be the 2 primary physical health factors affecting the quality of life; while the psychological health factors included body image disturbance and psychological stress in the form of anxiety, depression, emotional distress, fatigue, self-care, relationship issues, impaired mobility, and ability to participate in social activities.[40] Recent reviews have challenged the lifestyle-limiting "risk-reducing factors" such as IV placement, blood pressure monitoring, and blood draws in the affected arm. This recent data suggests no increased risk of lymphedema with these common procedures.[41]

Obesity—specifically a BMI $\geq$ 30 kg/m2 at breast cancer diagnosis—is the only independent risk factor for the development of lymphedema.[34,42] Emerging data support that monitored, low-impact exercise is actually beneficial in reducing the risk and symptoms of lymphedema. Additionally exercise improves the quality of life and can help with weight loss goals which decrease the risk and severity of lymphedema.[34,43,44]

Lymphedema treatment has expanded in recent years and includes a patient-specific regimen that is in line with their goals. The mainstay of lymphedema treatment is Complete Decongestive Therapy. This includes lymphatic massage, physical therapy, and compression stockings with surgical intervention being limited to those who fail medical management. The two microsurgical techniques that are most widely used are vascularized lymph node transfer and lymphaticovenous anastomosis. The indication for vascularized lymph node transfer is complete blockage and loss of lymph nodes in a patient who has failed conservative treatment.[45] Lymphaticovenous anastomosis, initially described in 1969, is indicated when patients still have a functional lymphatic system with an underlying blockage and a venous system with intact valves (Brahma and colleagues). A meta-analysis by Basta and colleagues, compared LVA and VLN, demonstrating that both interventions are efficient in short-term outcomes; however, patients with VLN showed better long-term improvement with an increased likelihood of not needing to wear compression stockings.[33,46] In patients who are plagued by recurrent infection or failure of medical management, surgical interventions can be considered, although not widely used due to the morbidities and inability to show generalizable results.[47]

Preventative surgical options are being evaluated such as arm lymph node mapping at the time of surgery to try to find lymph nodes or sentinel lymph nodes away from those that drain the arm. Studied techniques include primary lymphovenous bypass performed at the time of axillary treatment. Again, initial findings are hopeful, but are not strong enough to make these operations commonplace.

Radiation

Radiation has evolved into a refined and precise process that is pivotal in breast cancer care. Radiotherapy techniques have continued to improve to minimize adverse effects such as cardiomyopathy and lung damage which occurred when radiation fields of early breast cancer protocols were much larger. This is especially significant now as the indications for radiation in breast cancer continue to expand.

Overall, radiotherapy is initially tolerated fairly well, but early toxicities and late complications greatly impact the quality of life of our patients. Often, the hyperacute side effects are immediately noticeable and include fatigue, skin changes (dermatitis), and breast edema. These effects are often limited to the duration of the treatment and resolve completely within 2 weeks of completion of radiation.

The indications for radiotherapy for local control continue to increase as the treatment of the axilla moves away from axillary dissection due to the morbid complication of lymphedema. However, while the morbidity is lower, there are still long-term effects of radiation that may become more significant as the treated population continues to grow.

Early and late pulmonary complications may occur following radiation therapy as portions of the lung lie within the radiation portals: anterolateral peripheral in the setting of breast and chest wall irradiation and the lung apex in the setting of supraclavicular irradiation. One early occurring syndrome of note is bronchiolitis obliterans organizing pneumonia or bilateral lymphocytic alveolitis. This is a rare entity with symptoms including cough, dyspnea, asthenia, and weight loss that responds well to corticosteroids, has a high recurrence rate, and an excellent prognosis, virtually never progressing or developing into chronic fibrosis.[48,49] More commonly, radiation pneumonitis can occur and is seen typically in 4 to 12 weeks following the completion of radiotherapy. Symptoms can include dry cough, dyspnea, and low-grade fever. Corticosteroids are the treatment of choice and maximal improvement can be expected within 48 months. Symptoms that persist beyond 48 months will not typically improve.[48,50] Lung fibrosis can be seen as early as 6 months, peaks at 2 years, and remains stable thereafter. This is associated with limited changes in pulmonary function tests, and when occurs is irreversible.[48,50]

Cardiac toxicity is associated with the radiation of the internal mammary chain which is increasingly included in the clinical target volume as it increases overall survival.[51,52] Cardiac toxicities as a result of breast cancer treatment include left ventricular dysfunction, congestive heart failure, pericarditis, myocardial ischemia, arterial hypertension, conduction abnormalities, atrial and ventricular arrhythmias, and thromboembolic disease with the major cardiovascular toxicity of radiation therapy being coronary artery disease.[52] Techniques of radiation including proton therapy, breath-holding, optimization of the beam angles, intensity-modulated radiotherapy, and prone positioning among others are being used to attempt to decrease the cardiac effects of radiation therapy.[51]

Advances in radiation therapy have led to more favorable outcomes and radiotherapy can be routinely used in those who choose implant-based or autologous reconstruction with high satisfaction. The longer the time interval between surgery and radiation, the less likely patients are to encounter wound healing complications following reconstruction surgery (wound dehiscence).[53] Capsular contraction is seen more commonly in those patients that have radiation directly to the permanent implant as opposed to the tissue expander, but this disparity is attributed to the capsulotomy performed at the time of exchanging the tissue expander for the permanent implant. Anecdotal evidence supports the use of acellular dermal matrices for breast reconstruction as well as fat grafting to correct contour deformities, but the benefits have not been studied in a controlled manner.[54] Skin fibrosis is seen in approximately 11% of patients and is associated with ptosis (grade $^2/_3$) or pseudoptosis, bra size >/ = cup C, and a decreased time interval from surgery to radiotherapy.[53] Telangiectasias and impaired cosmetic outcomes are also seen in late radiation toxicity and may significantly impact the quality of life of the patient.

Radiation fibrosis results in other side effects including the relatively rare complication of brachial plexus neuropathy, which is motor or sensory symptoms or physical signs with or without pain in a nerve-root distribution and may include paresthesias, hypoesthesia, hypoalgesia, dysesthesia, paresis, hyporeflexia, and muscle atrophy; this plexopathy is irreversible.[48] Fibrosis may also lead to shoulder stiffness requiring physical therapy to alleviate this fibrosis, but again, is also irreversible.

Hyperbaric therapy (HBOT) has been studied in the Netherlands as a means to alleviate late radiation toxicity and is approved by insurance in the Netherlands for different tumor sites. Late radiation toxicity is primarily characterized by breast/chest wall pain, breast and/or arm edema, fibrosis, impaired arm movement, telangiectasia, and impaired cosmetic outcome following breast cancer treated with radiotherapy.[55] Batenburg and colleagues describe the reduced pain, breast and arm symptoms, and improved quality of life following hyperbaric treatment of late radiation toxicity.[55] In 1005 patients, pain scores improved from 43.4 to 29.7 at 3 months post-HBOT; breast symptoms decreased from 44.6 to 28.9 and arm symptoms decreased from 38.2 to 27.4; all of these being significant ($P < .05$). There were minimal side effects with the most prevalent being myopia and mild barotrauma.[55]

SUMMARY

To improve the quality of life for our patients, it is essential to recognize the side effects of breast cancer treatment, identify root causes of nonspecific symptoms, and understand cancer survivorship and the anxiety, self-image, and interpersonal relationship issues that patients experience. Comprehensive counseling begins at diagnosis and includes knowing available resources and appropriate treatment at each step along our patients' breast cancer journey. The number of breast cancer survivors will continue to grow and our understanding of life after breast cancer treatment must keep pace to maximize the quality of life in survivorship.

REFERENCES

1. Cristian A. Breast cancer and gynecologic cancer rehabilitation. 2021 [Online]. Available: https://www.clinicalkey.com.au/dura/browse/bookChapter/3-s2.0-C20 180032375. Accessed date May 25, 2022.
2. Jiralerspong S, Goodwin PJ. Obesity and Breast Cancer Prognosis: Evidence, Challenges, and Opportunities. J Clin Oncol 2016;34(35):4203–16. https://doi.org/10.1200/JCO.2016.68.4480.
3. Chlebowski RT, et al. Weight loss and breast cancer incidence in postmenopausal women. Cancer 2019;125(2):205–12.
4. Integrative Medicine: Search About Herbs | Memorial Sloan Kettering Cancer Center. Available at: https://www.mskcc.org/cancer-care/diagnosis-treatment/symptom-management/integrative-medicine/herbs/search. Accessed May 26, 2022.
5. Simapivapan P, Boltong A, Hodge A. To what extent is alcohol consumption associated with breast cancer recurrence and second primary breast cancer?: a systematic review. Cancer Treat. Rev 2016;50:155–67.
6. Coletta AM, Basen-Engquist KM, Schmitz KH. Exercise Across the Cancer Care Continuum: Why It Matters, How to Implement It, and Motivating Patients to Move. Am Soc Clin Oncol Educ Book 2022;42:1–7.
7. Campbell KL, et al. Exercise Recommendation for People With Bone Metastases: Expert Consensus for Health Care Providers and Exercise Professionals. JCO Oncol Pract 2022;18(5):e697–709.

8. Moving Through Cancer," Moving Through Cancer. Available at: https://www.movingthroughcancer.com. Accessed May 26, 2022.

9. Kingsberg SA, Simon JA. Female Hypoactive Sexual Desire Disorder: A Practical Guide to Causes, Clinical Diagnosis, and Treatment. J Womens Health 2020; 29(8):1101–12.

10. Kim L. Hypoactive sexual desire disorder: How do you identify it and treat it? Women's Healthc 2019. Available at: https://www.npwomenshealthcare.com/hypoactive-sexual-desire-disorder-how-do-you-identify-it-and-treat-it/. Accessed July 16, 2022.

11. Dupree B. The American Society of Breast Surgeons | ASBrS," The American Society of Breast Surgeons Fellows Webinars, Surveillance and Survivorship. 2021. https://www.breastsurgeons.org/resources/videos?v=214. Accessed May 25, 2022.

12. Gass J, et al. Breast Cancer Survivorship: Why, What and When? Ann Surg Oncol 2016;23(10):3162–7.

13. Fann JR, et al. Major depression after breast cancer: a review of epidemiology and treatment. Gen Hosp Psychiatry 2008;30(2):112–26.

14. Hermelink K. Chemotherapy and Cognitive Function in Breast Cancer Patients: The So-Called Chemo Brain. JNCI Monogr 2015;51:67–9.

15. McDonald BC, Conroy SK, Ahles TA, et al. Alterations in Brain Activation During Working Memory Processing Associated With Breast Cancer and Treatment: A Prospective Functional Magnetic Resonance Imaging Study. J Clin Oncol 2012; 30(20):2500–8.

16. Pomykala KL, de Ruiter MB, Deprez S, et al. Integrating imaging findings in evaluating the post-chemotherapy brain. Brain Imaging Behav 2013;7(4):436–52.

17. Raji MA, et al. Risk of subsequent dementia diagnoses does not vary by types of adjuvant chemotherapy in older women with breast cancer. Med Oncol Northwood Lond Engl 2009;26(4):452–9.

18. Bai L, Yu E. A narrative review of risk factors and interventions for cancer-related cognitive impairment. Ann Transl Med 2021;9(1):72.

19. Bhatnagar B, et al. Chemotherapy dose reduction due to chemotherapy induced peripheral neuropathy in breast cancer patients receiving chemotherapy in the neoadjuvant or adjuvant settings: a single-center experience. SpringerPlus 2014;3(1):366.

20. Mols F, Beijers T, Vreugdenhil G, et al. Chemotherapy-induced peripheral neuropathy and its association with quality of life: a systematic review. Support Care Cancer 2014;22(8):2261–9.

21. Stubblefield MD, et al. NCCN Task Force Report: Management of Neuropathy in Cancer. J Natl Compr Cancer Netw J Natl Compr Canc Netw 2009;7(Suppl_5). https://doi.org/10.6004/jnccn.2009.0078. S-1-S-26.

22. Stubblefield MD, McNeely ML, Alfano CM, et al. A prospective surveillance model for physical rehabilitation of women with breast cancer. Cancer 2012;118(S8): 2250–60.

23. Tofthagen C. Patient Perceptions Associated With Chemotherapy-Induced Peripheral Neuropathy. Clin J Oncol Nurs 2010;14(3). E22–E28.

24. Gutiérrez-Gutiérrez G, Sereno M, Miralles A, et al. Chemotherapy-induced peripheral neuropathy: clinical features, diagnosis, prevention and treatment strategies. Clin Transl Oncol 2010;12(2):81–91.

25. Zwart W, Terra H, Linn SC, et al. Cognitive effects of endocrine therapy for breast cancer: keep calm and carry on? Nat Rev Clin Oncol 2015;12(10). https://doi.org/10.1038/nrclinonc.2015.124. Art. no. 10.

26. Peddie N, Agnew S, Crawford M, et al. The impact of medication side effects on adherence and persistence to hormone therapy in breast cancer survivors: A qualitative systematic review and thematic synthesis. The Breast 2021;58:147–59.
27. Franzoi MA, et al. Evidence-based approaches for the management of side-effects of adjuvant endocrine therapy in patients with breast cancer. Lancet Oncol 2021;22(7). https://doi.org/10.1016/S1470-2045(20)30666-5. e303–e313.
28. Kagan R, Kellogg-Spadt S, Parish SJ. Practical Treatment Considerations in the Management of Genitourinary Syndrome of Menopause. Drugs Aging 2019; 36(10):897–908.
29. Andersen KG, Kehlet H. Persistent Pain After Breast Cancer Treatment: A Critical Review of Risk Factors and Strategies for Prevention. J Pain 2011;12(7):725–46.
30. Larsson IM, Ahm Sørensen J, Bille C. The Post-mastectomy Pain Syndrome—A Systematic Review of the Treatment Modalities. Breast J 2017;23(3):338–43.
31. Gärtner R, Jensen M-B, Nielsen J, et al. Prevalence of and Factors Associated With Persistent Pain Following Breast Cancer Surgery. JAMA 2009;302(18): 1985–92.
32. Chhabra A, Roy Chowdhury A, Prabhakar H, et al. Paravertebral anaesthesia with or without sedation versus general anaesthesia for women undergoing breast cancer surgery. Cochrane Database Syst Rev 2021;2. https://doi.org/10.1002/14651858.CD012968.pub2.
33. Pappalardo M, Starnoni M, Franceschini G, et al. Breast Cancer-Related Lymphedema: Recent Updates on Diagnosis, Severity and Available Treatments. J Pers Med 2021;11(5):402. https://doi.org/10.3390/jpm11050402.
34. McLaughlin S. The Valuable Ounce: Surgical and Radiation Oncology Considerations for Lymphedema Prevention," Lymphedema- Diagnosis and management. 2021. Available at: https://www.breastsurgeons.org/resources/videos?v=211. Accessed May 30, 2022.
35. Fleissig A, et al. Post-operative arm morbidity and quality of life. Results of the ALMANAC randomised trial comparing sentinel node biopsy with standard axillary treatment in the management of patients with early breast cancer. Breast Cancer Res Treat 2006;95(3):279–93.
36. Grada AA, Phillips TJ. Lymphedema: Pathophysiology and clinical manifestations. J Am Acad Dermatol 2017;77(6):1009–20.
37. Armer JM, et al. Lymphedema symptoms and limb measurement changes in breast cancer survivors treated with neoadjuvant chemotherapy and axillary dissection: results of American College of Surgeons Oncology Group (ACOSOG) Z1071 (Alliance) substudy. Support Care Cancer 2019;27(2):495–503.
38. McDuff SGR, et al. Timing of Lymphedema After Treatment for Breast Cancer: When Are Patients Most At Risk? Int J Radiat Oncol Biol Phys 2019;103(1):62–70.
39. Gillespie TC, Sayegh HE, Brunelle CL, et al. Breast cancer-related lymphedema: risk factors, precautionary measures, and treatments. Gland Surg 2018;7(4): 379–403.
40. Eaton LH, Narkthong N, Hulett JM. Psychosocial Issues Associated with Breast Cancer-Related Lymphedema: a Literature Review. Curr Breast Cancer Rep 2020;12(4):216–24.
41. Asdourian MS, et al. Association Between Precautionary Behaviors and Breast Cancer–Related Lymphedema in Patients Undergoing Bilateral Surgery. J Clin Oncol 2017;35(35):3934–41.
42. McLaughlin SA, et al. Trends in Risk Reduction Practices for the Prevention of Lymphedema in the First 12 Months after Breast Cancer Surgery. J Am Coll Surg 2013;216(3):380–9.

43. Kwan ML, Cohn JC, Armer JM, et al. Exercise in patients with lymphedema: a systematic review of the contemporary literature. J Cancer Surviv 2011;5(4): 320–36.
44. Schmitz KH, et al. Effect of Home-Based Exercise and Weight Loss Programs on Breast Cancer–Related Lymphedema Outcomes Among Overweight Breast Cancer Survivors: The WISER Survivor Randomized Clinical Trial. JAMA Oncol 2019; 5(11):1605–13.
45. Gasteratos K, Morsi-Yeroyannis A, Vlachopoulos NC, et al. Microsurgical techniques in the treatment of breast cancer-related lymphedema: a systematic review of efficacy and patient outcomes. Breast Cancer Tokyo Jpn 2021;28(5): 1002–15.
46. Basta MN, et al. Complicated breast cancer–related lymphedema: evaluating health care resource utilization and associated costs of management. Am J Surg 2016;211(1):133–41.
47. Brahma B, Yamamoto T. Breast cancer treatment-related lymphedema (BCRL): An overview of the literature and updates in microsurgery reconstructions. Eur J Surg Oncol 2019;45(7):1138–45.
48. Senkus-Konefka E, Jassem J. Complications of breast-cancer radiotherapy. Clin Oncol R Coll Radiol G B 2006;18(3):229–35.
49. Ducray J, et al. [Radiation-induced bronchiolitis obliterans with organizing pneumonia]. Cancer Radiother J Soc Francaise Radiother Oncol 2017;21(2):148–54.
50. Hanania AN, Mainwaring W, Ghebre YT, et al. Radiation-Induced Lung Injury: Assessment and Management. Chest 2019;156(1):150–62.
51. Taylor CW, Kirby AM. Cardiac Side-effects From Breast Cancer Radiotherapy. Clin Oncol R Coll Radiol G B 2015;27(11):621–9.
52. Caron J, Nohria A. Cardiac Toxicity from Breast Cancer Treatment: Can We Avoid This? Curr Oncol Rep 2018;20(8):61.
53. Hille-Betz U, et al. Late radiation side effects, cosmetic outcomes and pain in breast cancer patients after breast-conserving surgery and three-dimensional conformal radiotherapy : Risk-modifying factors. Strahlenther Onkol Organ Dtsch Rontgengesellschaft Al 2016;192(1):8–16.
54. Ho AY, Hu ZI, Mehrara BJ, et al. Radiotherapy in the setting of breast reconstruction: types, techniques, and timing. Lancet Oncol 2017;18(12):e742–53.
55. Batenburg MCT, et al. The impact of hyperbaric oxygen therapy on late radiation toxicity and quality of life in breast cancer patients. Breast Cancer Res Treat 2021;189(2):425–33.

Evidence-Based Guidance for Breast Cancer Survivorship

Elizabeth J. Cathcart-Rake, MD*, Kathryn J. Ruddy, MD, MPH

KEYWORDS

- Survivorship • Symptom management • Symptom control
- Side effects of chemotherapy • Side effects of endocrine therapy
- Breast cancer surveillance

KEY POINTS

Survivorship care encompasses the following:

- Control and management of side effects to cancer-directed therapy.
- Support for mental health concerns.
- Health and wellness promotion.
- Surveillance for breast and other cancers.
- Support for future fertility, if applicable.

INTRODUCTION TO BREAST CANCER SURVIVORSHIP

There are over 3.8 million breast cancer survivors in the United States, and this number is projected to increase by over 30% over the next decade due to advances in cancer screening and improvements In cancer therapeutics.[1,2] Cancer survivorship by definition starts immediately after a cancer diagnosis; the inclusivity of this term emphasizes the importance of supporting patients throughout the cancer continuum.[3] Cancer survivorship care consists of managing symptoms and side effects related to cancer and cancer-directed therapy as well as surveilling for recurrences and new primary cancers. Ideally, cancer survivorship care supports the overall health and wellness of a patient and a patient's caregivers throughout the cancer journey.

This guide discuss evidence-based recommendations regarding several aspects of cancer survivorship, focusing on long-term issues: management of lingering physical symptoms after completion of cancer-directed therapies, support for the emotional toll exacted by a cancer diagnosis and cancer therapies, monitoring and optimization of cardiac and bone health, general wellness promotion, reproductive considerations,

This article previously appeared in Surgical Clinics volume 37 issue 1 February 2023

Department of Oncology, Mayo Clinic, 200 First Street Southwest, Rochester, MN 55905, USA

* Corresponding author.

E-mail address: Cathcart-Rake.Elizabeth@mayo.edu

Twitter: @CathcartRake (E.J.C.-R.); @KathrynRuddyMD (K.J.R.)

Clinics Collections 14 (2024) 461–479

https://doi.org/10.1016/j.ccol.2024.02.021

surveillance strategies, care coordination, and mitigation of disparities in survivorship care. Although cancer survivorship also encompasses the management of acute toxicities of cancer-directed therapies as well as advanced care planning and end-of-life care, such topics will be not be covered in this review.

MANAGEMENT OF SYMPTOMS RELATED TO CANCER-DIRECTED THERAPY
Lymphedema

Lymphedema is a feared consequence of breast cancer surgery and radiation therapy and has prompted the development of new surgical and radiation oncology techniques aimed at decreasing the risk for this morbid condition. Rates of lymphedema differ greatly, from as low as 3% among women without nodal involvement of their cancer undergoing sentinel lymph node biopsies to 60% in women with significant nodal disease requiring both axillary lymph node dissection and axillary radiation therapy; incidence also greatly depends on diagnostic methodology and other patient characteristics (including body mass index [BMI], postoperative infection).[4] The timing of lymphedema onset also differs depending on surgical type but seems to peak between 12 and 30 months postoperatively.[5] Untreated lymphedema worsens with time. Although previous guidelines suggested that patients avoid such things as blood pressure checks and venipuncture on the side of their axillary surgeries, as well as wearing a compression garment during air travel, these cautions are not thought to be necessary based on data showing that following such guidance does not decrease risk for lymphedema.[6]

It is recommended that patients undergo presurgical limb measurements to decrease the risk for misdiagnosis postoperatively.[7] There is a lack of standardization in objective measurements, and so this may differ from site to site, but an increase in relative limb volume or weight-adjusted change by $\geq$ 10% is generally due to lymphedema.[4] Screening should continue every 6 to 12 months for a minimum of 2 to 3 years.[4] Unfortunately, despite the guideline recommendations for lymphedema surveillance, a paucity of providers with lymphedema-specific training remains.[8]

Mild-to-moderate lymphedema may be managed conservatively, with manual lymphatic drainage by a lymphedema therapist, followed by compression garments, self-performed manual lymphatic drainage, exercise, and skin care.[9,10] For patients with significant symptoms who are unable to attend clinic regularly or need adjunctive treatments, intermittent pneumatic compression pumps may be used, although the data supporting this approach are mixed.[11]

Exercise may also improve lymphedema symptoms. One randomized trial of a year-long, facility-based weight lifting exercise program showed a 35% reduction in lymphedema symptoms.[12] Unfortunately, a subsequent study of a home-based resistance training program did not show significant improvements between the exercise and control group.[13]

There is great interest in surgical management of breast cancer-related lymphedema, but it is not yet clear which procedures benefit which patients. Surgical decision-making should be discussed among a multidisciplinary team with relevant expertise.[4]

Chemotherapy-Induced Peripheral Neuropathy

Chemotherapy-induced peripheral neuropathy is a common symptom affecting at least one-third of breast cancer survivors receiving taxane chemotherapy and includes numbness, tingling, burning pain, and/or sensorimotor disturbances, which typically starts in the tips of the toes and fingers and may progress into a stocking-

and-glove distribution. In some survivors, this may persist for years beyond chemotherapy completion (sometimes permanently) and contributes substantially to poorer quality of life.[14]

Despite numerous studies investigating potential therapies for chemotherapy-induced peripheral neuropathy, only one medication has been shown to be effective in decreasing neuropathy-related pain within the context of a large placebo-controlled clinical trial: duloxetine.[15] Preliminary data suggest a potential benefit for interventions such as exercise, acupuncture, and Scrambler therapy, but further evidence is needed.[16,17] Results of studies of other agents, including oral gabapentin/pregabalin, topical baclofen/amitriptyline/ketamine, oral tricyclic antidepressants, and oral cannabinoids, have been mixed.

Vasomotor Symptoms

Nearly 80% of breast cancer survivors receiving endocrine therapy experience vasomotor symptoms, such as hot flashes and night sweats, according to population-based studies.[18] Vasomotor symptoms secondary to endocrine therapy typically plateau after a few months of therapy; occasionally they can self-resolve, though many women experience such symptoms for years.

Conservative strategies for managing hot flashes include dressing in layers, avoiding foods that exacerbate symptoms (caffeine, alcohol, and spicy foods), using fans, or cool pillows at night. Although weight loss may help decrease hot flashes, exercise alone does not seem to be particularly effective.[19,20]

Menopausal hormone replacement therapy, the traditional treatment option for women with hot flashes and no history of cancer, has been associated with an increased risk of breast cancer recurrence and so should only be considered in very limited scenarios, for instance, in women with estrogen receptor-negative breast cancers who have undergone bilateral mastectomy.[21]

Several antidepressants, including selective serotonin reuptake inhibitors (SSRIs) and serotonin norepinephrine reuptake inhibitors (SNRIs), have been shown to significantly decrease hot flashes; specifically, including citalopram, escitalopram, and venlafaxine have been shown to be beneficial in this setting.[22–24] Oxybutynin has also been shown to decrease hot flashes, with minimal side effects, compared with placebo.[25] As these agents have not been studied head-to-head, the decision as to which medication to initiate first depends on patient comorbidities and preferences. For instance, patients with concurrent depression might consider citalopram, whereas those who are on other QTc-prolonging medications (eg, ribociclib) might consider oxybutynin. Gabapentinoids have also been shown to reduce hot flash severity; however, when gabapentin was compared with venlafaxine, patients preferred venlafaxine due to differences in their side effects.[26]

Two studies suggest that women receiving vitamin E at 200 IU twice daily report fewer hot flashes than those receiving placebo, though the effect size seems to be small.[27,28] Acupuncture also seems to decrease hot flashes, according to data from a randomized controlled trial; however, it has not been compared with a sham acupuncture intervention (rather, was compared with a usual care cohort).[29] A myriad of other interventions have been studied and may decrease hot flashes, from stellate ganglion block (an invasive procedure) to hypnosis (a mind–body approach), but further research to quantify benefits is needed.[30–34]

Genitourinary Symptoms of Menopause

Genitourinary symptoms of menopause (GSM), which include a wide range of concerns—vaginal dryness or discomfort, dyspareunia, urinary urgency, dysuria, and urinary tract infections—are common among breast cancer survivors and worsen quality of life. Although these symptoms are pervasive, discussions of GSM are infrequent due to the sensitive nature of the topic.[35,36] Although clinicians may worry that such discussions could make patients uncomfortable, most patients express a willingness and a wish to discuss GSM.[36,37]

Vaginal estrogen therapy use is controversial, because of the uncertainty as to its long-term safety, particularly in women with a history of estrogen-sensitive breast cancers. It seems that there is acute, systemic absorption from nearly all vaginal estrogen preparations, but it is not clear whether this small, temporary increase in estradiol exposure is enough to increase breast cancer recurrence in all populations of breast cancer survivors.[38] One case control study reported that local hormonal therapy did not seem to increase the risk of breast cancer recurrence among patients treated with tamoxifen, but further studies on the long-term safety of these medications are needed.[39] Vaginal dehydroepiandrosterone (DHEA), a topical hormonal preparation, in which a precursor hormone is transformed into androgen and then aromatized to form estrogen, appears to improve vaginal atrophy. A randomized clinical trial comparing two different doses of DHEA to plain moisturizer did not report significant improvements in vaginal dryness, but the higher dose of DHEA (6.5 mg) improved sexual health compared with the other arms, and there was no increase in estrogen levels among women who were concurrently taking aromatase inhibitors.[40]

Nonhormonal vaginal moisturizers (eg, Replens) have been shown to reduce vaginal dryness and genitourinary symptoms by 60%.[41–43] These moisturizers should be applied on a scheduled basis, at least several times per week for maximum benefit, and combined with as-needed use of lubricants and/or topical lidocaine before sexual activity. Hyaluronic acid-based vaginal gels also have been shown to significantly improve genitourinary symptoms. Breast cancer survivors who applied hyaluronic acid three to five times weekly to the vaginal introitus as part of one single-arm trial reported significant improvements in sexual function and genitourinary symptoms.[44] Microablative CO_2 laser therapy has shown promise in improving GSM among breast cancer survivors in both retrospective data and a pilot study, but rare case reports of vaginal scarring and fibrosis have tempered enthusiasm for this approach.[45–47] In addition, in one sham-controlled, double-blinded, randomized clinical trial of 90 postmenopausal women without a history of breast cancer, there were no significant differences between women receiving carbon dioxide laser therapy compared with sham treatment.[48] Further trials are being developed to determine the risks versus benefits of this potential therapy in breast cancer survivors.[49]

Cognitive Changes

Breast cancer survivors sometimes report changes in cognitive function, with deficits in word finding, memory, and attention.[50] This is traditionally referred to as "chemo brain"; however, even patients who do not receive chemotherapy at times report cognitive changes after surgery, radiation therapy, and/or endocrine therapy. One meta-analysis of cognitive function 6 months after chemotherapy reported that patients who were treated with chemotherapy performed mildly worse on neuropsychological testing than controls, particularly in verbal and visuospatial abilities.[51] A more recent study reported that all women with breast cancer who received endocrine therapy experienced a decline in self-reported cognitive function; this was worse in patients who received chemotherapy in addition to endocrine therapy at 3- and 6-month follow-ups, but it was not sustained at 1 year.[52] The effects of chemotherapy on cognitive functioning have also been noted on neuroimaging, including reductions in gray and white matter volume and different patterns of activation.[53,54] Several additional factors may increase the likelihood of cognitive changes in cancer survivors, including psychological distress, depression, and anxiety associated with cancer diagnoses and therapies, fatigue, menopause, and worsening comorbid conditions.[55]

As the causes for cognitive changes plaguing breast cancer survivors are multifactorial, preventive strategies and treatments require a multifaceted approach, including lifestyle modifications, focused on adequate sleep, exercise, including yoga, nutrition, and stress reduction.[56–58] For instance, a recent prospective cohort study found that patients with greater moderate-to-vigorous physical activity levels before and during chemotherapy were more likely to report better cognition and demonstrated better cognitive scores immediately and 6 months after chemotherapy completion.[57] One older, small study of breast cancer survivors reported benefits from electroencephalography biofeedback.[59] Other studies have implemented strategies such as cognitive rehabilitation and brain-training programs.[60,61] One recent trial of 167 patients reported that patients who were randomized to a computer-assisted cognitive rehabilitation program with a neuropsychologist had significantly improved scores on the Functional Assessment of Cancer Therapy-Cognitive Function score, higher quality of life, and an improvement in depression symptoms when compared with patients who underwent home cognitive self-exercises or phone follow-up.[60] Finally, small studies suggest that stimulants such as modafinil or methylphenidate might help to improve cognitive function and attention, but further investigations are warranted.[62,63]

Musculoskeletal Symptoms

Musculoskeletal symptoms, particularly aromatase inhibitor-associated musculoskeletal symptoms (AIMSS), occur in half of women on aromatase inhibitors, and have the potential to worsen quality of life and limit endocrine therapy treatment adherence.[64–66] AIMSS typically start within 1 to 2 months of aromatase inhibitor initiation and contribute to bilateral joint discomfort and stiffness in hands, wrists, and knees that improves with activity.

Non-pharmacologic approaches have been evaluated to determine effects of such strategies on reports of AIMSS. AIMSS seem to improve with exercise, according to a clinical trial that compared exercise to usual care.[67] High doses of omega-3 fatty acids (3.3 g) also seem to decrease AIMSS, compared with placebo, in women with a BMI of 30 or above.[68,69] Most convincing is the data for acupuncture in breast cancer survivors reporting AIMSS. In a multicenter, randomized controlled trial, patients receiving acupuncture had significant reductions in their joint pain compared with patients who received sham acupuncture and those who received waitlist control.[70] One pharmacologic agent, duloxetine, has also been found to decrease AIMSS, when compared with placebo, within the context of a randomized, double-blind clinical trial.[71]

Fatigue

Fatigue is commonly reported among breast cancer survivors due to a myriad of contributing factors; from surgery to medications to laboratory abnormalities to mental health concerns to other medical comorbidities, such that screening for fatigue is recommended at baseline, after completion of primary therapy, and then annually thereafter by both American Society of Clinical Oncology (ASCO) and the National Comprehensive Cancer Network (NCCN) clinical guidelines.[72,73] First, evaluations for causes for fatigue should be completed, including careful medication reviews, paying close attention to cancer-directed medications and nausea/sleep/pain medications, reviews of potential comorbidities such as cardiac dysfunction and insomnia, laboratory evaluations for electrolyte/liver/kidney function aberrations, endocrinopathies including thyroid function, and hematologic changes, as well as evaluations for mental health concerns, including depression. Treatments for fatigue largely depend on results of the evaluations for reversible contributory factors and treatments for those. However, in addition to this, physical activity, specifically moderate aerobic exercise that is tailored to each patient's functional status and comorbidities, is recommended.[72] Mind–body approaches, such as yoga, and mindfulness seem to decrease fatigue.[74–77] There is little evidence to support the use of stimulants, such as modafinil and methylphenidate, in breast cancer survivors who have completed their primary cancer-directed therapy; these are only to be considered if all other therapies have been tried and other comorbidities and causes are well managed.[72] American Ginseng (2000 mg daily of pure ground root) has been studied in a double-blind clinical trial that included patients who completed primary therapies for cancer. Patients who received ginseng had significantly improved fatigue scores, compared with patients who received placebo at 8 weeks.[78] Specific attention to the type, source, and strength of ginseng is important due to the lack of regulation of this agent by the Food and Drug Administration, and evaluations for potential medication interactions should also be completed, as it seems to inhibit the CYP3A4 pathway.[79]

Dermatologic Concerns

Patients undergoing therapy for breast cancer report several dermatologic concerns, including chemotherapy-related alopecia, eyebrow and eyelash loss, paronychia, and hand-foot syndrome. Although many of these toxicities resolve after completion of chemotherapy, this is not always the case. For instance, some patients report alopecia secondary to endocrine therapy, and radiation dermatitis can persist years after completion of radiation therapy. In addition, some breast cancer survivors are at increased risk for secondary skin cancers due to genetic predisposition or radiation exposure.

In general, treatments for these late dermatologic concerns have not been well studied. Endocrine therapy seems to cause recession of the frontal and parietal hairline in over one-third of breast cancer survivors on aromatase inhibitors and contributes to early discontinuation of endocrine therapy.[80,81] However, further prospective evaluations of this prominent clinical issue are needed. Topical minoxidil (2% and 5%) may be effective, with one retrospective study showing that 80% of users experienced moderate to significant improvement in thinning.[82] In addition, there is interest in studying low-dose oral minoxidil (1.25 mg), which might be more effective may alter hair texture less.[83]

Radiation dermatitis, characterized by changes in skin pigmentation, telangiectasias, and dermal fibrosis can continue months or years after radiation therapy. There are small studies of a variety of therapies, including oral pentoxifylline in combination with vitamin E or even laser therapy, but additional data are needed to inform an evidence-based approach to management of this issue.[84–87]

MENTAL HEALTH CONCERNS

Anxiety, depression, and insomnia are common diagnoses among patients diagnosed with breast cancer. There are several inciting causes for such diagnoses. A fear for recurrence may cause significant anxiety, some patients may experience depression, due to changes in their function, appearance, or symptoms as a result of any local or systemic cancer-directed therapy, and insomnia is a common side effect of many medications for cancer survivors, including steroids and endocrine therapy. In one recent matched cohort study investigating mental health-related outcomes in breast cancer survivors and age-matched controls (1:4 ratio of survivors to controls, with over 57,000 breast cancer survivors) across the UK National Health Service database, breast cancer survivors were significantly more likely to experience anxiety (hazard ratio [HR]: 1.33, 95% confidence interval [CI]: 1.29, 1.36), depression (HR 1.35, 95% CI: 1.32, 1.38), and sleep disorder (1.68, 95% CI 1.63, 1.73).[88,89] Although these HRs decreased over time, risks for anxiety persisted over 2 years, depression for 4 years, and sleep disorder persisted for 10 years, as compared with age-matched controls. Such symptoms were particularly common among younger breast cancer survivors.

Clinician discussions about breast cancer survivorship and common patient experiences can help relieve anxiety.[90] Additional strategies include cognitive behavioral therapy (CBT), which has been shown to be improve depression and anxiety among breast cancer survivors, with large effect sizes (pooled for depression −1.11, 95% CI −1.28, −0.94; pooled for anxiety −1.10, 95% CI −1.27, −0.93).[91] CBT has also been shown to significantly improve insomnia and can induce durable responses of 12 months.[92] Yoga and tai chi may also be of benefit.[93,94] Although many of the medications aimed at improving mental health concerns in women without breast cancer may be prescribed for patients with breast cancer diagnoses, including SSRIs and SNRIs, it is important to avoid interactions with cancer-directed therapies (eg, paroxetine and fluoxetine are contraindicated in patients taking tamoxifen). For breast cancer survivors with hot flashes, citalopram, venlafaxine, or escitalopram are often appealing pharmacologic treatments.[95–99]

HEALTH AND WELLNESS PROMOTION

Regular exercise is recommended for cancer survivors by the NCCN, the American Society for Clinical Oncology (ASCO), and the American Cancer Society.[8,100,101] Exercise, including yoga and tai chi, discussed above, help to decrease side effects from cancer-directed therapy, such as fatigue, anxiety/depression, physical function, and joint pain. Epidemiologic studies suggest exercise may be associated with reduced risks for breast cancer recurrence; one meta-analysis found that post-diagnosis physical activity was associated with over one-third reduction in mortality.[102,103] However, such studies are often difficult to interpret due to varying definitions of physical activity and cancer recurrence, as well as potential confounding variables, including patient comorbidities and disease-related factors.[102,104,105] Conclusions from randomized controlled trial data have been limited by small sample sizes; for instance, the Supervised Trial of Aerobic versus Resistance Training trial did not show statistically significant improvements in disease-free survival in women who underwent supervised exercise programs compared with usual care, although there was a trend toward improvement in breast cancer-related outcomes among some subgroups.[106] One recent study enrolled 1340 patients into the Diet, Exercise, Lifestyle, and Cancer Prognosis study, a prospective survey study of lifestyle and prognosis. Patients who met exercise guidelines before and 1 year after diagnosis experienced reductions in recurrence, particularly at 2-year follow-up (HR: 0.45, 95% CI 0.31, 0.65), and mortality (HR 0.32, 95% CI 0.19, 0.52).[107] Prospective trial data are greatly needed to clarify the amount and type of exercise that is optimal for breast cancer survivors; one recent meta-analysis suggested that 150 to 300 minutes per week of moderate-intensity physical activity or 75 minutes per week of vigorous-intensity physical activity is associated with lower mortality,[103] but another study reported that even small amounts of physical activity were associated with reduced mortality.[104]

A plant-healthy diet is also possibly beneficial. The Mediterranean diet and plant-based diets have been linked to lower risks for breast cancer in epidemiologic and observational studies, although it is not clear if these are indirect associations that result from the importance of BMI and other patient and disease-related factors.[108–110] Two randomized trials of dietary interventions among breast cancer survivors, the Women's Intervention Nutrition Study (WINS), focused on dietary fat reduction and the Women's Healthy Eating and Living Study, focused on increasing fruit and vegetable intake, did not report statistically significant reductions in mortality, though WINS identified a reduction in breast cancer recurrence rate with a low-fat diet.[111,112] There has also been interest in ketosis-related diets such as intermittent fasting, but evidence for benefit is limited; one epidemiologic study reported an association between prolonged nightly fasting lower breast cancer recurrence risk: among 2413 women, patients who fasted over 13 hours per night experienced a lower risk for breast cancer recurrence compared with women who fasted less than this amount of time.[113,114] Although theoretic concerns initially existed about soy consumption due to worries about soy's estrogenic properties, this has been largely disproven.[115] Prospective trial data are needed to clarify specific nutritional advice for breast cancer survivors.

Dietary supplements, particularly antioxidants, may decrease efficacy of cancer-directed therapies and have been associated with poorer survival; therefore, their use is discouraged.[116] Tobacco and alcohol are also discouraged because they increase risks of other medical problems (including other cancers), and because alcohol also increases risk of breast cancer recurrence.[117]

FINANCIAL TOXICITY

Between one-third and one-half of breast cancer survivors experience financial distress because of their diagnosis and treatment (due to out-of-pocket costs and loss of income).[118–120] Financial toxicity can influence patients' treatment decisions (eg, they may choose their local and systemic therapy based on cost and required time off work).[119–122] This issue is only becoming more salient as targeted therapies, such as abemaciclib, which cost thousands of dollars per year, emerge as long-term adjuvant treatment strategies. Unfortunately, financial disparities also contribute to disparate breast cancer outcomes: uninsured patients and Medicaid-insured patients have been shown to have a higher risk for death from breast cancer.[123] One qualitative study of the financial toxicity facing patients with breast cancer identified four specific issues that worsen financial distress and are actionable within a clinical context: (1) incorrect treatment expectations, (2) lack of provider conversation, (3) inability to identify resources, and (4) lack of social support.[120] Clinicians may help mitigate these issues by discussing how finances may influence treatment adherence, referring patients with concerns to social work and/or billing departments and connecting patients to peer support groups.[120]

SECOND CANCER SCREENING

The ASCO and the NCCN guidelines recommend that breast cancer survivors complete age-appropriate cancer screening for cervical, colon, lung, and breast cancers.[8,124] However, some breast cancer survivors are at higher risk for other malignancies due to genetic predispositions (mutations in BRCA1 or 2, ATM, CDH1, PALB2, RAD31 C or D, STK11, and TP53, among others) or shared risk factors, including environmental exposures, obesity, or cancer-directed therapies.[125] The presence of pathogenic genetic mutations may prompt additional risk reduction or surveillance strategies for other cancer types; for instance, patients with a BRCA 1 or 2 mutation might consider a risk-reducing prophylactic bilateral oophorectomy.

Breast cancer-directed therapies can increase risks for secondary malignancies. Alkylating agents and topoisomerase II inhibitors increase risks for treatment-associated leukemia, which typically occurs 5 to 7 years after chemotherapy. Thankfully, the incidence of this is relatively low at 1.8% (relative risk 1.53, 95% CI 1.14, 2.06), so specific surveillance strategies are not recommended.[126] Tamoxifen increases risk for endometrial cancer in women over 50.[127] Although surveillance endometrial ultrasound and biopsies are no longer recommended components of survivorship guidelines, abnormal uterine bleeding should prompt an expeditious gynecologic examination.[8]

SURVEILLANCE FOR BREAST CANCER RECURRENCE

Women with a history of breast cancer are recommended to undergo breast and chest wall examinations between one to four times yearly.[8] Women with residual breast tissue after breast cancer treatment are recommended to continue with annual three-dimensional mammograms, starting 6 to 12 months after radiation therapy. For BRCA mutation carriers or suspected carriers, women at over 20% lifetime risk for breast cancer either based on the Tyrer-Cuzick model or due to a genetic mutation or history of chest irradiation between ages 10 and 30 may consider additional surveillance imaging with MRI. Supplemental MRI may also be added to mammography in women with dense breast tissue, although risks for false positives, over-detection, and cost should be balanced with potential benefits.[128] Other strategies, such as contrast-enhanced digital mammography and molecular breast imaging can also be considered on a case-by-case basis, although the screening interval and optimal patient population for these techniques have not been well-defined.[129]

REPRODUCTIVE CONCERNS

Retrospective studies report that pregnancy does not seem to increase risks for breast cancer recurrence, and the IBCSG48 to 14/BIG8-13 (POSITIVE) trial is investigating the safety of pregnancy prospectively.[130] However, pregnancy rates in breast cancer survivors are significantly lower than in women without a history of breast cancer; in one study, less than 10% of young women with a history of breast cancer had a live birth within 10 years of diagnosis.[131] This is likely in part because young breast cancer survivors may experience premature amenorrhea and infertility secondary to chemotherapy, and endocrine therapy for 5 to 10 years can also impede pregnancy plans.

Contraception is recommended for premenopausal women undergoing teratogenic therapies, including adjuvant tamoxifen. For women with a history of hormone-sensitive breast cancers, traditional estrogen and progesterone-containing contraceptives are contraindicated, and the progestin intrauterine device may increase risk for breast cancer recurrence; therefore, nonhormonal strategies of contraception are recommended.[132–135] The copper intrauterine device, two forms of barrier contraceptives, or sterilization of the patient of the patient's partner are all potential strategies to prevent pregnancy. As tamoxifen is a teratogen and ovarian suppression combined with aromatase inhibitors impedes ovulation, it is recommended that women stop endocrine therapy for at least 3 months before attempts at conception.

CARDIAC/OTHER HEALTH CONCERNS

Breast cancer survivors have been shown to have higher rates of hypertension and diabetes than matched controls.[136] This is at least partially due to shared risk factors of breast cancer and cardiovascular disease, including obesity, age, diet, and physical inactivity, but also sometimes due to cardiotoxicities of breast cancer-directed therapies, including (but not limited to) anthracycline-based chemotherapy.[137] Breast cancer survivors should be made aware of the risks for cardiovascular disease and should undergo routine screening for hypertension, diabetes, and hyperlipidemia, as recommended by the US Preventive Services Task Force. Smoking cessation and physical activity should be strongly encouraged.

OSTEOPOROSIS

Osteoporosis and resulting bone fractures are possible complications of endocrine therapy and chemotherapy. Therefore, breast cancer survivors are recommended to take in adequate calcium and vitamin D and undergo surveillance dual-energy X-ray absorptiometry scans at least every 2 to 3 years (especially if postmenopausal or receiving a treatment that can thin the bones).

Antiresorptive therapies should also be considered in women with osteoporosis or osteopenia, particularly because adjuvant zoledronic acid reduces risk of breast cancer recurrence.[138,139] The results of studies of the impact of denosumab on disease-free survival have been mixed, and a randomized, placebo-controlled, phase III trial of denosumab versus placebo did not report that denosumab improved bone metastasis-free survival.[140,141] Because of the risk of jaw osteonecrosis, all patients should have dental evaluation before starting zoledronic acid or denosumab (because risk for osteonecrosis of the jaw significantly increases if invasive dental work is needed soon after a dose).[142]

DISPARITIES IN SURVIVORSHIP

Disparities in cancer care related to geography, socioeconomic status, race, ethnicity, sexual orientation, and/or gender identity can impact the entire cancer care continuum including survivorship. One example of this is that Latina and Black women have higher rates of lymphedema than White women.[143] And Black breast cancer survivors report inadequate access to culturally appropriate posttreatment support services.[144] Rural breast cancer survivors are less likely to have access to mental health services,[145] whereas sexual minorities report higher rates of sexual side effects and social isolation after breast cancer and gender minorities report feeling that their oncology providers are unable to inform them adequately about how their cancer treatments may impact their gender-affirmation care.[146–148] Both the National Institute of Health and the ASCO recommend strategies for mitigating these disparities for the promotion of health equity.[149,150] Standardizing collection of data to identify disparities, increasing the number of clinicians working in at-risk communities, and supporting research aimed at addressing disparities are all necessary for improving access to equitable, quality survivorship care.

CLINICS CARE POINTS

- Duloxetine is the single intervention that has been shown to be effective in decreasing breast cancer chemotherapy-induced peripheral neuropathy pain. Duloxetine and acupuncture have also been shown to decrease the severity of aromatase inhibitor-induced musculoskeletal symptoms.

- Antidepressants may help to manage both vasomotor symptoms and mood changes associated with breast cancer and breast cancer-directed therapies. However, medication interactions can impact their use for some patients. Oxybutynin may be effective for patients with vasomotor symptoms who wish to avoid antidepressants.

- All breast cancer survivors should be counseled about late genitourinary effects from breast cancer-directed therapy. Survivors should be provided with recommendations as to how to manage such symptoms, including topical moisturizers (non-estrogenic preferred).
- A combination of a plant-healthy diet and regular aerobic and weight-bearing exercise has been shown to improve symptoms of cancer-directed therapy; furthermore, such strategies may even reduce risk for breast cancer recurrence.

DISCLOSURE

The authors have nothing to disclose.

REFERENCES

1. Siegel RL, Miller KD, Fuchs HE, et al. Cancer Statistics, 2022. CA: A Cancer J Clinicians 2022;72(1):7–33.
2. American Cancer Society. Cancer Treatment & Survivorship Facts & Figures 2022-2024. Atlanta: American Cancer Society; 2022.
3. National Cancer Institute. Office of Cancer Survivorship. Accessed2022.
4. McLaughlin SA, Brunelle CL, Taghian A. Breast Cancer-Related Lymphedema: Risk Factors, Screening, Management, and the Impact of Locoregional Treatment. J Clin Oncol 2020;38(20):2341–50.
5. McDuff SGR, Mina AI, Brunelle CL, et al. Timing of Lymphedema After Treatment for Breast Cancer: When Are Patients Most At Risk? Int J Radiat Oncol Biol Phys 2019;103(1):62–70.
6. Asdourian MS, Swaroop MN, Sayegh HE, et al. Association Between Precautionary Behaviors and Breast Cancer-Related Lymphedema in Patients Undergoing Bilateral Surgery. J Clin Oncol 2017;35(35):3934–41.
7. Tevaarwerk A, Denlinger CS, Sanft T, et al. Survivorship, Version 1.2021. J Natl Compr Canc Netw 2021;19(6):676–85.
8. Denlinger CS, Sanft T, Baker KS, et al. Survivorship, Version 2.2018, NCCN Clinical Practice Guidelines in Oncology. J Natl Compr Canc Netw 2018;16(10): 1216–47.
9. McNeely ML, Magee DJ, Lees AW, et al. The addition of manual lymph drainage to compression therapy for breast cancer related lymphedema: a randomized controlled trial. Breast Cancer Res Treat 2004;86(2):95–106.
10. Ezzo J, Manheimer E, McNeely ML, et al. Manual lymphatic drainage for lymphedema following breast cancer treatment. Cochrane Database Syst Rev 2015;(5):CD003475.
11. Shao Y, Qi K, Zhou QH, et al. Intermittent pneumatic compression pump for breast cancer-related lymphedema: a systematic review and meta-analysis of randomized controlled trials. Oncol Res Treat 2014;37(4):170–4.
12. Schmitz KH, Ahmed RL, Troxel AB, et al. Weight lifting for women at risk for breast cancer-related lymphedema: a randomized trial. JAMA 2010;304(24): 2699–705.
13. Schmitz KH, Troxel AB, Dean LT, et al. Effect of Home-Based Exercise and Weight Loss Programs on Breast Cancer-Related Lymphedema Outcomes Among Overweight Breast Cancer Survivors: The WISER Survivor Randomized Clinical Trial. JAMA Oncol 2019;5(11):1605–13.
14. Bandos H, Melnikow J, Rivera DR, et al. Long-term Peripheral Neuropathy in Breast Cancer Patients Treated With Adjuvant Chemotherapy: NRG Oncology/ NSABP B-30. J Natl Cancer Inst 2018;110(2).

15. Smith EM, Pang H, Cirrincione C, et al. Effect of duloxetine on pain, function, and quality of life among patients with chemotherapy-induced painful peripheral neuropathy: a randomized clinical trial. JAMA 2013;309(13):1359–67.

16. Loprinzi CL, Lacchetti C, Bleeker J, et al. Prevention and Management of Chemotherapy-Induced Peripheral Neuropathy in Survivors of Adult Cancers: ASCO Guideline Update. J Clin Oncol 2020;38(28):3325–48.

17. Childs DS, Le-Rademacher JG, McMurray R, et al. Randomized Trial of Scrambler Therapy for Chemotherapy-Induced Peripheral Neuropathy: Crossover Analysis. J Pain Symptom Manage 2021;61(6):1247–53.

18. Chang HY, Jotwani AC, Lai YH, et al. Hot flashes in breast cancer survivors: Frequency, severity and impact. Breast 2016;27:116–21.

19. Huang AJ, Subak LL, Wing R, et al. An intensive behavioral weight loss intervention and hot flushes in women. Arch Intern Med 2010;170(13):1161–7.

20. Daley A, Stokes-Lampard H, Thomas A, et al. Exercise for vasomotor menopausal symptoms. Cochrane Database Syst Rev 2014;11:CD006108.

21. Holmberg L, Anderson H. steering H, data monitoring c. HABITS' (hormonal replacement therapy after breast cancer–is it safe?), a randomised comparison: trial stopped. Lancet 2004;363(9407):453–5.

22. Loprinzi CL, Kugler JW, Sloan JA, et al. Venlafaxine in management of hot flashes in survivors of breast cancer: a randomised controlled trial. Lancet 2000;356(9247):2059–63.

23. Barton DL, LaVasseur BI, Sloan JA, et al. Phase III, placebo-controlled trial of three doses of citalopram for the treatment of hot flashes: NCCTG trial N05C9. J Clin Oncol 2010;28(20):3278–83.

24. Freeman EW, Guthrie KA, Caan B, et al. Efficacy of escitalopram for hot flashes in healthy menopausal women: a randomized controlled trial. JAMA 2011; 305(3):267–74.

25. Leon-Ferre RA, Novotny PJ, Wolfe EG, et al. Oxybutynin vs Placebo for Hot Flashes in Women With or Without Breast Cancer: A Randomized, Double-Blind Clinical Trial (ACCRU SC-1603). JNCI Cancer Spectr 2020;4(1):pkz088.

26. Bordeleau L, Pritchard KI, Loprinzi CL, et al. Multicenter, randomized, crossover clinical trial of venlafaxine versus gabapentin for the management of hot flashes in breast cancer survivors. J Clin Oncol 2010;28(35):5147–52.

27. Ataei-Almanghadim K, Farshbaf-Khalili A, Ostadrahimi AR, et al. The effect of oral capsule of curcumin and vitamin E on the hot flashes and anxiety in postmenopausal women: A triple blind randomised controlled trial. Complement Ther Med 2020;48:102267.

28. Barton DL, Loprinzi CL, Quella SK, et al. Prospective evaluation of vitamin E for hot flashes in breast cancer survivors. J Clin Oncol 1998;16(2):495–500.

29. Lesi G, Razzini G, Musti MA, et al. Acupuncture As an Integrative Approach for the Treatment of Hot Flashes in Women With Breast Cancer: A Prospective Multicenter Randomized Controlled Trial (AcCliMaT). J Clin Oncol 2016;34(15): 1795–802.

30. Othman AH, Zaky AH. Management of hot flushes in breast cancer survivors: comparison between stellate ganglion block and pregabalin. Pain Med 2014; 15(3):410–7.

31. Rahimzadeh P, Imani F, Nafissi N, et al. Comparison of the effects of stellate ganglion block and paroxetine on hot flashes and sleep disturbance in breast cancer survivors. Cancer Manag Res 2018;10:4831–7.

32. Walega DR, Rubin LH, Banuvar S, et al. Effects of stellate ganglion block on vasomotor symptoms: findings from a randomized controlled clinical trial in postmenopausal women. Menopause 2014;21(8):807–14.

33. Elkins G, Marcus J, Stearns V, et al. Randomized trial of a hypnosis intervention for treatment of hot flashes among breast cancer survivors. J Clin Oncol 2008; 26(31):5022–6.

34. Elkins GR, Fisher WI, Johnson AK. Clinical hypnosis in the treatment of postmenopausal hot flashes: a randomized controlled trial. Menopause 2013;20:291–8.

35. Cook ED, Iglehart EI, Baum G, et al. Missing documentation in breast cancer survivors: genitourinary syndrome of menopause. Menopause 2017;24(12): 1360–4.

36. Cathcart-Rake E, O'Connor J, Ridgeway JL, et al. Patients' Perspectives and Advice on How to Discuss Sexual Orientation, Gender Identity, and Sexual Health in Oncology Clinics. Am J Hosp Palliat Care 2020;37(12):1053–61.

37. Cathcart-Rake E, O'Connor JM, Ridgeway JL, et al. Querying Patients With Cancer About Sexual Health and Sexual and Gender Minority Status: A Qualitative Study of Health-Care Providers. Am J Hosp Palliat Care 2020;37(6):418–23.

38. Santen R. Vaginal administration of estradiol: effects of dose, preparation and timing on plasma estradiol levels. Climacteric 2015;18(2):121–34.

39. Le Ray I, Dell'Aniello S, Bonnetain F, et al. Local estrogen therapy and risk of breast cancer recurrence among hormone-treated patients: a nested case-control study. Breast Cancer Res Treat 2012;135(2):603–9.

40. Barton DL, Shuster LT, Dockter T, et al. Systemic and local effects of vaginal dehydroepiandrosterone (DHEA): NCCTG N10C1 (Alliance). Support Care Cancer 2018;26(4):1335–43.

41. Bygdeman M, Swahn ML. Replens versus dienoestrol cream in the symptomatic treatment of vaginal atrophy in postmenopausal women. Maturitas 1996;23(3): 259–63.

42. Mitchell CM, Reed SD, Diem S, et al. Efficacy of vaginal estradiol or vaginal moisturizer vs placebo for treating postmenopausal vulvovaginal symptoms: a randomized clinical trial. JAMA Intern Med 2018;178(5):681–90.

43. Loprinzi CL, Abu-Ghazaleh S, Sloan JA, et al. Phase III randomized double-blind study to evaluate the efficacy of a polycarbophil-based vaginal moisturizer in women with breast cancer. J Clin Oncol 1997;15(3):969–73.

44. Carter J, Baser RE, Goldfrank DJ, et al. A single-arm, prospective trial investigating the effectiveness of a non-hormonal vaginal moisturizer containing hyaluronic acid in postmenopausal cancer survivors. Support Care Cancer 2021; 29(1):311–22.

45. Pagano T, De Rosa P, Vallone R, et al. Fractional microablative CO2 laser in breast cancer survivors affected by iatrogenic vulvovaginal atrophy after failure of nonestrogenic local treatments: a retrospective study. Menopause 2018; 25(6):657–62.

46. Quick AM, Zvinovski F, Hudson C, et al. Fractional CO2 laser therapy for genitourinary syndrome of menopause for breast cancer survivors. Support Care Cancer 2020;28(8):3669–77.

47. Gordon C, Gonzales S, Krychman ML. Rethinking the techno vagina: a case series of patient complications following vaginal laser treatment for atrophy. Menopause 2019;26(4):423–7.

48. Li FG, Maheux-Lacroix S, Deans R, et al. Effect of Fractional Carbon Dioxide Laser vs Sham Treatment on Symptom Severity in Women With Postmenopausal Vaginal Symptoms: A Randomized Clinical Trial. JAMA 2021;326(14):1381–9.

49. Sussman TA, Kruse ML, Thacker HL, et al. Managing genitourinary syndrome of menopause in breast cancer survivors receiving endocrine therapy. J Oncol Pract 2019;15(7):363–70.

50. Boykoff N, Moieni M, Subramanian SK. Confronting chemobrain: an in-depth look at survivors' reports of impact on work, social networks, and health care response. J Cancer Surviv 2009;3(4):223–32.

51. Jim HS, Phillips KM, Chait S, et al. Meta-analysis of cognitive functioning in breast cancer survivors previously treated with standard-dose chemotherapy. J Clin Oncol 2012;30(29):3578–87.

52. Wagner LI, Gray RJ, Sparano JA, et al. Patient-Reported Cognitive Impairment Among Women With Early Breast Cancer Randomly Assigned to Endocrine Therapy Alone Versus Chemoendocrine Therapy: Results From TAILORx. J Clin Oncol 2020;38(17):1875–86.

53. Deprez S, Amant F, Smeets A, et al. Longitudinal assessment of chemotherapy-induced structural changes in cerebral white matter and its correlation with impaired cognitive functioning. J Clin Oncol 2012;30(3):274–81.

54. Deprez S, Vandenbulcke M, Peeters R, et al. Longitudinal assessment of chemotherapy-induced alterations in brain activation during multitasking and its relation with cognitive complaints. J Clin Oncol 2014;32(19):2031–8.

55. Hurria A, Somlo G, Ahles T. Renaming "chemobrain. Cancer Invest 2007;25(6): 373–7.

56. Galantino ML, Greene L, Daniels L, et al. Longitudinal impact of yoga on chemotherapy-related cognitive impairment and quality of life in women with early stage breast cancer: a case series. Explore (NY) 2012;8(2):127–35.

57. Salerno EA, Culakova E, Kleckner AS, et al. Physical Activity Patterns and Relationships With Cognitive Function in Patients With Breast Cancer Before, During, and After Chemotherapy in a Prospective, Nationwide Study. J Clin Oncol 2021;39(29):3283–92.

58. Hartman SJ, Nelson SH, Myers E, et al. Randomized controlled trial of increasing physical activity on objectively measured and self-reported cognitive functioning among breast cancer survivors: The memory & motion study. Cancer 2018;124(1):192–202.

59. Alvarez J, Meyer FL, Granoff DL, et al. The effect of EEG biofeedback on reducing postcancer cognitive impairment. Integr Cancer Ther 2013;12(6): 475–87.

60. Dos Santos M, Hardy-Leger I, Rigal O, et al. Cognitive rehabilitation program to improve cognition of cancer patients treated with chemotherapy: A 3-arm randomized trial. Cancer 2020;126(24):5328–36.

61. Von Ah D, Carpenter JS, Saykin A, et al. Advanced cognitive training for breast cancer survivors: a randomized controlled trial. Breast Cancer Res Treat 2012; 135(3):799–809.

62. Kohli S, Fisher SG, Tra Y, et al. The effect of modafinil on cognitive function in breast cancer survivors. Cancer 2009;115(12):2605–16.

63. Sood A, Barton DL, Loprinzi CL. Use of methylphenidate in patients with cancer. Am J Hosp Palliat Care 2006;23(1):35–40.

64. Crew KD, Greenlee H, Capodice J, et al. Prevalence of joint symptoms in postmenopausal women taking aromatase inhibitors for early-stage breast cancer. J Clin Oncol 2007;25(25):3877–83.

65. Henry NL, Giles JT, Ang D, et al. Prospective characterization of musculoskeletal symptoms in early stage breast cancer patients treated with aromatase inhibitors. Breast Cancer Res Treat 2008;111(2):365–72.

66. Henry NL, Giles JT, Stearns V. Aromatase inhibitor-associated musculoskeletal symptoms: etiology and strategies for management. Oncology (Williston Park) 2008;22(12):1401–8.
67. Irwin ML, Cartmel B, Gross CP, et al. Randomized exercise trial of aromatase inhibitor-induced arthralgia in breast cancer survivors. J Clin Oncol 2015; 33(10):1104–11.
68. Hershman DL, Unger JM, Crew KD, et al. Randomized Multicenter Placebo-Controlled Trial of Omega-3 Fatty Acids for the Control of Aromatase Inhibitor-Induced Musculoskeletal Pain: SWOG S0927. J Clin Oncol 2015;33(17):1910–7.
69. Shen S, Unger JM, Crew KD, et al. Omega-3 fatty acid use for obese breast cancer patients with aromatase inhibitor-related arthralgia (SWOG S0927). Breast Cancer Res Treat 2018;172(3):603–10.
70. Hershman DL, Unger JM, Greenlee H, et al. Effect of Acupuncture vs Sham Acupuncture or Waitlist Control on Joint Pain Related to Aromatase Inhibitors Among Women With Early-Stage Breast Cancer: A Randomized Clinical Trial. JAMA 2018;320(2):167–76.
71. Henry NL, Unger JM, Schott AF, et al. Randomized, Multicenter, Placebo-Controlled Clinical Trial of Duloxetine Versus Placebo for Aromatase Inhibitor-Associated Arthralgias in Early-Stage Breast Cancer: SWOG S1202. J Clin Oncol 2018;36(4):326–32.
72. Bower JE, Bak K, Berger A, et al. Screening, assessment, and management of fatigue in adult survivors of cancer: an American Society of Clinical oncology clinical practice guideline adaptation. J Clin Oncol 2014;32(17):1840–50.
73. Berger AM, Abernethy AP, Atkinson A, et al. NCCN Clinical Practice Guidelines Cancer-related fatigue. J Natl Compr Canc Netw 2010;8(8):904–31.
74. Hoffman CJ, Ersser SJ, Hopkinson JB, et al. Effectiveness of mindfulness-based stress reduction in mood, breast- and endocrine-related quality of life, and well-being in stage 0 to III breast cancer: a randomized, controlled trial. J Clin Oncol 2012;30(12):1335–42.
75. Kiecolt-Glaser JK, Bennett JM, Andridge R, et al. Yoga's impact on inflammation, mood, and fatigue in breast cancer survivors: a randomized controlled trial. J Clin Oncol 2014;32(10):1040–9.
76. Bower JE, Garet D, Sternlieb B, et al. Yoga for persistent fatigue in breast cancer survivors: a randomized controlled trial. Cancer 2012;118(15):3766–75.
77. Zetzl T, Renner A, Pittig A, et al. Yoga effectively reduces fatigue and symptoms of depression in patients with different types of cancer. Support Care Cancer 2021;29(6):2973–82.
78. Barton DL, Liu H, Dakhil SR, et al. Wisconsin Ginseng (Panax quinquefolius) to improve cancer-related fatigue: a randomized, double-blind trial, N07C2. J Natl Cancer Inst 2013;105(16):1230–8.
79. Posadzki P, Watson LK, Ernst E. Adverse effects of herbal medicines: an overview of systematic reviews. Clin Med (Lond) 2013;13(1):7–12.
80. Gallicchio L, Calhoun C, Helzlsouer KJ. Aromatase inhibitor therapy and hair loss among breast cancer survivors. Breast Cancer Res Treat 2013;142(2):435–43.
81. Moscetti L, Agnese Fabbri M, Sperduti I, et al. Adjuvant aromatase inhibitor therapy in early breast cancer: what factors lead patients to discontinue treatment? Tumori 2015;101(5):469–73.
82. Freites-Martinez A, Shapiro J, Chan D, et al. Endocrine Therapy-Induced Alopecia in Patients With Breast Cancer. JAMA Dermatol 2018;154(6):670–5.

83. Kuo AM, Reingold RE, Ketosugbo K, et al. Oral minoxidil fo rthe treatment of late alopecia in cancer survivors, Abstract #12022. Am Soc Clin Oncol Annu Meet 2022;2022.

84. Delanian S, Porcher R, Rudant J, et al. Kinetics of response to long-term treatment combining pentoxifylline and tocopherol in patients with superficial radiation-induced fibrosis. J Clin Oncol 2005;23(34):8570–9.

85. Jacobson G, Bhatia S, Smith BJ, et al. Randomized trial of pentoxifylline and vitamin E vs standard follow-up after breast irradiation to prevent breast fibrosis, evaluated by tissue compliance meter. Int J Radiat Oncol Biol Phys 2013;85(3):604–8.

86. Magnusson M, Hoglund P, Johansson K, et al. Pentoxifylline and vitamin E treatment for prevention of radiation-induced side-effects in women with breast cancer: a phase two, double-blind, placebo-controlled randomised clinical trial (Ptx-5). Eur J Cancer 2009;45(14):2488–95.

87. Rossi AM, Nehal KS, Lee EH. Radiation-induced Breast Telangiectasias Treated with the Pulsed Dye Laser. J Clin Aesthet Dermatol 2014;7(12):34–7.

88. Carreira H, Williams R, Dempsey H, et al. Quality of life and mental health in breast cancer survivors compared with non-cancer controls: a study of patient-reported outcomes in the United Kingdom. J Cancer Surviv 2021;15(4):564–75.

89. Carreira H, Williams R, Funston G, et al. Associations between breast cancer survivorship and adverse mental health outcomes: A matched population-based cohort study in the United Kingdom. Plos Med 2021;18(1):e1003504.

90. Smith SL, Singh-Carlson S, Downie L, et al. Survivors of breast cancer: patient perspectives on survivorship care planning. J Cancer Surviv 2011;5(4):337–44.

91. Ye M, Du K, Zhou J, et al. A meta-analysis of the efficacy of cognitive behavior therapy on quality of life and psychological health of breast cancer survivors and patients. Psychooncology 2018;27(7):1695–703.

92. Arico D, Raggi A, Ferri R. Cognitive Behavioral Therapy for Insomnia in Breast Cancer Survivors: A Review of the Literature. Front Psychol 2016;7:1162.

93. Mustian KM. Yoga as Treatment for Insomnia Among Cancer Patients and Survivors: A Systematic Review. Eur Med J Oncol 2013;1:106–15.

94. Ni X, Chan RJ, Yates P, et al. The effects of Tai Chi on quality of life of cancer survivors: a systematic review and meta-analysis. Support Care Cancer 2019;27(10):3701–16.

95. Stearns V, Johnson MD, Rae JM, et al. Active tamoxifen metabolite plasma concentrations after coadministration of tamoxifen and the selective serotonin reuptake inhibitor paroxetine. J Natl Cancer Inst 2003;95(23):1758–64.

96. Kelly CM, Juurlink DN, Gomes T, et al. Selective serotonin reuptake inhibitors and breast cancer mortality in women receiving tamoxifen: a population based cohort study. BMJ 2010;340:c693.

97. Desmarais JE, Looper KJ. Interactions between tamoxifen and antidepressants via cytochrome P450 2D6. J Clin Psychiatry 2009;70(12):1688–97.

98. Kerwin JP, Gordon PR, Senf JH. The variable response of women with menopausal hot flashes when treated with sertraline. Menopause 2007;14(5):841–5.

99. Loprinzi CL, Sloan J, Stearns V, et al. Newer antidepressants and gabapentin for hot flashes: an individual patient pooled analysis. J Clin Oncol 2009;27(17):2831–7.

100. Nutrition recommendations during and after treatment. American Society of Clinical Oncology 2022.

101. Rock CL, Thomson CA, Sullivan KR, et al. American Cancer Society nutrition and physical activity guideline for cancer survivors. CA Cancer J Clin 2022; 72(3):230–62.
102. Lahart IM, Metsios GS, Nevill AM, et al. Physical activity, risk of death and recurrence in breast cancer survivors: A systematic review and meta-analysis of epidemiological studies. Acta Oncol 2015;54(5):635–54.
103. Friedenreich CM, Stone CR, Cheung WY, et al. Physical Activity and Mortality in Cancer Survivors: A Systematic Review and Meta-Analysis. JNCI Cancer Spectr 2020;4(1):pkz080.
104. Lee J. A Meta-analysis of the Association Between Physical Activity and Breast Cancer Mortality. Cancer Nurs 2019;42(4):271–85.
105. Friedenreich CM, Shaw E, Neilson HK, et al. Epidemiology and biology of physical activity and cancer recurrence. J Mol Med (Berl) 2017;95(10):1029–41.
106. Courneya KS, Segal RJ, McKenzie DC, et al. Effects of exercise during adjuvant chemotherapy on breast cancer outcomes. Med Sci Sports Exerc 2014;46(9): 1744–51.
107. Cannioto RA, Hutson A, Dighe S, et al. Physical Activity Before, During, and After Chemotherapy for High-Risk Breast Cancer: Relationships With Survival. J Natl Cancer Inst 2021;113(1):54–63.
108. Toledo E, Salas-Salvado J, Donat-Vargas C, et al. Mediterranean Diet and Invasive Breast Cancer Risk Among Women at High Cardiovascular Risk in the PREDIMED Trial: A Randomized Clinical Trial. JAMA Intern Med 2015;175(11): 1752–60.
109. Tantamango-Bartley Y, Jaceldo-Siegl K, Fan J, et al. Vegetarian diets and the incidence of cancer in a low-risk population. Cancer Epidemiol Biomarkers Prev 2013;22(2):286–94.
110. Jochems SHJ, Van Osch FHM, Bryan RT, et al. Impact of dietary patterns and the main food groups on mortality and recurrence in cancer survivors: a systematic review of current epidemiological literature. BMJ Open 2018;8(2):e014530.
111. Hoy MK, Winters BL, Chlebowski RT, et al. Implementing a low-fat eating plan in the Women's Intervention Nutrition Study. J Am Diet Assoc 2009;109(4):688–96.
112. Pierce JP, Natarajan L, Caan BJ, et al. Influence of a diet very high in vegetables, fruit, and fiber and low in fat on prognosis following treatment for breast cancer: the Women's Healthy Eating and Living (WHEL) randomized trial. JAMA 2007;298(3):289–98.
113. Marinac CR, Natarajan L, Sears DD, et al. Prolonged Nightly Fasting and Breast Cancer Risk: Findings from NHANES (2009-2010). Cancer Epidemiol Biomarkers Prev 2015;24(5):783–9.
114. Marinac CR, Nelson SH, Breen CI, et al. Prolonged Nightly Fasting and Breast Cancer Prognosis. JAMA Oncol 2016;2(8):1049–55.
115. Fraser GE, Jaceldo-Siegl K, Orlich M, et al. Dairy, soy, and risk of breast cancer: those confounded milks. Int J Epidemiol 2020;49(5):1526–37.
116. Ambrosone CB, Zirpoli GR, Hutson AD, et al. Dietary Supplement Use During Chemotherapy and Survival Outcomes of Patients With Breast Cancer Enrolled in a Cooperative Group Clinical Trial (SWOG S0221). J Clin Oncol 2020;38(8): 804–14.
117. Rainey L, Eriksson M, Trinh T, et al. The impact of alcohol consumption and physical activity on breast cancer: The role of breast cancer risk. Int J Cancer 2020;147(4):931–9.
118. Irwin B, Kimmick G, Altomare I, et al. Patient experience and attitudes toward addressing the cost of breast cancer care. Oncologist 2014;19(11):1135–40.

119. Greenup RA, Rushing C, Fish L, et al. Financial Costs and Burden Related to Decisions for Breast Cancer Surgery. J Oncol Pract 2019;15(8):e666–76.
120. Gharzai LA, Ryan KA, Szczygiel L, et al. Financial Toxicity During Breast Cancer Treatment: A Qualitative Analysis to Inform Strategies for Mitigation. JCO Oncol Pract 2021;17(10):e1413–23.
121. Hershman DL, Tsui J, Wright JD, et al. Household net worth, racial disparities, and hormonal therapy adherence among women with early-stage breast cancer. J Clin Oncol 2015;33(9):1053–9.
122. Charlson JA, McGinley EL, Nattinger AB, et al. Geographic Variation of Adjuvant Breast Cancer Therapy Initiation in the United States: Lessons From Medicare Part D. J Natl Compr Canc Netw 2017;15(12):1509–17.
123. Niu X, Roche LM, Pawlish KS, et al. Cancer survival disparities by health insurance status. Cancer Med 2013;2(3):403–11.
124. Runowicz CD, Leach CR, Henry NL, et al. American Cancer Society/American Society of Clinical Oncology Breast Cancer Survivorship Care Guideline. J Clin Oncol 2016;34(6):611–35.
125. Sung H, Freedman RA, Siegel RL, et al. Risks of subsequent primary cancers among breast cancer survivors according to hormone receptor status. Cancer 2021;127(18):3310–24.
126. Patt DA, Duan Z, Fang S, et al. Acute myeloid leukemia after adjuvant breast cancer therapy in older women: understanding risk. J Clin Oncol 2007;25(25): 3871–6.
127. Fisher B, Costantino JP, Redmond CK, et al. Endometrial cancer in tamoxifen-treated breast cancer patients: findings from the National Surgical Adjuvant Breast and Bowel Project (NSABP) B-14. J Natl Cancer Inst 1994;86(7):527–37.
128. Bakker MF, de Lange SV, Pijnappel RM, et al. Supplemental MRI Screening for Women with Extremely Dense Breast Tissue. N Engl J Med 2019;381(22): 2091–102.
129. Shermis RB, Wilson KD, Doyle MT, et al. Supplemental Breast Cancer Screening With Molecular Breast Imaging for Women With Dense Breast Tissue. AJR Am J Roentgenol 2016;207(2):450–7.
130. Partridge AH, Niman SM, Ruggeri M, et al. Who are the women who enrolled in the POSITIVE trial: A global study to support young hormone receptor positive breast cancer survivors desiring pregnancy. Breast 2021;59:327–38.
131. Anderson C, Engel SM, Anders CK, et al. Live birth outcomes after adolescent and young adult breast cancer. Int J Cancer 2018;142(10):1994–2002.
132. Moorman PG, Havrilesky LJ, Gierisch JM, et al. Oral contraceptives and risk of ovarian cancer and breast cancer among high-risk women: a systematic review and meta-analysis. J Clin Oncol 2013;31(33):4188–98.
133. Morch LS, Skovlund CW, Hannaford PC, et al. Contemporary Hormonal Contraception and the Risk of Breast Cancer. N Engl J Med 2017;377(23):2228–39.
134. Dinger J, Bardenheuer K, Minh TD. Levonorgestrel-releasing and copper intrauterine devices and the risk of breast cancer. Contraception 2011;83(3):211–7.
135. Backman T, Rauramo I, Jaakkola K, et al. Use of the levonorgestrel-releasing intrauterine system and breast cancer. Obstet Gynecol 2005;106(4):813–7.
136. Kwan ML, Yao S, Laurent CA, et al. Changes in bone mineral density in women with breast cancer receiving aromatase inhibitor therapy. Breast Cancer Res Treat 2017;168(2):523–30.
137. Mehta LS, Watson KE, Barac A, et al. Cardiovascular Disease and Breast Cancer: Where These Entities Intersect: A Scientific Statement From the American Heart Association. Circulation 2018;137(8):e30–66.

138. Gnant M, Mlineritsch B, Schippinger W, et al. Endocrine therapy plus zoledronic acid in premenopausal breast cancer. N Engl J Med 2009;360(7):679–91.
139. Early Breast Cancer Trialists' Collaborative G. Adjuvant bisphosphonate treatment in early breast cancer: meta-analyses of individual patient data from randomised trials. Lancet 2015;386(10001):1353–61.
140. Coleman R, Finkelstein DM, Barrios C, et al. Adjuvant denosumab in early breast cancer (D-CARE): an international, multicentre, randomised, controlled, phase 3 trial. Lancet Oncol 2020;21(1):60–72.
141. Gnant M, Pfeiler G, Steger GG, et al. Adjuvant denosumab in postmenopausal patients with hormone receptor-positive breast cancer (ABCSG-18): disease-free survival results from a randomised, double-blind, placebo-controlled, phase 3 trial. Lancet Oncol 2019;20(3):339–51.
142. Kizub DA, Miao J, Schubert MM, et al. Risk factors for bisphosphonate-associated osteonecrosis of the jaw in the prospective randomized trial of adjuvant bisphosphonates for early-stage breast cancer (SWOG 0307). Support Care Cancer 2021;29(5):2509–17.
143. Barrio AV, Montagna G, Sevilimedu V, Gomez EA, Mehrara B, Morrow M. GS4-01. Impact of race and ethnicity on incidence and severity of breast cancer related lymphedema after axillary lymph node dissection: Results of a prospective screening study. Presented at San Antonion Breast Cancer Symposium. 2021.
144. Haynes-Maslow L, Allicock M, Johnson LS. Cancer Support Needs for African American Breast Cancer Survivors and Caregivers. J Cancer Educ 2016; 31(1):166–71.
145. Bettencourt BA, Schlegel RJ, Talley AE, et al. The breast cancer experience of rural women: a literature review. Psychooncology 2007;16(10):875–87.
146. Boehmer U, Ozonoff A, Timm A, et al. After breast cancer: sexual functioning of sexual minority survivors. J Sex Res 2014;51(6):681–9.
147. Brown MT, McElroy JA. Unmet support needs of sexual and gender minority breast cancer survivors. Support Care Cancer 2018;26(4):1189–96.
148. Taylor ET, Bryson MK. Cancer's Margins: Trans* and Gender Nonconforming People's Access to Knowledge, Experiences of Cancer Health, and Decision-Making. LGBT Health 2015;3(1):79–89.
149. Griggs J, Maingi S, Blinder V, et al. American Society of Clinical Oncology Position Statement: Strategies for Reducing Cancer Health Disparities Among Sexual and Gender Minority Populations. J Clin Oncol 2017;35(19):2203–8.
150. Lee Smith J, Hall IJ. Advancing Health Equity in Cancer Survivorship: Opportunities for Public Health. Am J Prev Med 2015;49(6 Suppl 5):S477–82.

Fertility and Sexual Health in Young Women with Early-Stage Breast Cancer

Marla Lipsyc-Sharf, MD[a], Ann H. Partridge, MD, MPH[b],*

KEYWORDS

- Fertility • Sexual health • Premenopausal • Breast cancer

KEY POINTS

- Fertility and sexual health are important concerns for young women with early-stage breast cancer. Optimal assessment and management of these concerns evolves throughout the care continuum from the time of diagnosis, through active treatment, and into survivorship care.
- Risk of infertility may be impacted by treatment regimens as well as patients' age, ovarian reserve, body mass index, smoking history, genetic mutations, and other factors.
- Data regarding safety of fertility preservation options as well as pregnancy after breast cancer are overall reassuring.
- Sexual health and well-being may be impacted by medications, surgery, radiation, and other physical and psychological challenges faced by patients with breast cancer.
- Treatment modalities for improving sexual health are improving and may include sexual health rehabilitation programs, medications, and other interventions.

INTRODUCTION

The incidence of breast cancer in young women is increasing, and over 10,000 young women are diagnosed annually in the United States alone.[1] Given their overall differences in developmental stage, health status, and life circumstances, young women have unique physical, mental, psychosocial, and sexual health concerns that significantly affect their oncologic and survivorship care. Initial treatment decisions, as well as care during and after treatment, can meaningfully impact patients' fertility and sexual health. Therefore, it is important to discuss and address these issues early and throughout each phase of treatment and into survivorship. Here, the authors

---

This article previously appeared in Surgical Oncology Clinics volume 32 issue 4 October 2023.
[a] Department of Medical Oncology, Dana-Farber Cancer Institute, 450 Brookline Avenue, Yawkey 1238, Boston, MA 02215, USA; [b] Department of Medical Oncology, Dana-Farber Cancer Institute, Harvard Medical School, 450 Brookline Avenue, Dana 1608-A, Boston, MA 02215, USA
* Corresponding author.
E-mail address: Ann_Partridge@dfci.harvard.edu

highlight the major considerations and potential interventions related to fertility and sexual health in young women with early-stage breast cancer at each stage of their breast cancer care.

FROM THE START: PRE-THERAPY CONSIDERATIONS
Assessing Fertility Goals and Risk of Ovarian Insufficiency

Discussion of fertility considerations is important at the time of diagnosis and throughout the care continuum to ensure patients can make decisions that align with their goals, preferences, and values (**Fig. 1**). For all young women in whom systemic therapy for breast cancer is recommended, oncology teams should assess fertility goals and risk of infertility as soon as possible. Appropriate counseling regarding risks of premature menopause, infertility, and fertility preservation is important for patients' physical health and quality of life. The risk of infertility is associated with the particular medications and regimens used for systemic cancer therapy as well as the patient's age, ovarian reserve, germline genetic mutations, body mass index (BMI), and smoking history.[2] The gonadotoxicity and premature ovarian insufficiency associated with systemic therapy for breast cancer are thought to occur via multiple mechanisms including impairment of ovarian follicles, follicular activation and depletion, and/or impact on ovarian blood supply.[2,3] Discussion regarding risk of premature ovarian insufficiency is important not only for assessing risk of infertility but also for assessing risk of premature menopause, which is associated with genitourinary and vasomotor symptoms, sexual dysfunction, reduction in bone density, and other potential long-term and late effects.[4]

Medications used to treat early-stage breast cancer, including chemotherapy, endocrine therapy (ET), targeted therapy, and immunotherapy, have varying levels of evidence regarding the risk of gonadotoxicity and premature menopause and there remain several areas of uncertainty. Although most studies investigating the effect of systemic therapies assess the risk of treatment-related amenorrhea (TRA), TRA is not synonymous with infertility.[3] Some women who resume regular menstruation after cancer treatment have very poor ovarian reserve and therefore experience infertility even with normal menstrual cycles. However, many women with longer term TRA

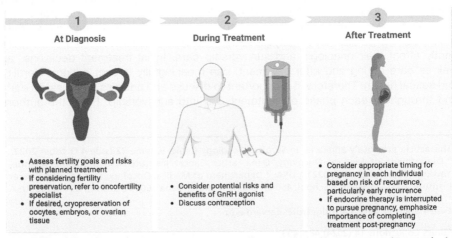

Fig. 1. Fertility considerations in young women with early-stage breast cancer. (*Created with BioRender.com.*)

attempting pregnancy will encounter fertility challenges, and because menstrual status is a straightforward and routine assessment for both patients and providers, this continues to be used as a surrogate for ovarian function and fertility. Importantly, most young women do recover ovarian function after systemic treatment of breast cancer; over 60% of women age 40 years and younger who are treated for early-stage breast cancer resume menstruation within 1 year, and over 80% resume menstraution within 2 years after diagnosis.[5] However, given the potential for ovarian insufficiency even in the setting of continued or resumed menses, it is important to discuss these risks as early as possible.

Currently, the most common chemotherapies used for early-stage breast cancer include cyclophosphamide, taxanes, anthracyclines, and carboplatin all of which increased the risk of TRA compared with treatment without chemotherapy. This risk also depends on other factors such as age at diagnosis.[2,3] Cyclophosphamide-based regimens seem to be associated with the highest risk of TRA, conferring over twice the risk TRA compared with chemotherapy regimens without cyclophosphamide, whereas anthracyclines were shown to increase the risk of TRA by about 39%.[6] Rates of TRA with taxanes were slightly better than with anthracyclines, increasing risk of TRA by about 24%.[6] Other data show that treatment with carboplatin and a taxane may less frequently cause TRA than treatment with cyclophosphamide-based regimens.[7] Dose-dense administration of chemotherapy is not thought to affect rates of TRA.[8] Importantly, some data suggest that amenorrhea is associated with better survival outcomes regardless of chemotherapy administered or estrogen receptor (ER)-positive status. This has motivated the currently unanswered question of whether optimal ovarian suppression could simultaneously allow for de-escalation of chemotherapy, improved ovarian function, and improved survival.[9]

The impact of newer targeted therapies on TRA is less well-studied. Existing data suggest that the most common targeted agent used for early-stage breast cancer, trastuzumab (an anti-human epidermal growth factor receptor 2 [HER2] therapy), does not significantly affect rates of TRA.[10] Trastuzumab emtansine (T-DM1), which is recommended for patients with early-stage HER2-positive breast cancer found to have residual disease after neoadjuvant chemotherapy, has been associated with a lower risk of TRA than paclitaxel and trastuzumab.[11] Additional analyses including pertuzumab (another anti-HER2 therapy) suggest that this agent similarly does not confer serious gonadotoxicity.[2,5] Other targeted therapies are currently approved for patients with high-risk early-stage breast cancers, including pembrolizumab, abemaciclib, olaparib, and neratinib. Effects of these agents on rates of TRA and infertility are unclear as menopausal and fertility outcomes are generally not assessed in the pivotal trials, and many studies assessing the potential impact of these agents on ovarian function are limited to preclinical data.[12] For example, early data show that immune checkpoint inhibitors may reduce the number and quality of oocytes and impact fertility through impairment of the hypothalamic–pituitary–gonadal axis.[13,14] As new targeted agents are incorporated into standard clinical practice for the treatment of early-stage breast cancer, it is critical to study the effect of these agents on ovarian function and fertility in premenopausal patients.

For the approximately 80% of patients diagnosed with breast cancer who have ER-positive disease, ET is the cornerstone of treatment and may be prescribed for 5 to 10 years. Premenopausal women are typically treated with tamoxifen, with or without ovarian function suppression (OFS) medication (ie, gonadotropin-releasing hormone [GnRH] agonist), or an aromatase inhibitor (AI) with OFS, depending on their level of risk, preferences, and tolerance. Overall, the use of ET with chemotherapy is known to increase the risk of TRA compared with treatment with chemotherapy without

ET.[15] Although tamoxifen is associated with an increased risk of TRA in premenopausal women, it likely does not impact ovarian reserve as it does not significantly affect levels of serum anti-Mullerian hormone (AMH) levels, which are indicative of ovarian reserve.[6] GnRH agonists (ie, leuprolide, goserelin, and triptorelin) are frequently used to further improve breast cancer outcomes in this setting. These medications suppress ovarian function during use, though are not thought to impair fertility, and effect on menses are generally temporary. Virtually all women under age 40 years treated with GnRH agonist alone resume menses when the treatment is stopped.[16] Data are limited regarding the effect of long-term treatment with AIs on menstrual function and fertility.[2] However, the combination of AI and OFS has been shown in recent years to improve survival over tamoxifen with or without OFS, particularly in patients with high-risk disease, so further understanding of the effect of combination GnRH agonist and AI on ovarian reserve and infertility is needed, despite a low likelihood of substantial impact given mechanisms of action.

Age is known to impact the risk of ovarian insufficiency with cancer treatment. Ovarian reserve decreases with age leading to greater risk of infertility. In the Young Women's Breast Cancer Study, a prospective cohort study of women age 40 years and younger diagnosed with breast cancer, although most patients (over 60%) resumed menses within 1 year after diagnosis, older age was associated with TRA.[5] Age more than 40 years has also been associated with TRA as has lower BMI.[3,5,15] In addition, low baseline serum AMH levels are associated with TRA and slower time to ovarian function recovery after chemotherapy.[17]

Particular consideration should be given to fertility preservation strategies for patients with germline breast cancer gene (BRCA) mutations, which affects approximately 10% of young women with breast cancer.[18] Limited available data have demonstrated lower AMH levels in women with a BRCA 1 mutation than women without germline BRCA mutation.[19] In addition to pursuing fertility preservation to mitigate the risks of infertility, women with germline BRCA mutations may elect to use assisted reproductive technology (ART), even when spontaneous conception is likely, to pursue preimplantation genetic testing to avoid passing the germline BRCA mutation to future children. All patients considering ART for any purpose should be referred to a fertility specialist for further evaluation and counseling, as existing data suggest that pregnancy and ART are safe in patients with BRCA mutations and do not confer differences in obstetrical risk or survival.[20,21]

Strategies for Fertility Preservation

Although many live births after breast cancer are the result of spontaneous pregnancies, patients who have undergone fertility preservation are more likely to become pregnant.[22] Oocyte/embryo or, less commonly, ovarian tissue cryopreservation is recommended for patients desiring fertility preservation.[23] Modern oocyte harvesting involves ovarian stimulation that can begin at any time in the menstrual cycle and lasts approximately 2 weeks.[2,3] In current practice, ovarian stimulation for fertility preservation in patients with breast cancer often includes an AI to minimize risks of rising estrogen concentrations during stimulation. Women who are intent on childbearing with a particular male partner (or using a sperm donor) may prefer to freeze embryos or both embryos and oocytes, whereas women who do not have a male partner or prefer not to freeze embryos for religious or other reasons may choose to freeze oocytes. Oocyte harvesting is typically recommended before initiation of systemic therapy.

Evidence on the safety of fertility preservation in patients with breast cancer is encouraging. Although historically there was concern that this delayed the time to cancer treatment, recent data suggest that the delay is quite short and does not impact survival.[24] Because ovarian stimulation transiently increases circulating estrogen, there has also been concern that oocyte harvesting might worsen the outcomes of patients with ER-positive breast cancers. However, fertility preservation does not seem to increase the risk of cancer recurrence or mortality, including in patients with ER-positive breast cancers.[2,3,22] Live birth rates after oocyte/embryo cryopreservation range from approximately 30% to 60%; younger age at the time of cryopreservation and a higher number of oocytes or embryos frozen are both associated with higher success rates.[2,3] For unknown reasons, a diagnosis of breast cancer is associated with worse oocyte quality compared with healthy women undergoing oocyte retrieval.[25] However, pregnancy rates overall are higher for breast cancer survivors who underwent fertility preservation than those who did not, so these strategies remain recommended for those patients who desire future biological children.[22]

Ovarian tissue cryopreservation is a less well studied and not widely available method of fertility preservation in which ovarian tissue is surgically removed, cryopreserved, and then transplanted back into the patient when conception is desired. Because ovarian stimulation is not necessary, only 2 to 3 days are needed before initiating systemic anticancer therapy. There is a theoretical risk that breast cancer metastatic to the ovaries would be reintroduced back into the patient after completion of anticancer therapy. Although there are no published accounts of this to date, ovarian tissue cryopreservation may not be the best method for patients with early-stage breast cancer with a high risk of recurrence.

The use of GnRH agonists for ovarian protection has been studied extensively. Given the ease of administration, these are often offered to premenopausal women undergoing chemotehrapy treatment for breast cancer in order to prevent ovarian insufficiency and limit the damage and depletion of ovarian follicles and therefore ovarian reserve. Although the potential mechanism of ovarian protection during cytotoxic chemotherapy is unclear and there is some controversy about the true benefits regarding GnRH for fertility preservation, several studies and meta-analyses show consistent efficacy and safety data for treatment with GnRH agonists for ovarian protection.[2,26,27] The largest meta-analysis to date studied 1231 patients receiving GnRH agonists alongside chemotherapy and found that patients receiving GnRH agonists had over 60% lower risk of premature ovarian failure and no significant difference in survival.[26] Given the uncertainty regarding efficacy for fertility outcomes, American Society of Clinical Oncology (ASCO) guidelines clearly recommend that coadministration of GnRH agonists should not be used in place of fertility preservation methods such as oocyte, embryo, or ovarian tissue cryopreservation.[23] The timing of treatment with GnRH agonist for ovarian protection may be important. Specifically, if patients undergo ovarian stimulation for oocyte or embryo cryopreservation, it is critical that GnRH agonist treatment is not started too soon after ovarian stimulation, as this can increase the risk of ovarian hyperstimulation syndrome. It is recommended that oncologists collaborate with patients' reproductive endocrinology teams to determine the earliest safe start time for GnRH agonists. Treatment with the GnRH agonist for ovarian protection is continued throughout the course of cytotoxic chemotherapy.

Surgical Considerations and Impact on Future Sexual Health

Most young women diagnosed with breast cancer have concerns about future sexual health and want information regarding how treatment may impact their sexual functioning and how to manage symptoms that arise. In initial counseling, it is important to discuss the risks and benefits of local therapy options with respect to sexual functioning. Although many young women with unilateral breast cancer are electing to have bilateral mastectomy, even in the absence of a known genetic predisposition to future breast cancer, young women treated with more extensive breast cancer surgeries have worse body image and overall sexual health than women treated with less extensive surgeries.[28,29] Specifically, women having bilateral mastectomies are at an increased risk of sexual dysfunction related to desire, excitation, lubrication, and orgasm compared with those having lumpectomy.[29] These effects were greater in women who did not undergo breast reconstruction. For women who did have breast reconstruction, autologous reconstruction was associated with improved breast satisfaction compared with implant-based or complex reconstruction.[30] Young women who have breast-conserving surgery have improved sexual functioning and better quality of life outcomes than women who underwent mastectomy with radiation. The mechanisms behind sexual dysfunction associated with mastectomy are likely multifactorial. It is possible that the loss of sensory nerves in the breast and nipple leads to loss of sexual stimulation that contributes to orgasm and libido. In addition, the impact of breast surgery on psychological health, including body image, likely affects sexual desire. As some women may value sexual health outcomes more than others, it is important to address these issues when discussing surgical planning as these risks and benefits may impact patients' decision-making.

IN THE THICK OF IT: MANAGEMENT DURING ADJUVANT TREATMENT
Assessment and Management of Sexual Health Challenges During Treatment

Many patients with breast cancer experience sexual dysfunction during treatment. Few patients report receiving any information regarding sexual health from their medical teams, and most welcome the opportunity to discuss sexual health considerations throughout the course of their treatment (**Fig. 2**). Overall, patients prefer to receive sexual health education from an oncology provider that is comfortable discussing sexuality as well as from written or online material. Assessment and discussion may

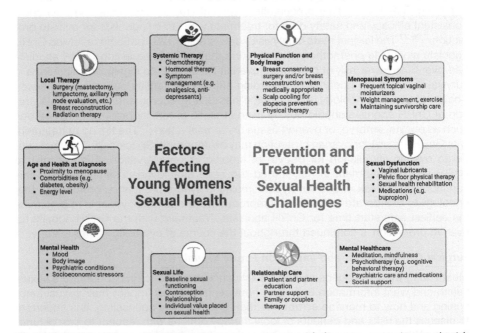

Fig. 2. Sexual health considerations in young women with breast cancer. (*Created with* BioRender.com.)

include topics such as sexual desire, contraception, comfort during sexual activity, orgasm, vaginal symptoms (including discharge and/or dryness), fatigue, and relationships, among others.

Patients with breast cancer who experience TRA have significantly more sexual side effects, including worse sexual interest, body image, and vaginal pain. In addition, most women with breast cancer have ER-positive disease and receive ET, which is also associated with sexual dysfunction. In particular, treatment with AI and OFS seems to be associated with more sexual side effects than treatment with tamoxifen with or without OFS.[31] Addressing the side effects of ET is important not only for patients' sexual and overall health but also to support their adherence to breast cancer treatment.[32] For women receiving ET in whom sexual side effects are significantly impacting their quality of life, we recommend discussing the risks and benefits of de-escalation. Although AIs with OFS are likely the most effective ET for risk reduction in high-risk ER-positive breast cancer, women with moderate to severe side effects may elect to switch to tamoxifen for risk reduction associated with fewer menopausal effects.[31]

Vaginal symptoms
Vaginal dryness, irritation, itching, and dyspareunia are common factors affecting sexual health in patients with breast cancer, particularly in those with TRA. The first line of treatment for these symptoms is the use of a topical nonhormonal vaginal moisturizer (including water-based, polycarbophil, and hyaluronic formulations).[33] Nonhormonal vaginal moisturizers have been found to reduce vaginal dryness and improve dyspareunia by over 60%, and overall have been shown to reduce sexual distress.[33] In cancer survivors, frequent application has been shown to increase efficacy, so moisturizers should be applied regularly, at least three times per week.

In the general population and in patients whose breast cancers do not express hormone receptors, treatment with topical vaginal estrogen is often recommended. However, the long-term safety of vaginal estrogen in women with a history of ER-positive breast cancer is not clear. Multiple studies have found that topical estrogen does have systemic absorption, and data on how this affects breast cancer outcomes are mixed.[34] A recent large Danish cohort study found that there was overall no increased risk of recurrence or mortality for patients treated for breast cancer that subsequently received vaginal estrogen.[34] However, in the subgroup receiving AIs, there was an increased risk of recurrence. Accordingly, vaginal estrogen can be a helpful tool though is used with caution and after thorough discussion with patients. If vaginal estrogen is prescribed, consideration should be taken to prescribe the lowest effective dose and, if possible, use vaginal softgels rather than tablets to limit systemic absorption.[35]

Research is ongoing to find additional safe and effective treatments for patients with breast cancer experiencing vulvovaginal atrophy. Topical dehydroepiandrosterone has been used for vaginal symptoms in patients taking ET for breast cancer, and there was no change in estrogen concentration for patients taking AIs.[36] Monthly vaginal micro-ablative CO_2 laser therapy with experts in this modality is also a promising option under study in breast cancer survivors. Ospemifene, an oral selective ER modulator, has been shown to improve symptoms of vulvovaginal atrophy in menopausal women, though the current data in patients with breast cancer are limited. For patients specifically reporting vaginal pain with penetration during sexual intercourse, the application of topical lidocaine before vaginal penetration can improve sexual distress and sexual dysfunction. In addition, though safety in patients with breast cancer has not been ascertained, the application of testosterone cream to the vagina and clitoris is being studied for improved sexual desire and function.

The intersection of psychosocial and sexual health

There is a clear relationship between psychosocial and sexual health challenges in patients with breast cancer. Most patients report that sexual dysfunction during and after treatment negatively impacts their mental health. The converse is also true: over half of patients with breast cancer experience anxiety and depression within 5 years of diagnosis, and these also affect sexual health and function.[32] In addition, intimate relationships are strained as patients experience significant life stressors and partners assume caregiving responsibilities, which add strain to sexual relationships. Some interventions traditionally used to improve mental and psychosocial health have been shown to improve patients' sexual health. Bupropion, an antidepressant, has also been shown to improve libido and sexual function in patients receiving treatment of breast cancer.[37] However, the most efficacious interventions in this setting are education, counseling, and cognitive behavioral therapy. Mindfulness, body awareness, and sexual health rehabilitation have also been shown to significantly improve sexual function and psychological distress in young patients with breast cancer receiving OFS. Referral to a professional with expertise in sex therapy should be considered when possible.

The Intersection of Physical and Sexual Health

Some interventions to address patients' physical health and symptoms (such as the use of selective serotonin reuptake inhibitors [SSRIs] or serotonin-norepinephrine reuptake inhibitors [SNRIs] for vasomotor symptoms, neuropathic pain, or aromatase-inhibitor musculoskeletal symptoms) have been associated with impaired sexual function.[32] However, these symptoms themselves may impair sexual functioning as well, so interventions may be tried and stopped if patients do not experience net benefit. Fatigue, poor body image, weight gain, and chemotherapy-induced alopecia are all known to impair patients' sexual health. Many non-pharmacologic interventions have been shown to improve fatigue, functional impairment, and quality of life in patients with breast cancer including exercise programs, cognitive behavioral therapy, acupuncture, acupressure, yoga, mindfulness, and martial arts.[32] There are also several efficacious interventions for weight loss in patients with breast cancer, and these include a combination of physical activity, nutritional changes, and behavioral therapy.[32] To prevent hair loss, scalp cooling systems are increasingly used by patients with breast cancer. Existing data suggest that this is a safe intervention, and efficacy for prevention of alopecia varies by chemotherapy regimen. Communicating these evidence-based strategies to patients is important for increasing utilization of these interventions that improve patients' health and well-being.

Contraception and Pregnancy During Adjuvant Treatment

Young women with breast cancer often have significant concerns about their fertility. For some, this may even affect their treatment choices or adherence.[38] Patients' desire for future pregnancy should inform providers' recommendations. In general, it is recommended that nonpregnant premenopausal women use contraception to avoid conceiving during active treatment of breast cancer. Contraception is an essential part of sexual health for women who do not desire current pregnancy or are receiving teratogenic medications. Chemotherapy administration during first trimester may impair healthy fetal development, and tamoxifen is a known teratogen. In women desiring future pregnancy, adjuvant zoledronic acid, a bisphosphonate that has been shown to improve disease-free survival in some patients with early-stage breast cancer, is generally avoided due to the long skeletal half-life and data suggesting adverse effects on pregnancy and neonatal outcomes. It is important for oncology providers to discuss contraception with their patients, as some patients may incorrectly assume that they are infertile during or after treatment and therefore decide not to use contraception. Hormonal oral contraceptives or intrauterine devices (IUDs) are avoided in patients with ER-positive breast cancers. Safe and effective methods of contraception include copper IUDs, barrier contraceptives, or sterilization of patients or their sexual partners.

Most data on the safety and success rates of pregnancy after breast cancer have focused on patients who have completed active adjuvant therapy. However, given the long duration of adjuvant ET, the recently reported POSITIVE trial was designed to assess the safety of temporary interruption of ET to attempt pregnancy in patients with a history of early-stage ER-positive breast cancer.[39,40] In this study, patients who received between 18 and 30 months of adjuvant ET stopped treatment, and 3 months later, attempted pregnancy. Patients remained off ET for up to 2 years during attempted conception, pregnancy, delivery, and, in some women, breastfeeding, with resumption of ET after this time to complete 5 to 10 years of adjuvant treatment. The initial trial results suggest that this strategy of interruption of ET does not compromise early breast cancer outcomes, and 43% of women used ART during trial participation.[39]

LIFE AFTER TREATMENT: POST-THERAPY CONSIDERATIONS
Fertility, pregnancy, and sexual health after breast cancer treatment

Although patients with breast cancer who underwent fertility preservation before treatment are ultimately more likely to become pregnant, pregnancy rates in these patients are lower than in women who have not had breast cancer.[22,41] This is likely multifactorial due to competing risks including disease recurrence, as well as infertility from systemic cancer therapies and increased age as pregnancy is delayed to allow for completion of systemic therapy. A large meta-analysis of over 8 million women showed that pregnant women with a history of breast cancer, especially those who received chemotherapy, have a higher risk of Cesarean Section, preterm birth, and low birth weight infants compared with the general population.[41] Interestingly, even after adjusting for confounders and clinicopathologic risk factors, breast cancer survivors with subsequent pregnancy had improved survival compared with breast cancer survivors without pregnancy. Importantly, patients with a history of ER-positive breast cancers who had a subsequent pregnancy did not have significantly different survival than those with no subsequent pregnancy.

The optimal interval between completion of breast cancer treatment and conception is not clear and may be individualized for each patient. Factors to consider include which treatments the patient received, their breast cancer biology and risk of recurrence, family planning goals, and their general health and well-being. Women who conceive within a year of completing chemotherapy are at an increased risk of preterm birth, so it is often recommended that most patients delay conception until at least 1 year after chemotherapy administration.[42] Patients receiving tamoxifen, a known teratogen, are generally advised wait at least 3 months after stopping before attempting conception, and the US FDA recommends waiting 9 months after tamoxifen based on animal data. It is unclear how long patients should delay conception after receiving AIs or targeted therapies. Women with ER-negative breast cancers have the highest risk of recurrence within the first 3 years after treatment, so many of these patients choose to delay pregnancy until after this interval. However, for patients with hormone receptor-positive breast cancers, the risk of recurrence persists for decades. The timing of pregnancy in these patients will likely depend on age and other clinicopathologic risk factors, whether ET will need to be interrupted, and patient desires and values.

The importance of sexual health care persists even after concluding active therapy for breast cancer. Treatment with chemotherapy and ET has been associated with lower rates of sexual activity and function long after the completion of therapy. Ongoing care of breast cancer survivors to manage sexual health challenges is essential to comprehensive long-term survivorship care.

CLINICS CARE POINTS

- It is critical to assess and address fertility and sexual health considerations at diagnosis and through survivorship.
- Future fertility interest and risk should be considered with all patients, and those interested should be referred to an infertility specialist for discussion and management of fertility preservation.
- Recommendations regarding timing of pregnancy should involve shared decision-making based on individual patient factors and available data.
- Patients should be counseled about the effects of cancer treatment on sexual health outcomes including libido, vaginal dryness and dyspareunia, and body image, as well as strategies for prevention and management of impairment.

FUNDING

Lipsyc-Sharf M., is supported by the Terri Brodeur Breast Cancer Foundation. Partridge A.H. is supported by Susan G. Komen and the Breast Cancer Research Foundation.

DISCLOSURES

AHP: Authorship for UpToDate. MLS: Honoraria from MJH Life Sciences.

REFERENCES

1. American Cancer Society, Breast Cancer Facts and Figures 2019-2020. Available at: https://www.cancer.org/content/dam/cancer-org/research/cancer-facts-and-statistics/breast-cancer-facts-and-figures/breast-cancer-facts-and-figures-2019-2020.pdf Accessed March 20, 2022.
2. Martelli V, Latocca MM, Ruelle T, et al. Comparing the Gonadotoxicity of Multiple Breast Cancer Regimens: Important Understanding for Managing Breast Cancer in Pre-Menopausal Women. Breast Cancer 2021;13:341–51. Dove Med Press.
3. Yildiz S, Bildik G, Benlioglu C, et al. Breast cancer treatment and ovarian function. Reprod Biomed Online 2022. https://doi.org/10.1016/j.rbmo.2022.09.014.
4. Rocca WA, Gazzuola-Rocca L, Smith CY, et al. Accelerated Accumulation of Multimorbidity After Bilateral Oophorectomy: A Population-Based Cohort Study. Mayo Clin Proc 2016;91(11):1577–89.
5. Poorvu PD, Hu J, Zheng Y, et al. Treatment-related amenorrhea in a modern, prospective cohort study of young women with breast cancer. NPJ Breast Cancer 2021;7(1):99.
6. Zhao J, Liu J, Chen K, et al. What lies behind chemotherapy-induced amenorrhea for breast cancer patients: a meta-analysis. Breast Cancer Res Treat 2014; 145(1):113–28.

7. Gast KC, Cathcart-Rake EJ, Norman AD, et al. Regimen-Specific Rates of Chemotherapy-Related Amenorrhea in Breast Cancer Survivors. JNCI Cancer Spectr 2019;3(4). https://doi.org/10.1093/jncics/pkz081.

8. Lambertini M, Ceppi M, Cognetti F, et al. Dose-dense adjuvant chemotherapy in premenopausal breast cancer patients; A pooled analysis of the MIG1 and GIM2 phase III studies. Eur J Cancer 2017;71:34–42.

9. Swain SM, Jeong J-H, Geyer CE, et al. Longer Therapy, Iatrogenic Amenorrhea, and Survival in Early Breast Cancer. N Engl J Med 2010;362(22):2053–65.

10. Lambertini M, Campbell C, Bines J, et al. Adjuvant Anti-HER2 Therapy, Treatment-Related Amenorrhea, and Survival in Premenopausal HER2-Positive Early Breast Cancer Patients. J Natl Cancer Inst 2019;111(1):86–94.

11. Ruddy KJ, Trippa L, Hu J, et al. Abstract P2-13-02: Chemotherapy-related amenorrhea (CRA) after adjuvant trastuzumab emtansine (T-DM1) compared to paclitaxel in combination with trastuzumab (TH) (TBCRC033: ATEMPT trial). Cancer Res 2020;80(4_Supplement). https://doi.org/10.1158/1538-7445.SABCS19-P2-13-02.

12. Cui W, Francis PA, Loi S, et al. Assessment of Ovarian Function in Phase III (Neo) Adjuvant Breast Cancer Clinical Trials: A Systematic Evaluation. J Natl Cancer Inst 2021;113(12):1770–8.

13. Winship AL, Alesi LR, Sant S, et al. Checkpoint inhibitor immunotherapy diminishes oocyte number and quality in mice. Nature Cancer 2022;3(8):1–13.

14. Garutti M, Lambertini M, Puglisi F. Checkpoint inhibitors, fertility, pregnancy, and sexual life: a systematic review. ESMO Open 2021;6(5):100276.

15. Lee S, Kil WJ, Chun M, et al. Chemotherapy-related amenorrhea in premenopausal women with breast cancer. Menopause 2009;16(1):98–103.

16. Bernhard J, Zahrieh D, Castiglione-Gertsch M, et al. Adjuvant Chemotherapy Followed By Goserelin Compared With Either Modality Alone: The Impact on Amenorrhea, Hot Flashes, and Quality of Life in Premenopausal Patients—The International Breast Cancer Study Group Trial VIII. J Clin Oncol 2007;25(3):263–70.

17. Su HC, Haunschild C, Chung K, et al. Prechemotherapy antimullerian hormone, age, and body size predict timing of return of ovarian function in young breast cancer patients. Cancer 2014;120(23):3691–8.

18. Guzmán-Arocho YD, Rosenberg SM, Garber JE, et al. Clinicopathological features and BRCA1 and BRCA2 mutation status in a prospective cohort of young women with breast cancer. Br J Cancer 2022;126(2):302–9.

19. Turan V, Lambertini M, Lee DY, et al. Association of Germline BRCA Pathogenic Variants With Diminished Ovarian Reserve: A Meta-Analysis of Individual Patient-Level Data. J Clin Oncol 2021;39(18):2016–24.

20. Condorelli M, Bruzzone M, Ceppi M, et al. Safety of assisted reproductive techniques in young women harboring germline pathogenic variants in BRCA1/2 with a pregnancy after prior history of breast cancer. ESMO Open 2021;6(6):100300.

21. Lambertini M, Ameye L, Hamy A-S, et al. Pregnancy After Breast Cancer in Patients With Germline BRCA Mutations. J Clin Oncol 2020;38(26):3012–23.

22. Wang Y, Tesch ME, Lim C, et al. Risk of recurrence and pregnancy outcomes in young women with breast cancer who do and do not undergo fertility preservation. Breast Cancer Res Treat 2022;195(2):201–8.

23. Oktay K, Harvey BE, Partridge AH, et al. Fertility Preservation in Patients With Cancer: ASCO Clinical Practice Guideline Update. J Clin Oncol 2018;36(19):1994–2001.

24. Greer AC, Lanes A, Poorvu PD, et al. The impact of fertility preservation on the timing of breast cancer treatment, recurrence, and survival. Cancer 2021; 127(20):3872–80.

25. Fabiani C, Guarino A, Meneghini C, et al. Oocyte Quality Assessment in Breast Cancer: Implications for Fertility Preservation. Cancers 2022;14(22). https://doi.org/10.3390/cancers14225718.

26. Lambertini M, Ceppi M, Poggio F, et al. Ovarian suppression using luteinizing hormone-releasing hormone agonists during chemotherapy to preserve ovarian function and fertility of breast cancer patients: a meta-analysis of randomized studies. Ann Oncol 2015;26(12):2408–19.

27. Lambertini M, Moore HCF, Leonard RCF, et al. Gonadotropin-Releasing Hormone Agonists During Chemotherapy for Preservation of Ovarian Function and Fertility in Premenopausal Patients With Early Breast Cancer: A Systematic Review and Meta-Analysis of Individual Patient-Level Data. J Clin Oncol 2018;36(19): 1981–90.

28. Rosenberg SM, Dominici LS, Gelber S, et al. Association of Breast Cancer Surgery With Quality of Life and Psychosocial Well-being in Young Breast Cancer Survivors. JAMA Surg 2020;155(11):1035–42.

29. Cobo-Cuenca AI, Martín-Espinosa NM, Sampietro-Crespo A, et al. Sexual dysfunction in Spanish women with breast cancer. PLoS One 2018;13(8): e0203151.

30. Dominici L, Hu J, Zheng Y, et al. Association of Local Therapy With Quality-of-Life Outcomes in Young Women With Breast Cancer. JAMA Surgery 2021;156(10): e213758.

31. Saha P, Regan MM, Pagani O, et al. Treatment Efficacy, Adherence, and Quality of Life Among Women Younger Than 35 Years in the International Breast Cancer Study Group TEXT and SOFT Adjuvant Endocrine Therapy Trials. J Clin Oncol 2017;35(27):3113–22.

32. Franzoi MA, Agostinetto E, Perachino M, et al. Evidence-based approaches for the management of side-effects of adjuvant endocrine therapy in patients with breast cancer. Lancet Oncol 2021;22(7):e303–13.

33. Loprinzi CL, Abu-Ghazaleh S, Sloan JA, et al. Phase III randomized double-blind study to evaluate the efficacy of a polycarbophil-based vaginal moisturizer in women with breast cancer. J Clin Oncol 1997;15(3):969–73.

34. Cold S, Cold F, Jensen M-B, et al. Systemic or Vaginal Hormone Therapy After Early Breast Cancer: A Danish Observational Cohort Study. JNCI: Journal of the National Cancer Institute 2022;114(10):1347–54.

35. Santen RJ, Mirkin S, Bernick B, et al. Systemic estradiol levels with low-dose vaginal estrogens. Menopause 2020;27(3):361–70.

36. Barton DL, Shuster LT, Dockter T, et al. Systemic and local effects of vaginal dehydroepiandrosterone (DHEA): NCCTG N10C1 (Alliance). Support Care Cancer 2018;26(4):1335–43.

37. Mathias C, Cardeal Mendes CM, Pondé de Sena E, et al. An open-label, fixed-dose study of bupropion effect on sexual function scores in women treated for breast cancer. Ann Oncol 2006;17(12):1792–6.

38. Sella T, Poorvu PD, Ruddy KJ, et al. Impact of fertility concerns on endocrine therapy decisions in young breast cancer survivors. Cancer 2021;127(16):2888–94.

39. Partridge AH NS, Ruggeri M, et al. GS4-09 Pregnancy Outcome and Safety of Interrupting Therapy for women with endocrine responsIVE breast cancer: Primary Results from the POSITIVE Trial (IBCSG 48-14/BIG 8-13).

40. Partridge AH, Niman SM, Ruggeri M, et al. Interrupting Endocrine Therapy to Attempt Pregnancy after Breast Cancer. N Engl J Med 2023;388(18):1645–56.
41. Lambertini M, Blondeaux E, Bruzzone M, et al. Pregnancy After Breast Cancer: A Systematic Review and Meta-Analysis. J Clin Oncol 2021;39(29):3293–305.
42. Hartnett KP, Mertens AC, Kramer MR, et al. Pregnancy after cancer: Does timing of conception affect infant health? Cancer 2018;124(22):4401–7.

Printed and bound by CPI Group (UK) Ltd, Croydon, CR0 4YY
03/10/2024
01040475-0005